Head and Neck Surgery
Volume 2

Head and Neck Surgery

in 3 volumes · 2nd completely revised edition

Coordinating Editor: H. H. Naumann
Edited by J. Helms, C. Herberhold, R. A. Jahrsdoerfer,
E. R. Kastenbauer, W. R. Panje, M. E. Tardy, Jr.

Volume 1: Face, Nose and Facial Skull
Edited by M. E. Tardy, Jr., E. R. Kastenbauer

Volume 3: Neck
Edited by W. R. Panje, C. Herberhold

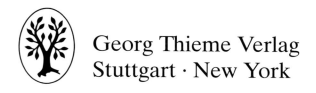

Georg Thieme Verlag
Stuttgart · New York

Thieme Medical Publishers, Inc.
New York

Volume 2:

Ear

Edited by R. A. Jahrsdoerfer, J. Helms

with contributions by:

E. A. Aguilar, III
D. E. Brackmann
W. Draf
K. Fleischer
B. J. Gantz
G. Geyer
B. Y. Ghorayeb
J. Helms

R. A. Jahrsdoerfer
F. Marguth
H. H. Naumann
V. Olteanu-Nerbe
M. Samii
A. Valavanis
E. Wilmes

772 illustrations

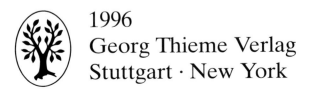

1996
Georg Thieme Verlag
Stuttgart · New York

Thieme Medical Publishers, Inc.
New York

Library of Congress Cataloging-in-Publication Data

Kopf- und Hals-Chirurgie. English
    Head and neck surgery / coordinating editor. H. H. Naumann :
edited by J. Helms... [et al.]. -- 2nd completely rev. ed.
        p. cm.
    Simultaneously published in German under title: Kopf- und
Hals-Chirurgie.
        Contents: v. 1. Face, nose and facial skull / edited by
M. E. Tardy, E. R. Kastenbauer. -- v. 2. Ear / edited by
R. A. Jahrsdoerfer, J. Helms. -- v. 3. Neck /edited by W. R. Panje,
C. Herberhold.
        ISBN 3-13-546902-6 (hardcover : v. 1)
        1. Head--Surgery. 2. Neck--Surgery. I. Naumann,
H. H. (Hans Heinz). 1919-   . II. Helms. J. (Jan), 1937-   .
III. Title.
        [DNLM; 1. Otorhinolaryngologic Diseases--surgery. 2. Face--
surgery. 3. Nose--surgery. 4. Skull--surgery. 5. Neck--surgery.
6. Ear--surgery. WV 168 K832 1995 a]
RD521.K6713   1995
617.5'1059--dc20
DNLM/DLC
for Library of Congress   95-11552
                                                                    CIP

Cover drawing by Renate Stockinger

© 1996 Georg Thieme Verlag, Rüdigerstraße 14,
70469 Stuttgart, Germany
Thieme Medical Publishers, Inc., 381 Park Avenue South,
New York, NY 10016

Typesetting by primustype Hurler GmbH, 73274 Notzingen

Printed in Germany by Neue Stalling, 26123 Oldenburg

ISBN 3-13-546802-X (GTV, Stuttgart)
ISBN 0-86577-660-1 (TMP, New York)   1 2 3 4 5 6

Medical Illustrators
Rudolf Brammer, Denzlingen, Germany
Robert J. Brown, Chicago, Ill, USA
Peter Cox, Herefordshire, England
Wolfgang Hanns, Denzlingen, Germany
Nancy Cliff Neumüller, Langenpreising, Germany
Taylor B. Randolph, New Orleans, LA, USA
Katharina Schumacher, München, Germany
Kirsten H. Siedel, Bernried, Germany

Translators German-English
Prof. Dr. P. M. Stell, Liverpool, England
Terry C. Telger, Fort Worth, Te, USA

Preface to the Second Edition

About twenty years have passed since the publication of the first German edition of *Head and Neck Surgery*. During that time the strategies and capabilities of head and neck surgery have been refined and have undergone some major changes. During this same period a new generation of surgeons has entered the operating suite, and international contacts in the medical field have burgeoned, creating an expanded base for the exchange and comparison of operative techniques. Accordingly, the editors and publishers solicited the input of this young generation of internationally oriented surgeons during the preparation of this new edition. One result has been the almost simultaneous publication of the series in German and in English.

This concept made it necessary to modify the organization and coordination of the project. In addition to the coordinating editor, an American and a German editor were appointed to share equally the responsibility for each of the three volumes in the series.

The *fundamental goal* of the first edition has remained unchanged, however: to provide otolaryngologists and head and neck surgeons with detailed, up-to-date information on the current status of specific operative techniques in the field.

The head and neck region is unique; in no other part of the body do so many surgical specialties come together. While this results in a degree of overlap among the neighboring specialties, the trend toward ever-increasing specialization can engender a "specialty blindness" that can have disastrous consequences for the patient. Accordingly, a further goal of this new edition is to promote interdisciplinary transparency and provide an up-to-date review of established and successful operative techniques for head and neck pathology.

The editors hope that they have at least approached this goal by enlisting the services of a pool of experienced and internationally recognized authors. In some topics the multidisciplinary background of the contributors has led to repetitions in the text and, occasionally, to differences of opinion. This has been readily accepted and is not considered detrimental. After all, there is no one true medical doctrine, and the maxim that "many roads lead to Rome" applies equally well in medicine! The surgeon faced with a difficult decision will always benefit from knowing multiple pathways that lead to the same destination.

To assist the reader in using the volumes more efficiently, each chapter is arranged according to a consistent set of subheads. Discussions of the actual surgical techniques are underlined in grey for emphasis.

When several techniques are available, each author has been asked to describe his or her preferred techniques in detail and then list additional alternatives or modifications that may be useful in selected cases. In this way we hope to provide a selection of *proven* and *reliable* techniques for all eventualities and clarify any doubts the inexperienced reader may have in deciding which procedure is best for a particular problem.

Since *Head and Neck Surgery* is intended to furnish practical help at the operating table, little emphasis has been placed on providing comprehensive reference lists. The concise bibliographic listing at the end of each chapter is intended simply to introduce the reader to the literature that is available on a given topic.

The editors are indebted to the authors who, coming from widely different specialties, made this book possible by contributing not only their knowledge and experience but also their understanding and acceptance of the formal constraints and time limitations associated with its production. We also thank the many medical illustrators who expressed the authors' ideas so vividly through their artistic talents and intuition.

The publisher, Georg Thieme Verlag, merits special recognition and thanks for enthusiastically embracing the concept of this bilingual publication and seeing it through to completion. In this regard, together with Dr. Günther Hauff, we are indebted to the Thieme staff members who were closely associated with the fulfillment of this project: Mr. Achim Menge, Mr. Gert Krüger, Mr. Rainer Zepf, Mr. Gerd Schlesak, Dr. Harlich Kübler, and Dr. Richard Dunmur. Simultaneous publication of the book in two languages would not have been possible without the help of competent specialist translators. Thus, we also express thanks to Prof. P. M. Stell, M. D. (Liverpool, England) and Mr. T. C. Telger (Ft. Worth, Texas) for their conscientious efforts.

H. H. Naumann

Preface to Volume 2

At the time of publication of the first edition of this handbook (1972–1976), surgery of the ear had just experienced massive new impulses through the introduction of microsurgery. Since then, the new technical possibilities for *microsurgical hearing improvements* (stapedectomy, tympanoplasty) have undergone further development and mostly been accepted into standard practice. One of the objectives of this 2nd edition is to present the current status of curative and functional microsurgery of the ear.

In addition, surgery of the ear has expanded in several directions over the past years. Surgery of the lateral skull base not only in the context of *traumatology* but also for the treatment of *tumors of the temporal bone and its adjacent areas* has undergone appreciable improvements. As a result of the systematization of pathological findings in the temporal bone and/or lateral skull base (by U. Fisch amongst others), concrete indications for the various operative techniques have arisen which, in turn, have further helped to improve and stabilize the safety and success of these surgical interventions. This new orientation towards the boundaries of neurosurgery has passed its probationary period, its consequences have been accepted, in the cases of correct indications, by the neighboring disciplines, and ultimately has led to increasing cooperation between ear surgeons and neurosurgeons in the formulation of common indications and joint operative measures, thus improving the chances for the respective patients.

These advances could not have been realized without the concomitant progress in the precision and differentiation of the available and newly developed *diagnostic modalities* which is reflected in the increased accuracy of indications and prognoses. Examples of this are the current possibilities in computed and magnetic resonance tomography, interventional neuroradiologic diagnosis as well as audiology and neuro-otology to mention but a few.

Other fields of classical otosurgery have also benefited from these dramatic diagnostic advances. Again, we need only mention the indications and surgical techniques for the *correction of malformations*, especially in the middle ear region and *surgery of the facial nerve* in its intratemporal course.

In close relation to the last mentioned topic, a further objective of the present volume was to describe the current status of *plastic and reconstructive surgery* in the region of the external ear, especially since the principle of regionally anchored plastic surgery has entered and found its firm place over the past years for procedures in the ear region.

Since the 1970's completely new perspectives have resulted from the *implantation of electrodes in the inner ear (cochlear implants)* which have enabled bilateral deaf patients not only to appreciate sound impressions but also often to develop a satisfactory understanding of speech. The results are in part so promising and encouraging that a description of the state of the art and the operative possibilities and technological advances just had to be included in this book.

Although inflammatory otogenic endocranial complications have lost part of their devastating threats and have become rather seldom since the introduction of antibiotic agents, it is still important that the life-saving operative techniques developed for such situations be retained in the surgeon's arsenal and not be forgotten. Indications for these operations do occur occasionally and today's generation of ear surgeons must be able to recognize them and master the required procedures. This is important because no guarantee can be given that the protection provided by current antibiotics will not be negated by the further development of drug resistances. Accordingly, the classical operative strategies to combat this group of complications are also described briefly in this volume.

Also the editors of this volume are grateful to the publisher for allowing new illustrations of modern ear surgery to form an essential part of this volume. All of the participating medical illustrators are expressly thanked for their patience and expertise in the preparation of didactically meaningful drawings. The editors further thank the authors and Dr. Ulrike Schwab for their tireless help with the manuscript and proof corrections.

Charlottesville, VA
and Würzburg, Spring 1996

Robert A. Jahrsdoerfer
Jan Helms

Addresses

Eugenio A. Aguilar, III, M.D.
Clinical Associate Professor
Department of Otolaryngology-
Head and Neck Surgery
University of Texas Medical School
Houston, Texas 77030
USA

Derald E. Brackmann, M.D.
House Ear Clinic, Inc.
2100 West Third Street
Los Angeles, California 90057
USA

Professor Dr. med. Wolfgang Draf
Chairman of the Department of Otorhinolaryngology
Head, Neck and Facial Plastic Surgery
Klinikum der Stadt Fulda
Pacelliallee 4
36043 Fulda
Germany

Professor Dr. med. Konrad Fleischer
retired Chairman of the Department
of Otorhinolaryngology
Justus-Liebig-University, Gießen
Wartweg 24
35392 Gießen
Germany

Bruce J. Gantz, M.D.
Professor and Chairman
Department of Otolaryngology-
Head and Neck Surgery
University of Iowa Hospitals and Clinics
Iowa City, Iowa 52242
USA

Priv.-Doz. Dr. med. Götz Geyer
Chairman of Ear, Nose and Throat Clinic
Städtisches Krankenhaus Solingen
Gotenstraße 1
42653 Solingen
Germany

Bechara Y. Ghorayeb, M.D.
Clinical Associate Professor
Department of Otolaryngology-
Head and Neck Surgery
University of Texas Medical School
Houston, Texas 77030
USA

Professor Dr. med. Jan Helms
Chairman of the Department of Otorhinolaryngology,
Head and Neck Surgery
Julius-Maximilians-University, Würzburg
Josef-Schneider-Straße 11
97080 Würzburg
Germany

Robert A. Jahrsdoerfer, M.D.
Professor
Department of Otolaryngology-
Head and Neck Surgery
University of Virginia Medical Center
Charlottesville, Virginia 22908
USA

Professor Dr. med. Frank Marguth †
retired Chairman of the Clinic of Neurosurgery
Ludwig-Maximilians-University, Munich
Großhadern Medical Center
Marchioninistraße 15
81377 München
Germany

Professor Dr. med. Hans Heinz Naumann
retired Chairman of the Department
of Otorhinolaryngology
Head and Neck Surgery
Ludwig-Maximilians-University, Munich
Großhadern Medical Center
Marchioninistraße 15
81377 München
Germany

Priv.-Doz. Dr. Vladimir Olteanu-Nerbe
Clinic of Neurosurgery
Ludwig-Maximilians-University, Munich
Großhadern Medical Center
Marchioninistraße 15
81377 München
Germany

Professor Dr. med. Madjid Samii
Chairman of the Clinic
of Neurosurgery
Krankenhaus Nordstadt
Medizinische Hochschule Hannover
Haltenhoffstraße 41
30167 Hannover
Germany

Professor Dr. med. Anton Valavanis
Chairman of the Institute of Neuroradiology
Universitätsspital Zürich
Frauenklinikstraße 10
8091 Zürich
Switzerland

Professor Dr. Eberhard Wilmes
Chairman of the
Department of Ear, Nose and Throat
Städtisches Krankenhaus Schwabing
Kölner Platz 1
80804 München
Germany

Contents

1 Local Anesthesia of the Ear

Jan Helms

Local Anesthesia of the Ear   1
Bibliography   3

2 Plastic and Reconstructive Surgery of the Auricle

Eugenio A. Aguilar, III and Robert A. Jahrsdoerfer

Correction of Protruding Ears   5

Correction of Lop Ears 14

Reconstruction of the Helix 18

**Auricular Reconstruction for Congenital
Microtia** 22

Reconstruction of Earlobes 30
    Bibliography 33

3 Surgical Management of Congenital Ear Malformations

Robert A. Jahrsdoerfer and Eugenio A. Aguilar, III

Minor Malformations 35
    Middle Ear 38
    Postauricular Approach 42
    Ossicular Chain 44
    Labyrinthine Windows 44
    Ossiculoplasty 44
    Stapedectomy/Stapedotomy 46
    Malleus Head Fixation 46

    Malleus Bar 46
    Incus Fixation 46
    Vestibulotomy 47
    Early Complications 48
    Late Complications 49

Congenital Aural Atresia and Stenosis 50
    Bibliography 66

4 Surgery of the Outer Ear, Middle Ear, and Temporal Bone for the Removal of Disease and for Reconstruction

Jan Helms
Surgery for Removal of Disease 67
  Surgical Anatomy 67

Surgical Procedures on the External Meatus .. 67
  Removal of Reactive and Inflammatory
  Lesions 69
  Removal of Exostoses 70
  Removal of an Arachnoid Cyst in the
  External Meatus 73
  Partial Resection of the External Meatus
  (in Patients with Aseptic Bone Necrosis
  or Malignant Otitis Externa) 73

**Surgical Procedures on the Tympanic
Membrane** 75
  Paracentesis 75
  Insertion of a Ventilation Tube 77

**Surgical Procedures on the Tympanic Cavity
and Mastoid** 80
  Antral Drainage, Antrotomy, and
  Mastoidectomy 80
  The "Radical" Mastoid Cavity 85
  Surgical Treatment of Tympanosclerosis 102
  Surgical Treatment of Tympanic
  Fibrosis 105
  Removal of Tympanic Cholesteatoma 106

Surgical Correction of Stenosis or
Occlusion of the Eustachian Tube 108
Surgical Treatment of Tympanic Atelectasis
and Epidermal Overgrowth of the
Tympanic Cavity 108
Bibliography 109

Götz Geyer and Jan Helms
Reconstructive Surgery 110

Myringoplasty 110

Ossicular Chain Reconstruction 119
  Preparation of Ossicular Prostheses 119
  Common Anatomic Situations 119
  Malleus Handle 120
  Incus 120
  Incus and Stapes Superstructure 124
  Isolated Stapes Arch Defect 124
  Special Form of Tympanosclerosis 125
  Empty Tympanum and Deficient Middle
  Ear Function (Type IV Tympanoplasty) 126
  Inaccessible Oval Window Niche
  (Fenestration of the Promontory) 126

**Grafts and Implants for Ossicular Chain
Reconstruction** 128
Bibliography 129

5 Temporal Bone Trauma

Robert A. Jahrsdoerfer and Bechara Y. Ghorayeb

Surgery of External Canal Injuries 131
  Incidence 131
  Causes 131

Surgery of Tympanic Membrane Injuries 136
  Incidence 136
  Causes 136
  Immediate Therapy 137
  Delayed Therapy 137

Surgery of Ossicular Chain Injuries 139
  Incidence 139
  Causes 139
  Removal of Dislocated Incus 141
  Stapes Intact and Incus Dislocated 142
  Incus Intact and Stapes Fractured 142
  Incus and Stapes are Fractured/Dislocated . 142
  Perilymphatic Fistula Closure 143

Surgery of Facial Nerve Injuries 144
  Incidence 144
  Etiology 144
  Pathology 144
  Physical Examination 145
  Classification 146
  Transmastoid-Extralabyrinthine 149
  Middle Fossa Exploration 151
  Anastomosis 151
  Grafting with Greater Auricular Nerve 152

Surgery of Mastoid Injuries 154
  Incidence 154
  Causes 154
  Physical Examination 154
  Imaging 154
  Bibliography 157

6 Surgery for Tumors of the Middle Ear and Lateral Skull Base

Jan Helms

Surgery for Tumors of the Auditory Canal 159
    Benign Tumors 159
    Malignant Tumors 159
        Malignant Tumors Outside the Tympanic
        Membrane 159
        Malignant Tumors of the External
        Auditory Canal with Involvement
        of the Tympanic Membrane 162

**Surgery for Tumors of the Middle Ear
and its Surroundings** 166

Subtotal Petrosectomy with Preservation
of the Labyrinth 166
Supralabyrinthine Subtotal Petrosectomy
with Preservation of the Labyrinth or
with Labyrinthectomy 171
Subtotal or Total Petrosectomy, with Facial
Nerve Transposition or Resection, and
Transposition of the Internal Carotid Artery .. 178
Malignant Tumors of the Middle Ear 196
Bibliography 205

7 Surgery of the Intracranial Facial Nerve Proximal to the Stylomastoid Foramen

Wolfgang Draf

Clinical Findings 207
Site-of-Lesion Determination 208
Electrical Testing 208
Radiologic Studies 208
Absolute Indications 209
Relative Indications 210

***Surgical Options for Lesions of the Intracranial
and Intratemporal Portions of the Facial Nerve*** . 211

Basic Methods 212
    Surgical Segmental Anatomy of the Facial
    Nerve 212
    Obtaining Graft Material for Nerve
    Reconstruction 212
    Technique of Nerve Anastomosis 214

Special Methods 215
    Simple Nerve Exploration 215
    Facial Nerve Decompression and
    Neurolysis 216
    Classic Transmastoid Facial Nerve
    Decompression 216

Decompression of the Geniculate Ganglion
through the External Auditory Canal 218
Complete Meatolabyrinthine –
Tympanomastoid Exposure of the Facial
Nerve 220
Vascular Decompression of the Facial
Nerve in the Cerebellopontine Angle 220

**Facial Nerve Surgery from the Cerebello-
pontine Angle to the Stylomastoid Foramen** .. 221
    End-to-End Anastomosis in the
    Cerebellopontine Angle 221
    Intracranial-Intratemporal Anastomosis 221
    Facial Nerve Reconstruction in the Internal
    Auditory Canal 222
    Transtemporal Extradural Approach 222
    Translabyrinthine Approach 224
    Tympanomastoid Reconstruction 225
    Intratemporal-Extratemporal
    Reconstruction 226
    Concluding Remarks 227
Bibliography 228

8 Operations for Stapedial Ankylosis

Hans H. Naumann and Eberhard Wilmes

Stapedectomy 230
    Anesthesia 232
    Partial Stapedectomy 238
    Complete Stapedectomy 240
    Closing Stages of Partial or Complete
    Stapedectomy 244

Procedure for a Thick Footplate or an
Obliterated Oval Window Niche 245
Procedure for a Narrow Oval Window
Niche 246
Otosclerosis Around the Round
Window 246

Fixation of the Ossicular Chain at
Several Points 247
Ossified Tendon of the Stapedius
Muscle 248
Congenital Anomalies of the Ossicular
Chain 248

Intraoperative Complications 248
Revision Surgery 248

Fenestration 254
One-Stage Endaural Procedure 254
Bibliography 261

9 Surgical Management of Otogenic Intracranial Complications

Konrad Fleischer

**Otogenic Extradural Abscess and Otogenic
Meningitis** 263
Causes and Routes of Extension 263
Extradural Abscess 266
Meningitis 266

Otogenic Brain Abscess 267
Pathogenesis, Causes, and Location 267

Otogenic Sinus Thrombosis 271
Pathogenesis and Course 272
Bibliography 276

10 Surgery of the Labyrinth and Internal Auditory Canal for Disequilibrium

Jan Helms

Endolymphatic Sac Surgery 277

Labyrinthectomy 283

Transtemporal Neurectomy 285

Translabyrinthine Neurectomy 293
Bibliography 300

11 Removal of Acoustic Neuroma through the Retrosigmoid (Lateral Suboccipital) Approach

Madjid Samii

**Acoustic Neuroma (Lateral Suboccipital
Approach)** 301
Indications 301
Operative Technique 303

Modifications 306
Postoperative Complications 310
Bibliography 311

12 Acoustic Tumor Removal: Middle Fossa and Translabyrinthine Approaches

Derald E. Brackmann

Middle Fossa Approach 313

Translabyrinthine Approach 328

Hemostasis and Closure 338
Bibliography 340

13 Basic Aspects of Neurosurgical Procedures in the Head Region

Frank Marguth and Vladimir Olteanu-Nerbe

Principles of Surgery 341
   Craniotomy and Craniectomy 342
   Burr Hole Trephination 352

Specific Operations 358

Head Injuries 358
   Epidural Hematoma 358
   Subdural Hematoma 358

Cerebrospinal Rhinorrhea 359
   Transcranial Intradural Approach 360

Cranial Infections 360
   Cranial Osteomyelitis 360
   Epidural Abscess 360
   Subdural Abscess 362
   Brain Abscess 363

Nerve Repair 365
   Technique of Nerve Repair 365
   Interfascicular (Perineural) Repair 365
   Direct (Epineural) Repair 366
   Autogenous Nerve Bypass (Dott's
   Technique) 366
   Cranial Nerve Anastomoses 367
   Cross-Facial Nerve Grafting 368

Tumors of the Skull Base 368

Endovascular Procedures 368
   Devascularization of Highly Vascular
   Tumors 368
   Traumatic Carotid Cavernous Fistula 369
Bibliography 370

14 Cochlear Implant

Bruce J. Gantz

Diagnosis and Preoperative Evaluation 371
Indications 372
Operative Technique 375

Postoperative Care 384
Bibliography 386

15 Interventional Neuroradiology for Tumors of the Temporal Bone

Anton Valavanis

Introduction to Embolization Techniques 387
   Balloon Occlusion of the Internal Carotid
   Artery 389

Bibliography 393

Index 401

1 Local Anesthesia of the Ear

Jan Helms

For a general introduction to anesthesia in otorhino-laryngologic surgery, see Volume 1, Chapter 1.

Preoperative Assessment and Interview

Before the decision is made to use local anesthesia for surgery on the ear, it must be ascertained whether there are factors that would contraindicate or restrict the use of local anesthetics. Accordingly, the patient is questioned about existing allergies to local anesthetics, and it is determined whether he or she has experienced any previous adverse reactions to local agents used in surgical procedures. During the preoperative interview, the patient is briefly informed about the proposed anesthetic procedure, advised that hypersensitivity reactions, though rare, cannot be entirely ruled out, and that the anesthetic will cause dulling of consciousness, but the patient will be responsive during the operation with a high level of analgesia.

Indications

Local infiltrative anesthesia is appropriate for surgical procedures on the middle ear and mastoid in the majority of adult patients. The primary election of general anesthesia is advised in children, in adults considered poor candidates for local anesthesia due to emotional factors, in patients with heavy scarring in the operative area, and in patients considered to have very extensive, florid inflammatory disease.

Principle

The patient should have a good night's sleep on the eve of the operation. A hypnotic or sedative is prescribed if necessary.

A combination of sedative agents is administered about 1 h before surgery to allay apprehension.

After the patient has been positioned on the operating table, an intravenous line is established (usually in the arm), and continuous drip infusion is initiated. This line is essential, as it provides a route for administering emergency medications should the need arise.

Just before injection of the local anesthetic, analgesics are administered through the i.v. line to reduce the tension pain that accompanies infiltration of the operative field.

The area is infiltrated with approximately 4–8 ml of the local anesthetic solution, which contains epinephrine to induce local vasoconstriction and decrease intraoperative bleeding.

Since the local anesthetic takes some time to diffuse into the proposed operative area, it should be injected prior to skin preparation and draping. At least 10 min should elapse following administration of local anesthesia before the operation itself is begun.

Our local anesthetic of choice is 1% Ultracain (carticaine) with 1:200,000 Suprarenin (epinephrine), which is supplied in 5–ml ampules. Epinephrine may be added independently to the anesthetic agent, but the ready–to–use ampules avoid error and confusion.

Preparations

In preparation for surgery under local anesthesia, the patient is advised not to eat or drink, similar to the restriction observed for general anesthesia. In this way the anesthesiologist can safely proceed to general anesthesia if the local agent proves inadequate.

Premedication

Premedication in adults is administered by intramuscular injection. A combination of 50 mg meperidine, 50 mg promethazine, and 0.5 mg atropine yields good results in a normally nourished adult with a body weight of approximately 70 kg. The premedication is administered 1 h before surgery. About 5 min before anesthetic infiltration of the operative field, an analgesic (e.g., 30 mg pentazocine) is injected through the i.v. line. If the patient is still fairly wide awake, an additional 5–10 mg diazepam is given intravenously.

Infiltration Technique

The external ear and its surroundings are infiltrated according to the distribution of the sensory nerves supplying the auricle and the middle ear. These nerves must be completely blocked by the local anesthesia.

The auricle is pulled forward, and a 1–ml subcutaneous depot is placed in the postauricular crease at the level of the opening of the external auditory canal. While anesthetic is injected, the needle is advanced anteriorly between bone and the auricular cartilage, raising a visible soft–tissue wheal in the intertragic incisure which bulges toward the opening of the auditory canal. This upper part of the operative field is infiltrated with a total dose of about 1.5–2 ml.

With the needle still in the primary insertion site, the tip is moved below the opening of the ear canal, and again 1.5–2 ml anesthetic is injected while the needle is advanced. If a postauricular incision is planned, an additional ¹/₂ ml of anesthetic is deposited subcutaneously at each of several points on the proposed line of incision (Fig. 1.**1**).

The external auditory canal itself is infiltrated from 4 points on its roof, floor, anterior wall, and posterior wall. Since the meatal skin at those sites is normally delicate with very little subcutaneous tissue, the bevel of the needle should be advanced in direct contact with, and parallel to, the underlying bone (Fig. 1.**2**).

The injection sites are located about 1 cm medial to the suprameatal spine. Approximately 0.5 ml of local anesthetic is injected while maintaining bone contact, at each of the 4 sites. The solution should be injected at a relatively high pressure to force it between the bone and periosteum, so it is best to use a 2–ml syringe. Larger syringes may not generate the necessary pressure.

The injection does not always reach the tympanic bone at the anterior meatal wall but may be deflected by the tragus cartilage or may penetrate it, leading to infiltration of a large, preauricular soft–tissue area. This

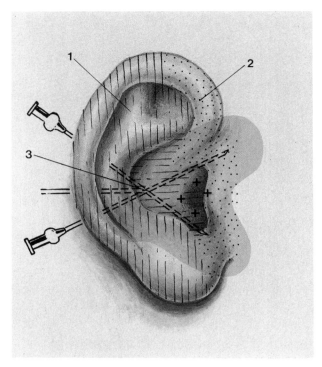

Fig. 1.**1**   Diagram of the area to be anesthetized, showing the corresponding distribution of the sensory nerves and the technique of postauricular infiltration, with distension of the soft tissues in the intertragic incisure
1   ⦀ C_2C_3 (N. auric. magn.)
2   ∴ N. V (N. auriculotemporalis)
3   ≡ N. VII, IX, X (R. auricularis N. X)

is not a problem in terms of analgesia, but occasionally it induces a facial nerve paralysis that lasts for about 4 h. It is desirable to infiltrate the anterior meatal wall at a point slightly higher and more medial than at the other 3 injection sites. This helps to ensure that local anesthetic will reach the anterior tympanomeatal angle.

Modifications

The above technique can be modified by injecting greater amounts of local anesthetic into a larger area around the ear, but this reduces the efficacy of the anesthesia. Neither should the local anesthesia be administered after the area has been prepared and draped, due to the temptation to proceed with surgery rather than give the solution time to diffuse.

Landmarks and Pitfalls

Essential landmarks are the postauricular crease, the intertragic incisure, and the suprameatal spine. Penetration of the tragus cartilage during infiltration of the

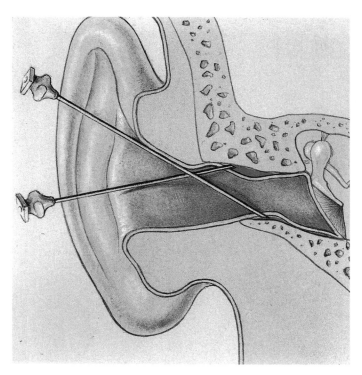

Fig. 1.**2**   Technique of endaural infiltration. The needle bevel is in contact with the bone

anterior meatal wall should be avoided if possible to avert transient facial nerve palsy. Since there are dehiscences in the cartilage, however, and the anesthetic can diffuse forward through the connective–tissue boundary between the anterior meatal wall and the tympanic bone, transient compromise of facial nerve function will occasionally occur despite proper application of the local anesthetic.

Rules, Hints, and Common Errors

Epinephrine should be added to the local anesthetic solution. We have had good results using 1% Ultracain with 1:200,000 Suprarenin. The anesthetic takes 10–15 min to diffuse adequately throughout the operative field when administered in accordance with the above recommendations. Some pressure is needed to force the solution between the bone and periosteum in the extenal auditory canal, and a syringe with a 2–ml capacity (rather than 5 or 10 ml) should be used to generate the necessary pressure. A fine–gauge needle (e.g., No. 14 or 27 gauge) is preferred due to the thinness of the

meatal skin. Failure to advance the needle tip to bone at the injection sites results in inadequate infiltration deep within the ear canal.

Postoperative Care

The sedative and analgesic medications administered prior to local anesthesia will cause the patient to sleep for several hours after the operation. The patient should remain in the operating room until protective reflexes have returned and he is responsive to verbal communications.

Postoperative Complications

Very rarely, allergic reactions may develop as postoperative complications and must be managed appropriately. Another rare complication is transient facial nerve palsy lasting 3–4 h caused by local preauricular infiltration of the facial nerve and surrounding tissues. If facial nerve palsy is noted postoperatively, the surgeon should be notified so that he can determine whether the paralysis has been caused by the operation. Palsy induced by the action of the local anesthetic does not require further treatment.

Functional Sequelae

The only sequelae relating to the local anesthesia that may be troublesome for the patient are allergic phenomena. If this type of sequela is observed, the patient should be thoroughly apprised of the problem so that future adverse reactions can be avoided.

Alternative Methods

The alternative to local anesthesia is general anesthesia.

Bibliography

Auberger H G, Niesel H C. Praktische Lokalanaesthesie-regionale Schmerztherapie. Stuttgart: Thieme; 5th edn, 1990.
Plester D, Hildmann H, Steinbach E. Atlas der Ohrchirurgie. Stuttgart: Kohlhammer; 1989, pp. 12–13.

2 Plastic and Reconstructive Surgery of the Auricle

Eugenio A. Aguilar III and Robert A. Jahrsdoerfer

Correction of Protruding Ears

Diagnosis and Preoperative Evaluation

The protruding ear is a defect which when correctly repaired can be a source of happiness for the patient and his or her family. It is an operation which requires that the plastic surgeon has some degree of artistic finesse. The operation may be one of the most satisfying that a plastic surgeon may perform. It can also be one of the most vexing.

While the diagnosis is self evident (Fig. 2.1), an analysis of the problem requires knowledge of auricular anatomy. The auricle grows at a rate that is usually predictable when adjusted to the patient's age. The angle of the ear to the head should be 15–30 degrees (Fig. 2.2). An angle greater then 30 degrees produces a protruding ear, a deformity most patients wish to have corrected (Fig. 2.3).

Preoperative evaluation should include photographs in the frontal, oblique, lateral, and rear views to record and allow categorization of the defect, and to provide a baseline for comparing the results of the reconstruction. The patient and family should be informed preoperatively of possible complications.

Indications

The indications for otoplasty are often clear cut. An angle greater than 30 degrees warrants correction. Psychological problems associated with the protruding ear can be significant. The best age for surgery is 5–6 years. At this age the child has not yet been exposed to intense peer ridicule for this common deformity. Also, at this age the size of the patient is adequate to tolerate any postoperative manipulation.

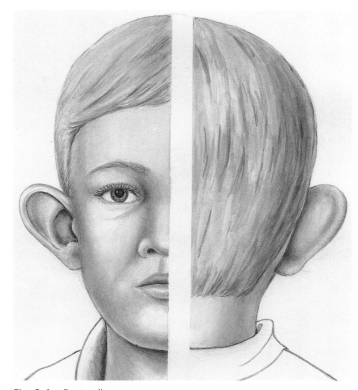

Fig. 2.1 Protruding ears.

Goals of the Operation

The goal of the operation is to reduce the angle of the ear relative to the head to 15 degrees, while maintaining a normal appearance to the pinna. There should be a definite antihelix, and the curve of the helix should be gentle and without breaks.

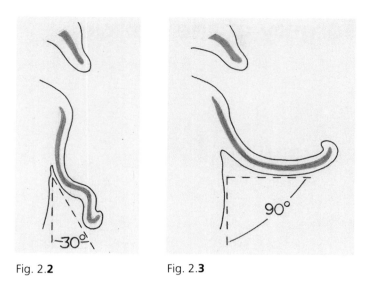

Fig. 2.**2**   Fig. 2.**3**

Fig. 2.**2**   Angle between head and auricle should normally be between 15 and 30 degrees.

Fig. 2.**3**   Pre-op angle is close to 80–90 degrees.

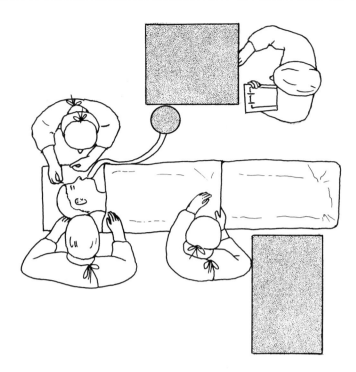

Fig. 2.**4**   Operating room positions.

Preparation for Surgery

The positions of the operating personnel are outlined in Figure 2.**4**, and the instruments in Figure 2.**5**. The patient should be sterilely prepped and draped with the head in a neutral position. This allows the head to be turned in order to infiltrate local anesthesia, and also allows manipulation of the head during surgery.

Anesthesia

In children, general anesthesia is preferred. This should be augmented with local anesthesia containing a vaso-constrictor. The local solution should be injected into the posterior and anterior surfaces of the auricle (Fig. 2.**6**). Local anesthesia with i.v. sedation is a good technique for older children and adults (see Chapter 1, Anesthesia).

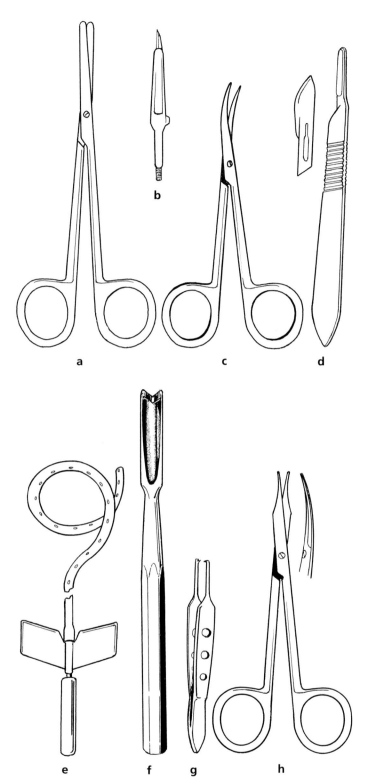

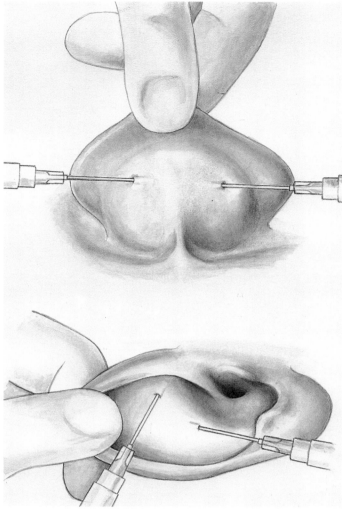

Fig. 2.**6**   Infiltration of local anesthetic in the posterior and anterior surface.

Fig. 2.**5**   Instruments for surgical procedure:
a: Metzenbaum scissors
b: Beaver 75/15 knife
c: curved iris scissors
d: no. 10 blade knife
e: drain
f: gouge
g: Bishop forceps
h: tenotomy scissors

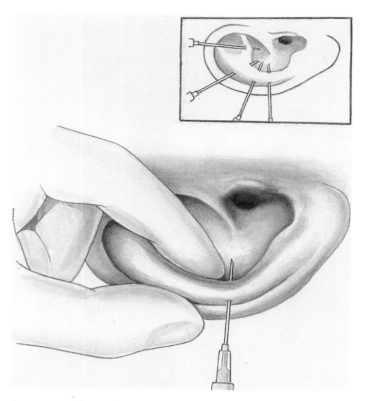

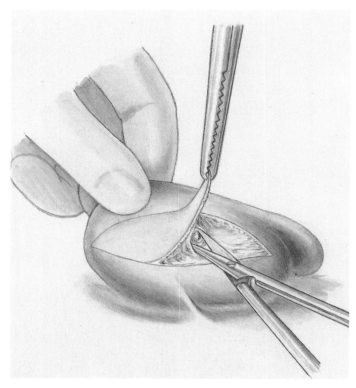

Fig. 2.**7** Marking of the anterior portion of the ear with needles and methylene blue.

Fig. 2.**8** Removal of posterior skin.

Operative Technique

The operative technique is determined by careful preoperative examination and by having a plan of action that will give to the ear a form and position as normal as possible by prudent excision of cartilage and excess tissue. The helical rim (Fig. 2.**7**) may be bent back and marked so that the surgeon understands the degree of flexion necessary in the antihelical fold. Once the ear has been properly marked, an incision is made in a previously outlined area in the postauricular skin and removal of skin is performed (Fig. 2.**8**). The previously marked cartilage is then readily seen (Fig. 2.**9**).

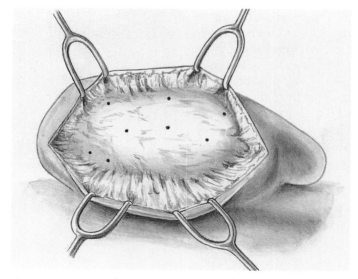

Fig. 2.**9** Removal of tissue and exposure of cartilage.

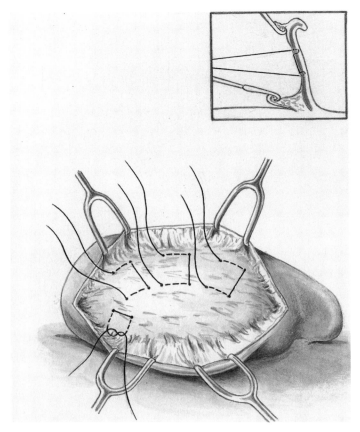

Fig. 2.**10** Identifying methylene blue marks and placement of Mustarde sutures.

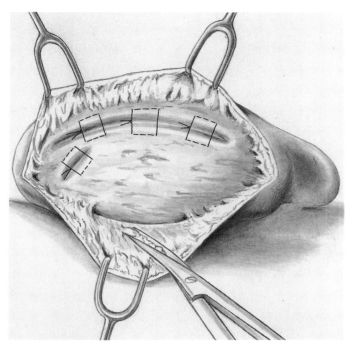

Fig. 2.**11** Dissection of postauricular skin off mastoid periosteum.

Atraumatic sutures of PDS or Ethibon are introduced into the cartilage as Mustarde mattress sutures, taking care to avoid puncture of the anterior skin (Fig. 2.**10**). Once the sutures have been placed, a dissection of the postauricular area (Fig. 2.**11**) over the mastoid periosteum is performed. Excision of conchal cartilage is performed, if necessary (Fig. 2.**12**).

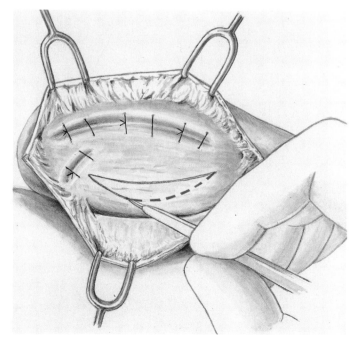

Fig. 2.**12** Conchal excision.

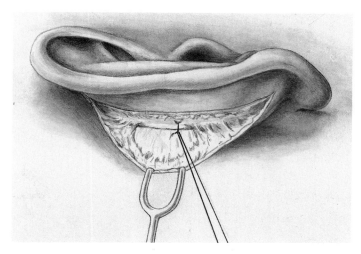

Fig. 2.**13**   Conchal–mastoid sutures.

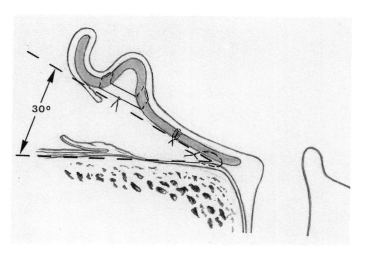

Fig. 2.**14**   Conchal–mastoid sutures anterior vs. posterior pull and effect on external canal.

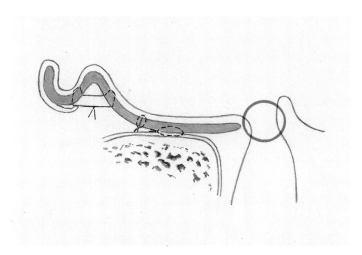

Fig. 2.**15**   Conchal–mastoid sutures anterior vs. posterior pull and effect on external canal.

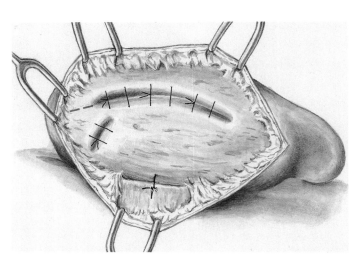

Fig. 2.**16**   Fossa triangularis.

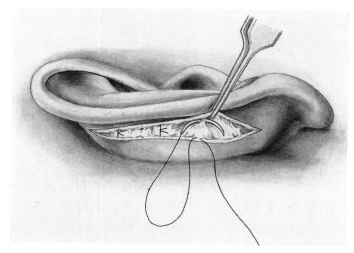

Fig. 2.**17**   Closure of subcutaneous and skin layers.

A conchal mastoid suture allows the concha to be rotated posteriorly to within 30 degrees of the lateral surface of the head (Fig. 2.**13**). Figures 2.**14** and 2.**15** illustrate the effect of this rotation on the overlying helical angle and on the external os of the canal. Occasionally, incisions for the antihelix should extend to the fossa triangularis to mimic a superior and inferior crus (Fig. 2.**16**). Closure of subcutaneous and skin layers should be performed meticulously as a layered closure (Fig. 2.**17**). A drain will be unnecessary if there is good hemostasis. A postoperative view of the completed auricle is seen in Figure 2.**18**.

The Pitanguy technique is demonstrated in Figures 2.**19**, 2.**20**, and 2.**21**.

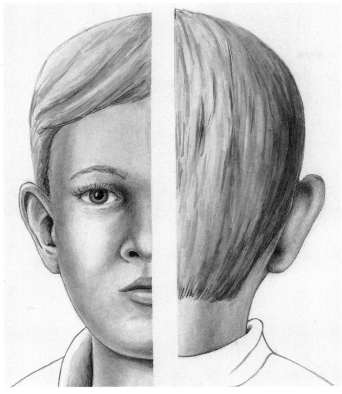

Fig. 2.**18**   Postoperative view.

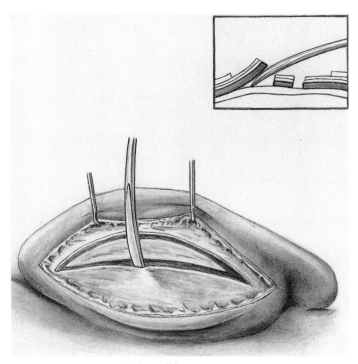

Fig. 2.**19**   Pitanguy technique (1).

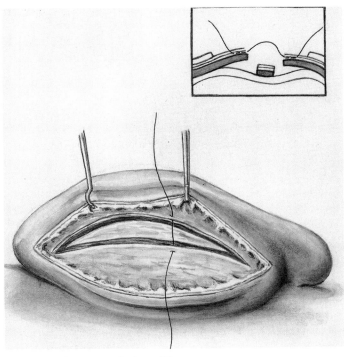

Fig. 2.**20**   Pitanguy technique (2).

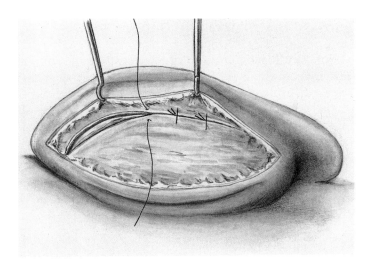

Fig. 2.**21**   Pitanguy technique (3).

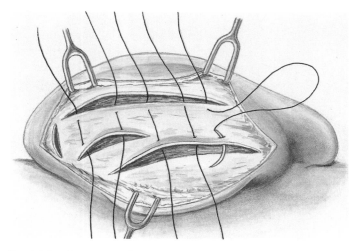

Fig. 2.**22**   Converse technique (1).

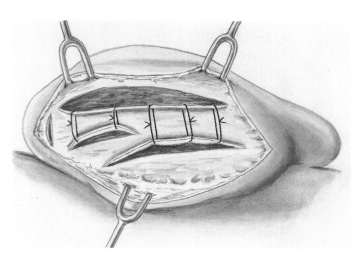

Fig. 2.**23**   Converse technique (2).

Figures 2.**22** and 2.**23** show the technique of Converse, in which numerous cartilaginous incisions are made to allow the cartilage to bend more naturally and to reduce sharp edges in the anterior portion of the ear.

The surgical dressing consists of a pressure type bandage with small pre- and postauricular dressings and a small fluff dressing to add minimal pressure to the underlying ear.

Surgical Landmarks and Danger Points

Major landmarks include the overall angle of the auricle from the head (should be less than 30 degrees), the fossa triangularis, and the conchal bowl. The depth of the conchal bowl should be noted and a decision made preoperatively whether resection of the bowl will be necessary, or if a conchal mastoid suture by itself will be sufficient. If the fossa triangularis is missing, it should be surgically created (see Fig. 2.**16**).

Rules, Tips, and Pitfalls

The greatest pitfall encountered in this surgery is pinching of the ear, a condition in which the antihelix is too narrow and causes a distortion of the normal curvature of the helix (Fig. 2.**24**).

If sutures are placed too near the surface of the skin, or if undermining has been done carelessly, necrosis of

the skin may occur (Fig. 2.**25**). The need for meticulous hemostasis is important to avoid hematoma formation. Overzealous retraction of the mid-portion of the ear may result in a "telephone" deformity (Fig. 2.**26**). Lastly, a conchal mastoid suture that is placed too far anterior, i. e. too close to the os of the external ear canal, may cause closure of the canal (Furnas, 1968).

Postoperative Care

If adequate hemostasis has been achieved, drains may be unnecessary. Drains should be placed only after careful consideration, since a drain represents one more area through which bacteria may enter the wound in a retrograde fashion, thereby increasing the chance of a postoperative infection. The dressings should be placed in a snug fashion without excessive pressure.

Postoperative Complications

Postoperative complications may be either minor or severe. Complications may be avoided by the judicious use of perioperative antibiotics, careful prepping of the surgical field, and meticulous surgical technique. Hemostasis with electrocautery is necessary at every step of the operation. Attention to sterility is of utmost importance. Handling of soft tissue must be done delicately. Antibiotics in the postoperative period should be continued for at least one week to lessen the possibility of infection.

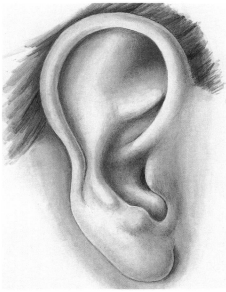

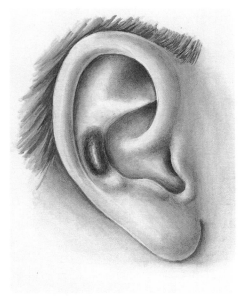

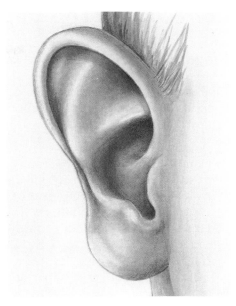

Fig. 2.**24**   Pinching of ear.   Fig. 2.**25**   Necrosis of skin.   Fig. 2.**26**   Telephone deformity.

Complications can be divided into early and late categories. *Early complications* include hematoma formation which is usually found in the postauricular space. The operative site should be carefully inspected on the first postoperative day, as this is the time when most hematomas can be readily drained without sequelae. If a hematoma is untreated for more than one week, infection and cartilage necrosis may occur. The presence of a hematoma may be suggested early on by postoperative pain out of proportion to that usually associated with the operation. The usual postoperative pain incurred in this surgery can be readily treated with mild analgesics.

Late complications involve severe pinching of the auricular cartilage with deformity of the overlying auricle. A second, more devastating loss, is skin necrosis secondary to improper handling of soft tissue, excessive stress on the auricle, or packing which is too tight. Skin loss should be treated with antibiotic ointment and closely followed. Frequently, if the necrotic skin is covered with antibiotic ointment on a daily basis, the underlying cartilage will survive and the skin will slowly regenerate. Another late potential complication is a "telephone" deformity as previously noted. This is secondary to excessive tension on the mid portion of the auricle and too little tension on the upper and lower poles of the auricle.

Sequelae

The most dreaded complication is chondritis with loss of auricular cartilage. This may occur as late as three months postoperatively. To avoid this complication, perioperative antibiotics should be administered.

Stitch abscesses may be a problem. Frequent postoperative visits in the first 2–3 months will lessen the chances of occult complications.

Correction of Lop Ears

Diagnosis and Preoperative Evaluation

There are several classifications of auricular defects. A concise classification initially proposed by Tanzer is as follows:

1) Anotia.
2) Complete hypoplasia (microtia):
   a) with atresia of the external auditory canal,
   b) without atresia of the external auditory canal.
3) Hypoplasia of the middle third of the auricle.
4) Hypoplasia of the superior third of the auricle:
   a) constricted cup or lop ear,
   b) cryptotia,
   c) hypoplasia of entire superior third.
5) The prominent ear.

Other classifications take into account even more detail (Rogers, 1968; 1974. Aguilar, 1988; 1992). The serious student of auricular deformity should review these classifications. By definition, lop ear involves reduction of the normal configuration of the upper third of the scapha and helix. There may be variations of the cup ear deformity, but all include a constricted helix as the major problem (Figs. 2.**27** and 2.**28**).

Indications

The greater the severity of the lop ear, the more difficult is the surgery. The age for surgery is approximately 5–6 years, particularly if extra cartilage is to be harvested from the rib cage.

Goal of the Operation

The goal of the operation is to change the lop ear to an ear that appears normal. Increasing the size of the ear is not necessarily the most important goal of the operation and takes second place to restoring a natural–looking ear. The long–term goal is the permanency of the results.

Preparation for Surgery

Photographs should be taken preoperatively. Full face, lateral, oblique, and posterior views should be taken to document the deformity. A surgical plan and a possible need for auricular cartilage from the ribs should be determined preoperatively.

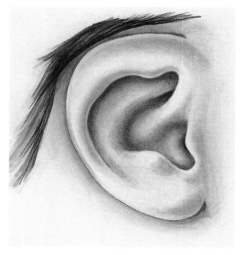

Fig. 2.**27**   Appearance of lop ear.

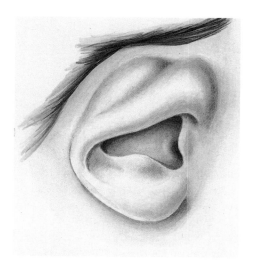

Fig. 2.**28**   Appearance of more severe lop ear.

Anesthesia

Auricular surgery in children is best performed under general anesthesia. Local anesthesia requires a very cooperative child. The length of the surgical procedure is also a factor. Local anesthesia with a vasoconstrictor agent should be used in conjunction with general anesthesia to aid in hemostasis. In those cases where the skin flaps to be elevated are extremely large, consideration should be given to avoiding the use of epinephrine as this may compromise the blood supply to the distal flap.

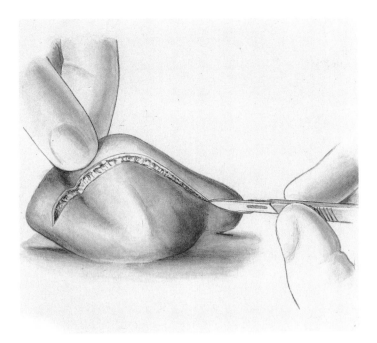

Fig. 2.**29**   Cosman technique — incision.

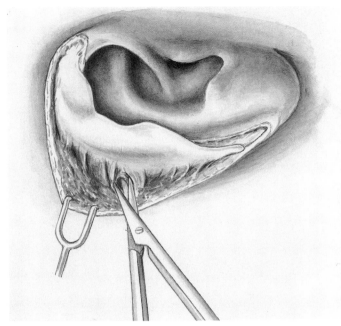

Fig. 2.**30**   Cosman technique — undermining.

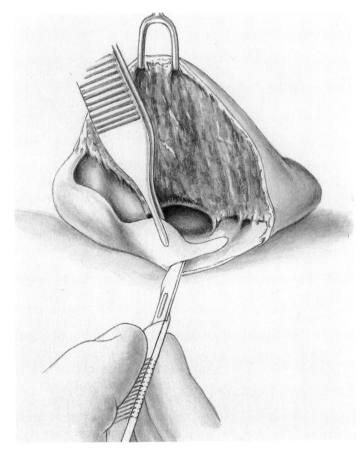

Fig. 2.**31**   Cosman technique — identification of helical rim.

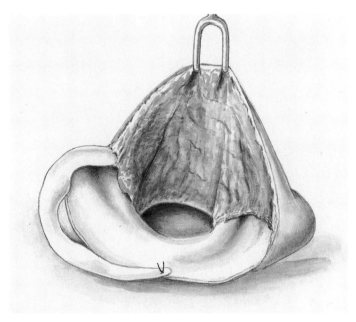

Fig. 2.**32**   Cosman technique — rotation of helical rim.

Operative Technique

The method for construction of the moderate lop ear is best illustrated by the Cosman technique. The postauricular incision is entered and wide undermining is carried out until the entire cartilage is bare (Figs. 2.**29** and 2.**30**). Identification of the lidded helical rim is made. The entire helical rim is separated except for its anterosuperior attachment. The helical rim is then rotated superiorly to add height (Figs. 2.**31** and 2.**32**).

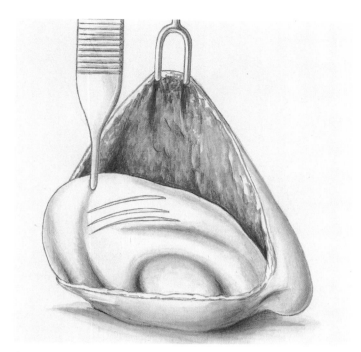

Fig. 2.**33** Scoring of scapha.

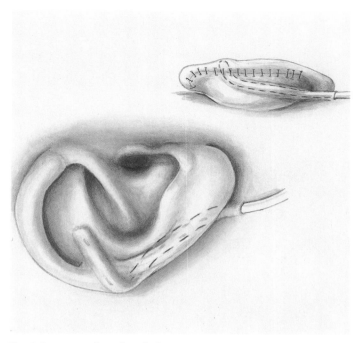

Fig. 2.**34** Use of suction drain.

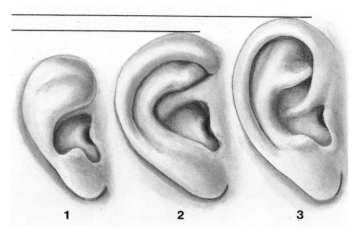

Fig. 2.**35** Root of helix position:
1: before operation,
2: after operation,
3: normal ear.

Prior to this, scoring of the scapha cartilage is undertaken, or mattress sutures are placed, in order to give an antihelical fold (Fig. 2.**33**). Once the rim is transposed, the overlying skin is checked for length. If more skin is needed, a split–thickness skin graft may be required posteriorly. A suction drain is used to coapt the skin to the underlying framework (Fig. 2.**34**). Mattress sutures (Mustardé, 1963) are usually needed to position the antihelical fold in its proper location. The position of the helical root should remain the same as preoperatively but the actual height of the helix should be improved. Note that it is difficult to maintain full height with this technique as compared to the normal side. However, a 50% improvement over the previous deformity may be experienced (Fig. 2.**35**).

Weerda uses a similar method but rotates the entire helical rim 180 degrees and then resutures it in place (Figs. 2.**36** and 2.**37**).

Surgical Landmarks and Danger Points

The root of the helix is of utmost importance. It should not be displaced from its original preoperative position. The scapha is usually not well formed. There is also a concomitant lack of an antihelical fold. These issues should be addressed prior to surgical correction.

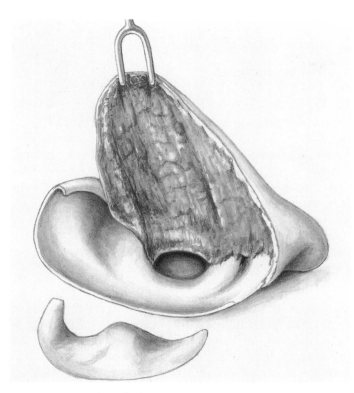

Fig. 2.**36**   Weerda technique.

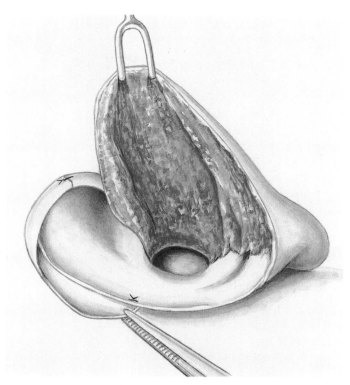

Fig. 2.**37**   Weerda technique.

Rules, Tips, and Pitfalls

It is important to use a sufficient width of helical rim. The rim itself may actually be reversed if the strength of the cartilage permits. The use of a suction drain is important. Sutures through the skin into the cartilage should be avoided because of the risk of chondritis.

Postoperative Care

Postoperative suction drains are recommended and should be removed when there is minimal drainage. Bandages should be light. Perioperative antibiotics are administered and continued for at least one week postoperatively.

Postoperative Complications

Possible complications include infection and hematoma. While these are treated if they occur, the use of perioperative antibiotics should lessen the risk of infection.

Reconstruction of the Helix

Diagnosis and Preoperative Evaluation

Reconstruction of the helix is usually necessary secondary to tissue loss from trauma, or from a resection due to cancer. It is incumbent upon the plastic surgeon to recognize the extent of the defect and to tailor the operation to suit the needs of the patient. If only the helix is missing, a piece of cartilage may be attached to the scapha component already present and covered with a local skin flap.

Indications

It is helpful to divide the loss of a helix into two categories:

(1) less than 1/3 of the helix involved and
(2) greater than 1/3 of the helical rim involved. The goal of the operation is reconstruction of the helix with as normal a contour as possible.

Goals of the Operation

The goal of the operation is the presence of symmetry and maintaining comparable size with the opposite ear.

Preparation for Surgery

As in other areas, preparation for surgery should include preoperative photographs and liberal skin markings so that the patient understands the extent of the operation. The contralateral ear should be examined for donor cartilage which may be used in reconstruction of the ear. Rib cartilage is also an excellent source of donor tissue.

Anesthesia

Usually, helical reconstruction lends itself well to local anesthesia. The anesthetic agent of choice is Xylocaine with 1:100,000 epinephrine. Adequate regional block in this area can be attained, especially if the lesion is small. General anesthesia is required if surgery includes harvesting of rib cartilage, or a large segment of auricular cartilage.

Operative Technique

Standard surgical prepping is performed with attention to sterile technique and meticulous surgical handling of the soft tissues. Figures 2.**38** and 2.**39** illustrate the upper third loss and the middle third loss of the helix, respectively. In planning the reconstruction of such defects, the surgeon must opt for the simple over the complex when allowed to do so. As shown in Figure 2.**40**, when a middle third defect exists, caused by excision of tumor or trauma, often the simplest solution is to rotate the upper and lower segments together. This will leave a smaller ear, but aesthetically the results are superior to any attempted major flap work.

As seen in Figure 2.**41**, defects of the upper third are somewhat more difficult to reconstruct, and there is frequently no easy solution to this problem. These cases may require the harvesting of composite cartilage or rib cartilage to create a helix. Carving the costal cartilage is somewhat easier for the experienced surgeon, and implanting it beneath the skin in the immediate postauricular area is a good solution. Repair of this defect requires a second stage elevation with a split–thickness skin graft to the posterior aspect of the ear (Fig. 2.**42**).

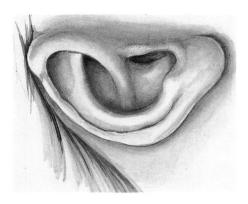

Fig. 2.**38**   Upper third loss of helix.

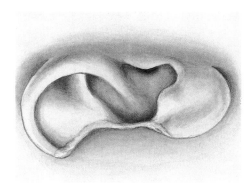

Fig. 2.**39a**   Middle third loss of helix.

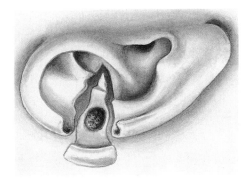

Fig. 2.**39b**   Middle third loss of helix.

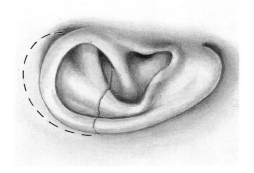

Fig. 2.**40**   Rotation of upper cartilage.

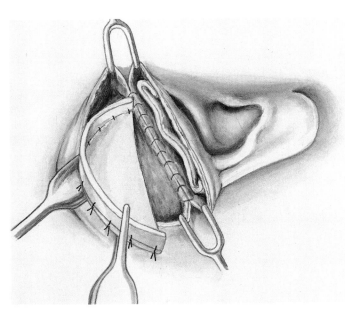

Fig. 2.**41**   Implantation of costal cartilage.

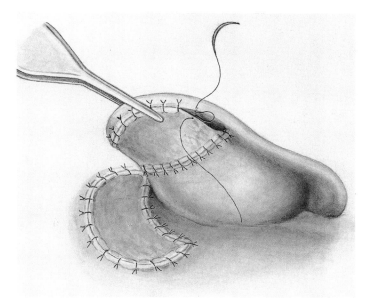

Fig. 2.**42**   Elevation of cartilage and placement of skin graft posteriorly.

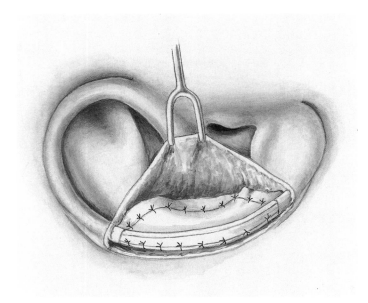

Fig. 2.**43** Implantation of cartilage — middle third.

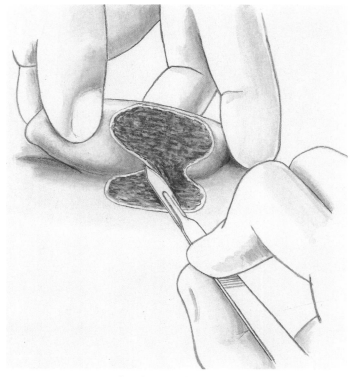

Fig. 2.**44** Elevation of middle third.

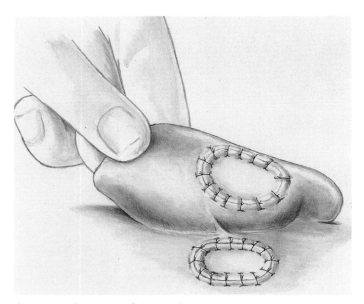

Fig. 2.**45** Placement of skin graft posteriorly.

Figure 2.**43** illustrates the implantation of a cartilage graft in the middle third followed by elevation and placement of a skin graft posteriorly (Figs. 2.**44** and 2.**45**).

Surgical Landmarks and Danger Points

Figure 2.**46** shows the use of local tubes and flaps. This maneuver should be avoided as it leaves extensive scarring and compromises the adjacent skin flaps which may be later used for reconstruction.

Suction drains should be used to coapt the skin to the underlying cartilage (Fig. 2.**47**).

Mattress sutures through both skin and cartilage should be avoided as the risk of chondritis is high.

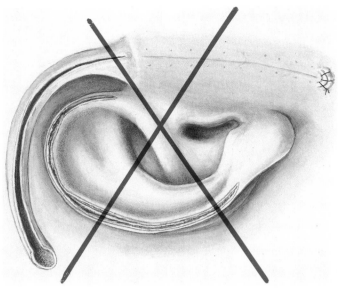

Fig. 2.**46**   Avoid local flaps and tubes.

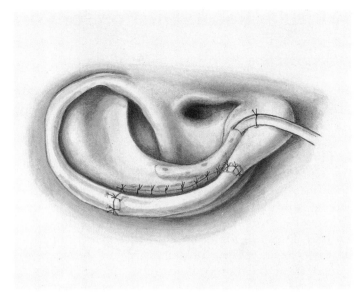

Fig. 2.**47**   Use of suction drain important.

Postoperative Care

Bandage dressings should be lightly placed to avoid pressure on the overlying skin.

Postoperative Complications

Postoperative complications are rare and are usually limited to bleeding, hematoma, or necrosis of skin and cartilage. As necrosis of skin and cartilage is closely associated with mattress sutures, they should be avoided.

Auricular Reconstruction for Congenital Microtia

Diagnosis and Preoperative Evaluation

Congenital microtia is an obvious malformation. The preferred classification includes three grades of microtia (Fig. 2.**48**). Audiologic evaluation is paramount before the child is subjected to reconstructive surgery of the auricle. This includes a behavioral audiogram if the child's age permits, or an auditory brainstem response test if the child is very young. In the case of bilateral aural atresia, the child should have already been fitted with a bone-conducting hearing aid. A high resolution CT scan of the temporal bones is recommended at about age 5. Lastly, informed consent should be obtained from the family before beginning any staged procedure for auricular reconstruction of congenital microtia. The family should have realistic expectations regarding the outcome.

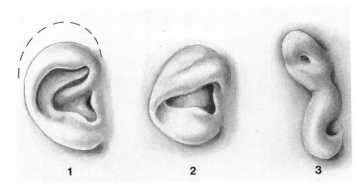

Fig. 2.**48**   Drawing of 3 grades of microtia:
1: grade I,
2: grade II,
3: grade III.

Indications

Surgery is begun at age six years. Bilateral microtia and atresia cases should be started earlier (age 5) if possible so that the atresia may be corrected sooner. At age 6, the size of the patient is sufficient to provide enough costal cartilage for the ear reconstruction. Also at age 6 the child can usually tolerate the postoperative care and he or she is psychologically ready to have corrective surgery. Peer ridicule concerning the size and differences of a child's ears has not yet intensified at this age.

Goals of the Operation

The short–term goals are to plan and effect a series of operations that will begin to restore the external ear to a normal appearance. The long–term goal is total replacement of the microtic vestige by the new auricle.

Preparation for Surgery

Preoperative photographs are important as well as template preparation. Figure 2.**49** shows the template outline on the opposite ear to determine the size of the auricular framework. Figure 2.**50** shows the suction drain and the special instruments used to sculpt the cartilaginous framework.

The stages of operation are as follows (Aguilar, 1989; 1991):

Stage I   — Auricular cartilage is harvested from the rib cage, sculpted, and implanted as the framework for the new ear.
Stage II   — Transposition of the lobule with excision of any superior microtic vestige.
Stage III   — Reconstruction of the tragus.
Stage IV   — Elevation of the auricle.

The stages may be performed three months apart, but should be attempted no sooner than this. Atresia repair is performed after stage IV when external ear reconstruction is complete. Although atresia repair can be done anytime after stage II, we have found that the final result is better if all stages are first completed by the plastic surgeon.

Anesthesia

Each stage of the auricular reconstruction should be performed under general anesthesia as the independent steps are lengthy and may require a prolonged surgical time.

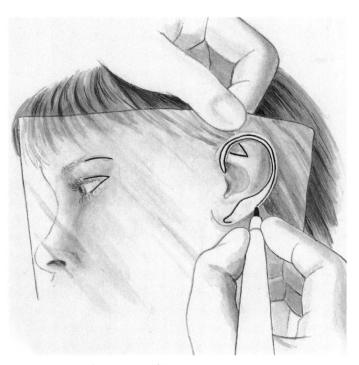

Fig. 2.**49**   Template preparation.

Operative Technique

A. Stage I

The procedure outlined here is the technique of Brent. He must be considered the foremost authority on ear reconstruction in the world. This is an excellent operation which gives predictable results in qualified hands. There should be a commitment by the surgeon to do this operation regularly, as his or her skill will increase as more experience is gained.

The patient's rib cage is shown in Figure 2.**51**, and the template is superimposed on the rib anatomy to demonstrate that area from which the ribs are harvested. The site is usually the 6th, 7th, and 8th ribs of the side opposite the microtic ear.

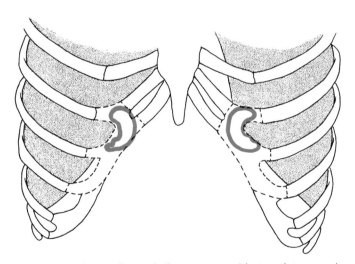

Fig. 2.**51**   Patient's ribs and rib anatomy with template superimposed.

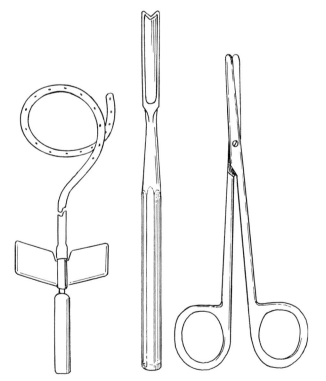

Fig. 2.**50**   Drain and special instruments.

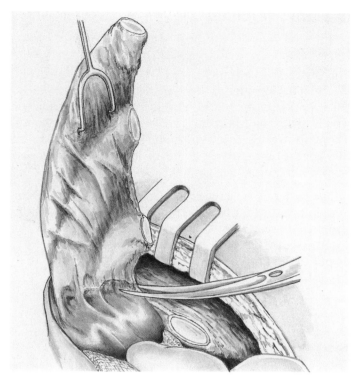

Fig. 2.**52**   Rib dissection with pleura demonstrated.

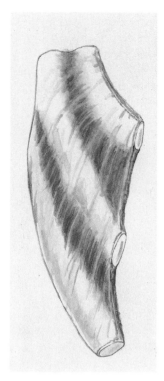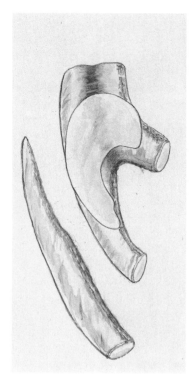

Fig. 2.**53**   Fig. 2.**54**

Fig. 2.**53**   Demonstrating 3 rib piece.

Fig. 2.**54**   Breakdown of ribs into component parts and carving of scapha.

The rib dissection is undertaken with preservation of the underlying pleura and the perichondrial layer of the ribs (Fig. 2.**52**). Once the three rib segment is removed as shown in Figure 2.**53**, the ribs are split. The 8th rib is set aside for later carving to make the helical rim, and the 6th and 7th ribs are left joined for the scaphal carving (Fig. 2.**54**).

Usually the 8th rib is carved first to allow for gentle bending of the cartilage to position it on top of the scaphal complex, and the scaphal complex is trimmed as outlined on the ribs earlier (Figs. 2.**54** and 2.**55**). This part of the procedure is time–consuming and requires the most artistic talent of the surgeon. It should not be approached lightly. Many hours of practice are necessary before the surgeon begins carving live cartilage.

Figure 2.**56** demonstrates the joining of ribs 6 and 7 to the 8th rib using a wire suture. Once the union is complete, the complex is ready to accept more carving to achieve the detail necessary to create an ear which has good form. Further sculpting (Fig. 2.**57**) is done to create the antihelical sulcus and the fossa triangularis.

Once the graft is sculpted, attention is turned to the microtic ear. Vestigial cartilage is removed, and wide undermining with placement of the sculpted cartilaginous

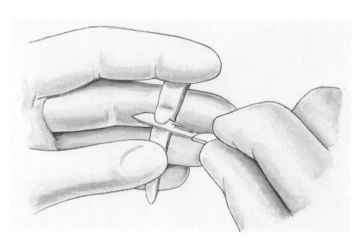

Fig. 2.**55**   Carving of helix.

implant is accomplished. Suction drains are placed to allow coaptation of the skin to the underlying cartilage (Figures 2.**58**–2.**60**). The dressings remain in place for 4–5 days. The suction drain is removed on postoperative day 3 or 4 depending on the amount of drainage.

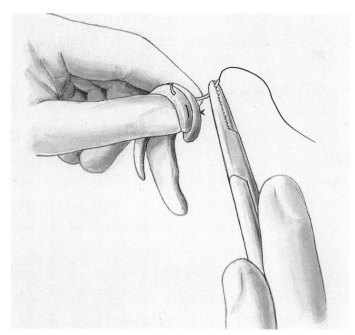

Fig. 2.**56**   Wiring of framework.

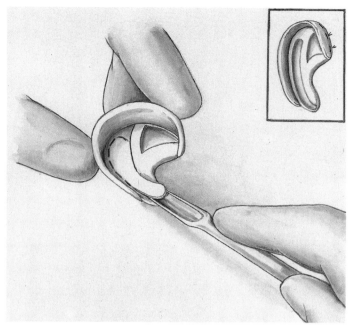

Fig. 2.**57**   Carving of fossa triangularis.

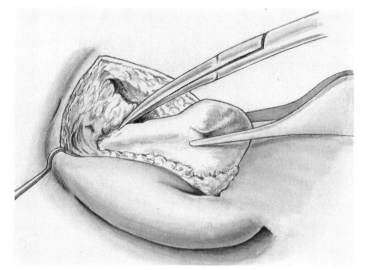

Fig. 2.**58**

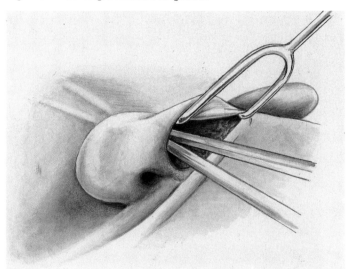

Fig. 2.**59**

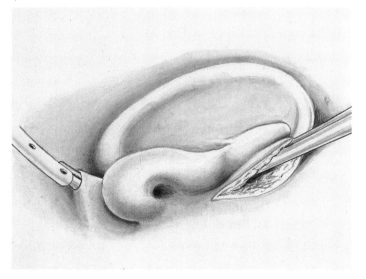

Fig. 2.**58**   Preparation of microtic ear with removal of vestigial cartilage.

Fig. 2.**59**   Wide undermining.

Fig. 2.**60**   Placement of implant and drain.

Fig. 2.**60**

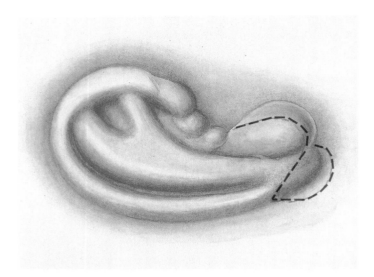

Fig. 2.**61**   Transposition of lobule — planning.

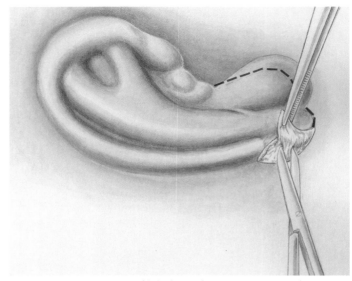

Fig. 2.**62**   Transposition of lobule — donor area preparation.

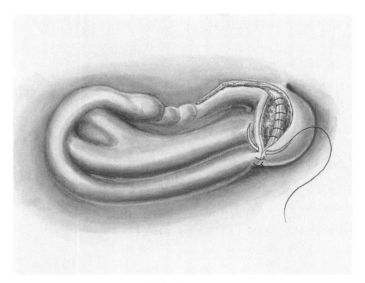

Fig. 2.**63**   Transposition of lobule.

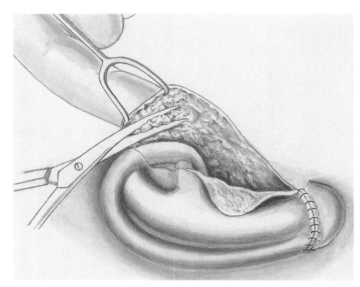

Fig. 2.**64**   Removal of microtic skin.

B. Stage II

Once the Stage I procedure has been completed, it is followed by transposition of the microtic segment to create a new earlobe. As the upper portion of the microtic ear still remains, it must be trimmed and transposed to expose the detail of the upper pole (Fig. 2.**61**).

Attention to the lower segment of the microtic ear centers around creating an inferiorly–based pedicle that can be swiveled onto the framework and spliced in the appropriate position to give the patient an ear that is complete (Figs. 2.**62**–2.**64**). The position of the pedicle remains a question of artistic interpretation by the surgeon. The surgeon must make the final decision as to where it should be placed. This can be difficult to master and requires extensive practice to excel in this stage.

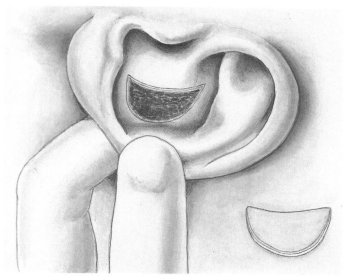

Fig. 2.**65**   Harvesting of composite graft.

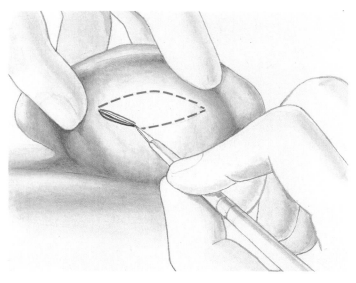

Fig. 2.**66**   Closure of donor site and skin graft harvest.

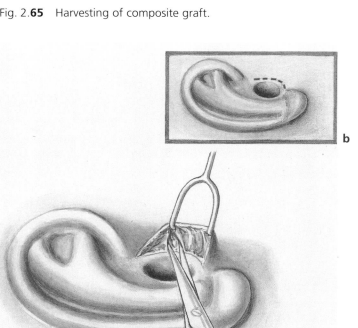

b

a

Fig. 2.**67 a**   Preparation of reconstructed side with planned incision.   **b** Undermining anteriorly.

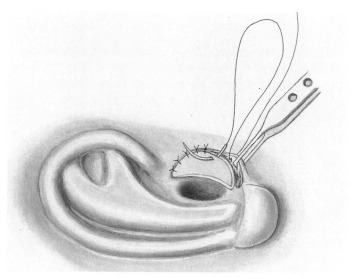

Fig. 2.**68**   Placement of composite graft.

C. Stage III

This stage involves harvesting a composite graft for creation of the tragus. Figure 2.**65** shows the donor site composite graft and Figure 2.**66** illustrates closure of the donor site and harvesting of the skin graft in the postauricular area.

The incision for reconstruction of the tragus is shown in Figures 2.**67 a** and **b**. The composite graft is placed on end with the anterior portion of the incision (Figs. 2.**68** and 2.**69**) and sutured with 6.0 Prolene. Placement of the skin graft is accomplished with an absorbable chromic suture (Fig. 2.**69**). The composite graft is advanced anteriorly by placing a stay suture and the skin graft is sutured to the posterior portion of the incision (Fig. 2.**70**).

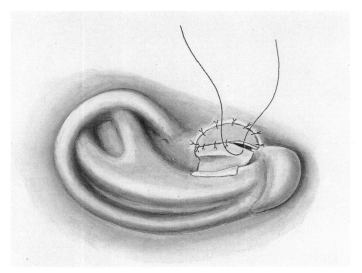

Fig. 2.**69**   Placement of skin graft.

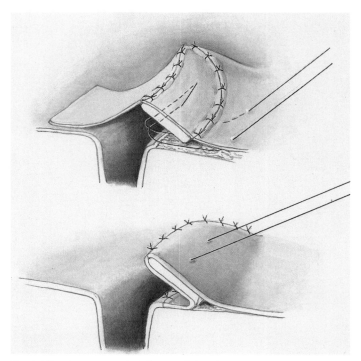

Fig. 2.**70**   Stay suture holding graft in place.

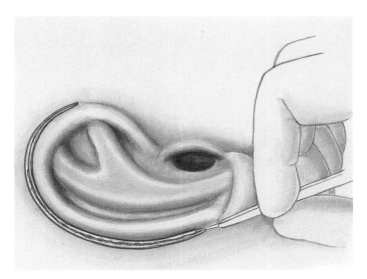

Fig. 2.**71**   Incision for elevation.

D. Stage IV

This stage is the culmination of the entire procedure. It involves elevation of the auricle on the side of the head and coverage of the posterior surface of the ear with a skin graft. Figure 2.**71** shows the incisions necessary to effect the elevation. The elevation proceeds as in Figures 2.**72**–2.**75**. The auricle may be advanced as far forward as necessary. Wide undermining of the skin flap posteriorly is important to allow the skin flap to be advanced. The skin graft is taken from the buttocks and covers the posterior portion of the auricle. A dressing stent consisting of interface and xeroform packing is placed over the skin graft and tightened with bolsters. The stent remains in place for 5 days.

Surgical Landmarks and Danger Points

Surgical landmarks are important in this procedure as in no other. The harvesting of the rib cartilage with the preservation of the pleura is a procedure that requires surgical dexterity. The surgeon must be cognizant of a possible abnormal course of the facial nerve in children with congenital microtia. The face should be observed for any twitching which may indicate stimulation of the facial nerve during the surgical dissection.

Rules, Tips, and Pitfalls

The potential for a pleural tear is high and the surgeon should be prepared to handle this complication in the postoperative period.

- The elevated postauricular flaps in Stage I should be thin and care should be taken to avoid injuring the deeper, superficial temporalis fascia.

- Transposition of the lobule should be done within the context of the overall framework structure.
- Carrying over too much posterior skin should be avoided as this will cause the lobule to protrude at an undesirable angle from the side of the face.
- Sufficient cartilage should be harvested to add height in creating a new tragus.
- The overlap of skin in the composite graft should be of adequate size to camouflage the edge of the graft.

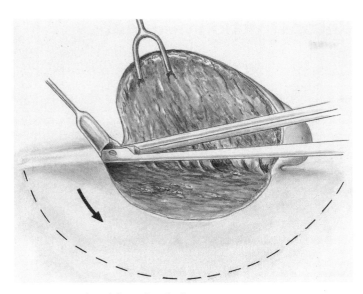

Fig. 2.**72**   Undermining of scalp flaps.

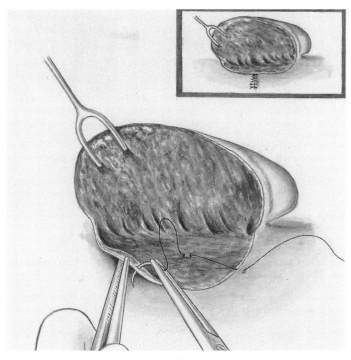

Fig. 2.**73**   Advancement of scalp flaps.

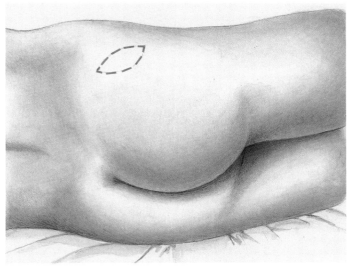

Fig. 2.**74**   Planning of skin graft.

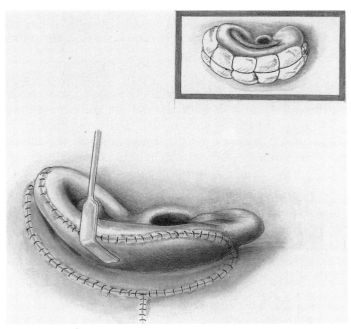

Fig. 2.**75**   Placement of skin graft and bolsters.

- Elevation of the auricle is performed in a manner whereby most of the normal scalp immediately behind the ear remains intact. This allows the skin graft to be placed directly on the posterior aspect of the reconstructed ear. The newly formed postauricular sulcus is thus composed of 50% skin graft and 50% postauricular scalp skin. While this may not be possible in every case, the attempt should be made nonetheless. The cartilage framework should be protected at every step of the operation. Care is taken to prevent inadvertent cartilage exposure.

Postoperative Care

All skin sutures are removed 4–5 days postoperatively. Suction drainage is used only in the first stage and the drain is usually removed on the fourth postoperative day. Postoperative antibiotics are used in every patient following each stage of the operation.

Postoperative Complications

Postoperative complications can be serious. Postoperative complications following Stage I include pneumothorax, pneumomediastinum, chest wall deformities, and hypertrophic scarring.

Serious complications may occur in the area where the cartilage is to be implanted. These involve necrosis of the overlying skin with exposure of the rib cartilage as well as chondritis with loss of cartilage framework. These complications can be devastating to the family and the patient and should be avoided by careful placement of the auricular framework.

Stage II may be complicated by necrosis of the lobule flaps. As this is an inferiorly–based flap, the blood supply may be compromised by twisting or torquing. If the flap is handled meticulously, this complication should be avoided. Sutures should be removed on the third or fourth postoperative day.

Stage III and Stage IV complications may include skin necrosis, infection, and hematoma.

Reconstruction of Earlobes

Diagnosis and Preoperative Evaluation

The absence of an earlobe is an obvious deformity. There are usually two reasons why an earlobe is missing: (1) congenital microtia or (2), traumatic amputation (Fig. 2.76). An oversized earlobe may require a reduction (Fig. 2.77).

Goal of the Operation

The goal of the operation is to create an earlobe that closely resembles a normal earlobe. Symmetry and balance with the opposite ear are important.

Preparation for Surgery

In planning for surgery, preoperative photographs are essential. Careful markings should be made of the various steps in the technique so that the family understands what the surgeon is attempting to do.

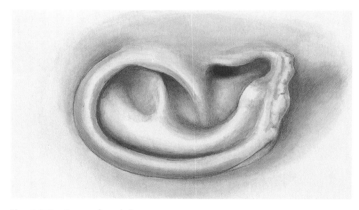

Fig. 2.**76**   Loss of earlobe.

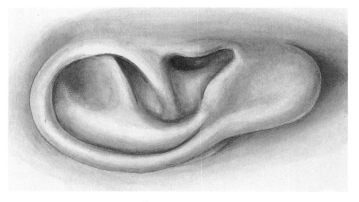

Fig. 2.**77**   Increased size of earlobe.

Anesthesia

This operation is well suited to local anesthesia. However, this choice depends on the patient's age, size, and temperament. General anesthesia may be used if necessary.

Operative Techniques

The technique for earlobe reconstruction for congenital microtia has already been outlined under microtia repair. An operative technique favored by Brent uses a cartilage graft that is harvested from the conchal bowl of the contralateral ear. This graft is rotated as appropriate to give the proper form for the earlobe, but it is implanted beneath the skin (Figs. 2.**78**–2.**80**). Once the cartilage is implanted, a period of time is allowed to pass and then the entire complex is elevated. A skin graft is subsequently placed behind this to complete the separation from the postauricular area. This method is preferred over local flaps as the scar is well hidden in the post–lobular area, and the adjacent skin is not affected.

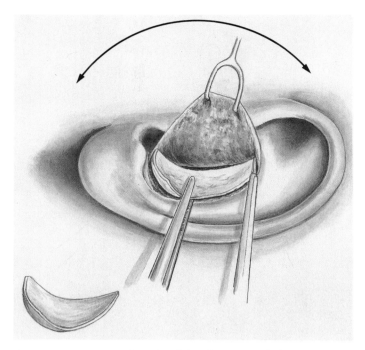

Fig. 2.**78**   Reconstruction of earlobe via Brent technique.

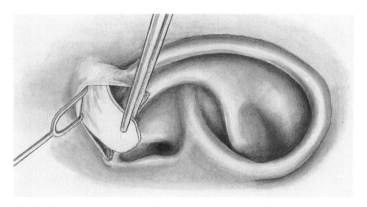

Fig. 2.**79**   Reconstruction of earlobe via Brent technique.

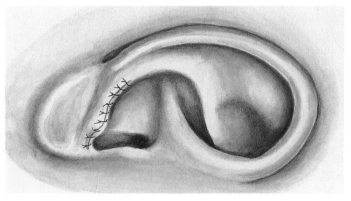

Fig. 2.**80**   Reconstruction of earlobe via Brent technique.

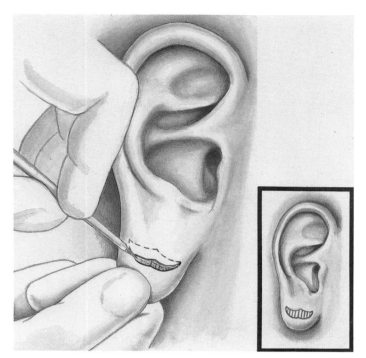

Fig. 2.**81**   Reduction of earlobe (1).

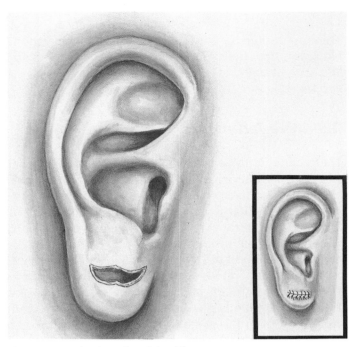

Fig. 2.**82**   Reduction of earlobe (2).

Operative techniques for reduction of earlobes are outlined in Figures 2.**81** and 2.**82**. This particular incision leaves a scar that mimics the natural crease of the lobe and is camouflaged well.

Modifications

Figures 2.**83** and 2.**84** show an alternate technique for reconstruction. The method of Gavello (Gersuny, 1962) is illustrated and is a standard procedure yielding predictable results.

Surgical Landmarks and Danger Points

As the facial nerve may have an aberrant course in children with a congenital ear malformation, care must be taken when undermining skin in this area. The parotid capsule should not be entered.

Rules, Tips, and Pitfalls

Earlobe reconstruction generally requires light bandages with minimal pressure. Steristrips may be used. A suction drain is rarely necessary.

Postoperative Complications

The two most common complications are: (1) infection and (2) necrosis of the pedicle flaps. The flap should be handled gently and carefully. Perioperative antibiotics are used routinely.

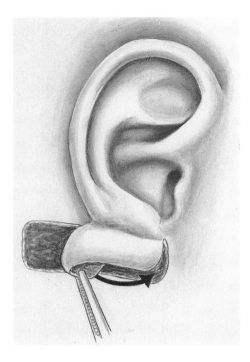

Fig. 2.**83**   Gavello technique (1).

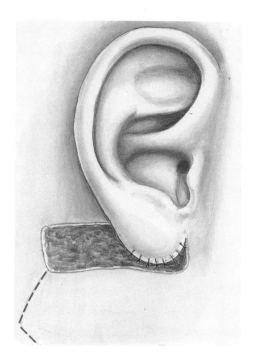

Fig. 2.**84**   Gavello technique (2).

Bibliography

Aguilar III E, Jahrsdoerfer R. The surgical repair of congenital microtia and atresia. Otolaryngol Head Neck Surg 1988; 98: 600.

Aguilar III E. Auricular reconstruction. Arch Otolaryngol Head Neck Surg 1989; 115: 1417.

Aguilar III E, Jahrsdoerfer R. The role of the plastic surgeon in microtia repair. In: Plastic and Reconstructive Surgery of the Head and Neck, Stucker F, ed. Philadelphia: BC Decker Inc; Vol 126, p 621, 1991.

Aguilar III E. Classification of auricular congenital deformities. In: Facial Plastic and Reconstructive Surgery, Papel I, Nachlas N, eds. St. Louis: Mosby Year Book; 1992, p. 532.

Brent B. The correction of microtia with autogenous cartilage grafts: II. Atypical and complex deformities. Plast Reconstr Surg 1980; 66: 13.

Brent B. Reconstruction of the ear. In: Plastic Surgery: A Concise Guide to Clinical Practice, Grabb W, Smith J, eds, 3rd ed. Boston: Little Brown Co; 1980, p. 299.

Brent B. Total auricular construction with sculpted costal cartilages. In: The Artistry of Reconstructive Surgery, Brent B, ed. St. Louis: CV Mosby Co; 1987, p. 113.

Brent B. Reconstruction of the auricle. In: Plastic Surgery, McCarthy J, ed. Philadelphia: WB Saunders Company; Vol 3, 1990, p. 2094.

Converse J. Reconstruction of the auricle in 2 parts. Plast Reconst Surg 1958; 21: 150.

Converse J. Reconstruction of the auricle in 2 parts. Plast Reconst Surg 1958; 22: 230.

Cosman B. Repair of the constricted ear. In: The Artistry of Reconstructive Surgery, Brent B., ed. St. Louis: CV Mosby Co; 1987; 99.

Furnas D. Correction of prominent ears by concha-mastoid sutures. Plast Reconst Surg 1968; 42: 189.

Gersuny. In: Plastische Operationen an der Nase und an der Ohrmuschel, Šerçer A, Mündnich K, eds. Stuttgart: Thieme; 1962; p. 364.

Mustardé J. The correction of prominent ears using simple mattress sutures. Br J Plast Surg 1963; 16: 170.

Pitanguy I, Flemming I. Plastic operations on the auricle. In: Head and Neck Surgery, Naumann H, ed. Philadelphia: WB Saunders; 1982.

Rogers B. Microtic, lop, cup, and protruding ears: four directly inheritable deformities? Plast Reconst Surg 1968; 41: 208.

Rogers B. Anatomy, embryology and classification of auricular deformities. In: Symposium on Reconstruction of the Auricle, Tanzer R, Edgerton M, eds. St. Louis: CV Mosby Company; 1974; p 3.

Tanzer R. An analysis of ear reconstruction. Plast Reconst Surg 1963; 31: 16.

Tanzer R. Congenital deformities. In: Reconstructive Plastic Surgery, Converse J, ed. Philadelphia: WB Saunders, 1977; p 1671.

Weerda H. Reconstructive surgery of auricle. Facial Plast Surg (International quarterly monographs) 1988; 399.

3 Surgical Management of Congenital Ear Malformations

Robert A. Jahrsdoerfer and Eugenio A. Aguilar III

Introduction

Congenital malformations of the ear are classified into major and minor groups. Major malformations are those in which there is stenosis or atresia of the external ear canal and the auricle will usually show some degree of microtia. In minor malformations the congenital problem is largely limited to the middle ear. An external ear canal is present and a tympanic membrane can be identified although one or both structures may be abnormal in size, shape, and position.

Minor Malformations

Minor congenital ear malformations frequently involve the stapes/facial nerve axis. An arrest of development in this area may result in a displaced and bare facial nerve and secondary anomalies of the stapes and oval window. These may range from a mild fixation of the stapes footplate to a congenital absence of the stapes and oval window. It is important that the surgeon be aware that the hearing problem may be congenital, and one should be mentally prepared to deal with an ossicular malformation if encountered.

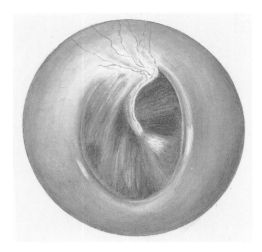

Fig. 3.**1**   Imprint of curved malleus handle on ear drum.

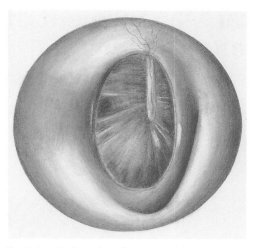

Fig. 3.**2**   Malleus handle encroaching upon anterior ear canal wall.

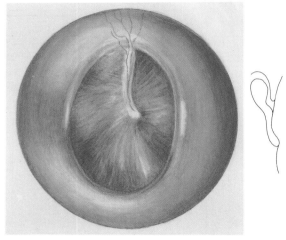

Fig. 3.**3**   Tip of malleus handle tenting tympanic membrane.

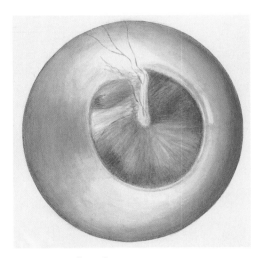

Fig. 3.**4**   Malleus bar.

Diagnosis and Preoperative Evaluation

Inspection of the Tympanic Membrane

This is performed as an office procedure using the operating microscope. The size and shape of the tympanic membrane are noted. A small eardrum is a clue that a congenital problem may exist. Ossicular landmarks are observed.

- Is there a curve to the imprint of the malleus in the ear drum (Fig. 3.**1**)?
- Does the malleus handle appear to encroach upon the anterior ear canal wall (Fig. 3.**2**)?
- Does the tip of the malleus handle at the umbo appear to protrude through the tympanic membrane (Fig. 3.**3**)?
- Are there any unusual bony bridges to suggest a "malleus bar" — an abnormal strut of bone from the malleus neck to the posterior bony anulus (Fig. 3.**4**)?

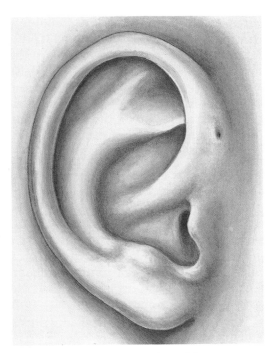

Fig. 3.**5**   Preauricular pit on lateral face.

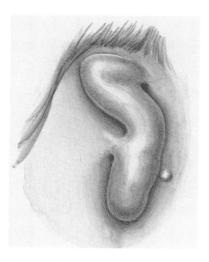

Fig. 3.**6**   External ear malformation.

Gross Inspection of Patient

The examiner should search for subtle indications which may indicate a congenital ear malformation.

- Is there a preauricular pit (Fig. 3.**5**)? Is the external ear oddly shaped (Fig. 3.**6**)?
- Does the ear canal slant superiorly?
- Are there other congenital anomalies involving the face and head?
- Is there a facial weakness or paralysis (Fig. 3.**7**)?
- Is the patient's hearing impaired?
- All are *"soft"* signs that should make the examiner mindful of the possibility that one is dealing with a congenital middle ear problem.

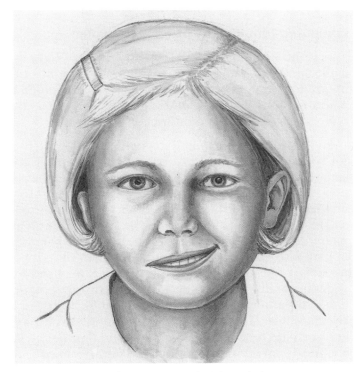

Fig. 3.**7**   Patient with preoperative facial paralysis.

Audiologic Evaluation

A complete audiologic evaluation is performed. This includes air and bone thresholds for pure tones, speech reception threshold, speech discrimination, and tympanometry. The stapedial reflex should be routinely tested as stapes fixation and other stapes anomalies are common in minor ear malformations. Auditory brainstem response testing should be done in patients in whom behavioral testing is not possible.

No patient should be operated until the surgeon is convinced beyond a reasonable doubt that adequate cochlear function is present in both ears. If this cannot be determined to the satisfaction of the surgeon or the audiologist, surgery should be deferred. The patient should continue to use a hearing device for amplification and be re–evaluated for hearing purposes at a future date.

Computed Tomography of Temporal Bones

This is the single most important study available to the clinician. While computed tomography is imperative in major malformations, i. e. aural atresia, its use in minor malformations is still essential, particularly when the tympanic membrane is malformed or opaque.

High resolution computed tomography will yield useful, often critical, information on the status of the stapes, labyrinthine windows, the incus/malleus complex, and the course and size of the facial nerve. More importantly, it will show if the inner ear is malformed and may warn of a potential *spinal fluid gusher*. Perilymphatic or spinal fluid gushers are much more common in patients with a minor malformation than they are in patients with aural atresia. The CT scan may show a widening or dilatation of the inner ear structures, particularly the internal auditory canal, vestibule, or semicircular canals. These findings may be noted despite normal cochlear function. Any inner ear malformation, including isolated widening of the lateral semicircular canal, should disqualify the patient for surgery.

Middle Ear

Jugular Bulb, Carotid Artery, Congenital Cholesteatoma

Careful preoperative inspection in the office setting using the operating microscope will usually alert the examiner to a middle ear malformation.

Vascular malformations of the middle ear include a persistent stapedial artery, an anomalous internal carotid artery, and a high and uncovered jugular bulb. A *persistent stapedial artery* is usually diagnosed after a tympanomeatal flap has been raised. An *anomalous in-ternal carotid artery,* on the other hand, is commonly seen through a transparent tympanic membrane. It presents as a pink, or pinkish-red, mass pressing against the medial surface of the tympanic membrane (Fig. 3.**8**). Pulsations of the blood vessel may be seen and the artery may blanche with each pulsation. Objective tinnitus may be heard on auscultation over the ear or high in the neck. Digital compression of the carotid artery in the neck abolishes the tinnitus.

A *high, uncovered jugular bulb* will commonly present as a bluish dome–shaped mass in the lower third of the middle ear (Fig. 3.**9**). It may or may not press against the medial surface of the tympanic membrane. On rare occasions, the jugular bulb will present at a level sufficiently high in the middle ear to encroach upon the ossicular chain and cause a conductive hearing loss (Steffen, 1968). It is important to know that most iatrogenic injuries to an uncovered jugular bulb occur because the surgeon is not cognizant of its presence, or the jugular bulb is obscured by a dense, scarred tympanic membrane. The bulb is thereby vulnerable during myringotomy or when turning a tympanomeatal flap.

The only other middle ear vascular lesion which offers a serious consideration in the differential diagnosis is *glomus tumor, either tympanicum or jugulare* (Fig. 3.**10**).

Small Tympanic Membrane

A tympanic membrane that is smaller than normal may presage a congenital ear malformation — particularly if the malleus handle is close to the anterior bony ear canal wall. While small ear drums are usually found in association with canal stenosis, they may on occasion be found in the presence of a normal ear canal. If the drum is small, the anulus is often incomplete. This finding may not be appreciated until one attempts to raise a tympanomeatal flap. A large chorda tympani nerve, or a deviation in its course, may also be seen.

Abnormal Ossicular Landmarks

In the normal ear, the imprint of the malleus handle on the tympanic membrane is readily seen, and a portion of the long arm of the incus is often appreciated through a transparent ear drum. The stapes is usually not well seen through an intact drum. In a congenital middle ear malformation, the ossicular landmarks may be distorted. The malleus handle may be short, blunt, curved anteriorly, or project lateral to the tympanic membrane at the umbo. An abnormal bony bar, or bridge, may be connected to the malleus neck or handle. Occasionally, a partial atretic plate is present medial to the drum (Fig. 3.**11**). It is difficult to appreciate an abnormality of the incus behind an intact tym-

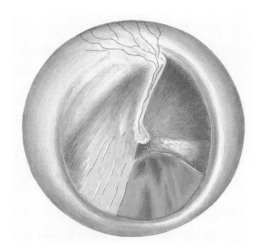

Fig. 3.**8**   Anomalous internal carotid artery pressing on medial surface of tympanic membrane.

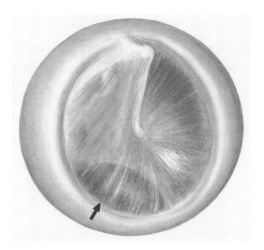

Fig. 3.**9**   High, uncovered jugular bulb seen through the tympanic membrane.

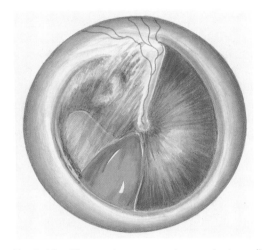

Fig. 3.**10**   Glomus tumor pressing against medial surface of tympanic membrane.

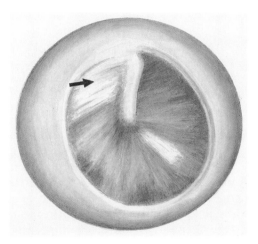

Fig. 3.**11**   Tympanic membrane with partial atretic plate.

panic membrane. However, the experienced examiner will know how far into the middle ear the incus long arm should project. Failure to see an incus long arm may mean it is foreshortened, or even absent. An isolated malformation of the incus is rare.

Indications

There are two absolute indications for operating on a congenitally malformed ear. One, there must be audiologic evidence of good cochlear function, and two, there must be no inner ear abnormality on high resolu-

tion CT scanning. Some ear surgeons may operate despite radiographic evidence of a malformed internal auditory canal (Rizer et al., 1989). If this is the only inner ear abnormality found on CT scanning in a patient with a bilateral malformation, then to operate or not is a judgement call on the part of the surgeon. However, it should be remembered that a widening or dilatation of the inner ear structures on CT may herald an abnormal communication between the inner ear and the subarachnoid space. If the stapes is manipulated in a patient with these findings, a *perilymphatic gusher* may ensue.

Goal of the Operation

Surgery in a patient with a congenital ear malformation has the potential to restore hearing to normal or near normal levels, particularly if the malformation is uncomplicated, i.e. congenital stapes ankylosis. The more complex the middle ear problem, the less chance there is of achieving normal hearing. Successful surgery in a hearing–impaired patient with a bilateral malformation often will allow the hearing aid to be discarded.

Preparation for Surgery

Same date admit: On the day prior to surgery, the patient is given a complete history and physical examination, routine blood work is obtained, and the ear is inspected one last time. Usually these studies are done as an outpatient procedure.

The patient is admitted to the day surgery unit of the hospital early on the morning of surgery having had nothing to eat or drink since midnight if general anesthesia is to be used. A liquid breakfast may be allowed if the surgery is to be performed under local anesthesia and sedation.

Pediatric anesthesiologist must be available: It is important to remember that children with congenital ear malformations may be syndromic, i.e., Treacher Collins syndrome (Fig. 3.**12**), hemifacial microsomia (Fig. 3.**13**), Pierre Robin syndrome, and have a hypoplastic mandible and a small oral cavity. Moreover, the neck may be short and thick as in Klippel–Feil syndrome or Down syndrome (Fig. 3.**14**). It is therefore imperative that a pediatric anesthesiologist who is expert in pediatric airway problems be present. If it is impossible to visualize the larynx, the intubation will be blind or must be performed under endoscopic control. In this situation, great care must be taken to avoid inadvertent extubation during the operation. The need for an emergency tracheotomy is rare but should be recognized as a distinct possibility.

Instruments

In addition to the usual instruments for ear surgery, it is important to have an electric hand drill available. As much as 3–4 mm of posterosuperior bony ear canal may need to be drilled away for adequate exposure of the oval window niche. Additionally, a fine drill should be available for footplate work, i. e. vestibulotomy.

Insofar as the facial nerve is commonly displaced in congenital ear malformations, it may be prudent to place electrodes for facial nerve monitoring.

Anesthesia

General endotracheal anesthesia: General endotracheal anesthesia is commonly used as most patients undergoing surgery for a congenital middle ear malformation are children. Even if the patient is an adult, general anesthesia is preferable because the duration of surgery is often unpredictable.

No urethal catheter: We no longer routinely place a urethal catheter, even if the case is posted to last five hours. Parents have convinced me that the single, most frequent complaint by their child is the postoperative burning and stinging on micturation following the use of a urethal catheter. This often is followed by urinary retention which requires a second catheterization. It is recommended that intravenous fluids be given in moderation to prevent bladder distention.

Local anesthesia: Occasionally local anesthesia may be used in the adolescent child or in the adult. This should be restricted to those cases in which the duration of surgery will be two hours or less. Even if local anesthesia is used, an anesthesiologist should be available to give general anesthesia, or intravenous medication, as needed.

Nitrous oxide: Nitrous oxide anesthesia may be used if the surgery requires that only a tympanomeatal flap be raised. If the tympanic membrane requires grafting, it is best to avoid nitrous oxide, or discontinue its use 45 minutes prior to grafting to lessen the risk of ballooning.

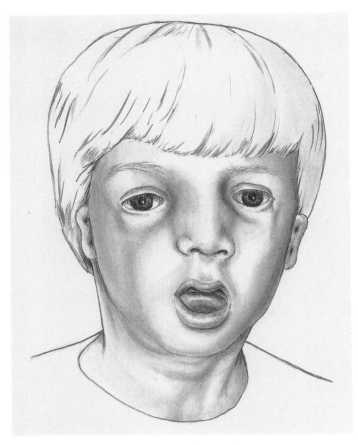

Fig. 3.**12**   Patient with Treacher Collins syndrome.

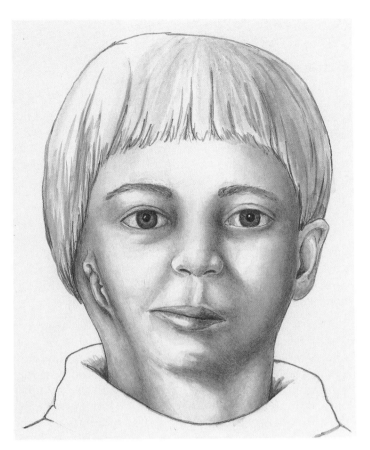

Fig. 3.**13**   Patient with hemifacial microsomia.

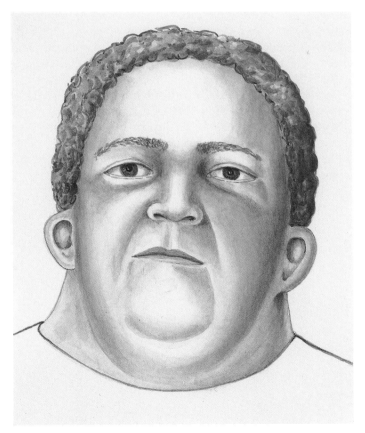

Fig. 3.**14**   Patient with Klippel–Feil syndrome.

Operative Technique

Postauricular Approach

A postauricular approach is used routinely. The incision is made in the postauricular crease and carried medially to the mastoid cortex. Temporalis fascia is harvested, spread on a Petri dish, and allowed to dry for later use as a tympanic membrane or oval window graft, if needed.

The posterior external ear canal skin is incised from 6 to 12 o'clock for exposure of the medial ear canal (Fig. 3.**15**). A self–retaining retractor holds the external ear anteriorly. The type of tympanomeatal flap to be raised depends on the size of the drum and how much bone will be drilled away posterior and superior. We prefer a large, inverted "V"–shaped flap (Fig. 3.**16**).

The tympanomeatal flap is raised. The surgeon should be alert for a chorda tympani nerve that exits the bone *lateral* to the anulus but still courses medial to the drum. This often warns of a congenital middle ear malformation. The middle ear is entered and the posterior part of the tympanic membrane with skin flap attached is reflected forward to expose the middle ear. Bony overhang may need to be removed by using a curette or power drill (Fig. 3.**17**). The chorda tympani nerve should be preserved. Once adequate exposure of the middle ear is obtained, a careful assessment is made of the problem. Particular attention is given to any soft–tissue tubular structure as this may be a displaced facial nerve. If the nerve is displaced it is usually naked (Fig. 3.**18**). On occasion the facial nerve may run in a bony trough across the promontory and be covered by middle ear mucosa (Fig. 3.**19**). It is camouflaged in this location and vulnerable to injury by an unwary surgeon. Beware of a large chorda tympani nerve (Fig. 3.**20**). This may not be the chorda at all, but rather a bare facial nerve suspended across the middle ear.

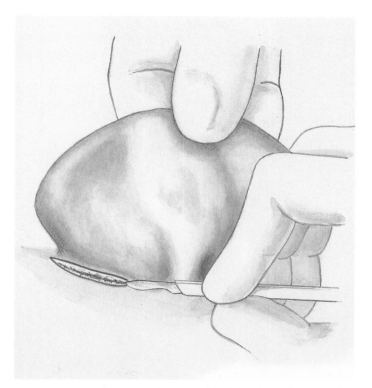

Fig. 3.**15**   Posterior external ear canal incision through postauricular approach.

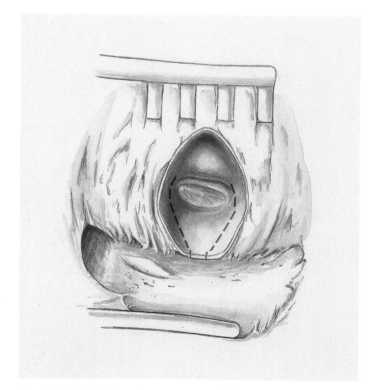

Fig. 3.**16**   "V"–shaped tympanomeatal flap.

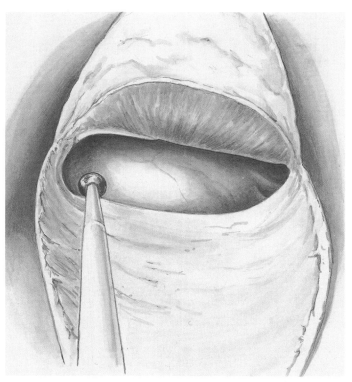

Fig. 3.**17**   Posterior bony canal wall overhang removed.

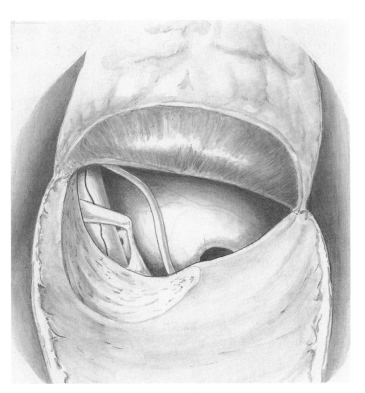

Fig. 3.**18**   Displaced and uncovered facial nerve.

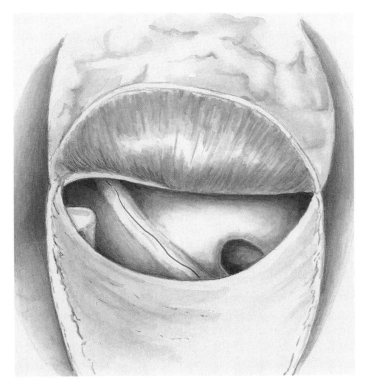

Fig. 3.**19**   Facial nerve in bony trough crossing promontory.

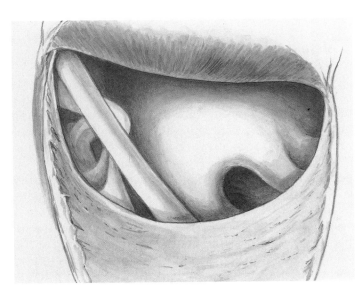

Fig. 3.**20**   Large chorda tympani nerve.

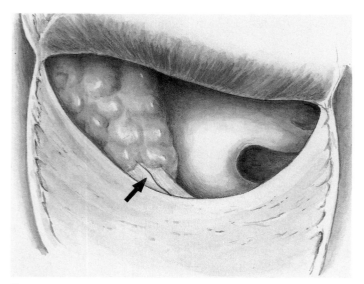

Fig. 3.**21**   Adipose tissue in middle ear.

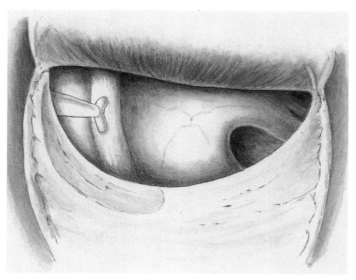

Fig. 3.**22**   Stapes remnant imbedded in bare facial nerve.

Other soft–tissue masses within the middle ear should give the surgeon a reason to pause. Adipose tissue found in the middle ear will signal a congenital middle ear malformation and may conceal a bare and displaced facial nerve (Fig. 3.**21**). Ectopic salivary gland tissue (choristoma) may do likewise. To reiterate, one should always watch for a displaced facial nerve when dissecting extraneous soft tissue within the middle ear.

Ossicular Chain

The ossicular chain should now be examined. The surgeon should note the location, shape, and mobility of the malleus and incus. Are there any bony struts fixing these structures? Next, the stapes should be investigated. If the facial nerve is displaced inferior to the stapes, this ossicle will never be normal. While the superstructure may have some shape and form to identify it as a stapes, and also be attached to a mobile footplate, it will never be completely normal. In the early embryonic development of the stapes/facial nerve axis, the facial nerve influences the final shape and position of the stapes, not the reverse. A dangerous situation is to find a stapes remnant apparently imbedded in a soft–tissue structure (Fig. 3.**22**). The senior author has seen two patients in whom the soft–tissue structure, in reality the facial nerve, was dissected in an attempt to gain better exposure of the oval window. In both patients, a facial nerve paralysis was incurred. Four similar cases have been reported recently (Welling et al., 1991).

Labyrinthine Windows

It is important to remember that a malformation affecting the stapes/facial nerve axis will often affect the oval window. The oval window may be absent or only partially formed. If a primitive stapes is found free–hanging from the incus, or fixed to the facial canal, the oval window will be commonly underdeveloped or absent (Fig. 3.**23**). A displaced facial nerve may obscure the area where the oval window is normally found. If this is the case, the nerve may be rolled slightly to determine the presence or absence of an oval window. Any major rerouting of the facial nerve — 6 mm or more — in the middle ear may result in a temporary facial paralysis. This possibility must be carefully explained to the patient or parents in preoperative counseling.

Ossiculoplasty

Once the surgeon has evaluated the middle ear and is secure in the assessment and his/her ability to correct the problem, ossiculoplasty may logically follow. It is important to stress that if the ossiculoplasty does not present a risk/benefit ratio in favor of the patient, the operation should probably be terminated. There is nothing wrong with aborting the effort and withdrawing from the case. Remember that the patient can usually wear a hearing device and get along quite well. This may be preferable to the surgeon taking an unnecessary risk of incurring a sensorineural hearing loss from overly aggressive oval window surgery.

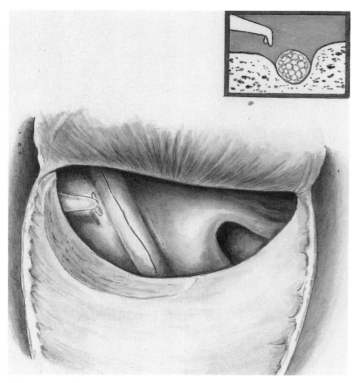

Fig. 3.**23**   Absent oval window.

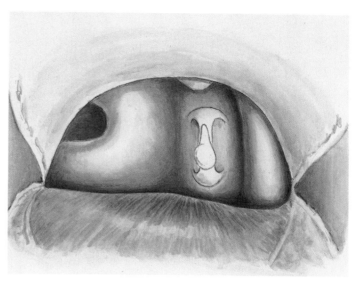

Fig. 3.**24**   Failure of stapedial anulus to differentiate.

The most common congenital middle ear malformation is stapes fixation. This occurs when part or all of the stapedial anulus fails to differentiate (Fig. 3.**24**). The diagnosis is made by inspecting the footplate margin under high magnification after stapes fixation has been confirmed. If only a small segment of the footplate anulus has failed to develop the surgeon may scratch a groove into that area with a sharp ear pick (Fig. 3.**25**). Often this will suffice in freeing the footplate. Refixation does not usually occur as this is endochondral bone with poor powers of regeneration. Remember that one is not dealing with otosclerosis: in otosclerosis refixation is common but this is not so in congenital stapes ankylosis.

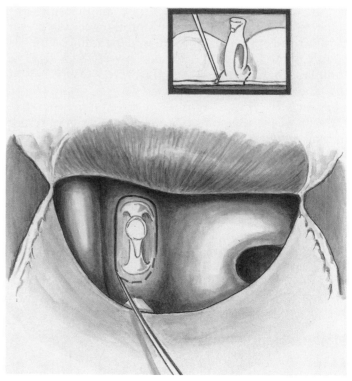

Fig. 3.**25**   Scratching a groove in bony anulus of footplate.

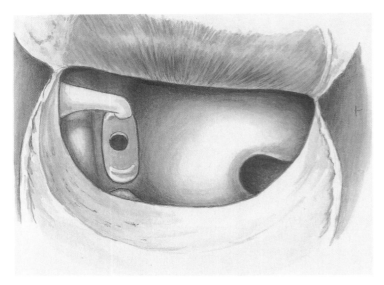

Fig. 3.**26**   Stapedotomy.

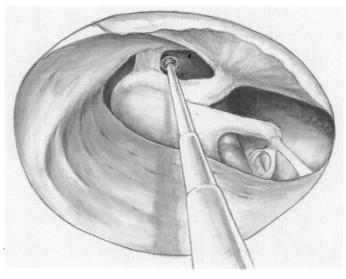

Fig. 3.**27**   Malleus fixation in anterior attic.

Stapedectomy/Stapedotomy
(See also Chapter 8)

Another alternative is to perform a stapedectomy or stapedotomy, as is the surgeon's preference. We prefer to retain the option of doing either depending on the exposure of the footplate. If a good view can be had of the footplate, a *stapedotomy* is performed (Fig. 3.**26**). If the footplate is poorly seen, we prefer to do a *stapedectomy*. It must be reiterated that a preoperative CT scan of the temporal bone is of utmost importance in a suspected congenital middle ear malformation. If a widened internal auditory canal, semicircular canal, or vestibule is noted, there is a high likelihood of a peri-lymphatic gusher once the integrity of the footplate is violated. If a stapedectomy or stapedotomy is performed, the surgeon should be prepared to use a stapes prosthesis of unusual length. Often the distance between incus and oval window, or malleus and oval window, is greater than normal requiring the use of a prosthesis 6 mm or more in length. Much smaller stapes prosthesis, 3.0 or 3.5 mm, are occasionally needed.

Malleus Head Fixation

One can usually determine the mobility of the stapes footplate independent of malleus fixation. It is important not to be trapped into believing that the problem is solely a fixed stapes, only to note that other ossicles are fixed after the stapes has been removed. While malleus head fixation can occur concurrently with a fixed stapes, this is usually *not* the case.

A fixed malleus head (or neck) can be addressed in the following manner: One, an *atticotomy* is performed and the bony bridge between the malleus and anterior or superior attic wall drilled away to free the ossicular chain (Fig. 3.**27**). Thin silastic sheeting must be interposed otherwise the fixation can recur. Two, the malleus may be nipped at the neck, superior to the attachment of the tensor tympani tendon, the incus removed, and an incus strut (autograft or homograft) positioned between the malleus neck and the stapes head (Fig. 3.**28**). Additionally, a partial ossicular replacement prosthesis may be fitted from the stapes to the drum.

Malleus Bar

A malleus bar is a term coined by Professor Nomura to describe a bar of bone from the malleus neck to the posterior bony anulus (Nomura et al., 1988) (Fig. 3.**4**). The bar fixes the malleus, and the ossicular chain, in place. This bony malformation is one of the simplest to correct but requires careful drilling at a slow speed to avoid vibratory trauma to the inner ear. Do not be lulled into thinking that the bony bar is the only reason the ossicular chain is fixed. It may be immobile from other points of fixation.

Incus Fixation

Primary incus fixation is rare.

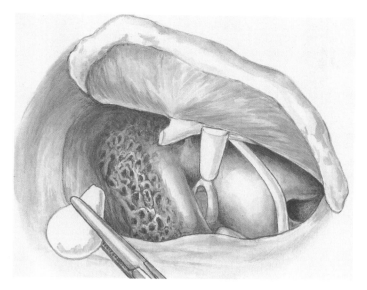

Fig. 3.**28**   Interposed incus strut.

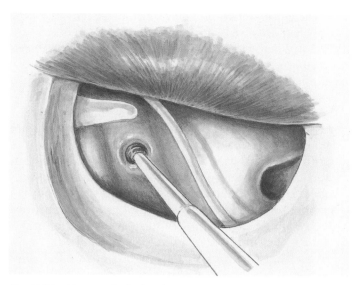

Fig. 3.**29**   New oval window being drilled.

Vestibulotomy

If the oval window is absent or poorly developed, a *vestibulotomy* may be performed. This entails drilling a new opening into the vestibule (Fig. 3.**29**). It may not be readily apparent where one should drill the opening. It is best to search for a bluish depression, or partially formed footplate, which affords some recognition of a landmark to locate the vestibule. Drilling should be done where one perceives the vestibule to be, even if the facial nerve is inferior to that site. It is best to attempt to saucerize a new oval window rather than drill a deep cylindrical opening. In the latter situation, the only choice of a stapes prosthesis is a piston, while in the former situation, other choices of stapes prosthesis are available (see also Chapter 4). We prefer to use a tissue graft (fascia) over a saucerized vestibulotomy before connecting the prosthesis.

Whenever a new oval window is drilled the postoperative hearing results are uneven. We have created oval windows de nova in 21 patients. Of this group, one patient sustained a profound and irreversible sensorineural hearing loss.

Plester prefers to drill a new oval window more anteriorly. He refers to his technique as a *promontorial window* (Plester et al., 1983). The bone over the promontory is saucerized to the level of the endosteal membrane of the cochlea. The window connects with the basal turn of the scala vestibuli.

Modifications

Endaural Approach

The endaural approach, rather than postauricular, is an alternative route to the middle ear.

Surgical Landmarks and Danger Points

- *Abnormal chorda tympani nerve:* Watch for an abnormal chorda tympani nerve as this will often indicate other middle ear malformations.
- *Search for the facial nerve:* The facial nerve can only be protected with confidence after it has been positively identified.

● *Use caution when working around the stapes:* Not only is there a risk of inner ear injury from overly aggressive stapes manipulation, there is a risk of a *perilymphatic gusher.* A gusher results from a direct communication of the perilymphatic space with the subarachnoid space (Fig. 3.**30**). In this situation the perilymphatic space contains cerebrospinal fluid under pressure. If the footplate is manipulated it may "blow", releasing cerebrospinal fluid into the middle ear and external ear canal. Should this occur, it is important that the surgeon remain calm. Most catastrophes, i. e. dead ears, occur when the surgeon indiscriminately packs the oval window (and therefore the vestibule) with a plug of soft tissue or other material to stem the flow of fluid.

To address the problem, one should elevate the head of the operating table thirty degrees and allow the spinal fluid reservoir to deplete itself. This takes approximately 15 to 20 minutes. When the flow has ebbed, the stapedectomy repair can be performed in a controlled fashion. A firm oval window seal of soft tissue bolstered by a prosthesis secured to the incus must be used. While hearing results are variable, this technique will best avoid trauma to the inner ear.

Rules, Tips, and Pitfalls

● Drill away the posterosuperior bony external ear canal wall before entering the middle ear (Fig. 3.**31**). If the anulus is raised first, essential landmarks may be obscured by the bony overhang of the posterior and superior ear canal wall.
● *Facial nerve monitor:* While it is often advantageous to use a facial nerve stimulator or monitor, the best safeguard is positive identification of the facial nerve in the middle ear.
● *Oval window:* Drilling a new oval window increases the risk of cochlear damage.
● *Fenestration:* Avoid fenestrating the horizontal semicircular canal. This is not a physiologic solution to a hearing problem. If fenestration is required we prefer a vestibulotomy rather than entering into the vestibular system.
● *Wire prosthesis:* Avoid the use of a wire prosthesis on the malleus (Fig. 3.**32**). While wire from the malleus neck or handle to the footplate may give a good short–term hearing improvement, the risk is high that it will subsequently transect the malleus neck or handle and extrude through the tympanic membrane.

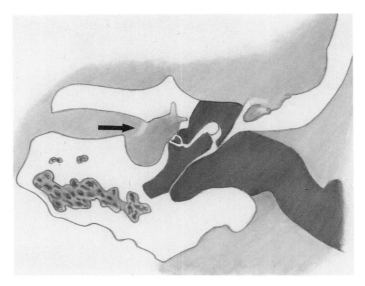

Fig. 3.**30**   Subarachnoid space connected to perilymphatic space.

Postoperative Care

● If the vestibule has been opened, use the same precautions one would routinely take for a stapedectomy (see also Chapter 8). We request that the patient avoid nose blowing for the first 7–10 days.
● The patient may be discharged on postoperative day one or two. If persistent postoperative vertigo from labyrinthine irritation is present, the patient should remain hospitalized until this has resolved.
● All ear canal packing and sutures are removed one week postoperatively.
● A second ambulatory care visit is scheduled 3–4 weeks postoperatively. At this visit the ear is cleaned and an audiogram is obtained.

Postoperative Complications

Early Complications

Facial nerve paralysis, facial nerve weakness: Immediate postoperative facial nerve paralysis or paresis signifies that the nerve has been injured. This may occur from inadvertent and *unrecognized* injury, from accidental but *recognized* injury, or from deliberate manipulation of the nerve, i.e., rerouting.

Infection: Early postoperative infection may occur despite the use of prophylactic antibiotics. All packing should be removed at the first sign of infection and the wound cultured. Immediate postoperative infections are often *Staphylococcus aureus* and early treatment should include coverage for this organism until positive identification is made on culture.

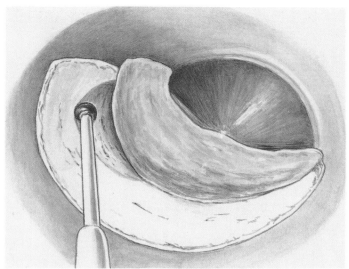

Fig. 3.**31** Posterosuperior bony external ear canal wall drilled prior to entering middle ear.

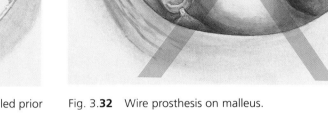

Fig. 3.**32** Wire prosthesis on malleus.

Persistent vertigo: Any dizziness or vertigo, particularly if accompanied by nystagmus, usually indicates a labyrinthine injury. If the vertigo does not abate within 3–4 days, the patient should be reassessed for inner ear injury to include perilymphatic fistula.

Sensorineural hearing loss

Fluctuating hearing: A fluctuating hearing loss may indicate a perilymphatic fistula, loose prosthesis at the incus level, or slippage of a prosthesis in the oval window niche.

Late Complications

Facial nerve paralysis/weakness: If the surgeon *knows* the nerve is intact but that it was bruised or stretched, there should be some return of facial function within 3 months. If the surgeon is unsure of the integrity of the facial nerve, or there has been no return of function in 3 months, exploration is indicated. A simple way to follow the early return of facial nerve function is to monitor the stapedial reflex.

Infection: Persistent infection must always be cultured and the sensitivity of the organism to antibiotics determined. Often the offending organism will be a Gram–negative bacterium, i.e., *Pseudomonas aeruginosa.* The treatment of this organism in adults has been simplified by the advent of the oral antibiotic ciprofloxicin.

Persistent vertigo: Persistent vertigo is a bothersome and serious problem and must be investigated. Audiologic and vestibular function testing is required and an imaging study (MRI) is often feasible to rule out other

possible reasons for the patient's symptoms. If the vertigo becomes incapacitating and cannot be controlled by medication, a neurotologic procedure may be indicated, i.e., vestibular nerve section, with the approach dependent on the presence or absence of serviceable hearing.

Sensorineural hearing loss — permanent

Sequelae

- An audiogram is obtained at 3–4 weeks postoperatively.
- Postoperative hearing results are less predictable for congenital stapes fixation than for otosclerosis.
- An initial good hearing result may fade with time. Re–exploration may be indicated.

Alternate Techniques

Hearing Device

As most of these patients will have a conductive hearing loss, or at least a conductive component to a mixed hearing loss, they are usually good candidates for a hearing or listening device. If the preoperative work–up indicates that the patient is not a good candidate for surgery, the patient is counseled that a hearing device may be of help.

Congenital Aural Atresia and Stenosis

Congenital aural atresia and stenosis occurs in 1/10,000 births. Unilateral atresia is six times more common than bilateral atresia. Microtia is usually found in concert with aural atresia although the external ear, on occasion, may be normal. If the auricle is well formed, the atresia may go undiagnosed for months, even years.

Diagnosis

Appearance of External Ear

The observation that a newborn has congenital microtia (Fig. 3.**33**) should immediately place the infant in a high–risk category. Appropriately, a careful otologic examination, preferably using the operating microscope, should be undertaken. In addition, it is imperative that an estimation of the hearing be obtained. Auditory brainstem response (ABR) testing is performed within the first few days of life. Multichannel simultaneous recording of the ABR is carried out with both air conduction and bone conduction stimuli. The appearance of a Wave I ipsilateral to the stimulus is evidence of hearing acuity in that ear. If the results are inconclusive, the infant is tested again in one month. Although it is uncommon, one will occasionally discover a sensorineural hearing loss in the normal–appearing ear of a child with unilateral microtia/atresia. If there exists any doubt as to the hearing thresholds, a hearing device should be placed. While this may be only a temporary placement, it is better to err on the side of amplification than to fail to aid a hearing–impaired child in the early critical years.

The examiner may note other clues which suggest a congenital ear malformation:

- Are preauricular tags present? Is the external ear poorly formed? Do other craniofacial anomalies exist? Is the mandible small, the lateral face flat?
- The examiner must be alert to subtle clues which may help him make the diagnosis of atresia or stenosis in the presence of a normal–appearing external ear.

One must inquire if there is a family history of ear malformations. In the author's experience of evaluating 1500 patients with congenital ear disease, only 5% were syndromic. An additional 5% had a positive family history of an isolated ear malformation. Ninety percent of the cases appeared to be new mutations.

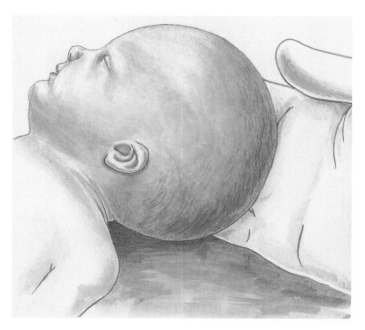

Fig. 3.**33**   Congenital microtia in a newborn.

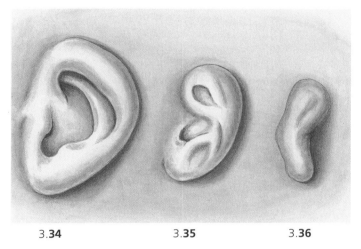

3.**34**   3.**35**   3.**36**

Figs. 3.**34**–3.**36**   Grade I microtia, Grade II microtia, and Grade III microtia.

Preoperative Evaluation

It is our philosophy that atresia repair should follow microtia repair. This means that if the external ear needs to be reconstructed, the plastic surgeon goes first. This is no longer a negotiable point and we will refuse to operate any patient who fails to accept this recommendation. However, not every patient with congenital atresia requires external ear reconstruction. Patients with

Grade III microtia (Fig. 3.**36**) always do. Patients with Grade II microtia may need parts of the auricle revised (Fig. 3.**35**), and patients with Grade I microtia (Fig. 3.**34**), in which the external ear is fairly well formed, may have the atresia repaired without the need for plastic surgery intervention. Grade II microtia sometimes presents a dilemma. The plastic surgeon may believe that in order to improve the appearance of the ear an auricular amputation is first required followed by implanting sculptured rib cartilage. Usually, those patients with Grade II microtia will opt to forego plastic surgery and proceed with the atresia repair directly. They will be satisfied with a small, but fairly well–formed auricle and a chance for hearing improvement.

If the plastic surgeon is to operate first, the child must have attained sufficient growth to enable adequate rib cartilage to be harvested for the ear implant. This usually requires the child to be 6–8 years of age. Insofar as atresia surgery follows microtia repair, this means that the otologic surgeon will usually operate at least 6 months after the plastic surgeon, or when the child is about 7 or 8 years of age. In patients with bilateral atresia/microtia we accelerate the process and try to operate at least one ear prior to the time the child starts school. As the hearing results are usually predictable, and assuming the absence of significant complications, there is no rationale for waiting until the child is a teenager or young adult and can share in the decision making process.

Audiometric Studies

It is essential that behavioral audiometric testing be done to assess the hearing acuity. Behavioral audiometry is difficult before age 3 and often impossible before age 2. By age 4 or 5 years, valid responses can be obtained routinely for each ear even in the presence of masking noise.

ABR

Auditory brainstem response (ABR) testing is also used at this age to complement behavioral testing.

Computed Tomography

At about age 5, high resolution CT scanning of the temporal bones is done. This is the single most important study performed on the child with atresia and will determine his/her candidacy for surgery. The protocol we use images the temporal bone in the 30° (Fig. 3.**37**) axial and the 105° (Fig. 3.**38**) coronal planes. This technique produces life–sized images without loss of resolution. Simply magnifying the images is inadequate. Three–dimensional reconstructions of the temporal bone surface anatomy are routinely made (Fig. 3.**39**).

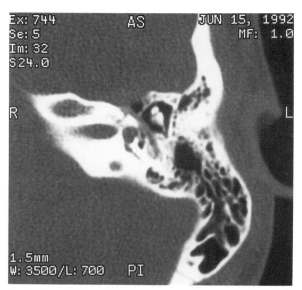

Fig. 3.**37** High resolution computed tomography of the temporal bone in the 30° axial plane.

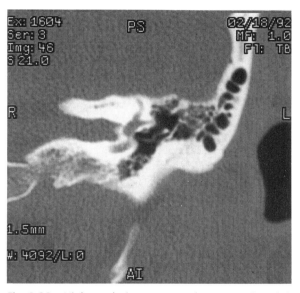

Fig. 3.**38** High resolution computed tomography of the temporal bone in the 105° coronal plane.

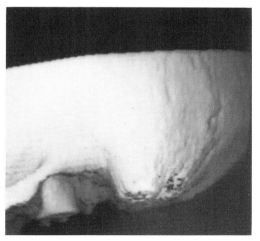

Fig. 3.**39** Three–dimensional computed tomographic reconstruction of the temporal bone.

Indications

Main Indications

There are two absolute indications for operating on a patient with congenital aural atresia: (1) audiometric evidence of inner ear function and (2) imaging evidence of a normal inner ear. We believe that any developmental anomaly of the bony inner architecture places the patient at risk of a perilymphatic gusher.

Secondary Indications

Grading scale: We have developed a grading scale based on the temporal bone findings on computed tomography and on the appearance of the external ear (Table 3.**1**). In this grading scheme the presence of a stapes has much clinical significance and is assigned 2 points. All other parameters are assigned 1 point. Ten points is a perfect score. It is our conservative nature that no patient gets a score of 10. A grade of 9/10 indicates that the patient is an very good candidate to have the ear opened for hearing purposes. A grade of 5 or less indicates that the patient is not a candidate for surgery (Table 3.**2**). Most patients upon whom we operate grade out at 7/10 or 8/10, which means that they are fair to good candidates for surgery. A rating of 8 points, for example, translates to an 80% chance of restoring hearing to normal or near–normal levels through surgery. Normal or near–normal hearing is defined as a postoperative speech reception threshold of 15–25 dB. In cases of bilateral aural atresia we may relax our criteria and operate at least one ear in which a grade of 5 was assigned. In unilateral cases the patient must grade out at 6 or above in order to be operated.

Infection and/or *Cholesteatoma:* There are times when surgery is mandated in congenital aural atresia despite a poor grade. If the patient has infection (Fig. 3.**40**) or cholesteatoma involving the atretic ear (Fig. 3.**41**), surgery is indicated. In these instances, hearing is not the primary reason for operating. Indeed, most cases with cholesteatoma will have advanced disease in which the middle ear structures have been destroyed.

Table 3.**1** Surgery of congenital aural atresia (rating scale – 10 point total).

Parameter	Score
stapes present	2
oval window open	1
middle ear space	1
facial nerve	1
malleus/incus complex	1
mastoid pneumatized	1
incus-stapes connection	1
round window	1
appearance external ear	1

Table 3.**2** Surgery of congenital aural atresia (rating scale).

Rating	Type of candidate
10	excellent
9	very good
8	good
7	fair
6	marginal
5 or less	poor

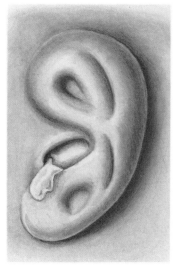 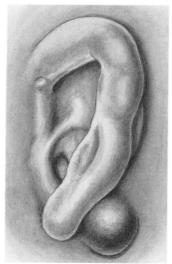

Fig. 3.**40**   Fig. 3.**41**

Fig. 3.**40** Presence of infection in a congenital atresia (repaired).

Fig. 3.**41** Cholesteatoma with abscess in congenital stenosis.

Goal of the Operation

In bilateral congenital aural atresia the goal of the operation is to obtain normal or near–normal hearing which will allow the patient to discard his or her hearing device. This postoperative hearing result is attainable in 80% of the patients selected for surgery.

In unilateral cases, our goal is to attain serviceable hearing through surgery which will allow improved sound localization and a better appreciation of speech in the presence of other noise.

Preparation for Surgery

Preoperative anesthesiology consultation: Approximately 20% of patients selected for surgery have other congenital anomalies involving the head and neck. Some of these malformations, i.e., mandibular hypoplasia, make general anesthesia hazardous. The service of an experienced anesthesiologist, knowledgeable in the care of craniofacial patients, is therefore required. An anesthesiology consult is routinely obtained preoperatively.

Admit morning of surgery: The patient is admitted the morning of surgery and taken directly to the operating room.

Position of patient: The patient is placed in the supine position with the ear to be operated facing up. The table is turned 45 degrees so the anesthesiologist is on the far side of the table from the surgeon and scrub nurse (Fig. 3.**42**).

Urethral catheter: Urethral catheterization is not routinely done. Our young patients have complained about this and the procedure has been discontinued. As the operation takes approximately 5 hours, fluid replacement is carefully controlled.

Special Instruments

The instruments used in atresia repair include routine middle ear and mastoid surgical instruments. A self–irrigating drill is used with a full range of cutting and diamond burrs. A facial nerve monitor is available in the operating room but not routinely used. However, we have no objection to its use if the surgeon so desires. Bipolar electrocautery (Fig. 3.**43**) is available and is advantageous if there is bleeding on or about the facial nerve. A video camera is connected to the microscope and television monitors are available in the operating room and also off-site. A dermatome (Zimmer) (Fig. 3.**44**) is necessary and should be a dedicated instrument to the operating room.

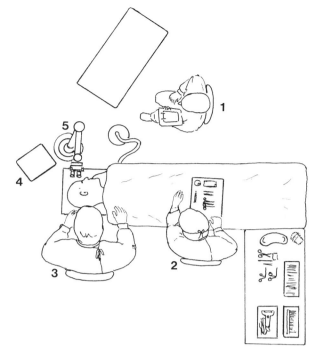

Fig. 3.**42**   Intraoperative position of patient.
1: anesthetist
2: nurse
3: surgeon
4: drill
5: operating microscope

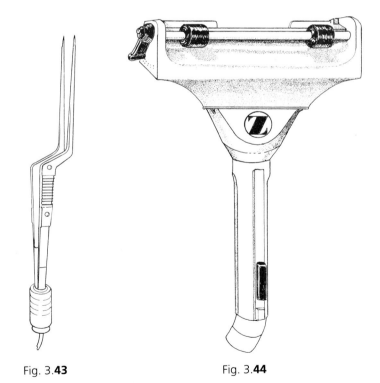

Fig. 3.**43**   Fig. 3.**44**

Fig. 3.**43**   Bipolar cautery.

Fig. 3.**44**   Zimmer dermatome.

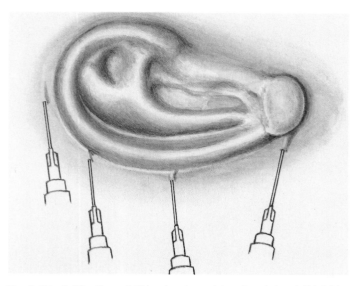

Fig. 3.**45** Infiltration of 1% xylocaine with epinephrine 1/50,000.

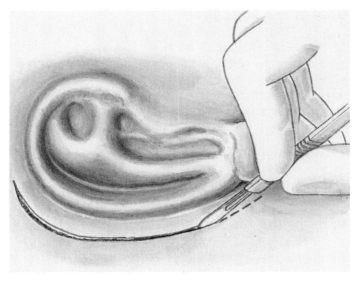

Fig. 3.**46** Postauricular incision for atresia repair.

Anesthesia

Surgery of congenital aural atresia is routinely done under general endotracheal anesthesia. Again, it is important to assign one of the better pediatric anesthesiologists to these children as they often have other craniofacial problems which make endotracheal intubation hazardous. While it is acceptable to use muscle–paralyzing agents in the case, their use should be discontinued if the surgeon wishes to use the facial nerve monitor. Even if the facial nerve monitor is not used, it is advisable to curtail paralyzing agents. A sudden twitch, or jump, of the face during drilling may warn of proximity to the facial nerve.

Intravenous fluids: The content and volume of intravenous fluids are left to the discretion of the anesthesiologist. As a urethral catheter is not used, replacement fluid therapy is moderated to avoid bladder distention.

Blood and blood products: Blood and blood products have never been used in any atresia case we have performed. Unless there are special circumstances to indicate possible bleeding, the typing and cross–matching of blood is not done.

Local anesthesia: Xylocaine 1% with epinephrine 1/50,000 is used. This is infiltrated into the soft tissue where the postauricular incision will be made, as well as into the soft tissue areas inferior and medial to where the new ear canal will be created (Fig. 3.**45**).

Nitrous oxide: The use of nitrous oxide is avoided. While we do not object to nitrous oxide being used during anesthesia induction, it is discontinued shortly

thereafter. We have also noted that even without nitrous oxide, the use of the ventilator produces a middle ear gas pressure which results in ballooning of the temporalis fascia graft used for the new tympanic membrane. We believe this is due to the increased partial pressure of nitrogen and oxygen in the blood. These gases are released into the middle ear through the mucosal capillaries and cause ballooning of the graft. This is not the result of increased middle ear pressure transmitted through the eustachian tube. This troublesome aspect of graft ballooning and displacement has been eliminated by asking the anesthesiologist to reduce the expired oxygen to less than 30%.

Operative Technique

The surgical repair of congenital aural atresia is planned as a *one-stage procedure*. This is made possible by the careful selection of cases on the preoperative rating scale. A low numerical rating, i.e., 5–6/10, would forewarn of a difficult reconstruction. For example, if one knows preoperatively that the patient lacks a stapes and/or oval window, the surgeon may decide to create a middle ear space and a new tympanic membrane initially and plan the vestibulotomy for a second stage. The reason for this stance is the inherent complexity in attempting to place a total ossicular replacement prosthesis between a newly drilled oval window and a newly created tympanic membrane. As there is instability at both ends of the prosthesis, as well as pressure on the prosthesis from packing in the ear canal, postoperative vertigo and dizziness would likely occur.

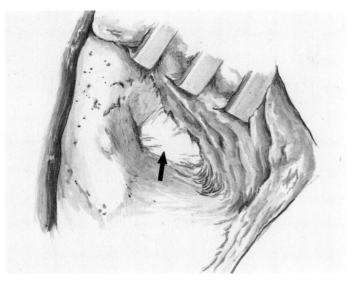

Fig. 3.**47**   Tympanic bone remnant.

Postauricular incision: A postauricular incision is used routinely (Fig. 3.**46**). While we have no concern about the use of an endaural incision, we believe a postauricular incision allows for better placement of the new meatus.

Fascia graft: Temporalis fascia is harvested through the postauricular incision. On occasion, temporalis fascia will be lacking, either on a congenital basis or from already having been harvested by the plastic surgeon. A "fan flap" technique is one in which the entire temporalis fascia is raised and turned down to cover a silastic external ear implant. This is done to help prevent extrusion. Unfortunately, this maneuver exhausts the supply of fascia for the ear surgeon who then must consider other options:
1) Temporalis fascia from the contralateral side;
2) Fascia lata from the leg;
3) Pericranium;
4) Homograft fascia from a parent.

If it is known in advance that the ipsilateral temporal fascia has been depleted, we routinely harvest fascia from the opposite side at the beginning of the procedure. The fascia is placed on a Petri dish, scraped to remove muscle tissue and occasionally fat, and allowed to dry.

Tympanic bone: In approximately 1/3 of cases with congenital atresia, a tympanic bone remnant will be identified (Fig. 3.**47**). Remember that aural atresia results when a tympanic ring fails to develop. A tympanic bone remnant is nothing more than an amorphous plaque of bone in the area where one would normally find an ear canal. As the surgeon reflects the perios-

teum off the anterior face of the mastoid cortex, he should search for a tympanic bone remnant. This will point the way to the middle ear which is located deep to the remnant. It is acceptable to bluntly dissect into the temporomandibular joint for a short distance. A caveat must be raised here, however. In 25% of atresia cases the facial nerve makes a sharp turn anteriorly at the level of the second bend to cross the middle ear and exit into the temporomandibular joint. If the surgeon is unaware of this possibility, he/she risks injury to the nerve before drilling has even begun.

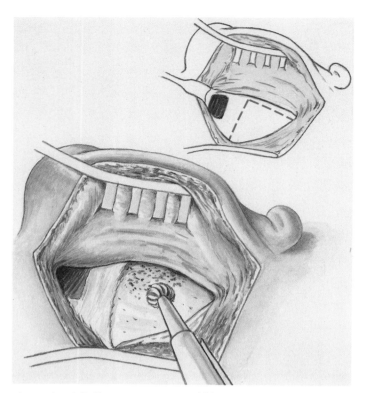

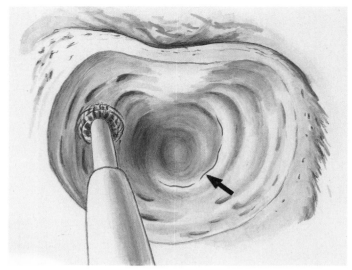

Fig. 3.**49** Displaced facial nerve (arrow).

Fig. 3.**48** Cribriform area on mastoid bone.

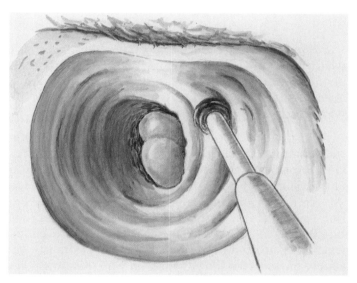

Fig. 3.**50** "Buttock sign" of fused incus/malleus.

Direct approach to the middle ear: If a tympanic bone remnant is identified, drilling is begun in that area. If a tympanic bone remnant is absent, drilling is begun in the cribriform area — that portion of the mastoid bone with multiple small cells (Fig. 3.**48**). The pathway for drilling is anterosuperior with a direct approach to the middle ear. Stay high and hug the tegmen as this best avoids a displaced facial nerve (Fig. 3.**49**). The tegmen may be thinned to identify the dura.

Stay out of the mastoid: There is no justification to indiscriminately drill out the mastoid air cells. This leaves a large, unsightly cavity that is prone to infection.

Watch for facial nerve: As drilling progresses medially, the first landmark encountered will be a fused incus/malleus in the epitympanum. This presents as two softly rounded hillocks separated by a medium cleft. This closely resembles the derriere of a baby and we have named this the *"buttock sign"*(Fig. 3.**50**). Gentle palpation will reveal some mobility, although rarely will the fused ossicles be fixed. Exposure of the middle ear is gained by systematically drilling away bone. The surgeon must keep a keen lookout for the facial nerve during this maneuver. Often the facial nerve is first recognized by a whitish band outlined against the pale yellow appearance of the atretic bone. Small blood vessels may be seen on the nerve's surface as the atretic bone is thinned (Fig. 3.**51**). The nerve is particularly at risk if it makes an acute bend anteriorly (25% of cases) and crosses the middle ear at the level of the round window (Fig. 3.**52**). The nerve also tracks laterally as it crosses the middle ear making it even more vulnerable to injury. The surgeon's vigil should never relax until the facial nerve has been positively identified. Only then can it be protected with confidence.

Drill away atretic plate: The dense bone of the atretic plate is thinned to eggshell thickness and gently picked away with a sharp elevator (dental excavator) (Fig. 3.**53**).

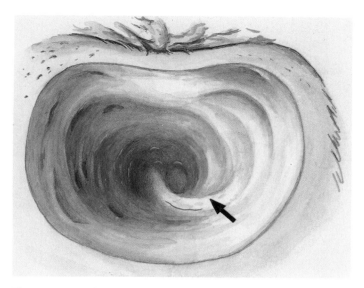

Fig. 3.**51**   Facial nerve as seen through thinned atretic bone (arrow).

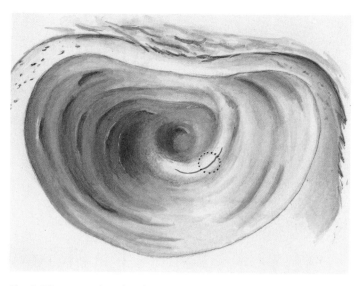

Fig. 3.**52**   Acute bend to facial nerve as it crosses the middle ear at the level of the round window (dotted circle).

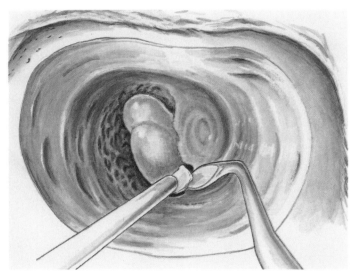

Fig. 3.**53**   A sharp elevator is used to pick away thinned atretic bone.

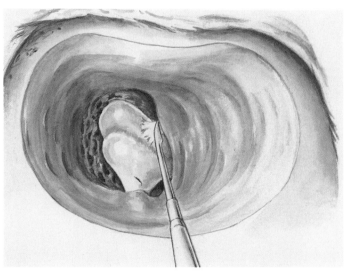

Fig. 3.**54**   A small S-59 Beaver blade used to incise the periosteum.

The ossicular chain is commonly fixed to the atretic plate at the level of the malleus neck. The fixation may be bony or by dense periosteum. Care must be taken in freeing the ossicular chain lest vibratory trauma be imparted to the inner ear. We prefer to use a sharp S 59 Beaver blade to incise the periosteum (Fig. 3.**54**). Once the ossicular mass is freed at the level of the malleus neck, it becomes highly mobile. This increases the risk of inner ear damage from drilling.

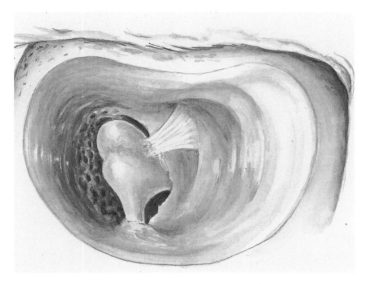

Fig. 3.**55** Broad band of periosteum from temporomandibular joint to malleus neck.

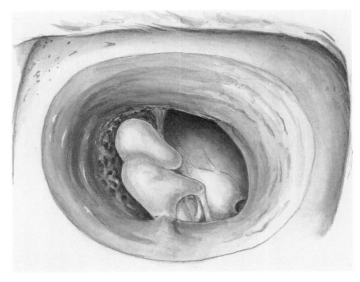

Fig. 3.**56** Malleus handle absent.

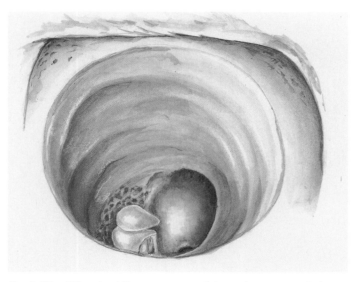

Fig. 3.**57** "Piggyback" appearance of incus long arm relative to malleus.

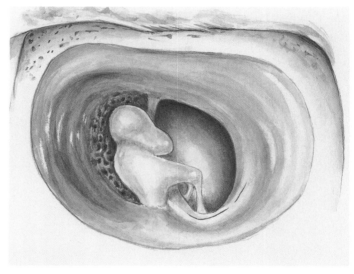

Fig. 3.**58** Sharp bend to facial nerve obscurring round window (vessel is under the thinned, bony canal).

A broad band of periosteum is frequently seen running from the temporomandibular joint to the malleus neck (Fig. 3.**55**). This courses through a defect in the bony wall separating the middle ear from the temporomandibular joint. The periosteal band is significant in that it must be discerned from the facial nerve and may be cut only after the latter has been positively identified. Inadvertent opening into the temporomandibular joint by drilling is usually inconsequential but should be avoided.

Open into middle ear: Once good exposure of the middle ear is achieved, the ossicular chain is carefully assessed. The malleus handle is often noted to be lacking (Fig. 3.**56**). The development of the incus long arm is variable. It may be short and blunt, or long and thin. Often it will be obscured by the malleus neck and will have a "piggyback" appearance relative to the malleus (Fig. 3.**57**). The development of the stapes is also variable. In most cases, the superstructure will be intact but smaller than normal. The close confines of the middle ear may make exposure of the stapes impossible. Sometimes, the presence or absence of stapes crura must be confirmed by gentle palpation with a right–angled hook because the surgeon cannot see the stapes. Every effort should be made to visualize the footplate, or at least a part of the anular rim. While stapes fixation is uncommon in congenital aural atresia, it does occur, and can only be diagnosed by observing the footplate while challenging the ossicular chain.

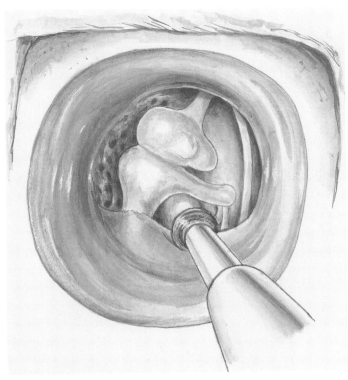

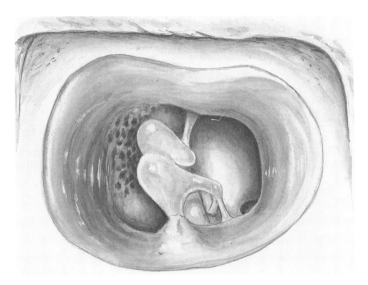

Fig. 3.**60** Attachments stabilizing fused malleus/incus.

Fig. 3.**59** Ossicular mass centered in approximate middle of new tympanic membrane.

If the stapes footplate is fixed, and the site of fixation can be demonstrated by a failure of the stapedial anulus to differentiate, the bony bridge between the footplate and oval window margin may be gently scraped with a sharp pick. As noted earlier, the bone in this location is endochondral bone and does not regenerate well. This means that if mobility is achieved, refixation will not likely occur. If mobilization of the stapes is not feasible, a stapedectomy/stapedotomy may be performed depending on the surgeon's preference. Remember that the footplate is smaller, about 1/2 normal size, and the distance between the incus long arm and the footplate is highly variable. Usually the distance is shorter in atresia patients and longer in non–atresia congenital middle ear malformations.

Labyrinthine windows: The labyrinthine windows should be inspected if possible. The size, shape, and degree of development of the oval window is assessed simultaneously with the inspection of the stapes. The round window may be inaccessible to inspection because of a sharply–bending facial nerve (Fig. 3.**58**). The round window can be adequately examined in only about 1/2 of atresia cases. It would be foolhardy to deliberately decompress the facial nerve in an attempt to see a concealed round window. Moreover, isolated round window closure is rare in congenital aural atresia.

Gain room peripherally: One must gain room peripherally by drilling away bone. Inferiorly, one is constrained by a sharply–bending facial nerve, anteriorly by the temporomandibular joint, superiorly by the tegmen, and posteriorly by the mastoid. Nonetheless, enough bone should be removed to enable the placement of a new fascia tympanic membrane measuring 1.0–1.5 cm in diameter. Also, by drilling away bone peripherally, the ossicular mass can be centered in the approximate middle of the new tympanic membrane (Fig. 3.**59**). If the ossicular chain is intact but malformed, and moves as a unit, it is left intact. There is no justification for dismantling the ossicular chain unless it is discontinuous. While some authors (Marquet et al., 1988) advocate the use of homograft tympanic membranes, we do not support this premise. Remember that there is often no malleus handle to accommodate the homograft tympanic membrane. Additionally, one needs more room at the level of the eardrum for the fascia graft and split–thickness skin graft. Homograft tympanic membranes do not lend themselves to easy placement in atretic ears.

The fused incus/malleus complex derives its structural support from the fossa incudis (do not drill this bone away), the incudostapedial joint, and the anterior malleal ligament (Fig. 3.**60**). If any of these support attachments are disrupted, the ossicular mass may collapse onto the medial attic wall affecting the postoperative hearing result.

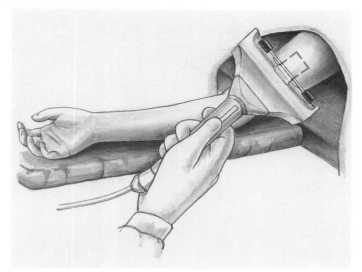

Fig. 3.**62**   Preparation of the skin graft.

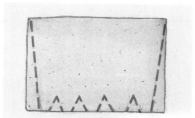

Fig. 3.**61**   Harvesting skin graft from upper arm.

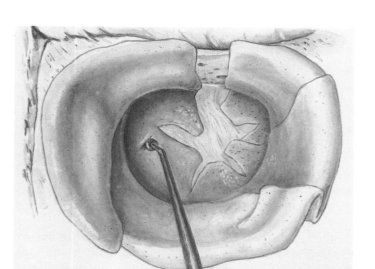

Fig. 3.**63**   Placement of skin graft in new bony ear canal.

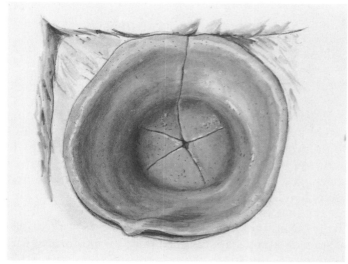

Fig. 3.**64**   Positioning of medial tabs of skin graft over the fascia graft.

At this stage of the operation, the soft tissue of the auricle is infiltrated with lidocaine containing epinephrine in preparation for the placement of the meatus. This will allow time for vasoconstriction (10–15 minutes) and the meatus may then be constructed in a dryer field.

Skin graft: A thin split–thickness skin graft measuring 0.010 inches in thickness is harvested from the medial aspect of the ipsilateral upper arm (Fig. 3.**61**). The dimensions of the skin graft are approximately 5×7 cm. The graft is placed on a cutting board, trimmed and notched (Fig. 3.**62**). The skin graft is placed into the new ear canal with the vertical slit facing anterior (Fig. 3.**63**). The notched tabs of the graft are reflected onto the fascia graft tympanic membrane (Fig. 3.**64**).

There are important points to remember in preparing the bony external ear canal and positioning the skin graft. Concerning the bony canal, if any large mastoid air cells appear to communicate with the new canal, they are plugged with soft tissue or bone chips. This is done to prevent skin from migrating into the large air cells and possibly causing a secondary cholesteatoma. The vertical slit in the skin graft is positioned anteriorly for the same reason, i.e., to prevent a free skin edge from migrating into the mastoid.

When preparing the skin graft on the cutting board, one will often notice that one edge of the graft is thinner than the other. The thin edge is best used at the level of the tympanic membrane, while the thicker edge is best suited for the meatus. Moreover, if the skin tabs are

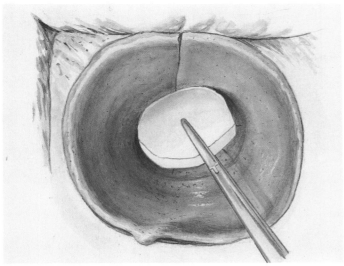

Fig. 3.**65**   Placement of silastic button.

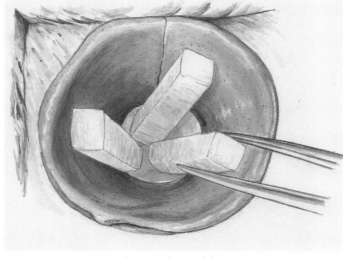

Fig. 3.**66**   Placement of Merocel ear wicks.

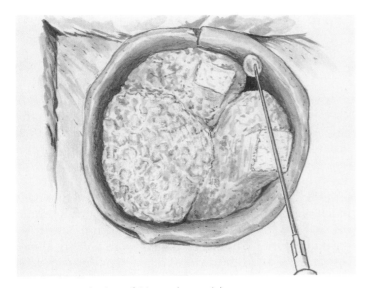

Fig. 3.**67**   Hydration of Merocel ear wicks.

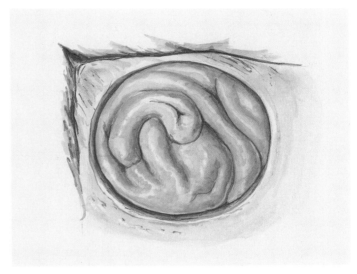

Fig. 3.**68**   Skin graft folded over Merocel.

thick at the drum level they will tend to curl and will be difficult to position.

Once the skin graft is satisfactorily positioned over the fascia, a silastic button 1.0 mm thick is cut to size and placed over the skin tabs (Fig. 3.**65**). This is a very important maneuver. It anchors the skin tabs in place and allows for the formation of a sulcus at the level of the anulus. This prevents blunting of the anterior and inferior sulci which would otherwise contribute to graft lateralization and compromise the postoperative hearing threshold. Graft lateralization was the single most frequent complication noted by De La Cruz in his atresia series (De la Cruz et al., 1985). Three or four Merocel ear wicks of the Pope type are cut to a length of 1 cm and strategically placed in the new bony external ear canal (Fig. 3.**66**). The wicks are hydrated with a steroid/antibiotic ear drop preparation (Fig. 3.**67**). After expansion of the wicks, the lateral edges of the skin graft are folded over the Merocel packing while attention is turned to the meatus (Fig. 3.**68**).

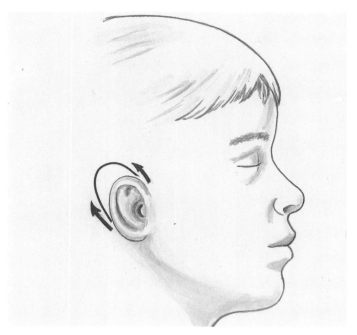

Fig. 3.**69**   Anterior and inferior location of reconstructed auricle on lateral face prior to repositioning.

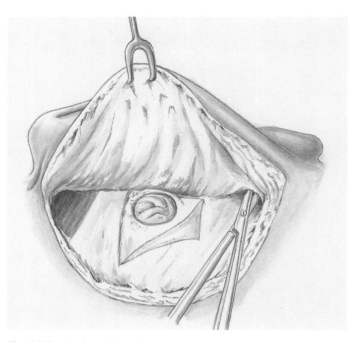

Fig. 3.**70**   Undermining skin anteriorly.

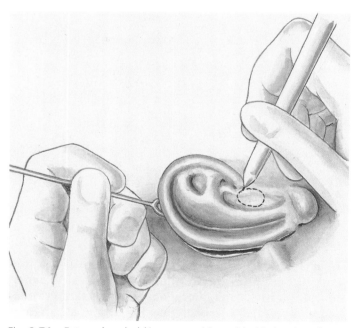

Fig. 3.**71**   External ear held in new position with skin hook and meatus outlined with marker.

Meatoplasty: At this junction, one can determine if the new meatus — not yet incised — will align with the new ear canal. Usually, the reconstructed auricle will be situated anterior and inferior on the lateral face (Fig. 3.**69**). It must be repositioned in a posterosuperior direction (Figs. 3.**70**–3.**73**). As the external ear is not tethered by an existing ear canal, it may be moved as much as 5 cm if necessary. This requires some undermining of soft tissue anterior to the auricle (over the parotid) (Fig. 3.**70**) and at times a minifacelift is indicated. Only after the external ear is mobilized should the new meatus be created (Fig. 3.**71**). An oval of skin and underlying soft tissue is sharply excised in the normal anatomic area on the auricle (Fig. 3.**72**). After confirming a good alignment of the meatus with the ear canal, the auricle is tacked into position with a 3.0 subcutaneous suture (Fig. 3.**73**). Usually an absorbable suture is used but if there is significant tension on the ear a nonabsorbable suture may be preferred. The lateral margin of the canal skin graft is identified, brought to the meatal skin and sutured with a running 5.0 nonabsorbable suture (Fig. 3.**74**). Merocel wicks are used to pack the lateral extent of the ear canal. The postauricular incision is closed with 3.0 absorbable subcutaneous sutures and a running 5.0 nylon suture for the skin. An optional "V" incision may be required to eliminate redundant skin (Fig. 3.**75**).

Surgical dressing: Sterile cotton is placed in the meatus and a mastoid dressing is applied in the customary manner.

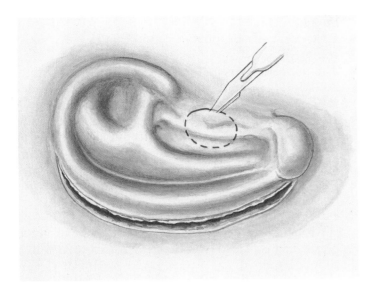

Fig. 3.**72**   Excision of external meatus.

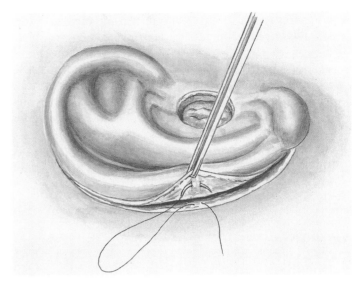

Fig. 3.**73**   Tacking of auricle.

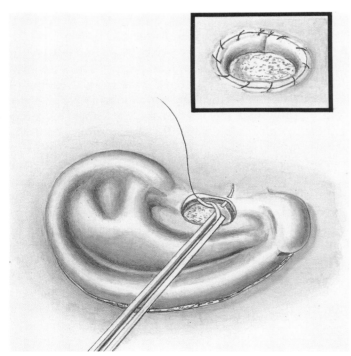

Fig. 3.**74**   Canal skin sutured to meatal skin.

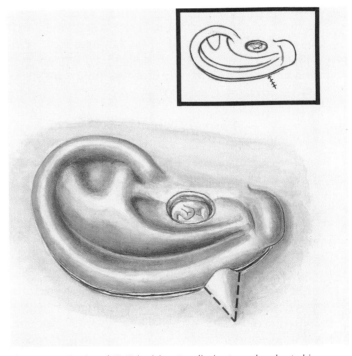

Fig. 3.**75**   Optional "V" incision to eliminate redundant skin.

Modifications

- Endaural incision.
- *Revision surgery* may be required for meatal stenosis, failure to achieve the desired hearing result, or slough of the skin graft over the tympanic membrane. Approximately 5% of cases will require revision surgery. If the meatus remains widely patent, one can perform the revision operation by a transcanal approach. Even if the skin graft has sloughed over the tympanic membrane, and a thick layer of granulation tissue has formed, this can be removed revealing an intact fibrous tympanic membrane beneath. One then needs only to regraft with split thickness skin.

Surgical Landmarks and Danger Points

- Cribriform area.
- Tympanic bone remnant.
- Temporomandibular joint.
- Temporal line.
- Drilling — stay high, hug tegmen.
- Air cell tracks should be followed to the attic, if possible.
- The body of the incus, actually the fused incus/malleus complex, is often the first landmark encountered.
- Facial nerve: Always be alert for this important structure.

Rules, Tips, and Pitfalls

- Facial nerve: The facial nerve is often first seen as a whitish structure encased in dense pale yellow atretic bone.
- Stay out of the mastoid.
- Center ossicular mass in middle of new tympanic membrane.
- Position thin skin tabs over fascia tympanic membrane.
- Size of meatus: In reconstructing Grade III microtia in which the anatomic area of the meatus consists of soft tissue only and no cartilage, the new meatus must be twice normal size in anticipation of stenosis. The opening may stenose 50% in the first month. Thereafter, stenosis slows and often arrests at an aperture of 4 or 5 mm. Infiltrating the meatal soft tissue with a long–acting steroid may be beneficial. If there is conchal cartilage present (Grade II microtia), stenosis is usually not a problem. The new meatus need only be slightly larger than normal.

Postoperative Care

- The patient may be discharged on the 1st or 2nd postoperative day.
- Postoperative prophylactic antibiotics are used routinely.
- The mastoid dressing is removed prior to discharge. Antibiotic ointment and cotton is placed in the meatus.
- *Donor site dressing:* The dressing over the donor site is removed on the first postoperative day leaving in place only the patch of scarlet red dressing. This is kept dry and will spontaneously slough in two weeks.
- *Avoid water in ear and on skin graft donor site:* Initially, no water should come in contact with the new ear canal or donor site. When showering, a plastic cup is held firmly over the ear against the head, and a plastic bag is placed over the arm and secured with a rubber band.
- Remove all sutures and packing at 1 week: The first postoperative outpatient visit is at one week when all sutures, Merocel ear packing, and the silastic button, are removed. The ear canal is flooded with a steroid/antibiotic ear drop preparation which is allowed to remain in place for 5 minutes. Thereafter, the patient uses ear drops, 5 drops b.i.d. for 1 week. The ear canal is left open to the air.
- *Debride skin graft at 3–4 weeks:* A second outpatient visit is scheduled four weeks postop. The skin graft will present as a thick, dark crust from shedding of the outer layer. This is carefully debrided (Fig. 3.**76**), preferably as a dry cast of the ear canal, revealing healthy pink skin beneath. An audiogram is obtained on this visit.
- *Ear cleaning every 6–12 months:* Thereafter, the patient must be seen every 6–12 months indefinitely for mechanical cleaning of the ear canal. The new skin lacks "memory" and does not migrate as in normal ears. This requires that the desquamated layer of epithelium be removed under the microscope on a periodic basis. Failure to do so may result in crusts which are prone to infection.

Postoperative Complications

Facial nerve paralysis: Facial nerve paralysis is an omnipresent potential complication in congenital atresia surgery. In 25% of cases, the nerve will be out of position and vulnerable to injury. Additionally, the nerve is often bare in the middle ear. The surgeon must, therefore, be ever mindful of this important neural structure.

In our series of almost 700 surgical cases, a postoperative facial paralysis/paresis was noted 6 times. Five of

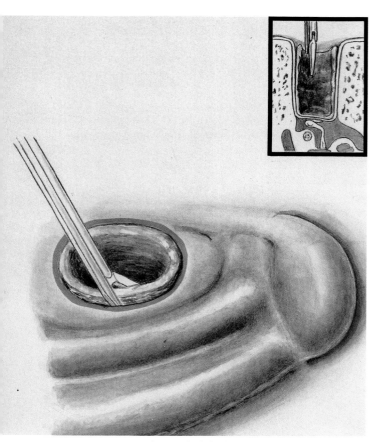

Fig. 3.**76** Outpatient skin graft debridement.

Despite the high frequency sensorineural hearing loss in a small percentage of patients, thresholds through the speech range are normal or near normal.

Infection: Infection has not been a problem. We attribute this to the judicial use of prophylactic antibiotics and ear drops postoperatively. To our knowledge, no patient actively being followed has a draining ear.

Temporomandibular joint: Temporomandibular joint swelling is a rare and temporary postoperative complication. The complaint is difficulty in chewing and resolves in a few weeks. Presumably, the swelling results from the proximity of the TMJ to the reconstructed middle ear or external ear canal.

Meatal stenosis: Meatal stenosis occurs predominantly in patients who have a Grade III microtia and in whom there is no conchal cartilage. The strategic placement of a cartilage ring to impede stenosis has not been of long–term benefit. We continue to seek ways to alleviate this problem.

Late onset of progressive conductive hearing loss due to graft lateralization: This is not a significant problem in our series and occurs in less than 2% of patients. We attribute our success to the careful placement of a silastic button to create a sulcus inferiorly and anteriorly. In addition, the placement of the fascia graft wherein the ossicles are higher than the lateral graft probably has a salutary effect.

Sequelae

Hearing results: Eighty percent of carefully selected patients will attain a postoperative speech reception threshold of 15–25 dB.

Follow-up: Follow-up visits with careful cleaning of the ear under the operating microscope must be scheduled every 6–12 months indefinitely. However, about 10% of patients never seem to accumulate significant epithelial debris or crusting and may be seen less frequently.

Graft lateralization: This is a potential problem.

Progressive meatal stenosis.

Restrictions: Postoperatively patients are allowed to swim. The only condition we place on swimming is that the patient must use alcohol ear drops (1–2 drops) after each swimming outing. If the skin graft is too thin it will withstand environmental abuse (water) poorly, and may subsequently slough.

these cases antedated the routine use of high resolution CT scanning which we began in 1982. In these 5 cases, the facial nerve was found to course over the oval window, or over the area where a new oval window was to be drilled, and was purposely rerouted. This action resulted in a temporary facial paralysis/paresis lasting as long as three months after which full normal function returned. Since 1982, only once have we been surprised by a postoperative facial nerve paralysis. This occurred when the facial nerve did not bend but coursed vertically through the middle ear. It was bruised by the drill. There was a full and normal recovery in 3 weeks. *No patient in our series has a permanent facial nerve paralysis or weakness.* Three patients sustained a permanent facial nerve injury from surgery done elsewhere.

Sensorineural hearing loss: A high frequency sensorineural hearing loss occurs in 5–10% of cases, presumably from vibratory trauma to the inner ear from drilling. However, the loss typically occurs at 6–8 kHz and is beyond the customary speech range. Discrimination scores remain good, i.e., 85–95%. Even when the inner ear shows evidence of a more extensive surgical insult, it may recover with time.

Alternate Techniques

Reconstruction of ear canal to accommodate ear level hearing aid: This technique is reserved for those patients in whom preoperative CT imaging has shown a poorly developed middle ear not amenable to ossicular reconstruction. The conductive hearing loss is usually maximum (60 dB) and the auricle must be lifted off the lateral face to create a retroauricular sulcus.

Reconstruction of ear canal to accommodate in–the–ear aid: For patients in whom there has been a partial restoration of hearing through surgery, an in–the–ear aid will help if the conductive hearing loss is moderate, i.e. 35 dB.

Implantable bone conducting hearing aid: This is reserved for those atresia patients who are otherwise not candidates for surgery.

Bone anchored hearing aid: This is also reserved for those atresia patients who are otherwise not candidates for surgery.

Bibliography

De la Cruz A, Linthicum F, Luxford W M. Congenital atresia of external auditory canal. Laryngoscope 1985; 95: 421.

Marquet J F, Declau F. Congenital middle ear malformations. Acta Oto-rhino-laryng belg 1988; 42: 117.

Nomura Y, Nagao Y, Fukaya T. Anomalies of the middle ear. Laryngoscope 1988; 98: 390.

Plester D, Katzke D. The promontorial window technique. Laryngoscope 1983; 93: 824.

Rizer F M, Lippy W H, Schuring A G, Emami A. Perilymph gushers in stapedectomy: predictive factors and surgical results. Trans Pacific Coast Ophthalmol Otolaryngol 1989; 62.

Steffen T N. Vascular anomalies of the middle ear. Laryngoscope 1968; 78: 171.

Welling D B, Glasscock M E, Gantz B. Avulsion of the anomalous facial nerve at stapedectomy. Laryngoscope 1992; 102: 729.

4 Surgery of the Outer Ear, Middle Ear, and Temporal Bone for the Removal of Disease and for Reconstruction

Surgery for Removal of Disease

Jan Helms

Since the second half of the nineteenth century, the capabilities of ear surgery have constantly expanded as the anatomy and pathophysiology of otologic diseases have become better understood. Discoveries in hygiene and microbiology, the development of antibiotics and new anesthesiologic procedures, and technological innovations in instrumentation have contributed to these advances. The present chapter deals with surgical methods for the eradication of non–tumorous, otologic diseases and defect reconstruction.

Surgical Anatomy

The knowledge of anatomy that is necessary for petrous bone (temporal bone) surgery can be derived from suitable textbooks and handbooks dealing with the anatomy and especially the surgical anatomy of the ear. Moreover, it is essential for students to practice surgical procedures on actual petrous bone specimens. These specimens should be deep-frozen after they are removed. Storage in formalin or other fixatives alters the consistency of the tissue, making it difficult to transfer practiced skills to the patient. The practice specimens are thawed in running water before use and can be repeatedly deep–frozen and reused.

Informing the Patient

Informed consent for ear surgery involves explaining the procedure, estimating the chances for a given outcome (e.g., the complete eradication of cholesteatoma or a noticeable hearing gain), and pointing out tran

sient or permanent deficits that may follow the operation. Besides the general risks of anesthesia and wound healing problems with hematoma formation, the patient should be informed about other potential risks such as displacement or deformation of the auricle, hearing loss, tinnitus, vertigo, and facial paralysis.

Given the possibility of litigation, it is advisable to make a brief, handwritten notation of each of these points as they are covered. To avoid needless distress, the patient should be reassured that the incidence of these complications is in the order of 1 to 0.1%, so they are unlikely to occur.

Surgical Procedures on the External Meatus

Preoperative Diagnostic Measures

Inspection

The best instrument for examining the external acoustic meatus is the binocular operating microscope. The examination includes inspecting the entrance to the meatus, removing any cerumen accumulation, aspirating liquid debris and secretions, and removing solid, adherent crusts.

Imaging Studies

Only rare conditions such as malignant otitis externa or a suspected malignant tumor in the ear canal would warrant imaging studies for the preoperative evaluation of meatal disease. The contours of the petrous bone are well defined by the classic Stenvers and Schüller X–ray projections. Standard and high–resolution CT scans offer additional diagnostic capabilities. Nuclear medicine studies may be used in selected cases to measure radionuclide uptake in a focal area of disease.

Indications

Surgical procedures on the external acoustic meatus may be performed for the purpose of removing foreign bodies, polyps, arachnoid cysts, and other lesions or for the treatment of meatal diseases such as otitis externa.

Polyps in the external meatus arise from the middle ear. They have a fleshy consistency and a reddish surface. Arachnoid cysts appear as pale, polyp–like soft tissue masses that project into the external meatus from above or from the posterosuperior quadrant. Very rarely they may develop spontaneously, but they most commonly follow previous otologic surgery. Exostoses in the external meatus (Fig. 4.**1**) narrow the canal lumen from the anterior or posterior side, and occasional pedunculated forms may hang from the roof of the canal. These lesions are distinguished by their hardness, which is easily recognized by probing with a blunt instrument under the operating microscope.

Principles of the Operation

Foreign bodies may be aspirated, extracted with small hooks, or if necessary fragmented and removed piecemeal while sparing the meatal skin (e.g., impression material left after the improper fitting of a hearing aid.)

All manipulations for the removal of meatal pathology should be performed under the operating microscope to minimize pain and tissue damage.

Preoperative Preparations

Most procedures on the external meatus are performed on an outpatient basis with the patient in a sitting position. The chair back should be reclined about 30° so that the head can lie comfortably against the head rest. This provides adequate immobilization for manipulations under the operating microscope. Necessary instruments such as suction tips, small hooks, snares, and delicate grasping forceps are placed within reach of the examiner; in most cases an assistant is not required.

If procedures on the external meatus go beyond cleaning, extracting foreign bodies, or taking a small biopsy, the preoperative preparations are the same as those for surgery of the middle ear. The patient is posi-

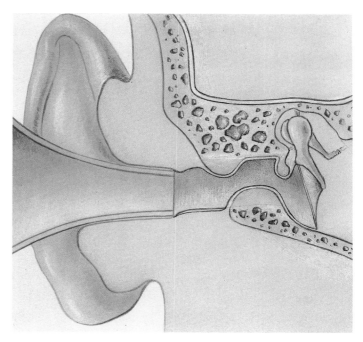

Fig. 4.**1**

tioned supine on the operating table. The head is supported on a rubber ring or other contoured rest so that, once positioned, the head will remain in place without additional fixation. The instrument stand is placed at the head of the operating table, and the instrument nurse sits opposite the surgeon. The microscope is positioned over the patient in such a way that it does not restrict the surgeon's freedom of movement, including elbow movements. Suction irrigators, bipolar cautery, and drilling instruments are brought into the operating field from the foot of the table so that their cables and hoses will not interfere with orderly work at the instrument table.

Short–term antibiotic prophylaxis is provided by giving a single i.v. dose about 30 min before the start of the operation.

The ear itself is prepared by thorough cleaning of the meatus under the operating microscope on the eve of the operation.

Instruments

Use of the operating microscope is recommended for the removal of foreign bodies in the ear canal. Small hooks and forceps, delicate snares, an ear curet, and high–capacity suction should also be available.

Anesthesia

In most cases neither local nor general anesthesia is required for the removal of freshly impacted foreign bodies. But if prolonged manipulations have already been made in an attempt to retrieve the object, local anesthesia should be administered by infiltrating anesthetic solution about the ear. General anesthesia is occasionally required, especially in children unable to remain quiet during a prolonged extraction attempt or in adults requiring removal of a firmly adherent impression material or adhesive substance.

Removal of Reactive and Inflammatory Lesions

The removal of reactive and inflammatory lesions of the external meatus employs instruments and anesthetic procedures like those used in surgery of the middle ear. Local anesthesia is satisfactory for most circumscribed lesions. But if adequate infiltration cannot be achieved, as in a patient with obliterative exostoses, the surgery should be performed under general anesthesia supplemented by local infiltration.

A limited instrument set is employed. A standard ear tray contains the following components:

2   Sponge–holding forceps
2   Mosquito forceps
1   Needle holder
2   Backhaus towel clips
1   Four–prong hook, small
1   Two–prong hook, small
1   Handpiece for suction tips
8   Suction tips, short (2 of each size)
2   Self–retaining retractors, 3 prong (postauricular)
2   Self–retaining retractors, 2 prong (endaural)
2   Lempert–type endaural retractors (1 each for right and left ear)
1   Nasal speculum (endaural incision)
1   Scissor with sharp points
1   General–purpose forceps
3   Aural specula, assorted sizes
1   Eustachian tube probe
3   Different drill–aspirators (with breaker plate)
1   Periosteal elevator, large
2   Scalpels
1   Rosen elevator
2   Different House curets
2   Ring curets
1   Antrum retractor
3   Silver suction–irrigators
1   Soft suction tube
1   Knife–elevator with straight round blade
1   Knife–elevator with angled round blade

1   Sickle knife
1   Curved needle
4   Different right–angle hooks
1   Reinforced right–angle hook
2   Different 45° hooks
1   Perforator (for stapes surgery)
1   Fork
1   Plexiglas plate (for preparation of cartilage, etc.)
2   Small dishes
1   Water basin
1   Small cupped forceps
1   Large cupped forceps
1   Alligator forceps
1   Belluci ear scissor
1   Malleus head nipper
2   Different stapes crimping forceps
Precut strips of silicone film (0.5×4 cm, rounded on one side, 0.125 mm thick)
2   Small dissecting pledgets
Large and small compresses
Large and small rolled packs

Also: 1 power drill (40,000 rpm) with matching handpiece and assorted burrs: round cutting burrs (rose burrs) of Vidia steel, pear burrs, disk burrs, and diamond burrs; 1 bipolar cautery; and high–capacity suction.

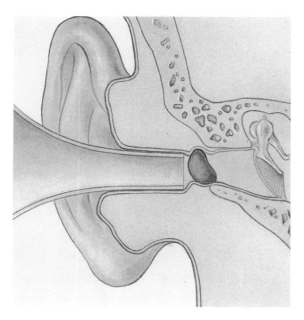

Fig. 4.**2**

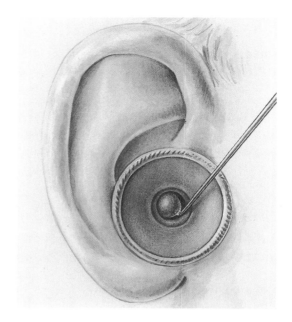

Fig. 4.**3**

Operative Technique

Removal of Foreign Bodies

The best instrument for removing a foreign body from the (usually pediatric) external meatus (Fig. 4.**2**) is a small hook (Fig. 4.**3**), which is passed behind the foreign body, rotated, and gently pulled outward. Grasping instruments tend to push the foreign body deeper into the meatus. Fine snares are best for detaching and removing firmly adherent crusts (Fig. 4.**4**). These lesions should not be forcibly washed off or peeled away, as this would damage the epithelial lining of the meatus.

Removal of Polyps

Polyps grow by extension from the middle ear into the external meatus. Often it is difficult to appreciate the pathology in cases where previous ear surgery has been performed. Polyps may arise from the mastoid cavity or from the roof of the meatus. Removal, which is preceded by infiltration of a local anesthetic solution with a vasoconstrictor, is accomplished by grasping the polyp with a suction tip and progressively reducing the lesion while holding the sucker in contact with the polyp surface (Fig. 4.**5**). If necessary the polyp can be removed with a fine cup forceps, which makes it easier to identify the origin of the polyp. The removal is carried only as far as necessary to ensure the unobstructed drainage of secretions from the middle ear or polyp base into the external meatus. More extensive tissue removal should be attempted only in a formal operative setting. If the pedicle passes toward the stapes, rem-

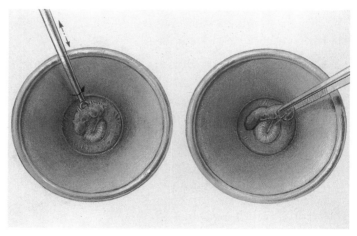

Fig. 4.**4**

nants of it should be left behind. If the patient experiences whirling vertigo during manipulation of the polyp, a labyrinthine fistula may be present, and further measures should be deferred until the polyp can be definitively removed by extirpative surgery.

Removal of Exostoses

Exostoses in the ear canal (Fig. 4.**6**) are removed through an endaural incision (see pp. 110–111). Pedunculated exostoses are removed by applying a gouge to the base. The skin is held aside, and the exostosis is removed (Fig. 4.**7**).

Most exostoses on the anterior wall of the meatus are broad–based. Cutting and diamond burrs are used to re-

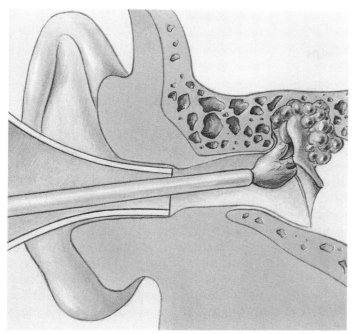

Fig. 4.**5**

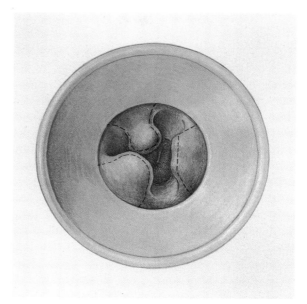

Fig. 4.**6**

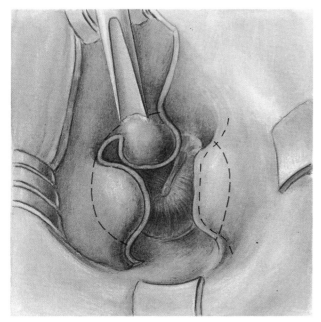

Fig. 4.**7**

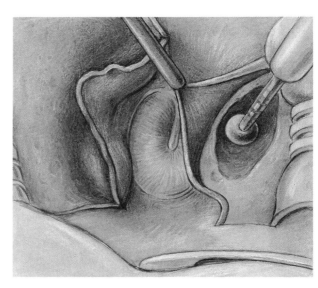

Fig. 4.**8**

duce the exostosis while avoiding damage to the overlying skin. The skin is opened with a horizontal H–shaped incision along the anterior wall of the meatus, placing the transverse limb of the incision over the summit of the exostotic mound.

The outer skin flap is reflected outward, and drilling proceeds on the plane between the meatal skin covering the exostosis and the anterior side of the meatus, behind the temporomandibular joint (Fig. 4.**8**). The burr should not touch the soft tissues of the joint. On ap-

proaching the periarticular soft tissues, the surgeon changes to a diamond burr to lessen the risk of periosteal injury and provide better tactile feedback for recognizing when the soft tissues have been reached.

Bone removal is continued until all of the tympanic anulus can be seen after replacement of the skin. The tympanic membrane itself is not touched during the resection. Relatively small burrs can be used in the anterior tympanomeatal angle to avoid touching the surface of the membrane, which could cause hearing loss.

The operation concludes by replacing the meatal flaps in their original position. Free skin flaps are replanted. Then the external meatus is completely lined with strips of silicone film 4 cm long, 5 mm wide, and about 0.1 mm thick. This lining prevents granulation tissue ingrowth into the endaural packing while promoting fibroblast proliferation and the formation of connective tissue directly on the bone. It also speeds the rate of epithelialization. Tetracycline–impregnated gelatin sponge has proven excellent for packing the lumen of the ear canal. The packing remains in place for three weeks.

Modifications

Exostosis removal with cutting and diamond burrs can lead to healing problems if a faulty drilling technique is used. A common error is deficient irrigation, allowing excessive heat generation in the bone with the formation of a necrotic focus of indeterminate size. If the site cannot be continuously irrigated during drilling, even broad–based exostoses can be removed manually with a gouge. In this case the surgeon must keep in mind the hazards of the gouge technique, which were frequently described in older textbooks of otologic surgery. The risks include inadvertent opening of the mastoid, damage to the tympanic membrane, partial or complete ossicular dislodgement caused by slipping of the gouge, and possible facial nerve damage due to careless gouge use in proximity to the nerve.

Landmarks and Pitfalls

If the burr touches the tympanic membrane or the malleus handle during the removal of exostoses in the external canal, postoperative hearing loss can result. Thus, the plane of the tympanic membrane is a critical landmark during this type of surgery, and the burr should be controlled so that it does not touch the drum. The best way to keep the burr from running or skipping on the bone is by keeping the field wide, shallow, and beveled rather than making a "hole" in the bone with the burr.

The approximate location of the temporomandibular joint can be estimated from the position of the tympanic membrane and the skin at the meatal opening and especially on the anterior canal wall. If the exostosis is associated with a narrow meatus, the lumen should be slowly enlarged with the diamond burr to ensure

that the temporomandibular joint is not entered and that any perforation of the periosteum on the anterior canal wall will be confined to a small area.

Rules, Hints, and Common Errors

The exostosis that is the easiest to dissect should be removed first to create working space within the ear canal. Generally this will be a pedunculated exostosis with a posterior or posterosuperior base. The posterior meatal skin should be removed as a single, large, free flap to create room for maneuvering the drill. If a pedicled meatal skin flap is raised, it is likely to become wrapped around the drill and sustain greater damage than when it is removed as a free flap. The freely replanted meatal skin should heal as well as a pedicled flap. The anterior meatal skin flap is reflected laterally outward and should be as large as possible, since the flap that is reflected toward the tympanic membrane is often reduced somewhat by the drilling.

As mentioned, the removal of the exostoses should be of adequate extent to afford a complete view of the anulus. This should be confirmed before packing is inserted into the meatus. The canal is packed after the skin flap has been replaced or replanted and after the entire canal has been lined with silicone strips.

Postoperative Care

The packing is left in the meatus for about three weeks. Finally it is suctioned out, and the silicone strips are elevated from the skin and removed. No antibiotics are required other than the preoperative prophylactic dose. However, if severe otitis externa was present between the tympanic membrane and the bulk of the exostoses prior to surgery and showed little or no preoperative improvement, the preoperative therapy should be continued for one week based on antibiotic sensitivity results. The ear should be checked regularly after the surgery—at least once a day initially—so that any infection of the meatal packing, postoperative bleeding, or other problems can be promptly detected and controlled.

Postoperative Complications

After the removal of exostoses, troublesome infections may arise due to bacterial colonization deep within the external meatus. This is manifested by increasing ear pain starting on about the third or fourth postoperative day, with liquefaction of the packing. The ear canal should be suctioned clear of this material while the silicone film is left in place. The packing is replaced by gelatin sponge impregnated with an aminoglycoside antibiotic. Frequent packing changes (e.g., every two days) are required.

Functional Sequelae

If the exostoses were sufficiently removed to expose the full circumference of the anulus, and if the replaced or replanted meatal flaps heal satisfactorily, the external meatus should be indistinguishable from a normal ear canal by one to two months after the surgery. Meatal stenosis is very rare following exostosis removal by the technique described.

Removal of an Arachnoid Cyst in the External Meatus

See postoperative complications after cholesteatoma removal, page 85.

Partial Resection of the External Meatus (in Patients with Aseptic Bone Necrosis or Malignant Otitis Externa)

Aseptic necrosis of bone is managed by complete removal of the affected bone. This condition is marked by the presence of a craterlike bone area, denuded of meatal skin, in front of the tympanic membrane (Fig. 4.**9**). The approach is similar to that for the eradication of cholesteatoma (see page 85). Healthy areas of meatal skin surrounding the necrotic bone are removed as free flaps to allow for extensive drilling and burring without harming the meatal skin. All of the aseptic bone is burred away, and the wound bed is smoothed with diamond burrs. Constant irrigation is necessary to avoid overheating of the bone and consequent problems of wound healing. The pieces of skin removed at the start of the operation are replanted close to the tympanic membrane. The external meatus is packed and lined with silicone strips in the usual manner. Exposed bone that could not be covered with meatal skin is completely covered with silicone. The canal is packed for three weeks with tetracycline–impregnated gelatin sponge.

In patients with *malignant otitis externa*, we recommend preoperative antibiotic sensitivity testing *(Pseudomonas aeruginosa)* as well as a complete medical examination. The resection of the diseased bone is more extensive but follows the same basic technique as in aseptic necrosis. Functionally important structures such as the facial nerve, jugular vein, and internal carotid artery are identified and preserved. In contrast to aseptic necrosis, the wound following the extirpation of malignant otitis externa is closed loosely, and multi-

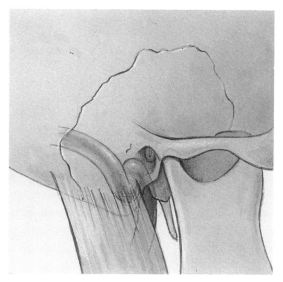

Fig. 4.**9**

ple drains are placed in the soft tissues adjacent to the petrous bone.

Modifications

Aseptic bone necrosis in the external auditory meatus is a very circumscribed process, so it is rarely possible to modify the procedure described above.

In the treatment of *malignant otitis externa*, the extent of the ear incision and neck approach are modified according to the extent of the disease. Modern neuroradiologic and nuclear medicine studies are of some use in determining the direction of spread. If the disease has progressed far into the petrous pyramid and below the skull base, a subtotal petrosectomy (see Chap. 6, p. 178) is occasionally necessary and will generally require sacrifice of the middle ear.

Not infrequently, multiple operations are necessary for the complete eradication of malignant otitis externa. Measures for reconstructing the opened or partially destroyed middle ear should be deferred until the primary infectious process has been successfully cleared.

Malignant otitis externa is now treated largely by medical, not surgical, means.

Landmarks and Pitfalls

In the treatment of *aseptic necrosis*, the tympanic membrane should be preserved, i.e., there should be no trauma to the middle ear. After the involved bone has been resected into healthy tissue, constant irrigation must be maintained as the surgical cavity is smoothed with a diamond burr. Otherwise the burr would overheat the bone and create necrotic foci that would necessitate further surgery. If it appears desirable to line the bony bed completely with skin, but the free flap of meatal skin is deficient for this purpose, complete coverage can be obtained by augmenting the meatal skin with split–thickness skin grafts 0.2–0.3 mm thick taken with a dermatome from the hairless area just behind the auricle. "Manual" graft outlining with a scalpel would yield full–thickness grafts that are predisposed to otitis externa.

In the treatment of *malignant otitis externa* involving extensive bone resection, attention must be given to the course of the facial nerve. The best sites for identifying the nerve are in the healthy mastoid portion of the nerve and in the soft tissues below the stylomastoid foramen. When these segments have been visualized, the bone resection can be performed without damaging the nerve. If it has been necessary to resect the base of the styloid process, then the jugular vein and internal carotid artery should be identified in the neck before any further dissections are performed. These structures are located just medial to the styloid process.

Rules, Hints, and Common Errors

Aseptic bone necrosis in the external meatus is apt to recur following an inadequate resection of the affected bone. The resection should be performed with sharp burrs, as this makes it easier to differentiate healthy from diseased bone; this is far more difficult to accomplish when a diamond burr is used. If the resection cavity in the bone is not completely lined with strips of silicone film, it is likely that granulation areas will form, necessitating a protracted course of postoperative treatment.

Malignant otitis externa is managed by resecting the diseased bone and establishing adequate drainage of the surrounding soft tissues. Inadequate soft–tissue drainage is a common error. Assorted sizes of suction catheters of the type used by anesthesiologists make effective drainage tubes. Also, perforations should be placed along the plastic tubes to allow an optimum drainage of secretions. It may be helpful to flush the drains with hydrogen peroxide or a similar solution during the first few days after surgery.

Postoperative Care

The postoperative regimen for aseptic bone necrosis is identical to that following the removal of exostoses (see page 72).

Postoperative care in *malignant otitis externa* is prolonged and complex. Besides twice daily dressing changes, a successful regimen includes effective control of the underlying diabetes and measures for general health improvement. The services of a well–equipped laboratory should be enlisted to monitor the patient's diabetic metabolic parameters as well as other data that affect wound healing, such as the protein and mineral balance including the trace elements copper, zinc, and selenium. Findings may indicate a need for replacement therapy. Most cases also require treatment with aminoglycoside antibiotics, which should be given in adequate doses. Drug monitoring is recommended and should indicate concentrations of 5–12 mg/liter. The medication should be continued for at least one week.

Postoperative Complications

Uncomplicated healing generally follows the adequate resection of aseptic bone necrosis. With malignant otitis externa, healing problems and recrudescence are common in cases where the disease has been suppressed but not eradicated. Secondary resections should be performed only if the disease process could not be adequately controlled at initial surgery. In rare cases the disease may spread to involve the meninges, central portions of the skull base, and additional cranial nerves, implying a significantly poorer prognosis. The successful management of these cases requires close cooperation with internists, neurologists, and microbiologists.

Functional Sequelae

The surgical treatment of aseptic bone necrosis results in a large external canal that occasionally extends below the tympanic membrane. The self–cleansing mechanism of the ear is occasionally impaired. Outpatient ENT follow–up examinations and periodic cleaning of the operative field under the microscope are recommended for these cases.

Auditory disturbances and facial nerve dysfunction occasionally occur as sequelae to the treatment of malignant otitis externa. Given the advanced age of these patients and their relatively high surgical risk (diabetes), later reconstructive operations should be performed sparingly in this population.

Alternative Methods

Purely conservative treatment methods have been repeatedly tried for aseptic bone necrosis as well as malignant otitis externa. In cases where rapid progression is noted, especially of malignant otitis externa, a nonoperative strategy should not be maintained for too long, as this would necessitate much more extensive extirpative surgery later on.

Surgical Procedures on the Tympanic Membrane

Paracentesis

Preoperative Diagnostic Measures

Before paracentesis is performed, the ear should be inspected, cleaned, and tested for auditory function. Neuroradiologic imaging studies are rarely necessary in selecting patients for this type of surgery.

Indications

Paracentesis may be used for decompression of middle ear effusion, in selected patients with acute otitis media, or to prepare for the insertion of a ventilation tube (see page 77).

Principle of the Operation

Paracentesis involves the creation of a temporary opening in the tympanic membrane in order to aspirate fluid from the middle ear and ventilate the middle ear space. A myringotomy incision 2–3 mm long is made through all the layers of the tympanic membrane.

Preoperative Preparations

The external meatus is mechanically cleaned under the operating microscope in preparation for paracentesis. If an infection of the middle ear is present, perioperative antibiotic use should be considered. Perioperative antibiotics are unnecessary if neither the meatus nor the middle ear show evidence of infection.

Instruments

Paracentesis is performed under the operating microscope through an aural speculum. A sharp myringotome is used that will incise rather than tear the tympanic membrane. A large–gauge suction tube is needed for the removal of thick mucus.

Anesthesia

Paracentesis for the treatment of a seromucous middle ear effusion in adults is usually performed without an anesthetic. Brief general anesthesia is recommended in children. If the tympanic membrane is inflamed, local anesthesia should be used even in adults.

Operative Technique

The speculum is positioned to give a clear view of the tympanic membrane, especially its anterior quadrants. The incision is made in the anteroinferior quadrant or the lower part of the anterosuperior quadrant, in front of the umbo (Fig. 4.**10**). A radial incision is preferred, as it is believed to heal more rapidly.

Modifications

Various incisions for paracentesis have been described in the literature (Fig. 4.**11**). Manipulations in the posterior quadrants of the tympanic membrane are more likely to traumatize the ossicular chain or jeopardize the floor of the tympanic cavity, where an occasional high–sited jugular bulb may be encountered.

Landmarks and Pitfalls

Structures at risk during paracentesis are the auditory ossicles and structures that can bleed profusely, such as a high–sited jugular bulb or glomus tumor.

Rules, Hints, and Common Errors

A common error is to place the myringotomy in the posterior quadrants of the tympanic membrane rather than anteriorly at the level of the umbo.

Aspiration through a myringotomy cannot clear the middle ear of all secretions. One must be careful when attempting to expel a mucous plug from the eustachian tube by applying positive pressure to the external meatus, because there may be bony dehiscences in the tegmen tympani that have but a thin dural cover. This can allow the sudden transmission of air to the cranial cavity, posing a serious threat to the patient.

Postoperative Care

No special care regimen is necessary after paracentesis. Decongestant nose drops or perhaps antiedematous agents should be given to improve eustachian tube function. Maneuvers to ventilate the middle ear through the eustachian tube (e.g., Otovent, Otobar) are recommended after the tympanic membrane has healed.

As long as the myringotomy opening is present, water should be kept out of the external meatus. Thus a petrolatum cotton wad should be stuffed into the ear canal when the patient swims, showers, etc.

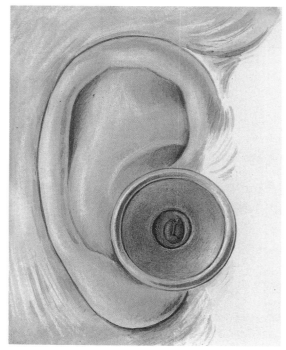

Fig. 4.**10**

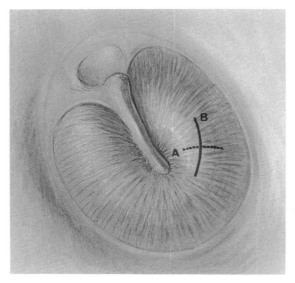

Fig. 4.**11**
A: incision for paracentesis
B: alternative

Postoperative Complications

Rarely, paracentesis may become complicated by an infection of the middle ear or a persistent perforation. A middle ear infection should be managed conservatively.

If a tympanic membrane perforation persists for more than six months after paracentesis, a tympanoplasty is indicated.

Functional Sequelae

The myringotomy will usually heal within a few days without sequelae.

Alternative Methods

Transtympanic air insufflation with a needle through the intact tympanic membrane offers an alternative to paracentesis in selected cases, especially when there is deficient ventilation of the middle ear following tympanoplasty. A long, thin cannula is introduced through the anterior half of the tympanic membrane, and a small amount of air is injected into the obstructed lumen of the tympanic cavity. The benefit is only temporary. A nonabsorbable gas such as sulfur hexafluoride may be instilled if desired (Koch).

Antrotomy (see page 80), while frequently discussed as a measure for improving middle ear ventilation, is not considered an alternative to paracentesis. The prolonged conservative treatment of a middle ear effusion is potentially hazardous in that the pars tensa of the tympanic membrane may gradually atrophy and necessitate an eventual myringoplasty. When signs of tympanic membrane atrophy become apparent, paracentesis should no longer be delayed, and a ventilation tube should be inserted if required.

Insertion of a Ventilation Tube

Preoperative Diagnostic Measures

The need for a ventilation tube is confirmed by inspection of the tympanic membrane and, if necessary, by tympanometry. The nasopharynx should also be inspected, especially in children and adults with no signs of systemic infection, and obstructions should be investigated. In children with cleft deformities, the differential diagnosis should be made in consultation with an oral surgeon.

Indications

The insertion of a ventilation tube is indicated for recurrent pediatric middle ear effusions following adequate adenotomy, in children with cleft palate, and in adults with nasopharyngeal tumors. A ventilation tube is occasionally inserted for adhesive processes in the middle ear and for the treatment of Ménière's disease, in which case the tube may serve only to ventilate the middle ear cleft or may additionally provide a route for the instillation of ototoxic medications.

Principle of the Operation

The ventilation tube is inserted to provide for extended drainage and aeration of the middle ear space, independent of the function of the eustachian tube.

Preoperative Preparations

The preparations are the same as those for paracentesis (page 75).

Instruments

For commercial, and occasionally for medical reasons as well, myringotomy tubes are produced in a variety of designs. Ideally, the tube should have a maximal inside diameter and minimal outside diameter. Usually it should be retained in the tympanic membrane for 6 to 12 months, but much longer–term placement is required in patients with cleft palate and in adults with pharyngeal tumors.

A gold–plated tube is advantageous for most ordinary purposes, as it combines a small outside diameter with a large inside diameter. An atrophic tympanic membrane will provide a very weak hold for the ventilation tube, and a metal tube that has been spontaneously and prematurely extruded should be replaced by a plastic T–tube with self–expanding intratympanic side arms (Fig. 4.**12**).

Anesthesia

In adults, the ventilation tube is inserted either without anesthesia or with local infiltration of the area around the tympanic membrane. Children are given a short–acting general anesthetic.

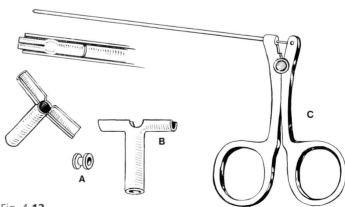

Fig. 4.**12**
A: gold tube
B: self–expanding tube
C: instrument for application

Operative Technique

As described under paracentesis, a myringotomy incision 2–3 mm long is made in the anterior part of the tympanic membrane. Seromucous material is aspirated from the middle ear. The metal ventilation tube is placed next to the myringotomy on the surface of the tympanic membrane, one edge of the inner flange is slid under one margin of the incision, and the rest of the flange is slipped through the incision (Fig. 4.**13**). A special insertion instrument is not needed with this technique. If a T–tube is used, the soft half tubes of the implant are grasped and passed through the myringotomy. Once they are fully inside the tympanum, the side arms spread out and bear against the inner surface of the tympanic membrane.

Modifications

A special introducer can be used to insert the ventilation tube into the tympanic membrane (Fig. 4.**12**).

Landmarks and Pitfalls

The myringotomy should be no longer than that required for paracentesis; this ensures that the incision will grip the tube securely. Tube placement in the posterior half of the tympanic membrane is reserved for special circumstances such as a prominent hump in the anterior canal wall blocking access to the anterior half of the membrane. During inspection of the ear, the surgeon should check for a high jugular bulb or glomus tumor in the hypotympanum, which could lead to profuse hemorrhage.

Rules, Hints, and Common Errors

The incision follows the same guidelines stated for paracentesis (page 76). Additionally, care is taken that the ventilation tube does not carry small tags of tympanic membrane tissue into the middle ear space. These small, displaced areas of keratinizing squamous epithelium on the inner surface of the tympanic membrane could create a nidus for cholesteatoma formation.

Tube placement in the posterior half of the tympanic membrane is associated with a higher risk than paracentesis in that area. The manipulations involved in tube insertion and the poor visibility of the tube end in the tympanic cavity pose additional risks of trauma to the ossicular chain. Attention should be given to these risks if anatomic obstructions necessitate tube insertion in the posterior part of the tympanic membrane.

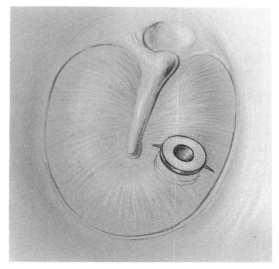

Fig. 4.**13**

Postoperative Care

A special postoperative regimen is not required, although the external meatus should be sealed with a petrolatum cotton wad during shampooing, showering, and swimming to keep water out of the ear.

Two to four weeks after tube insertion, a follow–up examination is conducted to verify the proper position and function of the tube. A short–term tube should remain in place for 6–12 months, but considerably longer ventilation is needed in patients with palatal clefts. Instrumental removal of the tube after the desired ventilation period is necessary only if a T–tube has been inserted. With all other tube designs, gradual spontaneous expulsion tends to occur as a result of epithelial migration on the tympanic membrane, and it is necessary only to remove the extruded device from the ear canal.

Premature spontaneous expulsion is managed either by reinserting the original tube or by inserting a T–tube, although this device is less favorable than a gold–plated tube in terms of its compatibility and fuction.

Postoperative Complications

The irritated condition of the middle ear during tube insertion occasionally gives rise to a prolonged postoperative aural discharge. Superinfection may also develop. Before the tube is removed for the purpose of stopping the discharge, a one–week trial of conservative treatment should be tried while the tube is still in place. A smear is taken and sent for bacteriologic analysis, and a broad–spectrum antibiotic is administered for one week. Meanwhile an anti–inflammatory agent such as

Celestamine ($2 \times \frac{1}{2}$ tablet for children, 2×1 tablet for adults) is also given. This can avoid the unnecessary removal of ventilation tubes. If the apparent intolerance does not respond to this conservative regimen, the tube should be removed so that the ear can heal.

This wait–and–see approach is recommended for standard gold–plated tubes and for standard commercially manufactured plastic tubes. If a homemade tube has been inserted, it should be removed without a trial of medical therapy. Plastic tubes shaped by heating contain tissue–incompatible compounds (monomers) that can incite a severe adverse reaction.

Rarely, a pale cholesteatoma causing no apparent irritation and visible behind the drum may be noticed several years after the insertion of a ventilating tube. The cholesteatoma is surgically removed as part of a tympanoplasty.

In very unfavorable cases the tube can provide a portal of entry for pathogenic organisms, especially if water enters the tympanic cavity from the external meatus through the indwelling tube. This may incite an acute otitis media, which in rare cases can lead to more extensive complications including meningitis.

Functional Sequelae

As long as the ventilation tube remains in the middle ear, hearing will be impaired to a mild degree. After normal expulsion or removal of the tube, the tympanic membrane will heal with the formation of a scar, usually very faint, that may undergo slight calcification. This is not associated with audiologic impairment.

The recurrence of seromucous middle ear effusion in children may necessitate repeated tube insertions. Normal epipharyngeal findings should always be documented in these cases, and training should be provided to promote nasal respiration. Habitual mouth breathers are prone to middle ear effusions even when the epipharynx and eustachian tube function appear normal.

Alternative Methods

Possible alternatives are procedures to restore eustachian tube function such as tubal drainage or tubal reconstruction. These procedures do not yield reliable results, however, so they are not appropriate for the treatment of chronic middle ear effusion. They should be used only in cases where tubal dysfunction has produced effects more severe than effusion, i.e., damage to the middle ear that is causing troublesome symptoms.

Surgical Procedures on the Tympanic Cavity and Mastoid

Antral Drainage, Antrotomy, and Mastoidectomy

Definitions

Antral drainage, antrotomy, and mastoidectomy can be performed as independent procedures to open the antrum and mastoid while preserving the posterior canal wall and, if necessary, to establish postauricular drainage. These procedures may also be done as part of extensive extirpative operations, serving to provide access to the ear, provide access for other parts of the operation, or establish a drainage route for the clearing of disease (Fig. 4.**14**).

Antral drainage involves drilling a channel about 1 cm in diameter from the mastoid cortex to the antrum.

Antrotomy involves a considerably broader opening of the mastoid and antrum. It includes opening the aditus as well as large mastoid cells.

Mastoidectomy involves a thorough exenteration of the mastoid in which all larger cells are opened and cleared. Ideally the mastoid is cleared "to the last cell."

Preoperative Diagnostic Measures

In most inflammatory diseases that necessitate resective surgery of the mastoid, the *history* and *inspection* of the external ear and external auditory meatus are of prime importance.

An elevated *white blood count* and an increased *ESR* are useful signs in patients who have not already received a prolonged, preliminary course of antibiotic treatment.

The *Schüller radiograph* demonstrates shadowing and haziness of the mastoid cells and provides information on the position of the middle fossa dura and the anterior border of the sigmoid sinus.

In exceptional cases, such as when intracranial complications are present, *magnetic resonance imaging* and *computed tomography* are also useful as preoperative studies.

Indications

The most common indications for antrotomy or mastoidectomy are acute, subacute, and chronic inflammations of the ear such as antritis or mastoiditis and its

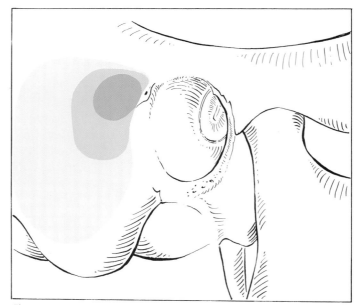

Fig. 4.**14**

complications. The procedures are rarely indicated for cholesterol granuloma or excessive mucus production in chronic suppurative otitis media.

Antrotomy and mastoidectomy are performed as separate parts of extirpative operations for the treatment of cholesteatomas, tumors, post–traumatic lesions, labyrinthine disease, and disease of the petrous apex, internal meatus, cerebellopontine angle or jugular foramen.

The purpose of an *antrotomy* is to establish effective drainage of the antrum and adjacent cell tracts. *Mastoidectomy* has as its goal the removal of all cellular septa and diseased soft tissues and bone from the antrum and mastoid.

Principle of the Operation

Antral drainage, antrotomy, or mastoidectomy involves establishing narrow or broad access to the antrum or to the antrum and mastoid from the mastoid cortex, depending on the extent of the underlying pathology.

Preoperative Preparations

Except in emergency situations, the patient (or guardian) is informed preoperatively about the nature of the disease, possible complications, the principle of the operation, the prospect of clearing the ear of disease, and the associated risks. The most appropriate anesthetic procedure is determined. Premedication may be given, depending on the type of anesthesia used, and antibiotic prophylaxis is administered 30 min before the start of the operation.

Fig. 4.**15**
A: surgeon
B: instruments
C: nurse
D_1: microscope (floor–mounted)
D_2: microscope (ceiling–mounted)
E: anesthesiology
H: suction, electronic monitors, infusion, irrigation
G: foot switches for bipolar electrocautery and drill

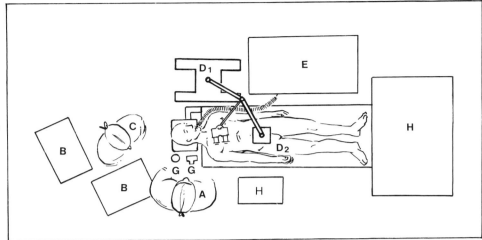

The patient is positioned supine (Fig. 4.**15**) with the head turned slightly to the opposite side. A 2–cm–wide strip of skin above and behind the ear is shaved, and a large, nonirritating adhesive strip is applied to keep the hair from falling into the wound area during the surgery and for the first few days after the operation.

Instruments

See page 69. As in any operation, the surgeon should select a proven instrument set that contains very few specialized instruments and can be used for a variety of surgical procedures when supplemented by a few additional instruments.

Anesthesia

General anesthesia is recommended for children and for patients with a very severe ear infection. If the antral drainage, antrotomy, or mastoidectomy is performed in an adult patient whose otologic disease has a less severe inflammatory component, local anesthesia is acceptable.

Operative Technique

The postauricular approach is recommended for surgery of the mastoid. The auricle is pulled forward, and the skin and subcutaneous tissue are incised along the postaural fold (Fig. 4.**16**). Applying light pressure to the back of the scalpel, the surgeon separates the soft tissues from the mastoid periosteum and from the temporalis fascia by semisharp dissection. The periosteum

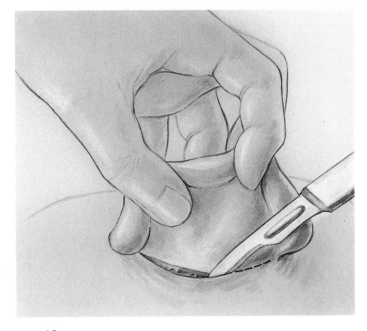

Fig. 4.**16**

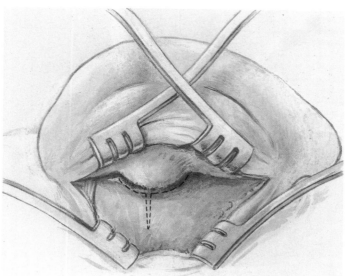

Fig. 4.**17**

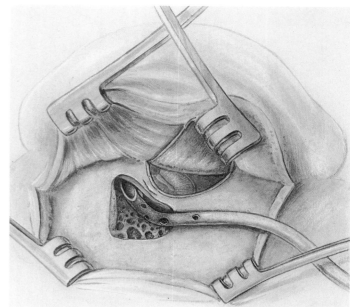

Fig. 4.**18**

is incised at the bony entrance to the meatus, just outside the suprameatal spine, carrying the incision from the posterior part of the roof to the floor of the meatus (Fig. 4.**17**). Also, a relaxing incision is made from the center of the posterior canal wall backward over the mastoid cortex. The postauricular periosteum and connective tissue are fashioned into a pair of triangular soft-tissue flaps, one superior and one inferior (broken lines in Fig. 4.**17**). The meatal soft tissues are now mobilized to the border of the bony meatal entrance. At this point the suprameatal spine can be identified as a landmark.

Drilling, burring, and grinding work in otologic microsurgery is performed with sharp bits, preferably using a small, hand-held drill and a slightly angled handpiece that has high-quality bearings and will accommodate relatively inexpensive bits. The optimum drilling speed of approximately 40,000 rpm should be used for all but a few applications, such as the control of hemorrhage. Continuous suction irrigation is maintained during drilling; this keeps the burr sharp, avoiding overheating of surrounding tissues, and allows very light pressure to be applied to the burr to avoid overloading and heating of the handpiece and drill.

For *antral drainage*, the proposed drainage tunnel in the anterosuperior part of the mastoid and the antrum should be at least 1 cm in diameter so that structures in proximity to the burr can be adequately identified. A high-speed rose burr of Vidia steel is used to drill through the mastoid cortex, which occasionally is very hard behind the suprameatal spine. Further bone work below the middle fossa dura is directed parallel to the axis of the external meatus with a disk or pear-shaped

burr. This helps to avoid uncontrolled plunging of the burr and produces a surgical cavity with smoother margins. If orientation is difficult, a medium-size diamond burr is used. Finally the lateral semicircular canal is exposed, and the antrum is drained (Fig. 4.**18**). The meatal exposure shown in the figure is purely for purposes of illustration; the meatus remains closed during the operation.

An *antrotomy* requires broader opening of the mastoid cortex (Fig. 4.**19**). The entrance to the bony cavity in the mastoid has a triangular shape whose sides are roughly parallel to the dura, the posterior canal wall, and the sigmoid sinus. The excavation is broader than for simple antral drainage and reaches the antrum just below the middle fossa dura. Large terminal mastoid cells near the sigmoid sinus and in the mastoid tip are also opened. Small or medium-size diamond burrs should be used when the aditus is reached, and further bone removal proceeds slowly and cautiously to avoid touching the incus with the burr. Drilling is paused intermittently so that polyps can be removed for vision and orientation. Overhangs in the epitympanum close to the ossicles are taken down as required to establish free access to the tympanum. Polyps in this region should be removed with extreme care, giving close attention to the position of the malleus and incus so that these ossicles are not inadvertently dislodged. If severe inflammation is present, we recommend the insertion of one or two medium-size plastic catheters for three to five days to provide for effective postoperative drainage of secretions. Extra side holes are placed in the catheters to improve drainage efficiency.

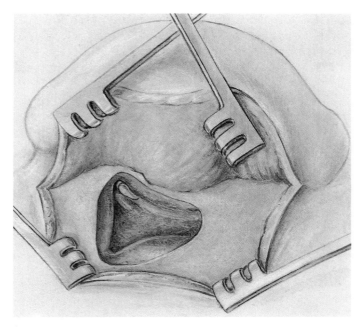

Fig. 4.**19**

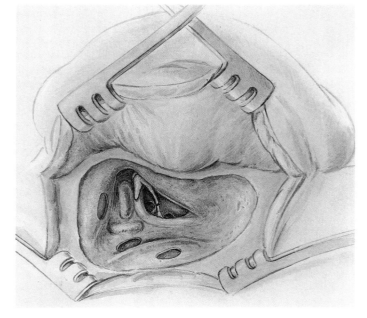

Fig. 4.**20**

The mastoid process is opened somewhat more broadly for a *mastoidectomy* than for an antrotomy. The posterior bony canal wall is thinned to about 1–2 mm using disk or pear burrs. The bone over the sigmoid sinus and over the posterior and middle cranial fossae is thinned until the peripheral mastoid cells are reduced to shallow indentations. As in antrotomy, the aditus region is smoothed down with a diamond burr until the incus and malleus head can be identified. The lateral semicircular canal and the solid bone over the posterior semicircular canal are freed from the overlying cells, and cells along the facial nerve are progressively opened below the lateral semicircular canal.

With purulent mastoiditis, the dura of the middle and posterior cranial fossae should be exposed at a circumscribed site to rule out epidural pus (Fig. 4.**20**). If necessary, the sigmoid sinus can also be exposed with a diamond burr at a circumscribed site, and a fine needle can be passed into the sinus to exclude thrombosis. Finally one to two medium–size drainage tubes with extra side perforations are inserted, as in antrotomy, and the wound is closed in layers. The triangular periosteal–connective tissue flaps raised at the start of the operation are sutured to the soft tissues at the meatal entrance on the posterior canal wall as a safeguard against meatal stenosis.

Modifications

Access to the tympanic cavity in a mastoidectomy can be expanded by excavating the angle between the facial nerve, the posterior part of the tympanic anulus and the chorda tympani, below and anterior to the tip of the short process of the incus. This, the most technically demanding part of a posterior tympanotomy (Jansen; Fig. 4.**20**, area in front of the facial nerve), is performed using small and medium–size diamond burrs. Portions of the incus are visible, so its boundaries can be estimated. The exposure of the lateral semicircular canal, incus, and tympanic portion of the facial nerve allows the surgeon to assess the position of the facial nerve below the lateral semicircular canal. If sufficient irrigation is provided as bone removal is carried forward toward the canal of the chorda tympani with sufficiently large diamond burrs, the chorda tympani can be identified as a white cord before the tip of the burr penetrates its canal. In this way the nerve can be preserved. To ensure adequate visualization of the tympanic cavity, the chorda–facial nerve angle is opened until the round window niche can be identified. This approach permits disease removal from the sinus tympani as well as other procedures such as cochlear implant insertion without opening the tympanic membrane. Further opening of the epitympanum in a lateral direction establishes access to the upper part of the tympanic cavity.

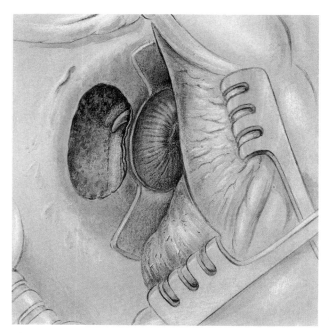

Fig. 4.**21**

Pathologic tissue on the malleus and incus is freed by dissection with a suitable instrument, such as a fine sickle knife, and removed with a fine grasping instrument (cupped forceps, alligator forceps) without exerting significant traction on underlying structures. If concomitant movements of the ossicles are observed, the maneuver should be halted and the pathologic tissue mobilized further until it can be removed without causing significant ossicular movement.

Another modification of antral drainage surgery is *atticoantrotomy* through the posterior canal wall (Fig. 4.**21**). The ear is opened with an endaural or postauricular incision, the posterior meatal skin is removed, and the antrum is opened while leaving intact the posterosuperior bony tympanic ring, called the "bridge" *(red)*. Additional removal of the bony tympanic ring establishes wide access to the aditus and to the antrum itself, giving a clear view of the ossicles and surrounding folds as well as any pathologic processes in that area. Because there is a postoperative risk of retraction formation with this technique, it is recommended only if the posterior canal wall is reconstructed at the end of the operation. This approach, then, is not recommended for the treatment of acute inflammatory disease, although it is very useful for the removal of small cholesteatomas that may necessitate resection of the "bridge" (page 84).

Landmarks and Pitfalls

Important landmarks for antral drainage, antrotomy, and mastoidectomy are the *suprameatal spine* and the *middle fossa dura*. If orientation is doubtful, the surgery should proceed along the dura to avoid dissecting too low on a plane that would jeopardize the facial nerve and labyrinth. The surgeon should dissect along the facial nerve and labyrinth only if he can clearly identify the lateral semicircular canal and can therefore estimate the position of the ossicles and facial nerve. If bone removal proceeds with continuous irrigation and good illumination, *the sigmoid sinus* is quickly recognized in the posterior part of the surgical cavity by its bluish–gray color. The burr should not touch the ossicles, especially the incus, during bone removal in the epitympanum, as this would transmit acoustic trauma to the inner ear.

Rules, Hints, and Common Errors

Diamond burrs should be used in proximity to the dura, sigmoid sinus, facial nerve, and labyrinth to avoid serious, immediate soft–tissue damage in the event that the bone covering the dura, nerve, and sinus is completely removed. It is dangerous to use burrs that are too small, for they can penetrate structures such as the facial nerve canal more easily and deeply, causing damage to underlying soft tissues. Larger burrs are safer because their movement is constrained by the margins of the bony opening. Constant irrigation is maintained to avoid overheating. This is particularly important when drilling about the facial nerve canal.

If injury occurs to the sigmoid sinus, a finger is immediately placed on the sinus to stop the bleeding until the scrub nurse can prepare a definitive hemostatic pack (e.g., Tabotamp). The foot of the operating table should be lowered slightly to reduce the intracranial pressure, but care should be taken that outside air is not sucked into the opened sinus (air embolism). When all preparations for definitive hemostasis have been made, the hemostatic pack is placed on the bleeding site in the sinus and pressed against the site with a dural allograft or moist neurosurgical cotton. The dural allograft may be tucked beneath the bony margins at the site of the injury. Neurosurgical cotton is held in place and kept moist for about 5 min and then slowly removed to confirm sinus hemostasis. The edges of the implanted dura are additionally secured with fibrin glue.

If less than a 5×5-mm area of dura has been exposed with no significant dural injury, the exposed area may be left alone. If the dura has been thinned or a larger bone area has been removed, allograft dura should be inlaid to back up the bony defect. Bone defects in the tegmen tympani larger than 1 cm should also be stabilized with hard materials or cartilage to avoid later dural prolapse.

Postoperative Care

The drainage tubes are left in place for two to five days. They are removed when significant discharge is no longer visible during the daily dressing change. The ear may be flushed initially with hydrogen peroxide or other antiseptic solution, but often this is unnecessary, and prolonged, repeated flushings tend to irritate the middle ear.

Postoperative Complications

Suppurative mastoiditis will recur if insufficient access was established to the middle ear, resulting in deficient drainage through the tube. Reoperation is advisable in these cases and should be supplemented by a prolonged course of postoperative antibiotics.

Functional Sequelae

With technically proficient drainage of the epitympanum, antrum, and mastoid, the disease should resolve completely without sequelae. If the ear heals well but a significant conductive hearing loss of more than 30 dB is noted, it is likely that the incus has been dislodged. A second operation to improve hearing should be deferred for at least six months after the initial surgery and preferably for one year.

Occasionally a postauricular hematoma will produce a low–set or prominent auricle that persists to some degree following partial reabsorption of the hematoma. After six months have passed, surgical correction of the deformity should be considered.

Alternative Methods

Long–term antibiotic therapy is occasionally viewed as an alternative to the surgical drainage of an inflammatory focus in the mastoid. This philosophy is encountered with some frequency in the treatment of children. In reality, though, antibiotic therapy is not an alternative to surgical treatment. It obscures the clinical picture and occasionally leads to abscess formation and complications such as labyrinthitis, sinus thrombosis, zygomaticitis, or Bezold's mastoiditis, all of which are avoidable by surgery.

The "Radical" Mastoid Cavity

Definitions

Treatment Options for Cholesteatoma

The successful treatment of cholesteatoma requires either the complete removal of the cholesteatoma matrix or free drainage of the matrix to the external meatus through a smooth drainage tract that is unobstructed by bony protrusions. In cases where the matrix has been excised, recurrent ingrowth of the matrix is prevented by sealing off its access to the mastoid.

The surgical establishment of drainage to the meatus is called the *open technique.* Its efficacy is optimized by surgically enlarging the meatal entrance. A *closed technique* is one in which the matrix is removed and measures are taken to prevent the further ingrowth of keratinizing squamous epithelium into the mastoid.

Surgical exenteration and drainage of the mastoid is technically easier to perform for cholesteatoma removal than for resective and reconstructive procedures. Cavities in the mastoid can be problematic, however, as they may incite a very prolonged and persistent aural discharge. A disproportion often exists between the large cavity and the relatively limited capacity for cavitary drainage. This "moist chamber" is predisposed to chronic infection. Measures can be taken at operation, therefore, to reduce the volume of a large cavity. But an open technique can be effective only if all surfaces reached by or accessible to the matrix can drain freely to the external ear canal. Thus, a cavity reduction is feasible by this definition only if a natural wall of the mastoid can be transposed toward the center of the cavity, i.e., the soft–tissue coverage of the mastoid cortex following a wide cortical resection.

Obliteration of the mastoid cavity by transposing local tissue or by the free implantation of various materials will inevitably cover over an area of actual or potential cholesteatoma involvement. This type of procedure is a closed technique, therefore, as are procedures in which the posterior wall of the external meatus is left intact.

The "Radical" Mastoid Cavity

The eradication of cholesteatoma by the creation of a "radical" mastoid cavity ("radical cavity") offers an effective means of establishing complete drainage of the mastoid to the external meatus.

Preoperative Diagnostic Measures

The ear is inspected with an operating microscope. Any crusts and polyps are removed, and the diagnosis of cholesteatoma is established. A Schüller radiograph is useful for defining the shape of the mastoid and the position of the dura and sigmoid sinus. Computed tomography is occasionally indicated.

Indications

A "radical cavity" for cholesteatoma removal is most suitable in patients with a small mastoid. The cavity in these cases is relatively small and is likely to undergo good epithelialization with reliable drainage and no recurrence of intracavitary infection. A closed technique is more suitable in patients with a large mastoid and a correspondingly extensive cholesteatoma to avoid troublesome postoperative discharges from the surgical cavities.

Formerly, a "radical cavity" was created in a fenestration procedure for the treatment of otosclerosis. There is little if any indication for this procedure today.

If the disease process is not a cholesteatoma but a tumor, for example, it is still important to create a large mastoid cavity with open drainage to the meatus, as in the treatment of cholesteatoma. But the extent of the resection goes beyond the cavity itself and, when a tumor is diagnosed, should encompass the tympanic membrane and occasionally the labyrinth and other structures.

Principle of the Operation

A basic principle in the treatment of cholesteatoma is to follow the lesion along its inherent growth direction, i.e., from the tympanic membrane through the epitympanum and antrum into the mastoid, following the cholesteatoma until all of its matrix can be seen. This entails removing all or part of the posterior canal wall. Overhangs on the roof of the surgical mastoid cavity that project toward the meatus and especially bony edges in the epitympanum should be polished down to create a smooth passageway from the surgical cavity to the external meatus. Once all bony overhangs and edges have been burred away, it can be determined whether the matrix has indeed been removed.

Occasionally this assessment can be made while smaller overhangs are still present. This is possible when the surgeon has been able to dissect all of the matrix from the bone in an intact, untorn condition. Matrix integrity can be checked under the operating microscope. If there is only a small mastoid with no significant

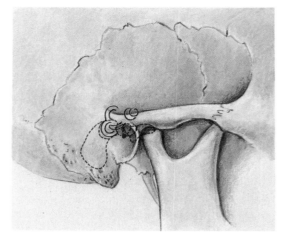

Fig. 4.**22**

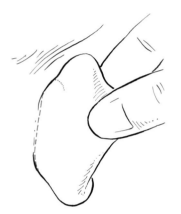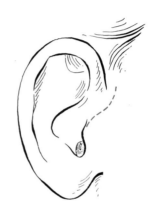

Fig. 4.**23**

cant cellularity behind the matrix, and if the floor of the surgically excavated mastoid cavity is above the floor of the external meatus, it is unnecessary to reduce the cavity or reconstruct the posterior canal wall. A "radical cavity" is created, and in this case the matrix lining of the cavity can be left alone. The matrix must be removed, however, if there is a possibility that there are still mastoid cells underlying the matrix and not just smooth bone.

If the mastoid is large, or if there are mastoid cells extending below the floor of the external meatus, the creation of a radical cavity will frequently lead to postoperative drainage problems with cavitary infection and associated complaints. Obliteration of at least the lower portion of the cavity or reconstruction of the posterior canal wall are recommended in these cases (see below).

The principle of cholesteatoma removal involves following the matrix until its extent can be reliably assessed (Fig. 4.22). Then the rest of the procedure is determined. If the mastoid is small, a radical cavity is created. In any other situation a closed technique is used.

As noted above, the creation of a radical mastoid cavity involves removing the posterior canal wall and creating a smooth junction between all cavity walls and the external meatus, with no palpaple bony edges or depressions. A postauricular incision is best for this purpose, but an endaural incision can also be used (Fig. 4.**23**).

Preoperative Preparations

See page 80.

Instruments

See page 69.

Anesthesia

Local or general anesthesia can be used when creating a "radical" mastoid cavity in adults. General anesthesia is usually indicated for children, less cooperative adults, and patients with severe inflammation or multiple previous operations.

Operative Technique

The ear is opened with a postauricular incision like that used for mastoidectomy (page 81) (Fig. 4.**24**). Additionally the meatal skin is incised about 3 mm inside the level of the suprameatal spine (broken line), and a lateral relaxing incision (dotted line) is made in the roof of the meatus at the upper end of the posterior wall incision. Self–retaining retractors are now inserted to give broad exposure of the mastoid cortex, external meatus, and tympanic membrane (Fig. 4.**25**).

Generally there will be a marginal tympanic membrane perforation or variable retraction of the pars tensa in which cholesteatomatous scales, polyps, or granulations can be seen. Accordingly, the meatus is incised along the approximate midline of the canal floor and posterior to the midline of the canal roof, the lower incision extending to a point just in front of the anterior edge of the marginal perforation (Fig. 4.**26**).

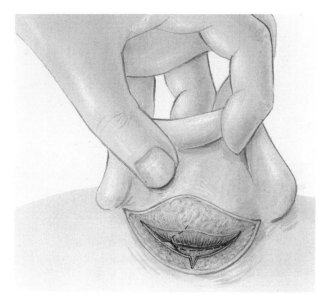

Fig. 4.**24**

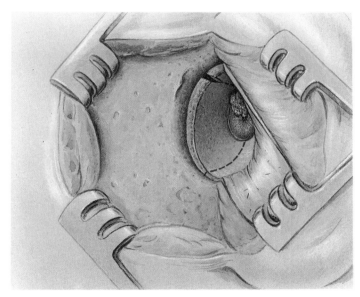

Fig. 4.**25**

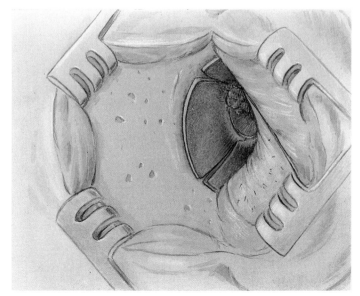

Fig. 4.**26**

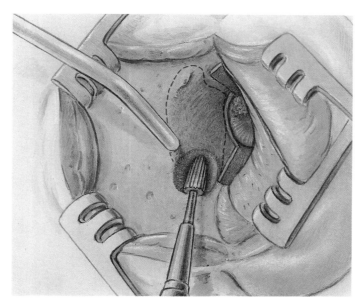

Fig. 4.**27**

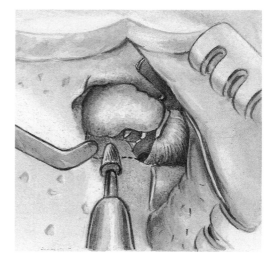

Fig. 4.**28**

A knife–elevator with a straight round blade is used to mobilize the delicate lower portion of the meatal flap for a distance of 1–2 mm along the incision. The surgeon should work slowly and deliberately in this area. The subcutaneous tissue on the roof of the meatus is quite firm, so this part of the flap can be dissected swiftly toward the tympanomastoid suture. The meatal flap is freed from the underlying bone with an angled knife–elevator and developed toward the tympanic anulus. Care is taken at this stage to keep the edge of the blade in contact with the bone while the suction tip is moved along behind the blade. This is important to avoid damage to the meatal skin. The meatal flap is developed to the anulus, divided about 1–2 mm outside the tympanic membrane, and removed as a free flap. The meatal flap should heal well when replaced, regardless of whether it is taken as a free flap or left based on the tympanic membrane. A free flap is preferred, however, because a pedicled flap might easily wrap around the sharp burrs that will be used to resect the canal wall.

First the meatal entrance is enlarged with a conical or pear burr, removing the suprameatal spine and surrounding bone (Fig. 4.**27**). This is continued until mastoid cells are just visible through the bone. The wide, funnel–shaped external ear canal provides access for further work in the region of the tympanic membrane and labyrinth.

Below the bony edge of the marginal tympanic membrane perforation are the incus, facial nerve, and lateral semicircular canal. Drilling and polishing should not cause additional damage to these structures beyond that already caused by the cholesteatoma.

The posterior tympanic spine and overlying bony edge of the marginal perforation are taken back with a cutting burr (Fig. 4.**28**) and medium-size diamond burr until the condition of the incus can be clearly assessed. If the incus is covered by cholesteatoma, it should be removed after opening the oval niche and separating the incudostapedial joint (Figs. 4.**29**, 4.**30**).

By disrupting the ossicular chain, this technique avoids the transmission of acoustic trauma to the inner ear. Also, removal of the incus or its remnants permits visualization of the facial nerve and the lateral semicircular canal so that these structures can be preserved.

The cholesteatoma is now tracked farther into the mastoid by progressive removal of the posterior canal wall with a cutting burr, preferably one of conical shape. The removal of mastoid cells and posterior canal wall is continued until all areas of the surgical cavity can be visualized. One should avoid burring behind a bony overhang that obstructs the surgeon's view. During this resection of the posterior canal wall, the cholesteatoma matrix should be progressively freed from its substrate in an intact condition; it should not be cut into fragments that become dispersed within the mastoid. Often a cholesterol granuloma of variable size is located behind the matrix in the mastoid (Fig. 4.**31**, 1 = cholesteatoma, 2 = cholesterol granuloma), making it easier to elevate the matrix. The surgeon progressively separates the cholesteatoma matrix from surrounding bone and tissues, carrying the dissection toward the antrum. The matrix is freed from all adherent surfaces, including the tegmen tympani, as far as the horizontal semicircular canal. At that point we recommend suctioning the debris from the matrix "sac" (Fig. 4.**32**) to facilitate dissection in the epitympanum.

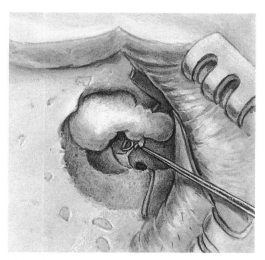

Fig. 4.**29**

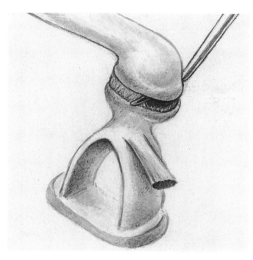

Fig. 4.**30**

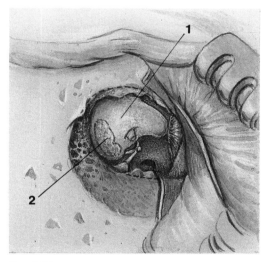

Fig. 4.**31**
1: cholesteatoma
2: cholesterol granuloma

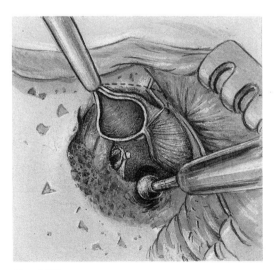

Fig. 4.**32**

If the mastoid is small and there are few cells behind the cholesteatoma matrix, the floor of the cavity is smoothed back to the external meatus, avoiding the "facial ridge." The position of the facial nerve can be reliably determined within the tympanic cavity. First sharp burrs and then diamond burrs are used to track the facial nerve from the middle ear to the floor of the external meatus, leaving a sufficient plate of bone covering the nerve. Next the lateral portions of the mastoid cavity and finally the upper portions are polished to create a perfectly smooth passage to the meatus that is free of bony ridges. Shallow cellular depressions in the area of the sinodural angle and above the labyrinth are polished smooth with medium–size diamond burrs.

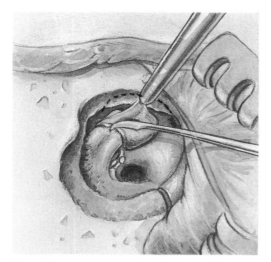

Fig. 4.**33**

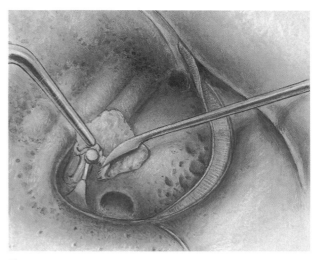

Fig. 4.**34**

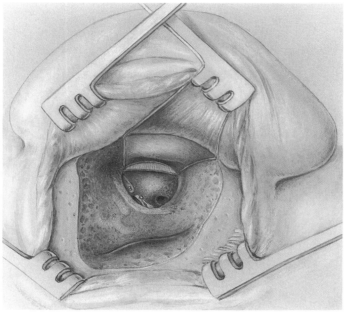

Fig. 4.**35**

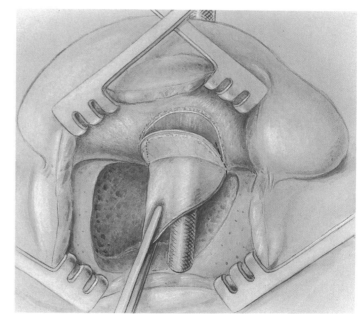

Fig. 4.**36**

Separation of the matrix from the lateral semicircular canal should proceed slowly and deliberately, with close attention given to the labyrinthine bone (Fig. 4.**33**). The most common site for a labyrinthine fistula is in the anterior part of the lateral semicircular canal bone. In most cases the matrix continues over the malleus head into the epitympanum. All bony projections in this area are ground smooth with a medium–size diamond burr, and the malleus head is resected. The tensor tympani tendon can be left intact to stabilize the position of the malleus. A large fold of mucosa between the tensor tympani muscle and the tegmen is divided to improve aeration of the epitympanum. The matrix is freed from the border of the tympanic membrane and is progressively mobilized from the sinus tympani. If the stapes is eroded, the matrix is dissected

toward the footplate using slow, small–amplitude movements of the dissector (Fig. 4.**34**).

It is important to preserve the continuity of the matrix, making certain that small remnants are not left behind. Vestigial matrix is most likely to be missed in the epitympanum, the oval window niche, and the hypotympanic recess. Finally the entire matrix is removed, and all bony margins and overhangs are smoothed to avoid trapping of keratinizing squamous epithelium following general re–epithelialization of the cavity (Fig. 4.**35**).

Procedures for reconstructing the ossicular chain and the posterior portions of the tympanic membrane are described elsewhere (see page 112). The meatal flap removed at the start of the operation is spread open over the labyrinthine block, and the entire cavity is lined with silicone strips.

To prevent the formation of a moist chamber in the "radical" mastoid cavity, the operation is concluded by widening the entrance to the meatus (Fig. 4.**36**). A crescent–shaped area of cartilage near the meatal entrance is excised from the posterior surface of the conchal cavity, and appropriate skin incisions are made to effect the desired enlargement of the meatal entrance.

A circular subcutaneous suture unites the posterior border of the newly formed meatal introitus with the triangular connective tissue–periosteal flaps developed at the start of the operation. The cavity is packed with doxycycline–impregnated gelatin sponge, and the skin is closed with continuous sutures. The result of this procedure is an enlarged meatal entrance (Fig. 4.**37**).

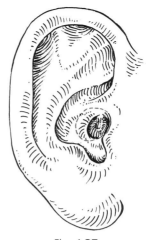

Fig. 4.**37**

Modifications

The creation of a "radical" mastoid cavity, especially in a large mastoid, is frequently followed by postoperative complications in the form of recurrent infections and aural discharge. Modifications of the above technique have been devised, therefore, in an attempt to reduce the volume of the cavity or eliminate the cavity problem altogether by reconstructing the posterior canal wall and establishing drainage of the cavity through the middle ear to the eustachian tube. In most cases reconstruction of the posterior canal wall with autologous auricular cartilage is preferred over the technically simpler option of cavity obliteration.

Cavity Reduction

If reduction of the cavity volume is desired with preservation of the "open technique" (in which all actual or potential sites of cholesteatoma involvement in the mastoid are open to the external meatus), cavity reduction can be accomplished only by transposing the lateral cavity wall inward. This is done by resecting the mastoid cortex and burring the posterior canal wall down to the level of the facial nerve. Additionally the mastoid apex lateral to the stylomastoid foramen is removed, and the posterior wall of the cavity is burred away from the mastoid cortex to the sigmoid sinus, leaving a plate of bone covering the sinus itself. The soft tissues covering the mastoid will then "fall" into the cavity lumen from the lateral side without obliterating matrix–involved areas.

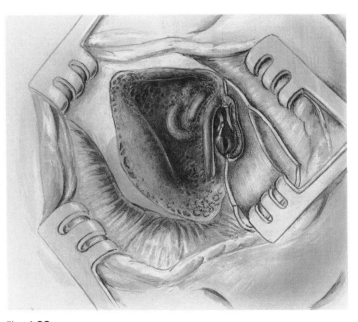

Fig. 4.**38**

This technique is more time–consuming than other procedures but is very effective (Fig. 4.**38**).

All other procedures for cavity reduction will invariably cover recurrence–prone areas on the cavity walls, so they must be classified as closed techniques.

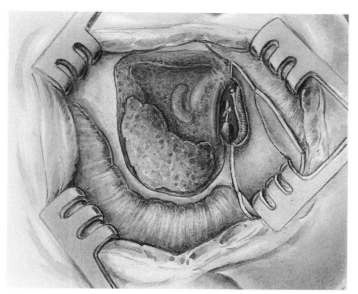

Fig. 4.**39**

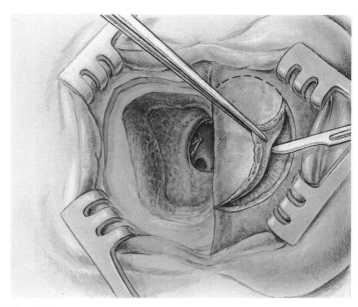

Fig. 4.**40**

After all of the matrix has been removed and all bony margins and overhangs have been smoothed down, various materials can be implanted to reduce the volume of the mastoid cavity. Good results have been obtained with cartilage chips, bone dust, and various hard materials such as porous implants. The material is implanted in the form of small particles (Fig. 4.**39**) that are firmly impacted into the cavity. In all cases pedicled tissue flaps should be used to establish soft–tissue coverage. Fibrin glue is occasionally helpful for securing the flaps and promoting their revascularization.

With passage of time, the implanted material tends to become visible below the overlying soft tissues due to atrophy of the soft–tissue envelope. Nevertheless, the keratinizing squamous epithelium that covers the mate-

rial provides an effective barrier to microorganisms as long as it is not damaged by overvigorous washing.

If cavity reduction is desired, it is helpful to place the initial soft–tissue incisions in a way that will produce sufficiently large and broad–based flaps in the area of the meatal entrance. Palva's technique is particularly useful; it involves elevating a periosteal–connective tissue flap on the mastoid cortex that is broadly based at the root of the auricle. This flap is transposed into the cavity at the conclusion of the operation. Its auricular base ensures a smooth contour below the auricle and at the meatal entrance, and it provides effective coverage of the sinodural angle and the lateral portions of the surgical cavity, which are more difficult to assess later, even when the operating microscope is used.

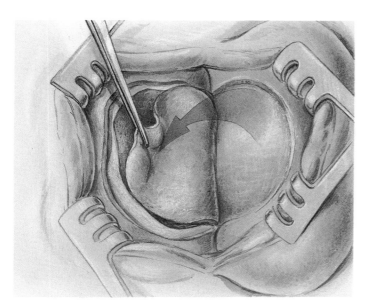

Fig. 4.**41**

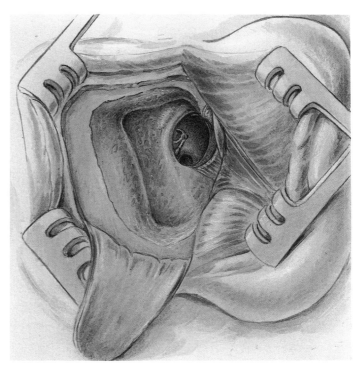

Fig. 4.**42**

If the need for cavity reduction is first appreciated at operation and it is too late to outline a Palva flap on the mastoid cortex, a reliable muscle–connective tissue flap of considerable thickness can be obtained from another local source, such as the forward–reflected auricle (Fig. 4.**40**). The connective tissue is elevated from the auricular periosteum and swung into the cavity (Fig. 4.**41**).

Another potential flap is based on the tip of the mastoid (Fig. 4.**42**). In contrast to the Palva flap, the range of this flap is insufficient to cover portions of the cavity near the labyrinth, but it is sufficient to raise the cavity floor (Fig. 4.**43**).

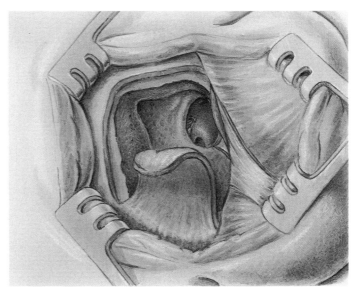

Fig. 4.**43**

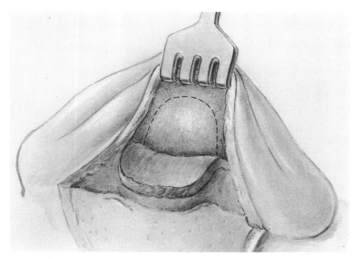

Fig. 4.**44**

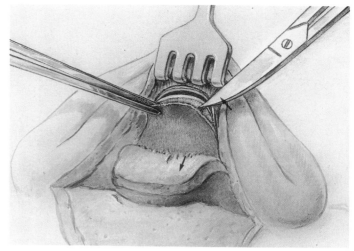

Fig. 4.**45**

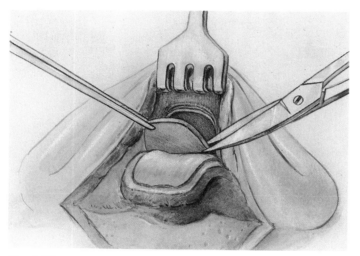

Fig. 4.**46**

Reconstruction of the Posterior Canal Wall

Auricular cartilage or other materials can be used to re-construct the posterior canal wall. The tympanic mem-brane may additionally require reconstruction with perichondrium or cartilage, so it may be necessary to ex-cise two large pieces of cartilage from the back of the auricle. With proper donor sites and removal tech-nique, this should not compromise the appearance of the auricle.

The ear is entered through a postauricular incision, the auricle is pulled sharply forward, and subcutaneous tissue is separated from the perichondrium by semi-sharp dissection (Fig. 4.**44**). This is done by angling the blade of the knife slightly away from the perichondrium while applying pressure to the back of the scalpel and using stroking movements to develop a plane of cleav-age without perforating the perichondrium (Hildmann).

A perichondrial flap of the desired size is outlined down to the cartilage surface, the cut edge is grasped with a fine forceps, and the perichondrium is progres-sively dissected from the cartilage with a closed, pointed scissors (Fig. 4.**45**). For removal of the car-tilage, the incision is extended to the skin on the front of the auricle, and this anterior skin is separated from the cartilage by semisharp dissection, using the operating microscope as required to avoid perforating the tissues (Fig. 4.**46**). The upper part of the auricular concha (cymba conchae) has a natural shape that is excellent for reconstructing the posterior canal wall. Additional, thinner pieces of cartilage can be harvested from the conchal cavity itself.

An endaural incision provides access for obtaining pieces of cartilage from the tragus. About 2 mm inside the border of the tragus, the skin is incised to the car-tilage (Fig. 4.**47**) and grasped with a forceps. The peri-chondrium is only loosely adherent to the subcu-taneous tissue in this area, and spreading scissor–blade dissection is used to expose the perichondrium on the meatal side of the tragus (Fig. 4.**48**). The peri-chondrium itself is grasped with a fine forceps, and the plane between the perichondrium and tragal cartilage is developed by spreading the blades of a thin, pointed scissors (Fig. 4.**49**). Lateral adhesions are easily freed. After the plane has been developed to a depth of about 1 cm, however, connective–tissue fibers passing through the cartilage to the front of the tragus become an obstacle, and some sharp dissection is required. A similar technique is used on the anterior side. Cartilage harvested from this area is thinner than that obtained from the auricle.

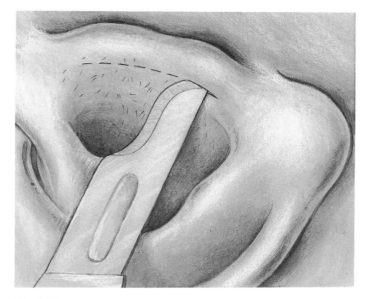

Fig. 4.**47**

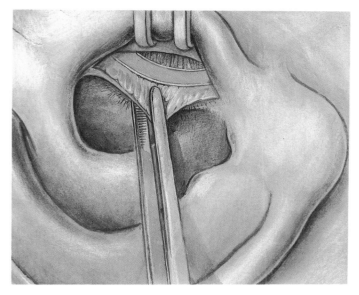

Fig. 4.**48**

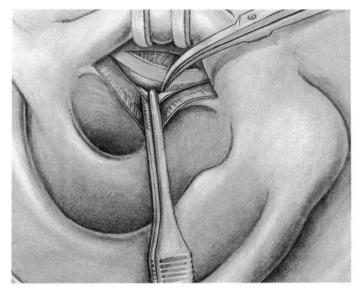

Fig. 4.**49**

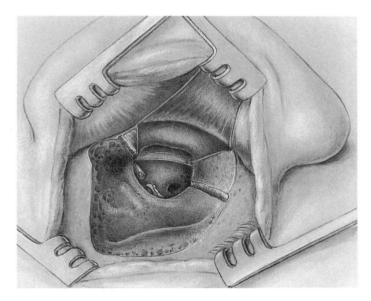

Fig. 4.**50**

For reconstruction of the posterior canal wall with cartilage, shallow grooves are cut in the roof of the surgical cavity and in its floor (Fig. 4.**50**). The cartilage is repeatedly trimmed and shaped so that it can be fitted into these grooves under a degree of tension. Thin cartilage strips are inserted to obliterate any remaining slit-like gaps between the cartilage and the petrous roof or meatus (Fig. 4.**51**). A precise fit is essential to avoid later retractions and ingrowth of meatal epithelium. The tympanic membrane and ossicular chain are also reconstructed. The arrow indicates the subsequent drainage route from the mastoid to the eustachian tube. The meatal skin, which is in partial contact with the bone of the canal floor or bony petrous roof and covers only half of the cartilage at most, is replanted, and the external meatus is completely lined with silicone film

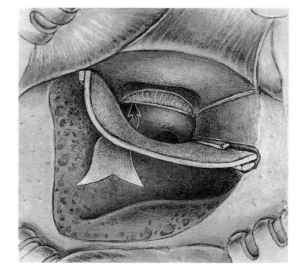

Fig. 4.**51**

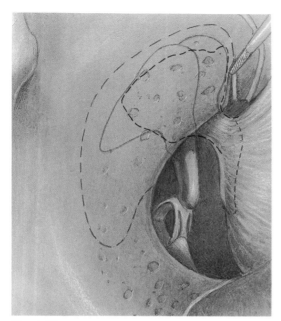

Fig. 4.**52**

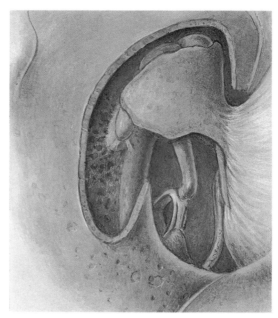

Fig. 4.**53**

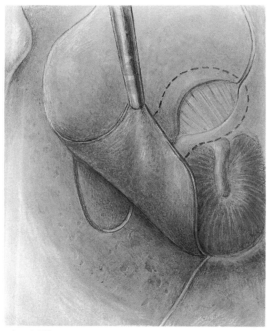

Fig. 4.**54**

and packed with antibiotic–impregnated gelatin sponge to promote the formation of a loose connective tissue layer on the bone and cartilage within a few days. Re–epithelialization occurs within several weeks after the packing is removed.

A special technique for reconstructing the posterior canal wall is the osteoplastic epitympanotomy of Wullstein. After removal of the posterior meatal skin, a portion of the meatal wall is outlined with a sharply tapered conical burr and removed for later replantation (Fig. 4.**52**). The cut proceeds laterally from the lateral attic wall, parallel to the dura, and from the lower part

of the "bridge", parallel to the facial nerve, so that the tip of the burr stays clear of underlying structures.

Removing the bone flap affords a clear view of the aditus and of the antrum itself (Fig. 4.**53**). The inner surface of the bone flap is freed of cholesteatoma matrix, and the cholesteatoma is resected. If all of the matrix can be removed, the bone flap can be replaced in its original position. The tympanic membrane perforation is repaired with an underlay graft, and residual gaps are obliterated with bone dust. The meatal skin is replanted in its original position (Fig. 4.**54**).

Another technique is to use a special microsaw (Feldmann) to excise and later replant a larger portion of the posterior canal wall.

The replantation of portions of the posterior canal wall is technically demanding. Because the extent of the cholesteatoma cannot be accurately determined preoperatively, the excised bone flap does not necessarily provide all the space needed for the clearing of disease. The removal of sufficient portions of the posterior canal wall with the burr ensures a better view of the underlying structures, can be adapted as required to intraoperative demands, and allows for effective reconstruction with cartilage plates.

Jansen's Intact Canal Wall Technique

The postoperative problems associated with the presence of a radical surgical cavity (sensitivity, drainage) prompted Jansen to develop a technique for the complete removal of a cholesteatoma while leaving the posterior canal wall intact. In the hands of a very experienced surgeon, this technique is effective for the eradication of cholesteatoma. It is technically demand-

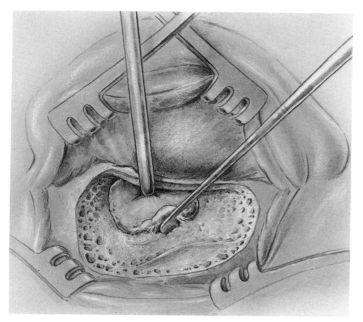

Fig. 4.**55**

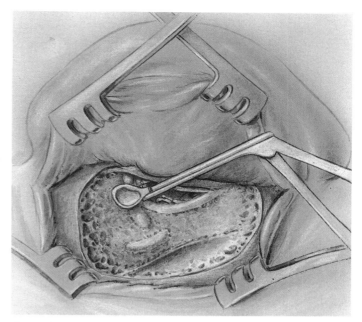

Fig. 4.**56**

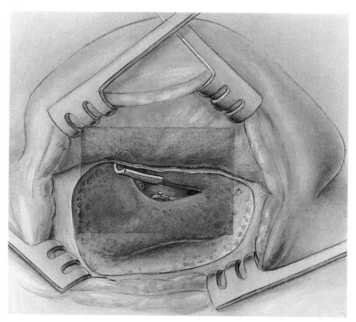

Fig. 4.**57**

ing and time–consuming, however, and inexperienced surgeons may expect up to a 50% recurrence rate of cholesteatoma.

The mastoid is opened and exenterated as in a mastoidectomy. The cholesteatoma matrix is dissected toward the marginal tympanic membrane perforation to avoid damaging the origin of the mass. Bony overhangs that obstruct the view of the epitympanum are repeatedly burred away until the cholesteatoma can be clearly seen. Meanwhile debris is suctioned from the marginal perforation to facilitate removal of the cholesteatoma sac and dissection in the mastoid (Fig. 4.**55**). The posterior canal wall is thinned to about a 1–mm thickness to obtain a satisfactory view of the epitympanum, the short process and body of the incus, and the malleus head. Once the epitympanum has been cleared of cholesteatoma, the chordofacial angle is drilled open until the tympanic anulus, chorda tympani, and facial nerve can be identified. At this stage the promontory and round window are fully visible in the field (Fig. 4.**56**), and the tympanic orifice of the eustachian tube can be inspected following extensive removal of the upper portion of the mastoid. This posterior approach gives access to the entire middle ear as well as the inner surface of the tympanic membrane so that perforations can be repaired and ossicular continuity re–established without resection of the posterior canal wall. This technique requires extensive removal of mastoid cortex at the sinodural angle, the resection of cells lateral to the ossicles above the meatal roof, and considerable thinning of the posterior canal wall to obtain the epitympanic exposure necessary for removing all of the cholesteatoma matrix.

To avoid the formation of retraction pockets with recurrence of the cholesteatoma, a cartilage underlay graft must be placed to back the superior and posterior portions of the tympanic membrane (Jansen) (Fig. 4.**57**). Also, the epitympanum must be widely opened to ensure that sufficient mastoid aeration is maintained after placement of the cartilage. Any bone defects in this region caused by cholesteatoma erosion or burring of the posterior canal wall should also be backed with cartilage to re–establish stability and prevent retraction.

The conclusion of this operation is the same as for mastoidectomy (q.v.).

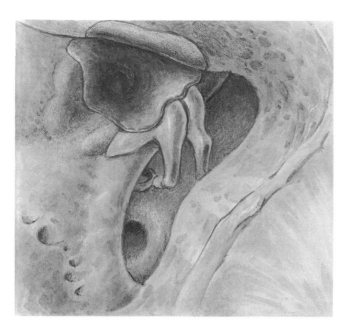

Fig. 4.**58**

Following a Cholesteatoma into the Petrous Apex

Invasion of the petrous apex is present in cases where the cholesteatoma has spread medially past the superior semicircular canal (Fig. 4.**58**). If hearing is intact, it should be considered whether this area can be removed by the transtemporal route (see Chapter 10 on Surgery of the Internal Auditory Canal) to preserve the function of the inner ear. This is feasible if the labyrinthine capsule has remained largely intact.

If the cholesteatoma has already invaded portions of the labyrinth, especially the superior and lateral semicircular canals, usually it will also have eroded portions of the cochlea and the posterior wall of the internal auditory canal. Rarely the matrix will spread out broadly toward the petrous apex, causing extensive erosion of the pyramid but only limited damage to the labyrinth. These extensions of the cholesteatoma matrix, which often are very delicate, should be slowly followed to ensure that they are not lost from the field of view. Usually this requires burring away additional portions of the labyrinth, preferably with a medium-size diamond burr, until all of the cholesteatoma in the petrous apex can be clearly visualized.

Closure of a Labyrinthine Fistula

When removing matrix from the labyrinthine block, especially from the lateral semicircular canal above the facial nerve, the surgeon should proceed slowly due to the frequency of labyrinthine fistulas in this region. Matrix is first removed from the surrounding surfaces, i.e., from the roof and medial wall of the epitympanum and antrum, before it is slowly and gently dissected from the surface of the labyrinthine bone.

If a glistening gray area is seen beneath the matrix, this means that the cholesteatoma has eroded the bone to such a degree that the perilymph is visible through it. At this point the surgeon switches to higher magnification and continues the dissection with fine, deliberate movements (Fig. 4.**59**) until the entire border of the thinned bony area over the perilymph can be identified (Fig. 4.**60**). The endosteum of the perilymphatic space is visible at the center of a typical labyrinthine fistula. The matrix can be separated from this endosteal surface and completely elevated. Bony edges are polished smooth (Fig. 4.**61**).

Bone dust is obtained from the mastoid cortex with a coarse, sharp burr, and a few drops of irrigating solution are added to make a paste (Fig. 4.**62**), which is applied directly to the fistula (Fig. 4.**63**). Perichondrium or meatal skin is then onlaid over the repair to cover the fistulous area with a superficial connective–tissue layer or, preferably, with epithelium.

If granulations are found in the fistulous area, they should be followed into the labyrinth and completely removed to gain access for the removal of underlying matrix. The fistulous opening is enlarged somewhat to obtain an adequate view. Then it is repaired with bone dust as described above and overlaid with perichondrium and meatal skin.

The functions of the auditory and vestibular apparatus are inevitably jeopardized in this situation. But if burring of the labyrinthine bone about the fistula is performed with a high–speed, delicately controlled diamond burr under continuous irrigation, and if the soft–tissue dissections are performed slowly and gently, hearing and perhaps even vestibular function can be preserved.

The operation is concluded as described above, regardless of whether a fistula is present. The repair of a labyrinthine fistula does not necessarily require an "open" technique, therefore.

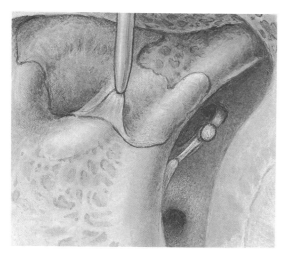

Fig. 4.**59**

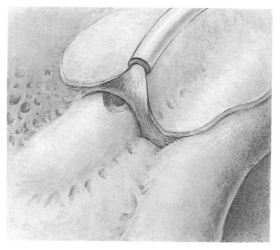

Fig. 4.**60**

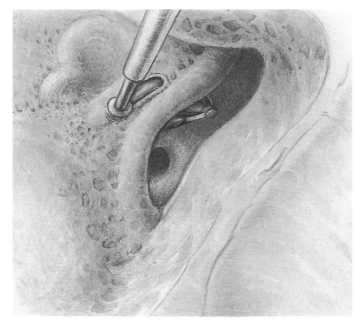

Fig. 4.**61**

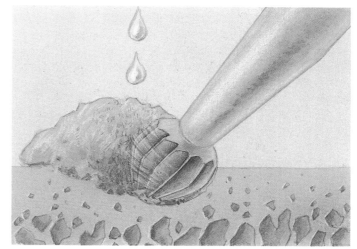

Fig. 4.**62**

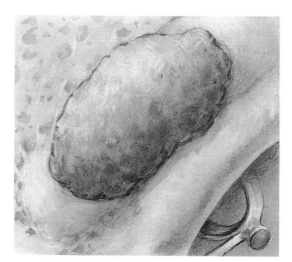

Fig. 4.**63**

Closure of a Bony Defect in the Roof of the Mastoid

If dura has been exposed due to bone erosion by the cholesteatoma, the matrix at that site should be dissected under high–power magnification. Occasionally this is difficult at the bone margins, where matrix fibers appear to blend intimately with the periosteum. Thus, the bony margin of the erosive defect should be drilled away with a medium–size diamond burr until grossly healthy dura can be seen.

This dura is mobilized by inserting the tips of suitably curved instruments into the space between the dura and bone, and a small dural allograft of the appropriate size is inserted into the space (Fig. 4.**64**). With a larger bony defect, the repair is further stabilized by inserting a cartilage, ceramic, or cement implant.

This closure is adequate if the cholesteatoma has been removed by a "closed" technique. If eradication of the cholesteatoma by an "open" technique is intended, involving the creation of a radical mastoid cavity, the site of the dural repair should be covered with a fully vascularized soft–tissue flap to promote epithelialization.

The above measures are recommended for bone defects larger than 0.5–1 cm in diameter. Otherwise the dura may eventually atrophy, allowing the prolapse of arachnoid or, rarely, brain substance (see Arachnoid Cyst, page 101).

Following a Bony and Dural Defect into a Brain Abscess

If the cholesteatoma is found to have eroded the bone and exposed a granulation–covered area of dura (usually in the roof of the pyramid), these granulations should be removed by applying gentle pressure and scraping them away to uncover a possible dural opening. If discharge of pus or debris is noted, the surgeon should proceed as described on page 98. The discharge of pus may signify the presence of a brain abscess (Fig. 4.**65**). In this case the dural defect should be slightly enlarged with bipolar cautery so that a drainage tube can be inserted into the abscess (Fig. 4.**66**). This tube is brought out through the mastoid to the postauricular incision. See also Chapter 9.

Neurosurgical consultation is sought during or immediately after the operation, and further operative and nonoperative management is planned in accordance with neuroradiologic and clinical findings. Occasionally it is wise to discontinue the operation pending neuroradiologic evaluation and continue the surgery at a later time.

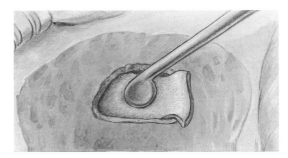

Fig. 4.**64**

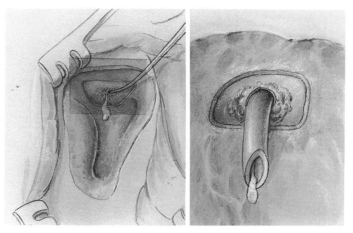

Fig. 4.**65**   Fig. 4.**66**

Landmarks and Pitfalls

Anatomic details should be identified early in operations for cholesteatoma, starting with larger, more superficial structures and then identifying deeper structures as they are encountered. The surgeon gives particular attention to structures that must be preserved, noting the position of the suprameatal spine, the course of the facial nerve, the position of the middle and posterior fossa dura, the sigmoid sinus, the semicircular canals, and the auditory ossicles. In every phase of the procedure, the surgeon should keep track of the course of the facial nerve by identifying the nerve at various points along its course. Burrs should not come into contact with the ossicles, as this would transmit acoustic trauma to the inner ear.

Rules, Hints, and Common Errors

A preoperative Schüller radiograph is obtained to define the position of the sigmoid sinus and middle fossa dura so that the surgeon can burr along these structures without damaging them. The cholesteatoma matrix itself should be slowly elevated from its substrate and dissected in one piece or several large pieces so that its continuity can be accurately assessed. This is especially important at obscured bony margins, cell walls, and overhangs to avoid leaving undetected cholesteatoma matrix at deep sites where it would promote recurrence. Some residual matrix may deliberately be left on smooth underlying bone to provide lining for a well-polished surgical cavity that communicates broadly with the external meatus; this will promote more rapid epithelialization of the cavity. The cavity can also be lined with split–thickness skin grafts (0.2–0.4 mm thick) to provide a further stimulus for epithelialization. These grafts can be taken from behind the ear, for example, using a dermatome rather than a scalpel, which tends to produce a graft with full–thickness components. Full–thickness skin is undesirable as a graft material, because it is susceptible to prolonged, recurrent dermatitis. Rapid epithelialization of the cavity can be further assisted by lining the entire cavity with silicone strips about 0.1–0.2 mm in thickness. This promotes the rapid formation of a connective–tissue covering on the exposed bone and prevents the ingrowth of granulation tissue into the meatal packing.

Postoperative Care

The external meatus is packed with antibiotic–impregnated gelatin sponge (rolitetracycline or doxycycline) for three weeks. If the patient does not notice a spontaneous "clicking" sound in the ear on swallowing, Valsalva maneuvers should be performed starting on the second postoperative day to maintain middle ear aeration. The sutures are removed on the sixth to eighth day, and a return visit is scheduled at three weeks for removal of the packing. The packing should be checked earlier, and if necessary changed, if it liquefies or emits an unpleasant odor (this should be checked by a family member during daily changes of the external dressing) or if the patient experiences significant pain.

A drain placed intraoperatively to decompress the mastoid should be removed after about three days or five days at the latest. Flushing the ear with 3% hydrogen peroxide or similar solution is occasionally useful but should be continued for no more than two or three days so that it will not interfere with healing.

Generally there is no need for postoperative antibiotic therapy beyond the perioperative "one–shot" prophylaxis, unless there are complications or other special circumstances that would warrant such therapy.

If labyrinthine damage is present, 0.5–1.0 g hydrocortisone is given intraoperatively by i.v. injection. Postoperative balance disturbances should be treated with a two– to three–day course of antivertiginous medication. On the fifth postoperative day, the patient should be started on graded exercises to train and improve the balance sense.

Postoperative Complications

Infection occasionally develops in the area of the incision along the postaural fold. In rare cases perichondritis may develop in this area, requiring appropriate treatment.

If the meatal packing liquefies or emits an unpleasant odor (an early sign of infection), it should be suctioned out, leaving the silicone sheeting in place, and replaced with a polyvalent antibiotic and antifungal ointment and a long gauze strip. The ointment is administered through tubing attached to a 5–ml disposable syringe; the tube is inserted through an aural speculum under the microscope, and the ointment is injected into the old operative field until it completely fills the cavity and external meatus. Finally the gauze strip is introduced into the ointment mass with a suitable applicator so that the ointment is apposed to all the surfaces of the operative field.

Postoperatively, Weber's tuning fork test (C2 and C3) is performed daily to assess audiologic function. Vestibular function is also tested by questioning the patient about dizziness and by using Frenzel glasses to check for nystagmus. If signs of labyrinthine dysfunction are noted in a case where the labyrinth was not opened at operation, labyrinthine irritation may have developed postoperatively, and it may be appropriate to initiate antibiotic coverage combined with anti–inflammatory medication (e.g., 0.5–1.0 g hydrocortisone).

If facial paralysis is present immediately after surgery and persists after local anesthesia has subsided, it must be assumed that the nerve was traumatized intraoperatively, and the ear should be reopened and inspected, preferably on the following day.

Serious complications in the form of an arachnoid cyst or cerebral prolapse may arise years after cholesteatoma surgery that involved the creation of a "radical" mastoid cavity. These complications cannot always be recognized at first sight, even when the previous history is known. The differential diagnosis includes polyposis, cholesteatoma recurrence, and cholesterol granuloma. An arachnoid cyst is recognized by its pulsations when viewed under the operating microscope. Cerebral prolapse presents a similar appearance in its early stages. Once the brain has fully herniated into a cavity, little or no pulsation is evident in the prolapsed tissue.

An arachnoid cyst, like an exposed area of dura (page 100), is backed with preserved dura and secured by onlaying a firm plate of cartilage or, preferably, bone replacement material.

The same technique is used to repair a cerebral prolapse. However, a true cerebral herniation through a relatively small dural defect should be resected before the dural defect is repaired. An attempt to reduce the herniated brain tissue will result in brain abscess. If necessary, the situation can be discussed pre– and intraoperatively with a neurosurgical colleague. The transtemporal approach (q.v.) has proven excellent for determining the appropriate site for resecting the herniated brain and for repairing the dural and bony defect.

Functional Sequelae

Hearing ability following extensive cholesteatoma removal is discussed in the section "Reconstructive Surgery", pages 110–129.

The sequelae of a moist chamber, with recurrent infection of the operative field, can follow the construction of a radical cavity, especially if the cavity is disproportionately large in relation to its entrance. Besides cleaning under the operating microscope, long–term measures should be instituted to help keep the chamber dry, such as regular forced–air drying of the cavity with a hair dryer. If necessary, the volume of the cavity can be reduced in a second procedure about one year after the initial operation. The patient should try to keep water out of the ear by stuffing a petrolatum cotton wad into the external ear canal during swimming or shampooing.

Alternative Methods

At present there are no effective conservative options for the treatment of cholesteatoma, so there are no alternatives to surgical eradication.

In borderline cases between a shallow tympanic membrane retraction and incipient cholesteatoma, a conservative trial of exercises to ventilate the middle ear (inflating a balloon with the nose, Valsalva maneuver, occasional use of a Politzer bag) may be beneficial, especially in children. This may be supplemented by a twice daily regimen of salicylate otic drops to remove keratin buildup in the ear. Children are told to avoid forceful sniffing. Besides causing a low intranasal pressure, this act can also produce negative pressure in the middle ear through a patent eustachian tube, leading rapidly to the development of an extensive retraction ("snuffle ear"). If sniffing is avoided, the tympanic membrane retraction may resolve completely within a period of weeks.

Surgical Treatment of Tympanosclerosis

Definition

"Tympanosclerosis" should be used as a clinical term only in cases where the pathologic process has caused hearing impairment. A calcium deposit in the tympanic membrane that is not associated with hearing loss is more properly characterized as a clinically nonsignificant myringosclerosis.

Preoperative Diagnostic Measures

The ear is examined and cleaned under the operating microscope, and the findings are documented.

Indications

Surgery is indicated in tympanosclerosis to repair a tympanic membrane perforation and improve hearing. Occasionally a cholesteatoma is concealed within the tympanosclerotic deposits and can be detected only by viewing through the perforation under high magnification. This finding is a definite indication for surgery.

Principle of the Operation

Surgical removal of the tympanosclerotic deposits should be sufficient to establish an adequate lumen in the middle ear space while allowing ossicular chain reconstruction and myringoplasty. A coexisting cholesteatoma, which may be difficult to detect, is eradicated as described earlier (page 86).

Preoperative Preparations

See page 80.

Anesthesia

Local anesthesia is usually satisfactory for the removal of tympanosclerosis, since all of the surgery is performed within the tympanic cavity. Some patients may require general anesthesia, however.

Operative Technique

If the tympanic membrane perforation can be plainly seen through the speculum, an endaural incision is used. This can be done in the majority of patients (Fig. 4.**67**). If visualization is difficult because an anterior perforation is obscured by the meatal wall or it is unclear whether there is a coexisting cholesteatoma, a postauricular incision is preferred.

When tympanosclerosis is present, the tympanic membrane perforation should be widely excised despite the technical difficulty. Calcific deposits that can impede the movement of the tympanic membrane, i.e., deposits located below the anterior half of the membrane, should be removed. This results in a thinned tympanic membrane remnant and occasionally in considerable enlargement of the perforation.

After the middle ear space has been entered by developing a tympanomeatal flap or perhaps removing a free flap of meatal skin, the lateral attic wall is taken back with a sharp (House) curet or burr until all of the oval window niche can be seen. If the incus is damaged or fixed, the incudostapedial joint is opened and the incus is removed. If the malleus itself is fixed, the malleus head is resected. Attempts have often been made to mobilize the incus and malleus in the epitympanum, but these measures have proven ineffective in the long term. Large tympanosclerotic deposits below the malleus handle, on the promontory, and near the tympanic tubal orifice should be removed in layers to the degree necessary to ensure adequate postoperative aeration. We do not advocate the resection of all accessible adherent disease, as this would cause excessive mucosal damage.

A special problem is posed by tympanosclerotic fixation of the stapes in the oval window niche. Mobilization can be attempted in these cases (Fig. 4.**68**) by removing the chalky but sometimes bone–hard tympanosclerotic deposits with small hooks, leaving the stapes in place, until the oval window niche appears clear except for the intact footplate. Stapes mobilization should not be forced if there appears to be an excessive risk of opening the oval window. This must be avoided, because histologic examination has confirmed the presence of bacteria in tympanosclerotic plaque, so even if the mucosa appears normal in a middle ear involved by tympanosclerosis, opening the oval window carries a high risk of inciting an infectious labyrinthitis. In most cases, however, the stapes can be mobilized with an acceptable degree of risk. Reconstruction of the ossicular chain and tympanic membrane are performed as described on pages 116–125. Perichondrium or cartilage is the material of choice for tympanic membrane reconstruction. Revascularization occurs more slowly in tympanosclerosis than in chronic suppurative otitis media, and the use of fascia is associated with a higher rate of recurrent perforation secondary to atrophy of the implant.

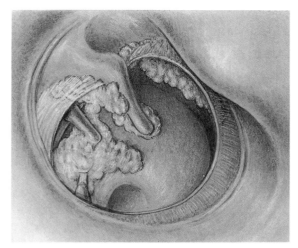

Fig. 4.**67**

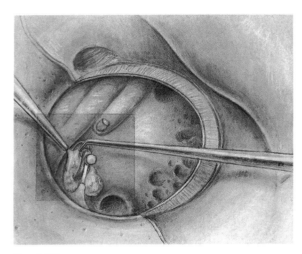

Fig. 4.**68**

Modifications

The ideal goal in otologic surgery is to clear the ear of disease and perform the reconstruction in the same sitting. This applies equally to the eradication of tympanosclerosis, despite knowledge that recurrent fixation of the mobilized stapes is common. This refixation need not occur, however, and it would be unnecessary to proceed with a routine second operation for definitive hearing improvement in these patients. It is appropriate to attempt a one–stage operation, therefore, and if hearing is deficient at one year, proceed with a second operation that was already discussed with the patient at the time of the initial surgery.

If the oval window niche was adequately cleared of disease in the initial operation, the second operation should consist of a stapedectomy with reconstruction of the sound–conducting apparatus by establishing a connection between the malleus handle and the oval window (see sections on Otosclerosis and Reconstructive Surgery of the Middle Ear, pages 110–126).

Landmarks and Pitfalls

Tympanosclerotic remodeling in the middle ear is not limited to the submucous connective tissue but also involves the underlying bone. In cases where tympanosclerosis has been present for years, this remodeling of the bony substrate may be so extensive that portions of the facial canal and even the promontory may come away when the tympanosclerotic deposits are removed. The deposits should be removed in layers, therefore, perhaps aided by the use of high–power magnification, so that at least a thin layer of hard tissue is left covering the facial nerve and cochlea.

The removal of tympanosclerotic plaque from the oval window niche is technically demanding and time–consuming. The surgeon should avoid opening the inner ear, especially when tympanosclerosis is severe, to avoid inciting labyrinthitis. If stapedial dislocation occurs with extravasation of perilymph, small pieces of lint–free connective tissue should be placed over the footplate. Postoperative antibiotic therapy is continued for 3–5 days, supplemented by 0.5–1 g hydrocortisone.

Rules, Hints, and Common Errors

Tympanosclerotic deposits should be removed to a degree that restores tympanic membrane vibration out to the anulus, creates a patent tympanic tubal orifice, establishes adequate clearance between the promontory and the umbo, and clears the oval window niche to a degree that will allow for possible stapedectomy at a later time. If a one–stage stapedectomy is performed,

total hearing loss is a danger due to bacterial contamination of the tympanosclerotic plaque. If the oval window niche is uninvolved by tympanosclerosis, or if stapes immobility is caused entirely by tympanosclerotic involvement of the stapedial tendon, hearing can be improved in the same sitting by mobilizing the stapes with resection of its tendon.

The use of perichondrium or cartilage is recommended for reconstructing the tympanic membrane due to the poor vascularity of the tympanosclerotically involved surrounding tissues.

If it has been possible to mobilize the stapes when removing the tympanosclerosis material from the oval window niche, but a perilymphatic fistula cannot be excluded with certainly, the anular ligament of the stapes should be covered with small, lint–free pieces of connective tissue as a safety precaution.

Textile lint from the operating room air can incite the formation of foreign body granulomas if the perilymphatic space has been opened.

Postoperative Care

The postoperative care regimen is the same as that following other types of tympanoplasty (see page 101).

Postoperative Complications

There are no special complications other than the possibility of labyrinthine damage after opening the oval window (page 238).

Functional Sequelae

A good hearing result should follow the successful and adequate removal of the tympanosclerosis and reconstruction of the tympanic membrane and ossicular chain. Conductive hearing loss may occasionally develop after about six months due to recurrence of the tympanosclerosis. These new deposits may have to be surgically removed to cure the conductive hearing deficit. The same applies to recurrent perforations.

Alternative Methods and Techniques

If the tympanosclerosis is very severe and repeated attempts have been unsuccessful in providing sufficient oval window clearance to restore acceptable sound transmission, fenestration of the horizontal semicircular canal can be discussed as an option.

Surgical Treatment of Tympanic Fibrosis

Definition

Tympanic fibrosis is a condition in which the lumen of the tympanic cavity has become filled with fibrous tissue strands, cholesterol granuloma, mucous cysts, and loose granulation tissue. The eustachian tube is occluded. In contrast to an adhesive process, the plane of the tympanic membrane remains in an essentially normal position.

Preoperative Diagnostic Measures

A detailed history is taken that includes questions about previous operations and any prior history of tuberculosis, both of which would imply a previous tubal obstruction. Tympanometric tests of tubal function are unreliable but still should be performed where needed. Transnasal endoscopic examination of the pharyngeal tubal orifice and computed tomography may be indicated.

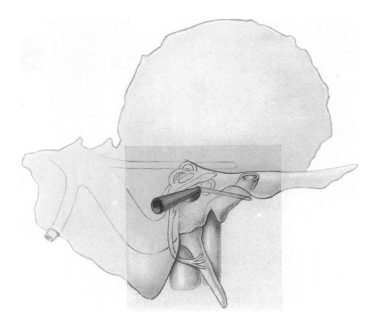

Fig. 4.**69**

Indications

The eradication of tympanic fibrosis may be attempted in patients with bilateral conductive hearing loss, although the outlook is poor for achieving successful middle ear aeration and long–term patency of the eustachian tube. There is a high probability that tympanic fibrosis will recur or that extensive adhesions will form during the first postoperative year.

Principle of the Operation

The operation should be performed in at least two stages. The first stage, which is painful and requires general anesthesia, serves to reestablish patency of the eustachian tube. If this is successful, the second stage follows a year later with ossicular chain reconstruction and, if necessary, grafting of the tympanic membrane.

Preoperative Preparations

The preparations are the same as those for ear operations previously described (see page 80).

Anesthesia

The requirements are basically the same as for other operations, although general anesthesia is recommended due to manipulations on the eustachian tube in proximity to the mandibular nerve.

Operative Technique

The ear is opened with a postauricular incision, and a tympanomeatal skin flap is raised on the posterior canal wall to permit inspection of the ossicular chain. If the chain is present, an additional incision is made in the tympanic membrane in front of the malleus handle to gain access to the tympanic tubal orifice. A heavy steel pick (Heermann) or suitably bent paranasal sinus probe is maneuvered with considerable force along the canal of the tensor tympani muscle (i.e., along the natural course of the eustachian tube) to open up the tube (Fig. 4.**69**). A crackling sound is heard as the bony tubal stenosis is opened. If the tubal stenosis is caused by soft tissues rather than bone, there is very little chance of establishing long–term patency for adequate ventilation.

A plastic catheter of approximately the same gauge as the previously used stylet (2–3 mm in diameter) is passed into the restored tubal lumen. The position of the catheter tip in the epipharynx is verified endoscopically; it should project about ¹/₂ cm past the pharyngeal tubal orifice. The tympanic end of the catheter is knotted to retain the catheter in the middle ear space and keep it from slipping into the pharynx during swallowing.

If insertion of the catheter proves difficult, the catheter can be threaded over an eustachian tube probe and introduced with the aid of the probe. An extra hole is placed next to the intratympanic knot so that the catheter can be threaded over the probe.

After optimum placement of the tubal catheter has been confirmed, the anterior half of the tympanic membrane is backed with perichondrium, and the tympanomeatal flap is returned. Standard meatal packing is inserted for three weeks.

Modifications

A bony stenosis of the eustachian tube can be opened through a Jansen–type posterior tympanotomy without opening the tympanic membrane. In this technique the mastoid and tympanomeatal angle are burred open as described previously for the removal of cholesteatoma (page 87). This gives access to the tympanic tubal orifice, which can be opened with diamond burrs. To assist orientation and ensure that the burr is properly directed, Jansen also suggests inserting a thin endoscope through the pharyngeal tubal orifice to provide a visible, lighted target toward which the surgeon can dissect. The tubal catheter, which also must be inserted with this technique, can be brought out through the mastoid to provide a route for drug instillation, for example, or for channeling drainage toward the mastoid.

Landmarks and Pitfalls

Whether the Heermann dilatation technique or Jansen burring technique is used to clear a bony occlusion of the eustachian tube, it should be kept in mind that the internal carotid artery courses below and medial to the tympanic tubal orifice, and that the tubal isthmus is located medial to the foramen ovale. It is important, therefore, to make a positive identification of the tympanic tubal orifice and to insert the stylet or direct the burr precisely along the natural course of the eustachian tube.

Rules, Hints, and Common Errors

There is little prospect for the successful opening of a soft–tissue tubal stenosis or occlusion. If the bony tubal isthmus has been surmounted and a palpable obstruction is then encountered in the soft–tissue portion of the tube, the operation should be discontinued. Even if tubal patency has been successfully restored by dilatation or burring and it is confirmed that the tubal catheter is within the pharyngeal eustachian orifice, an impatient attitude on the part of the patient may prompt the surgeon to remove the catheter prematurely, leading to rapid recurrence of the stenosis. The catheter should remain in place for at least six months and preferably for one year.

Postoperative Care

The postoperative regimen is the same that following other ear operations (page 101).

Postoperative Complications

Some patients may experience postoperative pain in the distribution of the mandibular nerve lasting several days or even a few weeks. The presumed source of this pain is hematoma forming near the surgically dilated tubal isthmus, directly adjacent to and below the foramen ovale. Conservative measures should be instituted to relieve the pain and hasten reabsorption of the hematoma.

Functional Sequelae

About one year after the initial operation, the eustachian catheter is removed through an incision made in front of the malleus handle under local anesthesia. Heavy granulations that have formed about the tube are also removed. The tympanic membrane is simply covered with silicone film, and the deep portion of the external meatus is packed for three weeks with antibiotic–impregnated gelatin sponge. The patient is told to perform a Valsalva maneuver several times daily, starting on the third postoperative day. If effective ventilation of the middle ear space is confirmed at six months by demonstrating an air crescent near the tympanic tubal orifice, it is appropriate to proceed with ossicular chain reconstruction. The risk of failure is still relatively high, however, for even if aeration near the tubal orifice has been confirmed, the necessary epithelialization of the other portions of the tympanic cavity cannot always be assured.

Alternative Methods

No alternative methods are available.

Removal of Tympanic Cholesteatoma

Definition

Tympanic cholesteatoma is one that is confined to the tympanic cavity. Usually it results from paracentesis or the placement of a ventilation tube. The ossicular chain is intact.

Preoperative Diagnostic Measures

A pure tympanic cholesteatoma is diagnosed from the history and the typical otomicroscopic finding of a white, spherical area below the anterior half of the tympanic membrane.

Indications

Surgical eradication is indicated.

Principle of the Operation

Surgical treatment involves opening the tympanic cavity and removing the cholesteatoma together with all of its matrix, which may be very delicate and difficult to identify.

Preoperative Preparations

The preparations correspond to those for other ear operations (page 80).

Anesthesia

General anesthesia is indicated for children; local anesthesia is adequate for adults (page 2).

Operative Technique

If all of the tympanic membrane can be seen, the surgery is performed through an endaural incision. Otherwise postauricular access is required. With cholesteatoma that is causing no apparent irritation, the matrix is elevated from the mucosa with blunt instruments after first opening the tympanic cavity and widely mobilizing the tympanic membrane and fibrous anulus, especially on the canal floor. In all dissections an effort is made to avoid tearing the cholesteatoma matrix. If the cholesteatoma is too large, the matrix is incised at a clearly visible site and its contents are partially aspirated. The area on the inner surface of the tympanic membrane should be watched closely during removal of the matrix, as it represents the cause of the cholesteatoma. Usually it is unnecessary to back the tympanic membrane with an underlay graft, since the dissections should not disrupt the integrity of the membrane. At the end of the procedure the meatal flap is returned to its original position. The ear canal is lined with silicone film and packed with antibiotic–impregnated gelatin sponge.

Modifications

If an extensive area of attachment is found on the inner surface of the tympanic membrane during dissection of the matrix, and all of the matrix cannot be reliably removed, this portion of the tympanic membrane may have to be resected along with the malleus handle. The ossicular chain and tympanic membrane are then reconstructed as described on pages 110–126.

Landmarks and Pitfalls

The greatest danger is leaving matrix on the inner surface of the tympanic membrane. If there is the slightest doubt in this regard, this area of the tympanic membrane should be resected.

Rules, Hints, and Common Errors

Manipulations of cholesteatomas in the middle ear should be performed slowly and gently to avoid opening the matrix. In doubtful cases the tympanic membrane should be mobilized further or partially resected.

Postoperative Care

The same rules apply as in other ear operations (page 72).

Due to the fragility of the matrix, it is entirely possible that remnants will be left behind. Thus, long–term follow–up examinations are recommended for a period of at least five years.

Postoperative Complications

Postoperative complications are not anticipated.

Functional Sequelae

The surgery typically produces a good hearing result with a normal appearance of the external ear and tympanic membrane. Residual cholesteatoma is a definite possibility, so long–term follow–up is required. Careless work during dissection of the cholesteatoma can dislodge the incus or dislocate the incudomalleolar joint, resulting in conductive hearing loss that will require a second operation.

Alternative Methods

No alternative methods are available.

Surgical Correction of Stenosis or Occlusion of the Eustachian Tube

See the section on Surgical Treatment of Tympanic Fibrosis (pages 105–106).

Surgical Treatment of Tympanic Atelectasis and Epidermal Overgrowth of the Tympanic Cavity

Definition

In *tympanic atelectasis* the atrophic tympanic membrane is collapsed against the promontory and other portions of the walls of the tympanic cavity, sometimes with modeling and variable rarefaction of the ossicular chain. This may be associated with the formation of retraction pockets, cholesteatoma, and even tympanic membrane perforation toward the eustachian tube.

Preoperative Diagnostic Measures

The diagnosis is made by inspection of the ear. As in the clinical diagnosis of cholesteatoma, it may be necessary to obtain a Schüller radiograph or CT scan.

Indications

If the atelectasis is circumscribed with no deep niche formation (see Sadé, for example, for the staging of atelectasis), a ventilation tube is inserted to confirm a normal gas composition and normal gas pressure in the middle ear. This procedure may be therapeutic, restoring the tympanic membrane to its normal position. If this does not occur, extensive surgical treatment is required, especially if retraction pockets have formed or adhesions have developed between the atrophic tympanic membrane and the promontory.

Principle of the Operation

With a circumscribed area of atelectasis, a ventilation tube is inserted to aerate the middle ear space and ensure a normal gas composition and gas pressure.

With extensive atelectasis associated with retraction pockets and adhesions between the atrophic tympanic membrane and the medial wall of the tympanic cavity, the adhesions must be cleared and the tympanic membrane reconstructed (assuming adequate ventilation). Because the atelectasis has a tendency to recur, the materials used to reconstruct the tympanic membrane should be able to effectively withstand a negative pressure in the middle ear. The cartilage reconstruction technique of Heermann, for example, is excellent for this purpose.

Preoperative Preparations

See page 80.

Anesthesia

See page 81.

Operative Technique

The technique of ventilation tube insertion is described on page 78.

Removal of the atrophied tympanic membrane follows the same technique used for removing a delicate cholesteatoma matrix as described on page 87.

Reconstruction of the tympanic membrane is described on pages 116–118.

Modifications

Various implants can be used for reconstruction of the tympanic membrane. Given the latent ventilation deficit in this situation, fascia and perichondrium are not as stable as cartilage. The insertion of a tympanic membrane homograft is one alternative to cartilage implantation. Another option is to use commercially available myringoplastic materials, which may consist of collagen or banked dura. On the whole, however, these materials appear to be less resistant to the chronic negative pressure in the middle ear than cartilage implants.

Landmarks and Pitfalls

These are the same as described on page 107.

Rules, Hints, and Common Errors

A particular problem in the surgical treatment of tympanic atelectasis is the need to completely separate the atrophic portions of the tympanic membrane from the medial boundary of the tympanic cavity while leaving no vestiges of keratinizing squamous epithelium in that area. The atrophic portions of the tympanic membrane must be mobilized without tearing. Usually a small, air-containing area of the tympanic cavity with a normal mucosal lining is found within the tympanic orifice of the eustachian tube. From there a small antrum hook, for example, can be used to separate the adhesion between the tympanic membrane and the promontory in the correct plane. Subsequent healing is aided by leaving a soft–tissue covering on the promontory and elevating only the epithelium of the tympanic membrane. This improves the chances of reestablishing a mucosa–like covering on the promontory.

The materials used for tympanic membrane reconstruction should have a high capacity for pressure resistance. Cartilage is excellent for this purpose. Maximum clearance should be obtained between the promontory and the reconstructed tympanic membrane to prevent the formation of new adhesions.

Postoperative Care

See page 72.

Postoperative Complications

See page 107.

Functional Sequelae

With favorable healing and the re–establishment of a tympanic lining similar to the original mucosa, normal hearing can result. Cartilage used to reconstruct the tympanic membrane will appear strange in subsequent examinations, and an inexperienced examiner may mistake the whitish material for a cholesteatoma. The thickness of the cartilage should cause negligible limitation of tympanic membrane function, however.

Alternative Methods

Tympanic atelectasis in older patients that is not associated with a detectable cholesteatoma or a perforation toward the eustachian tube may be considered a stable condition that does not necessarily require surgical treatment. The fitting of a hearing aid is a possible alternative to surgery in these patients, who will then require regular follow–up examinations every 6 to 12 months to allow for the prompt detection of cholesteatoma.

Bibliography

Donaldson J A, Duckert L G, Lambert P M, Rubel E W. Surgical Anatomy of the Temporal Bone. New York: Raven Press; 1992.

Fisch M. Tympanoplasty, Mastoidectomy and Stapes Surgery. Stuttgart: Thieme; 1994.

Heermann J. Thirty Years Cartilage Tympanoplasty. In: Long Term Results in Otology, Charachon et. al, eds. Amsterdam: Kugler; 1991; pp. 159–164.

Jansen C W. Intact Canal Wall for Cholesteatoma. Am J Otol 1985; 6: 3–4.

Lang J. Klinische Anatomie des Ohres. Heidelberg: Springer; 1992.

Nadol J B, Schuknecht H F, Surgery of the Ear and Temporal Bone. New York: Raven Press; 1993.

Plester D, Hildmann J, Steinbach E. Atlas der Ohrchirurgie. Stuttgart: Kohlhammer; 1989.

Sadeé J, Berco E. Atelectasia and secretory otitis media. Ann Otol Rhinol Laryngol 1976; 85 (suppl 25): 62–72.

Tos M. Manual of Middle Ear Surgery. Stuttgart: Thieme; 1993.

Wullstein H-L, Wullstein S R.: Tympanoplasty. Stuttgart: Thieme; 1990.

Reconstructive Surgery

Götz Geyer and Jan Helms

Myringoplasty

Preoperative Diagnostic Measures

A recurrent, odorless aural discharge is symptomatic of chronic suppurative mucosal disease, while fetid otorrhea is indicative of chronic bone suppuration (cholesteatoma). The ear is cleaned under the microscope (with a smear taken for microbiologic analysis), and the findings are documented with notation of the Bellucci classification, e. g. a rough estimation of proper healing depending upon the preoperative situation (infection, scarring, etc.). Drawings should be made of any pathologic changes that are found (location and size of a defect; condition of the tympanic membrane: inflammation, sclerosis, scarring, calcium deposit, displacement of the malleus handle; middle ear mucosa: thickening, inflammation, polyposis, suppuration). The Weber and Rinne tests (C2, C3) are performed and a threshold audiogram obtained to assess the severity of hearing loss. Schüller radiographs demonstrate the degree of pneumatization of the mastoid process. If necessary, more sophisticated imaging studies can be performed to obtain more detailed information on middle ear structures.

Indications

Tympanoplasty is the procedure of choice for chronic suppurative ear disease. The ear is cleared of chronic inflammatory disease, and hearing gain is achieved in most patients regardless of the size and location of the defect. If the patient is deaf on one side ("last ear" situation), one should be cautious in selecting the patient for a myringoplasty, and only an experienced surgeon should carry out the procedure. Coexisting morbidity should be considered in elderly candidates for myringoplasty, for even local anesthesia is associated with a degree of systemic risk.

Principle of the Operation

The middle ear is broadly opened using extended, largely standardized incisions of the meatal skin. Tissues that are diseased (e.g., polyps) or dystopic, keratinizing squamous epithelium are removed. The method of choice for tympanic membrane reconstruction is underlay grafting with autogenous tissue. The continuity of the ossicular chain is restored using ossicular autografts or homografts or alloplastic prostheses (see page 119).

Preoperative Preparations

See page 80.

Anesthesia

See Chapter 1, page 1.

Operative Technique

The principle of the myringoplasty is illustrated for a Wullstein type I tympanoplasty using an endaural incision (Figs. 4.**70** to 4.**81**).

Endaural Incision

Access to the external acoustic meatus is extended with an endaural incision from the crus of the helix to the tragus. Meanwhile the assisting nurse pulls the auricle backward, upward, and outward to keep the superior helical spine out of the line of incision. A nasal speculum is inserted to gain broader access to the meatal entrance. The skin and subcutaneous tissue are divided while preserving the temporalis fascia (Fig. 4.**70**). The incision is continued medially along the roof of the meatus, keeping the blade in contact with the bone. The skin of the posterior canal wall is incised from below upward about 3 mm medial to the meatal entrance. Both incisions are connected to form a triangular flap, and a periosteal elevator is used to develop the flap laterally over the helical spine (Fig. 4.**71**).

Removal of Temporalis Fascia

If the size of the tympanic membrane defect can be assessed, a suitable graft can be taken from the temporalis fascia during this stage of the operation. The endaural incision is spread open, and the fat and connective tissue over the temporalis fascia are elevated with a sharp periosteal elevator. The fascia is incised parallel to the zygomatic arch and separated from the muscle with a periosteal elevator using semisharp dissection (Fig. 4.**72**). The excised piece of fascia is stored in a moist container. Perichondrium is, however, a more reli-

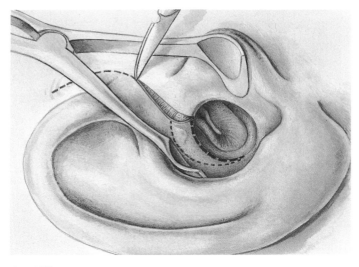

Fig. 4.**70**

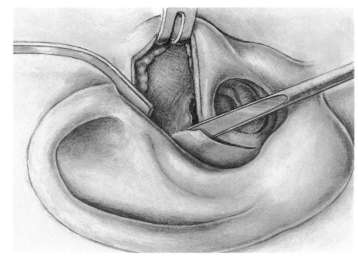

Fig. 4.**71**

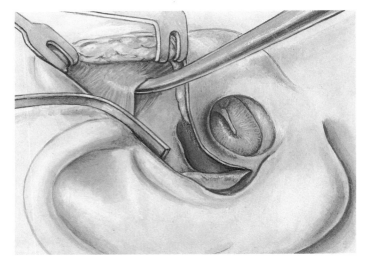

Fig. 4.**72**

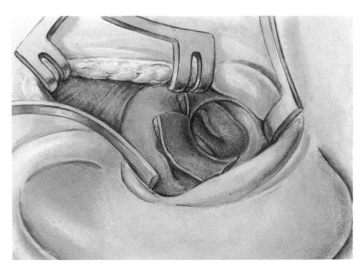

Fig. 4.**73**

able material for repairing a tympanic membrane per-foration (see Figs. 4.**44** to 4.**49**).

Exposure of the Tympanic Membrane Region

The soft tissues are retracted with self–retaining retrac-tors placed at right angles to each other, exposing the posterior wall of the meatal entrance. The meatal flap has already been outlined with incisions at 7 and 12 o'clock using a No. 15 scalpel (Fig. 4.**73**). This approach gives an adequate view of the posterior portion of the tympanic membrane and the entire ossicular chain. If more anterior portions of the middle ear need to be ex-posed intraoperatively, the incision can be extended up-ward and backward along the aural crease while the auricle is retracted downward. For defects located in the far anterior portion of the tympanic membrane, a postauricular incision is preferred.

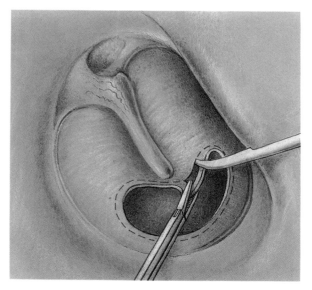

Fig. 4.**74a**

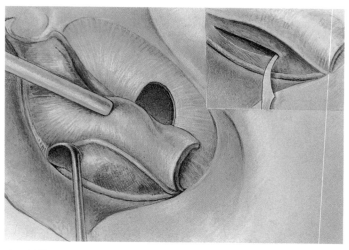

Fig. 4.**75**

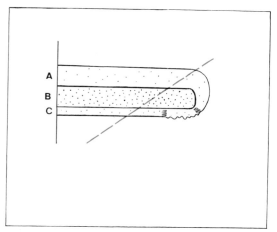

Fig. 4.**74b**
A: epithelium
B: pars tensa
C: mucosa

Preparation of the Recipient Bed

An incision is made encompassing the margins of the perforation before the tympanic membrane is freed from its bony ring. The edge of the perforation is incised with a sickle knife and retracted with a fine grasping forceps (Fig. 4.**74a, b**). As shown in Fig. 4.**74b**, the edge of the defect is beveled in a way that leaves intact surface epithelium (A) and creates a recipient bed with an enlarged contact area composed of freshened pars tensa (B) and mucosa (C).

With a subtotal or total defect, mucoperiosteum is additionally resected from the bony ring. A sickle knife is used to elevate the mucosa tangentially to the tympanic membrane remnant about 3 mm peripheral to its margin. This creates an enlarged recipient surface that will promote graft healing.

Opening the Middle Ear

The meatal flap, with its slight lateral taper, is elevated from the underlying bone, leaving a broad pedicle at the tympanic membrane (tympanomeatal flap). A knife–elevator with an angled round blade is used to elevate the anulus from the tympanic sulcus and incise the tense middle–ear mucosa (Fig. 4.**75**). The mobilized tympanomeatal flap is placed on the anterior half of the tympanic membrane.

A wide meatus will facilitate manipulations in the tympanic cavity. The posterior canal wall can be thinned with a conical cutting burr or diamond burr until the cells of the mastoid process are visible through the bone.

The lateral wall of the attic is taken down with a House curet until the structures of the oval window niche can be clearly seen. If necessary, the ossicular chain can be checked at this time for continuity and mobility (Fig. 4.**76**).

Reconstruction of the Tympanic Membrane

The moist, lint–free fascia is spread flat on the end of a periosteal elevator by the assisting nurse and passed into the operative field from below. It is grasped with a sickle–knife and suction tip (with shutoff), and in one motion it is slipped beneath the anterior half of the tympanic membrane (Fig. 4.**77**).

The anterior part of the graft should overlap the margins of the perforation by about 3 mm. It should broadly underlie the malleus handle and should appose smoothly to the medial surface of the tympanic membrane (Fig. 4.**78**). The posterior part of the graft is

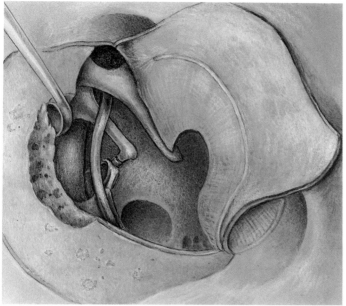

Fig. 4.**76**

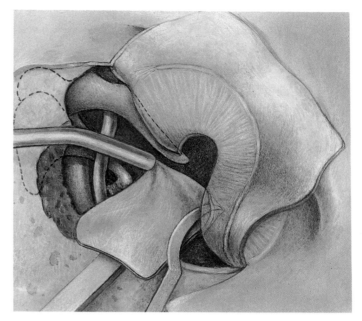

Fig. 4.**77**

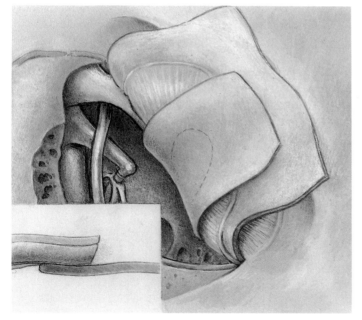

Fig. 4.**78**

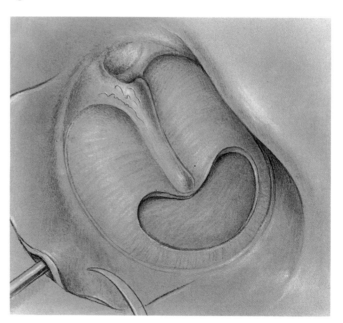

Fig. 4.**79**

placed against the meatal bone between the chorda tympani and tympanic membrane. When the tympanomeatal flap is replaced, care is taken to avoid trapping squamous epithelium between the skin and bone (Fig. 4.**79**).

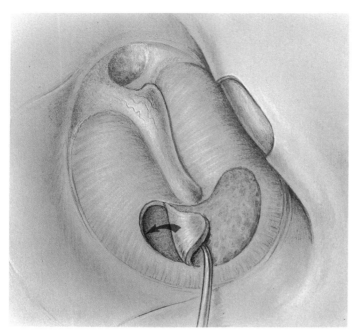

Fig. 4.**80**

A free skin graft can be fitted precisely into the residual epithelial defect as an aid to epithelialization (double–flap repair). The graft, free of cutaneous appendages, is taken from the anterior canal wall 3 mm lateral to the plane of the tympanic membrane (Fig. 4.**80**).

Meatal Packing and Wound Closure

Thin strips (40×5×0.1 to 0.2 mm) of silicone film, rounded at the front, are placed into the anterior tympanomeatal angle and positioned against the tympanic membrane remnant and the graft. The smooth silicone film stabilizes the graft position and reduces problems of wound healing. The external meatus is loosely packed with antibiotic–impregnated gelatin sponge so that as the packing swells slightly, it will press the graft into the middle ear space. The film overlaps the edges of the incision and thus prevents granulation tissue ingrowth into the packing. The wound is closed with continuous cutaneous sutures. Finally a slightly larger piece of gelatine sponge is placed into the meatal entrance to keep the small pieces of packing from falling out prematurely. Normally the outer ear dressing is removed on the second postoperative day and replaced with a protective ear patch, while the tamponade remains in place for 3 weeks.

Important Modifications

The authors basically prefer the underlay graft technique for myringoplasty. Modifications are therefore limited to the selection of various autograft materials. Homografts and xenografts are not used.

Perichondrium: Perichondrium may be obtained from the tragus (see Figs. 4.**44** to 4.**46**) when an endaural incision is used or from the back of the concha (see Figs. 4.**47** to 4.**49**) when a postauricular incision is used. This material is thicker than fascia and appears less susceptible to resorption or thinning in case of infection. Fashioning and placement are somewhat more difficult due to the thickness of the graft.

Perichondrium with cartilage: This material is obtained from the tragus or the back of the concha. The bradytrophic tissue is highly resistant to infection, does not shrink, and has a firm, resilient consistency. This eliminates the danger of retraction pocket formation in a poorly aerated middle ear. The presence of perichondrium on the cartilage promotes graft viability.

Cartilage: The functional properties of cartilage are as favorable as those of cartilage–perichondrium, but cartilage alone perhaps, makes for a less viable graft.

The selection of the graft material depends on the size of the defect and the nature and extent of the pathologic changes. Pericondrium is the material of choice for repairing a large tympanic membrane perforation. If there is a tendency toward graft adhesion, the stiffer, more resilient cartilage–perichondrial or cartilage (palisade technique of Heermann) graft is preferred. (Onlay technique, see page 118)

Landmarks and Pitfalls

Chorda Tympani

The chorda tympani nerve courses in mucosal folds and occasionally is loosely apposed to the tympanic membrane. Its site of emergence from the bone is variable. The chorda may be confused with the fibrocartilaginous anulus, especially if the tympanic structures are inflamed and difficult to differentiate. An effort should be made to spare the chorda, even though dividing the nerve in a chronically inflamed ear often does not cause permanent disability.

Ossicular Chain

If the high–speed burr touches the ossicular chain during enlargement of the meatus, it can cause acoustic trauma with sensorineural damage. Thus, it is safer to use a curet for bone removal in proximity to the ossicles (Fig. 4.**76**).

The stapedial tendon and, perpendicular to it, the long crus of the incus are identified as aids to identifying the stapes, which is preserved.

The entrance to the round window niche is located below the oval window niche and is separated from the oval window niche by a small bony prominence. The tympanic tubal orifice can be located by identifying the cochleariform process and following the tensor tympani semicanal forward and downward.

Facial Nerve

The facial nerve may approach the floor of the meatus very closely, especially in previously operated patients, and this must be considered when the meatal floor is burred down for widening the canal. Since the facial nerve is the most important structure for the patient that is encountered in otologic surgery, it should always be identified before any nearby structures are dissected. The nerve may be found next to the horizontal semicircular canal or more medially between the semicircular canal and the cochleariform process. This is a consistently more reliable "marker" than the stapes, which may be absent or displaced.

Rules, Hints, and Common Errors

Endaural Incision

If at all possible, the incision should spare the cartilage bordering on the intertragic notch as a precaution against auricular perichondritis.

Tympanomeatal Flap

If a large tympanomeatal flap (e.g., produced by incising the meatal skin too far laterally) interferes with dissection in the middle ear or if it threatens to wind around the burr, it is temporarily removed. Following the myringoplasty, the flap will overlap the lateral border of the graft but not overlie keratinizing squamous epithelium.

The chorda is freed from its mucosal folds and transposed to the undersurface of the tympanic membrane without stretching it. If the chorda obstructs the surgeon's view of the middle ear structures, it can be freed from its bony canal in a functionally intact condition by removing the underlying bone with a House curet or diamond burr.

The bony meatus is enlarged with a conical burr while constant irrigation with physiologic saline or Ringer's solution is maintained. Overheating can cause osteonecrosis and may damage the facial nerve.

Ossicular Chain

- Ossicular mobility is tested by slightly elevating the malleus handle. The *"round window reflex"* evoked by touching the ossicular chain is not always visible, so it is helpful to observe a fluid level (e.g., one or two drops of Ringer's solution in the hypotympanum) placed in the area of the round window membrane. The reliability of this "test" is occasionally overrated.
- A very gentle force should be applied to elevate the malleus handle. Excessive force can cause a malleus neck fracture (occasionally unnoticed) that will not heal spontaneously, disrupting normal sound transmission from the tympanic membrane to the rest of the chain. An incus transposition will yield better functional results in this situation (type III tympanoplasty with a stapes–to–drum reconstruction).
- Recurrent bouts of otitis media often cause distortion of the malleus handle, which becomes deflected toward the promontory. In this situation the tensor tendon can be divided to permit lateral displacement of the malleus handle. The graft can be placed below the malleus handle without fear of adhesions with the nearby promontory.
- Mucosal folds between the long crus of the incus and the malleus handle are divided so that the graft can cover a broad area below the malleus handle. Connective–tissue or mucosal adhesions between the malleus handle/tympanic membrane and the medial wall of the tympanic cavity are sharply divided. With extensive mucosal damage on the medial wall of the middle ear, a thin silicone disc or similar implant can be interposed to prevent adhesions between the tympanic membrane and the wall of the promontory.

Tympanic Membrane

Subtotal or Total Defect

- Remnants of tympanic membrane are usually present near the short process of the malleus and the fibrous anulus. The meatal skin flap is temporarily removed, and the circumferentially mobilized anulus is reflected laterally with the attached meatal skin. The groove of the bony limbus is widened and deepened to 2–3 mm with a diamond burr, especially the portion above the tympanic tubal orifice. Cartilage–perichondrial strips taken from the concha or tragus are then inserted at their narrow ends into the enlarged limbus; these implants spare the malleus handle and are oriented parallel to it, completely filling the area within the limbus. They are buttressed and supported by adjacent structures such as the tensor tympani canal. The strips behind the malleus handle may appose to the incus, and additional cartilage strips are placed in the epitympanum for support and to close residual defects ("palisade technique" of Heermann). The laterally reflected meatal skin is turned back over the cartilage strips, and the free meatal skin flap is reimplanted. A thin film of tissue adhesive may be applied to the surface of the myringoplasty to help stabilize its position.
- The perichondrial graft, which is highly resistant to trophic disturbances and may include cartilage elements, has proven almost equivalent to the individually applied cartilage strips. The graft is fully apposed to the undersurface of the malleus handle, and its margins appose broadly to the bony tympanic ring. As noted above, the laterally mobilized meatal skin is replaced in its original position.

Myringosclerosis

Poorly vascularized, calcium–containing areas of the tympanic membrane are an impediment to graft healing. The hard, submucosal residues that form after repeated episodes of otitis media are therefore removed. The epithelium over the calcium deposits is preserved and is laid smoothly over the graft.

Tympanic Membrane Atrophy

Large, atrophic, distensible scars in the tympanic membrane do not permit effective sound transmission to the ossicular chain. Excess scar tissue is excised, and the atrophic portions of the tympanic membrane are broadly underlaid with a suitable graft material such as perichondrium or cartilage–perichondrium. The atrophic epithelium can be glued to the graft with fibrin adhesive to form a smooth, continuous bond, but it will also adhere well to the graft spontaneously.

Proneness to Adhesions

If the promontory mucosa is undamaged, there is little chance that graft adhesions will form. If a mucosal lesion is present, a silicone disc 0.1 mm thick can be interposed so that it lies flat against the promontory wall. Tented or folded silicone film may cause a perforation of the grafted tympanic membrane. Starting on the second postoperative day, careful Valsalva maneuvers are performed to aerate the middle ear. The insertion of silicone sheeting is rarely indicated. I may be helpful when the reconstructed tympanic membrane contacts the promontory already under surgery.

Graft Stabilization

1) The moist, pliable perichondrial or fascial graft usually adheres well to be undersurface of the tympanic membrane. The graft should be large enough to allow for shrinkage, which is more a problem with fascia than with perichondrium (pure cartilage will not shrink).

2) If it appears that the graft will sag too far into the middle ear, it can be stabilized by making small incisions around it (Gerlach, 1972), finding small connective–tissue strands adherent to the graft, drawing them through the perforation with a fine suction tip (0.7 mm with shutoff), and pulling them outward with a fine alligator forceps (Fig. 4.**81**). Usually it is sufficient to stabilize the graft over the eustachian tube. Any granulation tissue that forms on the tympanic membrane with this technique can be cauterized during postoperative follow–up.

3) Alternatively, a properly positioned, unwrinkled graft can be secured by placing a drop of tissue adhesive on the surface of the graft and the margin of the tympanic membrane to prevent sagging or slipping of the graft.

- Before replacing the tympanomeatal flap, the surgeon makes certain that the graft is unwrinkled and correctly positioned on the tympanic membrane remnant. The portions behind the malleus handle can be assessed by gross visual inspection, and the position of the malleus handle can be tested by palpating it with an antrum retractor or Rosen elevator. If the graft slips out from under the malleus handle, a residual perforation may persist or there may be deficient contact between the malleus handle and the tympanic membrane. Figure 4.**82** shows a spontaneously healed tympanic membrane perforation in which the malleus handle has separated from the regenerative drum, causing impairment of sound transmission. This situation is managed in the same way as tympanic membrane atrophy (see above).
- If fibrin glue has been used, control of the perforation is especially necessary. The fibrin film can mislead an inexperienced surgeon. A perforation may seem to be nicely closed, but this is partly established

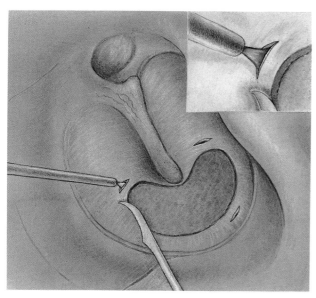

Fig. 4.**81**

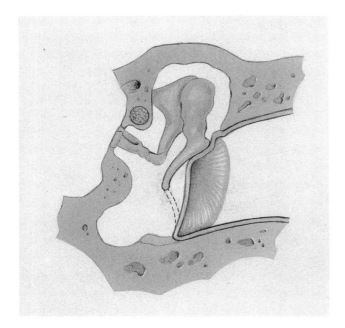

Fig. 4.**82**

only by the fibrin film which undergoes fibrinolysis after a few days. High rates of recurrent perforations can be expected.

- The anterior tympanomeatal angle should remain untouched or be reconstructed as a natural angle for better hearing.

Pre- and Postoperative Care

Preparation of the Operative Field

In patients with a heavy aural discharge, the external meatus and middle ear are irrigated three times daily for up to four days before surgery to reduce the local concentration of microorganisms. Physiologic saline, 0.02% Rivanol solution, or 0.3% hydrogen peroxide solution may be used. Systemic antibiotics are also administered in this situation.

Perioperative Prophylactic Antibiotics

Usually a "one-shot" prophylactic dose of a cephalosporin active against staphylococci is administered 30 min before the incision is made. Even with a middle ear discharge, the concentration of antibiotic dissolved in the meatal packing (e.g., tetracycline-impregnated gelatin sponge) is usually sufficient to provide an adequate local antibacterial action following surgery.

Hospitalization

Most patients are discharged one week postoperatively after removal of the cutaneous sutures. This allows time for the development, detection, and management of rare complications such as perichondritis, hematoma formation, abscess formation, or deep meatal infection.

Assessment of Labyrinthine Function

1) Bone conduction hearing is tested daily with C2 und C3 tuning forks (Weber test). A pure-tone audiogram (bone conduction hearing) is unreliable but may be done if the tuning fork tests are equivocal.
2) Frenzel glasses are used to test for spontaneous nystagmus and exclude vestibular dysfunction.

- Valsalva maneuvers are initiated two days after the operation. Forced aeration could cause displacement of the graft. Only a very brief, click-like aeration sound should be audible in the ear.
- In uncomplicated cases the dressing is changed on the second postoperative day.
- The packing, including silicone strips, is removed from the external meatus at three weeks. Usually it is sufficient to brush the canal with Castellani's solution (colored, without phenol; new fuchsin 1.0, 90% denatured ethanol 9.0, purified water 90.0, resorcinol 10.0, acetone 5.0), which provides a cleansing and drying action. If the external meatus is moist or if bits of gelatin sponge do not come away with the rest of the pack, it is helpful to instill a product such as Decoderm Trivalent ointment with a gauze strip. At one week the ear canal is completely cleaned and brushed with Castellani's solution.
Any granulation tissue at the incision site is mechanically removed and/or cauterized with 5% silver nitrate or other caustic solution.

Postoperative Complications

Facial Nerve Palsy

Local anesthetic may inadvertently be injected close to the facial nerve or into the exposed but unrecognized nerve, or the agent may diffuse into the nerve canal through sites of bone dehiscence. The palsy is transient and should resolve completely within a few hours.

Healing Problems

Wound healing problems can result from the introduction of bacteria into the incision site or from the persistence of resistant organisms in the meatus and middle ear. The wound is opened and irrigated with a solution such as 3% hydrogen peroxide, and appropriate antibiotic therapy is initiated.

If a deep ear inflammation develops accompanied by nystagmus and hearing impairment, the meatal packing should be removed without delay. It may be necessary to reopen the middle ear, depending on the severity of the clinical manifestations. Treatment is initiated with a broad–spectrum antibiotic that is appropriate for the infecting organisms. Adjunctive treatment with cortisone (e.g., 500 mg Solu–Decortin) for labyrinthine dysfunction is indicated in selected cases.

If small dehiscences are noted postoperatively in the tympanic membrane graft, it is reasonable to await spontaneous closure. This can be aided, for example, by placing cigarette paper over the site to stimulate wound reaction. Perforations can be repaired by performing a repeat myringoplasty after about one year.

Meatal stenosis may result from a faulty meatal incision or deficient epithelialization of the ear. An attempt is made to dilate the meatus with rubber foam or restore a normal canal lumen by means of free or regional skin transfers.

Functional Sequelae

The definitive hearing result with myringoplasty relies on an intact, mobile ossicular chain. If the chain can vibrate freely owing to an absence of graft adhesions and good contact between the grafted membrane and the malleus handle, sound conduction across the middle ear should be essentially normal.

Alternative Methods

Onlay Technique

An incision is made around the margin of the perforation, the epithelium is elevated from the tympanic membrane, and the graft is placed onto the pars tensa. Peripheral epithelial tags are apposed to the graft, which can additionally be covered with a skin graft from the anterior canal wall. With perforations that extend close to the limbus, deep cutaneous papillae may be divided when the epithelium is elevated. An anular cholesteatoma may form that causes "blunting" of the anterior tympanomeatal angle. Therefore the authors prefer the underlay technique.

Tympanic Membrane Homograft

The use of homografts is acceptable only if it can be established that the donor was free of transmissible disease or that the homograft material has been adequately processed and treated.

As with a subtotal or total defect, the meatal skin is dissected laterally from the bony limbus. Any keratinizing squamous epithelium that has grown deeply into the ear is removed. The homograft tympanic membrane (along with any ossicular components that may be required) is fitted into the bony limbus. The mobilized meatal skin is replaced, and the graft is stabilized with tissue adhesive. The external meatus is lined with silicone strips and packed.

Ossicular Chain Reconstruction

Preoperative Diagnostic Measures

See page 80.

Indications

Microsurgical techniques are available for reconstructing an ossicular chain that has been damaged as a result of chronic otitis media, trauma, tumor resection, or malformation. The functional results depend on the nature and extent of the ossicular defects and on otologic findings (e.g., aeration, intensity of inflammation or scarring, sclerosis, size of tympanic membrane perforation). Ossicular reconstruction is indicated in patients with an adequate cochlear reserve and a conductive impairment of about 20 dB or more, and occasionally it is indicated for lesser degrees of impairment.

Principle of the Operation

The middle ear is cleared of disease, and the tympanic membrane is reconstructed with an autograft. Missing ossicles are replaced with custom–sized autografts, homografts, or alloplastic implants that are compatible with the middle ear. No effort is made to reconstruct functioning joints between the ossicles. A one–stage ossiculoplasty yields satisfactory functional results in approximately two–thirds of patients.

Preoperative Preparations

See page 80.

Anesthesia

See page 81.

Operative Technique

Homograft ossicles are as compatible as autografts and function just as well (for limitations, see Tympanic Membrane Homograft on page 118). The authors prefer alloplastic prostheses owing to their unlimited availability and reduced rate of fixation by bony adhesions. This preference is reflected in the illustrations on operative technique. The patient's own ossicles should only be used when they are free of erosion and ostitis.

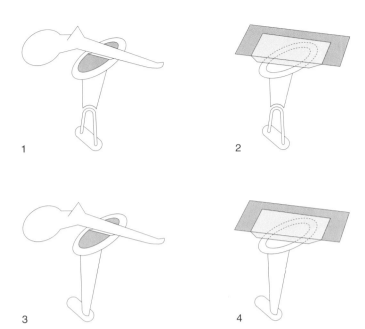

Fig. 4.**83**   Reconstruction of the ossicular chain.*
PORP: 1. Malleus handle present: stapes–to–malleus reconstruction
         2. Malleus handle absent: stapes–to–drum reconstruction
TORP: 3. Malleus handle present: columella
         4. Malleus handle absent: columella

Preparation of Ossicular Prostheses

The prosthesis is held between the thumb and forefinger or in a special forceps and is sculpted with a diamond burr under constant physiologic saline irrigation. The surface of organic ossicles should be disrupted as little as possible, since opened Haversian canals are predisposed to granulation tissue ingrowth leading to premature resorption of the implant.

Common Anatomic Situations

The most commonly encountered situation is a partially eroded incus. If the incus is definitely free of cholesteatoma and osteitis, it can be interposed between the stapes capitulum and the malleus handle, or an alloplastic prosthesis can be used (Fig. 4.**83**, 1, 2). If the stapes superstructure is absent, an alloplastic prosthesis is positioned between the malleus handle and the footplate (Fig. 4.**83**, 3, 4). If the malleus handle is absent, the myringoplasty is usually reinforced with a cartilage disc (Fig. 4.**83**, 2, 4)*.

The options for ossicular chain reconstruction are discussed in terms of the missing structures rather than clinical frequency.

---

* PORP = partial ossicular replacement prosthesis,
  TORP = total ossicular replacement prosthesis.

Malleus Handle

Only an intact handle of malleus that is securely coupled to the tympanic membrane will transmit sound normally. There may be an isolated fracture of the malleus handle (e.g., following a petrous fracture), shortening of the handle secondary to recurrent inflammation, or coupling of the handle to the tympanic membrane may become deficient during spontaneous healing of the membrane (Fig. 4.**82**). If the malleus handle is encased by cholesteatoma, it is removed. In every reconstruction of the malleus or its equivalent, a sufficient length of contact must be established between the malleus and drum.

Fractured Malleus Handle

In this situation the malleus handle is left alone, and a prosthesis is placed between the fragment on the umbo side (lower part of the tympanic membrane) and the incus. Sound striking the fragment on the attic side (upper part of the tympanic membrane) can be transmitted normally across the malleus remnant, incus, and stapes.

Shortened Malleus Handle

If the malleus handle has been shortened due to erosion or other pathology, a myringoplasty will not produce a satisfactory hearing gain. In this case the malleus handle is completely removed, and the tympanic membrane can be placed broadly against the exposed body and long process of the incus (type II tympanoplasty). With a deep middle ear space (e.g., intact canal wall), a gap may exist between the tympanic membrane and the remaining ossicular chain, and an interposition between the stapes capitulum and the reconstructed tympanic membrane or intact handle of malleus will produce better functional results (type III tympanoplasty Fig. 4.**83**, 1).

Deficient Contact between the Malleus and Tympanic Membrane

If lower portions of the tympanic membrane have lost contact with the umbo, sound striking the tympanic membrane cannot be transmitted effectively (Fig. 4.**87**). This is corrected by making longitudinal incisions in the tympanic membrane along both sides of the malleus handle and placing graft material (e.g., perichondrium) beneath the malleus handle and the margins of the newly created perforations.

Malleus Handle Encased by Cholesteatoma Matrix

If the malleus handle is overgrown by cholesteatoma matrix, the handle should be removed. If the malleus neck is also involved, the whole ossicle is removed, and the tympanic membrane defect is backed with a cartilage–perichondrial graft. The incus can be transposed or, if cholesteatoma involvement is suspected, an alloplastic prosthesis is placed between the stapes and the grafted tympanic membrane (Fig. 4.**83**, 2).

Malleus Handle Absent, Footplate Fixed

In cases with an absent malleus handle and fixed footplate, the footplate is partially or completely removed (see section on Otosclerosis for technique) and replaced with an overlapping piece of cartilage–perichondrium. This graft will function as a loose–fitting "cork" to seal the vestibule and prevent perilymphatic leak. This will stabilize the position of an alloplastic prosthesis placed with minimal tension between the tympanic membrane graft and the oval window niche.

Incus

Classic Type III Tympanoplasty (Fig. 4.**84**)

In a classic Wullstein type III tympanoplasty, sound transmission and protection are established by reconstructing the tympanic membrane (e.g., with a cartilage–perichondrial graft) and placing it in contact with the normal stapes. In a "radical" otosurgical cavity, the middle ear is well suited for this type of tympanoplasty (shallow middle ear), since the cartilage–overlapping perichondrium can be apposed to the horizontal semicircular canal and meatal floor in the plane of the new tympanic membrane. A good hearing result is achieved when the stapes capitulum projects above the semicircular canal, and a large cartilage disc can be permanently and securely coupled to the mobile stapes. With a deep middle ear space (e.g., intact canal wall), it is preferable to perform a stapes–to–drum reconstruction (see below).

Malleostapedopexy with a Wire (Fig. 4.**85**)

Stapes–to–malleus reconstruction with an interposed wire is recommended only in patients with a closed, sterile middle ear. Even with perfect surgical technique, there is a potential for stapedial dislocation. A tunnel is developed between the tympanic membrane and the middle third of the malleus handle. A steel wire 0.6 mm in diameter is cut to size, and the ends are fashioned into two open loops that will fit the malleus handle and stapes neck. The stapedial loop is placed around the stapes neck below the stapedial tendon. The opposite loop is passed through the tunnel over the middle third

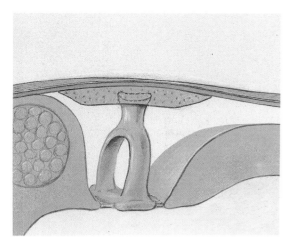

Fig. 4.**84**

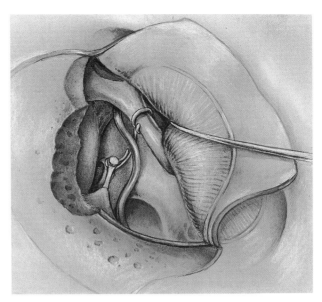

Fig. 4.**85**

of the malleus handle using a fork–shaped instrument. The position of the stapes is constantly observed during this part of the procedure. After the malleus loop has been placed on the handle, the stapedial loop is crimped in front of the anterior crus with a fine alligator forceps. This procedure is technically demanding, but the long–term hearing results are occasionally good.

This procedure is very useful for the training of beginners in temporal bone techniques. The fragility of middle ear structures is convincingly illustrated.

Incus Absent (Fig. 4.**83**, 1)

● *Tympanic Membrane Perforation:* The incus replacement follows repair of the tympanic membrane perforation, which usually coexists with an absent incus. It is functionally advantageous to place the prosthesis in direct contact with the malleus handle. With a large tympanic membrane defect, graft tissue may come between the prosthesis and malleus handle. The head of the prosthesis is notched with a burr so that it will engage the malleus handle securely even if there is interposed soft tissue.

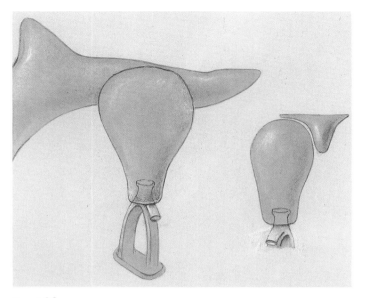

Fig. 4.**86**

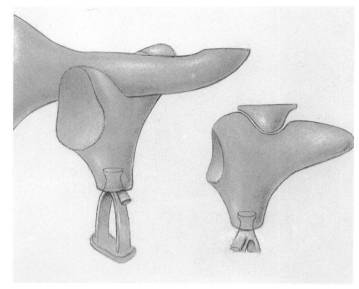

Fig. 4.**87**

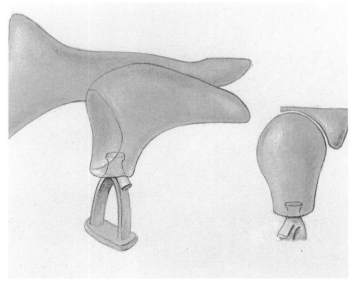

Fig. 4.**88**

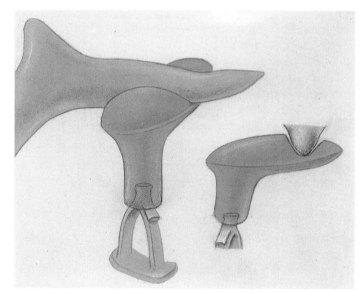

Fig. 4.**89**

- *Autograft or Homograft Prosthesis:* The long crus of the incus is divided and, under constant irrigation, a small cup is burred into the end of the crus to accomodate the stapes capitulum. If a malleus head is used as a prosthesis, the handle is divided at the malleus neck, and the cut surface is hollowed to receive the stapes capitulum (Fig. 4.**86**). If the body of the incus is fitted to the malleus handle, a transverse notch is burred into the incus body to stabilize the fit (Fig. 4.**87**). Alternatively, the incus body can be interposed in the same way as the malleus head for incus replacement (Fig. 4.**88**).
- *Alloplastic Prosthesis:* A notch is burred into the narrow side of the shaft of the incus replacement prosthesis to fit the stapes capitulum, and the head of the

prosthesis is hollowed to articulate with the malleus handle. The head of the prosthesis is given a rounded edge so that slight tilting of the implant will not damage the tympanic membrane. The individually sculpted prosthesis is positioned between the stapes and the middle third of the malleus handle under slight tension (Figs. 4.**89** and 4.**90**).

Incus and Malleus Absent (Fig. 4.**83**, 2)

Stabilizing material, such as a cartilage disc, is placed in the area of prosthesis contact to reinforce the tympanic membrane graft and prevent perforation. If a large cartilage–perichondrial graft is used to reconstruct the tympanic membrane, the cartilaginous portion of the

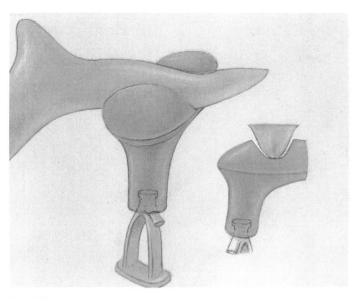

Fig. 4.**90**

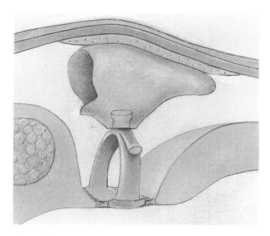

Fig. 4.**91**

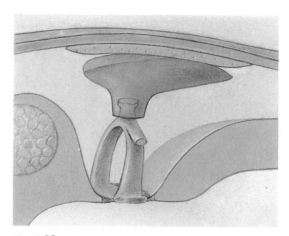

Fig. 4.**92**

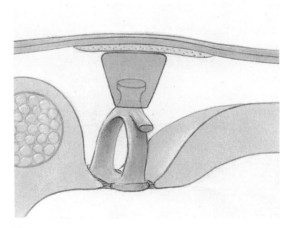

Fig. 4.**93**

graft is positioned over the oval window niche. The prosthesis should extend slightly past the anticipated plane of the tympanic membrane. This creates a slight tension that will stabilize the shaft of the prosthesis on the stapes capitulum. If too short, the prosthesis will separate from the stapes due to postoperative scar contraction of the reconstructed tympanic membrane.

- *Autograft or Homograft Incus:* The long crus of the incus can be placed below the reconstructed tympanic membrane to function as a substitute malleus. A small cup is burred into the narrow side of the short incus crus to receive the stapes capitulum. An equivalent prosthesis can be made by severing the long crus of the incus and drilling a depression in the stump to engage the stapes capitulum. The body of the incus is placed against the drum under slight tension (Fig. 4.**91**).
- *Alloplastic Prosthesis:* A socket for the stapes capitulum is drilled into the narrow side of the shaft of the prosthesis. The head of the prosthesis, which fits broadly against the drum, is rounded at its edges so that subsequent tilting of the implant will not irritate or perforate the drum (Figs. 4.**92** and 4.**93**).

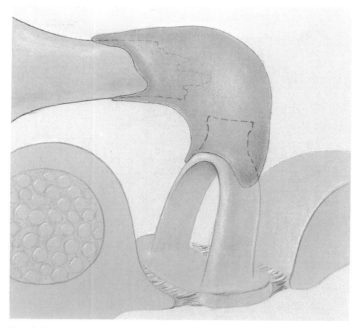

Fig. 4.**94**

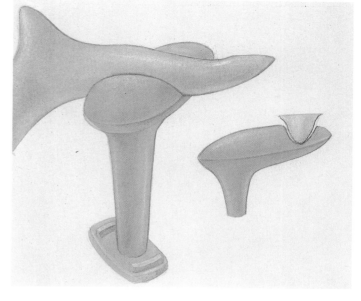

Fig. 4.**95**

Implant between the Stapes Capitulum and Incus Remnant

The rare isolated defect of the lenticular process can be bridged with ionomeric cement. The cement is applied as a viscous fluid that flows over the stapes capitulum and hardens to produce a functionally competent linkage between the stapes and the long crus of the incus (Fig. 4.**94**).

Incus and Stapes Superstructure

A columella can be implanted to establish continuity between the footplate and the malleus handle/tympanic membrane. Autograft and homograft implants are not well suited for this type of reconstruction. When in contact with the facial canal or promontory, they tend to form adhesions with adjacent surfaces that restrict the mobility of the implant.

Incus and Stapes Superstructure Absent (Fig. 4.**83**)

The prosthesis should be about 1 mm longer than the distance from the footplate to the plane of the tympanic membrane. A notch is cut in the head of the prosthesis to engage the malleus handle. The malleus handle is lifted slightly with a small right–angle hook, and the cap of the prosthesis is placed between the middle and upper thirds. The shaft of the prosthesis should exert a slight pressure on the footplate. A thinned footplate is reinforced with a flat cartilage disc to reduce the risk of prosthetic penetration into the vestibule. Alloplastic materials are best for columellar prostheses (Fig. 4.**95**).

A Y–shaped wire prosthesis is fashioned from 0.6 mm–gauge steel wire. A piece of connective tissue is tied around the end of the wire that engages the footplate (Fig. 4.**96**).

Malleus, Incus, and Stapes Superstructure Absent (Fig. 4.**83**, 4)

In a mobile footplate–only situation, the ossiculoplasty consists of implanting a prosthesis between the footplate and the tympanic membrane (Fig. 4.**97**). Occasionally the implant will tilt due to postoperative scarring and distortion of the graft. If the functional result is unsatisfactory, a second operation can be performed at about one year for definitive positioning of the prosthesis. There should be no further drum scarring or distortion after the revision.

Isolated Stapes Arch Defect

An isolated stapes arch defect can occur in patients with van der Hoeve's syndrome, tympanosclerosis, an aberrant facial nerve, or primary cholesteatoma, or it may be caused by trauma. In van der Hoeve's syndrome and tympanosclerotic fixation of the footplate, a stapedectomy is performed, and ossicular chain continuity is re-established with, for example, a platinum band–Teflon implant or other suitable prosthesis (see section on Otosclerosis, page 229). If the footplate is mobile and stapedectomy is not desired, one option is to shorten a prosthetic shaft made, for example, of ionomeric cement so that it will fit between the footplate

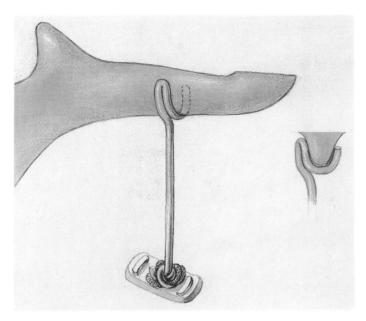

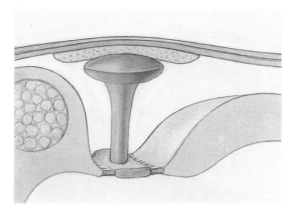

Fig. 4.**97**

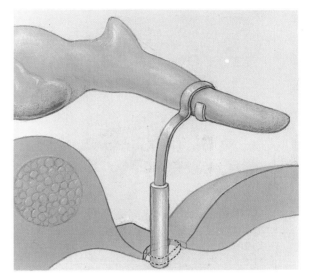

Fig. 4.**96**

and lenticular process under minimal tension. An indentation is drilled into the narrow side of the prosthesis to engage the lenticular process.

Special Form of Tympanosclerosis

In the case of a perforation in the tympanic membrane, the calcific plaques are removed, and the defect is repaired (see page 116). A fixed malleus head is resected, and the incus is interposed between the malleus handle and the mobile stapes (type III tympanoplasty). With sclerotic fixation of the stapes, the tympanosclerotic plaques are elevated from the oval window niche area using a needle and small hooks without damaging the anular ligament (risk of perilymphatic leak). A stapes fixed by sclerotic plaque is not primarily mobilized or removed due to the risk of deafness. With an otherwise mobile ossicular chain, a stapedectomy is performed about one year later (see section on Otosclerosis, page 229). A fixed malleus head and immobile incus are removed. A prosthesis composed of a platinum loop and Teflon piston, gold, titanium or steel wire (4.5–5.5 mm) is positioned in the oval window following stapedectomy or stapedotomy. A tunnel is developed between malleus and tympanic membrane, and the platinum loop is crimped around the middle third of the malleus handle (Fig. 4.**98**).

Fig. 4.**98**

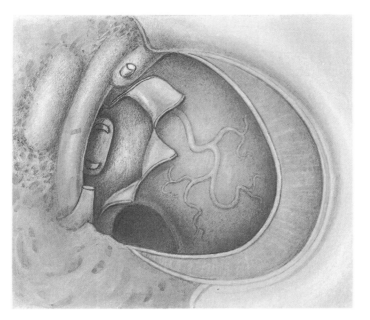

Fig. 4.**99**

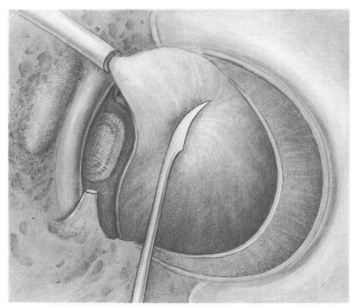

Fig. 4.**100**

Empty Tympanum and Deficient Middle Ear Function (Type IV Tympanoplasty)

A type IV tympanoplasty may be indicated in patients with a small, scarred middle ear space devoid of ossicles, an aeration tract to the round window, and perhaps an accompanying granulation process in the oval window niche (Fig. 4.**99**). A "radical" otosurgical cavity is usually present. The granulation tissue is removed from the empty oval window niche, and the footplate, annular ligament, and adjacent bone are covered with overlapping epithelium from the anterior meatal wall. A fascial graft is applied over the tympanic tubal orifice and round window niche, placing the graft beneath the margin of the tympanic membrane (Fig. 4.**100**). If the mucosal lining of the resulting small tympanum is deficient, a narrow strip of silicone film can also be placed between the round window niche and the tympanic tubal orifice.

Inaccessible Oval Window Niche (Fenestration of the Promontory)

If the footplate is inaccessible (e.g., due to an aberrant facial nerve or vascular anomaly), the tympanic membrane–ossicular complex can be coupled to the inner ear by fenestration of the promontory (Plester). The inner ear is located and identified above the scala vestibuli. At the level of the anterior stapes crus, a 3×3-mm area of mucosa is freed from the promontory, and the bone is thinned with a diamond burr until about 1 mm of endosteum is exposed (Fig. 4.**101**). A stapes prosthe-

sis is looped around the long crus of the incus or the malleus handle, depending on the position and condition of the ossicle (Fig. 4.**102**). The piston of the implant is positioned against the exposed cochlear endosteum under slight tension, indenting it by about 0.5 mm. If a tiny portion of the endosteum is opened during bone removal, this will not seriously jeopardize the inner ear. As in a stapedectomy, a lint–free piece of connective tissue is applied to seal the perilymphatic space. Textile particles can incite foreign–body granuloma formation.

Modifications

Tympanic Membrane–Ossicular Chain Homograft

For a total homograft reconstruction of the ossicular chain, it is recommended that the middle ear be free of infection and the banked tissue be hydrated for approximately 24 hours before use (see page 122). The footplate of the graft is placed against the intact, mobile endogenous footplate. Previously the meatal wall was reduced sufficiently to allow easy delivery of the homograft into the middle ear. Fibrin glue is used to help secure the position of the graft. Effective sound transmission with a favorable hearing result relies on an experienced surgeon applying expert technique. (Potential hazards include transmission of AIDS or Jakob-Creutzfeldt disease.)

Landmarks and Pitfalls

The landmarks and pitfalls of total ossicular reconstruction are basically the same as those described in the sec-

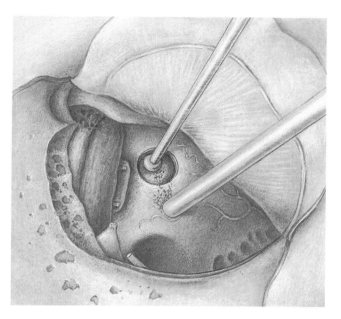

Fig. 4.**101**

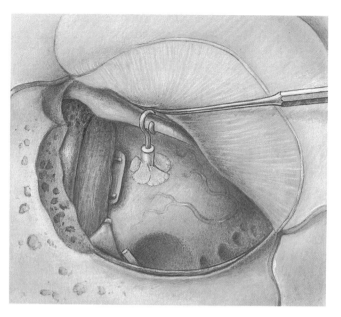

Fig. 4.**102**

tion on Myringoplasty, page 116. The condition of the ossicular chain must be evaluated before any manipulations are performed in the middle ear.

Incus

If the incus is removed, the incudostapedial joint must be completely disarticulated. The ossicles are always separated away from the pyramidal process, in line with the longitudinal axis of the stapedial tendon. This reduces the danger of stapedial dislocation.

Footplate

If the stapes superstructure is absent, the stability of the footplate should be assessed. The footplate may be thinned as a result of tympanosclerosis, cholesteatoma, or other disease. Before a prosthesis is placed upon it, the footplate can be reinforced if necessary with a cartilage disc to prevent perforation by the implant. The damping effect produced by interposed soft tissue will somewhat reduce the efficiency of sound transmission to the inner ear.

Vestibule

If the vestibule is opened, the adjacent squamous epithelium and granulation tissue are removed without delay. A small, noninfected connective tissue flap is used to seal the vestibule and prevent perilymphatic leak, and the middle ear is closed without reconstructing the ossicular chain. Adjunctive cortisone treatment (e.g., 500–1000 mg Solu–Decortin) is indicated.

Rules, Hints, and Common Errors

Tympanic Membrane, Malleus Handle

The head of the malleus can be left in place for a stapes–to–malleus or columellar reconstruction, although resection can occasionally improve ossicular chain mobility and antral ventilation. The tensor tendon and the anterior ligament of the malleus should be preserved, as they tend to prevent forward tilting of a prosthesis placed below the malleus handle.

Myringoplasty

If the prosthesis is placed directly against (below) the reconstructed tympanic membrane, the latter should be reinforced with a flat cartilage disc in the area of contact with the prosthesis. If the tympanic membrane has been reconstructed by cartilage–perichondrial grafting, the cartilage should not slip off the head of the prosthesis.

Preparation of the Implant

The surface of autograft or homograft ossicles should be left as intact as possible, since opened Haversian canals will promote granulation tissue ingrowth. Although the ossicles are among the hardest bones in the body, this can lead to early resorption of the graft.

The head of an alloplastic implant should be rounded at the edges. Otherwise, if the implant becomes tilted (e.g., due to scar contraction of the tympanic membrane graft), its sharp edge may cause trophic disturbances in the reconstructed membrane predisposing to perforation and extrusion.

If the original tympanic ring is still present, the necessary length of the prosthesis is easily determined. In the absence of a malleus handle and tensor tendon, the tympanic membrane or graft will tend to stretch within the tympanic ring during the postoperative period. When definitively positioned, the ossicular prosthesis should tent the reconstructed menbrane about $1/2$ mm laterally. If the tympanic ring is absent, it is more difficult to estimate the extent of postoperative scar contraction of the grafted membrane.

Stapes, Footplate

A columella that is too long may perforate the tympanic membrane, especially if the drum undergoes postoperative medial displacement. Only isolated instances of vestibular penetration by implants have been reported.

Meatal Packing

The external meatus is lined with thin ($40 \times 5 \times 0.1$ to 0.2 mm) silicone sheetings. The meatal packing, consisting of antibiotic–impregnated gelatin sponges, is placed loosely against the tympanic membrane. Swelling of the sponges in the postoperative period may press upon the drum, causing displacement of the prosthesis or even a more hazardous transmission of prosthetic pressure causing tilting of the stapes, displacement or penetration of the footplate, impingement of the Teflon piston on the saccule (e.g., in a malleovestibulopexy), or indentation of the cochlea by the piston (after fenestration of the promontory).

Postoperative Care

Postoperative measures are the same as those following a myringoplasty (see page 117).

Postoperative Complications

Immediate Postoperative Period

Tympanic membrane: The graft may become displaced, resulting in a residual perforation, or the graft may undergo partial or complete necrosis due to an insufficient recipient bed.

Footplate: Pressure from the prosthesis may displace the footplate, with associated vertigo and risk of deafness.

Longer–Term Complications

Tympanic membrane: The prosthesis may perforate the reconstructed membrane, especially with metal prostheses at the handle of the malleus.

Malleus handle: The prosthesis may become tilted due to scar tension in the tympanic membrane graft, for example, causing ossicular discontinuity and impaired sound transmission.

Incus: When a platinum prosthesis has been fixed to the incus (incudoplatinopexy), the platinum loop may erode the long crus of the incus, and the unstable loop will disrupt the path for sound transmission.

Stapes: A prosthesis that is too long, for example, can exert excessive pressure that will tilt the stapes.

Footplate: In rare cases the shaft of the prosthesis may penetrate the footplate, usually with no significant labyrinthine reaction.

Functional Sequelae

Permanent, effective aeration of the middle ear is essential for a good audiologic result after tympanoplasty. The smaller the ossicular defect that is bridged by the ossiculoplasty, the better the hearing results. Replacing the incus alone generally produces a better audiologic result than having to replace, say, the malleus, incus, and stapes superstructure. An incudoplatinopexy, malleovestibulopexy, or fenestration of the promontory will usually provide total correction of conductive hearing loss.

Alternative Methods

Tympanic membrane–ossicular chain homograft (see page 116–126).

Grafts and Implants for Ossicular Chain Reconstruction

See also Table 4.1.

Autograft ossicles are advantageous for ossicular chain reconstruction but may undergo bony fixation. They can be used only if they are completely free of inflammation and free of adherent keratinizing squamous epithelium. Bony tissue is partially resorbed, and cartilage may soften. Homograft ossicles are functionally equivalent to autografts, but there is always a potential for the transmission of infectious disease. Hydroxyapatite ossicles are an inexpensive bone substitute and can be sterilized, but resorption phenomena have been reported with these prostheses. Xenograft materials currently do not play a role in ossicular chain reconstruction.

In the diverse group of alloplastic materials, ossicles made of wrought gold or platinum appear to be proving

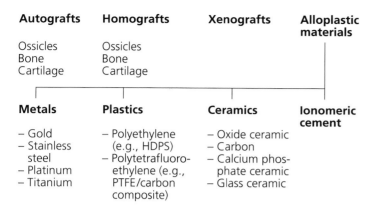

Autografts	Homografts	Xenografts	Alloplastic materials
Ossicles	Ossicles		
Bone	Bone		
Cartilage	Cartilage		

Metals	Plastics	Ceramics	Ionomeric cement
– Gold	– Polyethylene (e.g., HDPS)	– Oxide ceramic	
– Stainless steel	– Polytetrafluoroethylene (e.g., PTFE/carbon composite)	– Carbon	
– Platinum		– Calcium phosphate ceramic	
– Titanium		– Glass ceramic	

Table 4.**1**   Materials for ossicular chain reconstruction.

their value. They are equivalent to platinum band–Teflon prostheses for stapes replacement. Plastic implants are very rarely used in German–speaking countries, most notably because of their histologically confirmed tendency to incite a marked foreign–body reaction.

Inert aluminum oxide ceramic is distinguishing itself among the ceramic materials owing to its stability and biocompatibility. Dense calcium phosphate ceramics have the same composition as the mineral matrix of bone. They are biocompatible and appear to undergo only a minimal degree of resorption. Glass ceramics have proven to be compatible with the middle ear environment. Some materials, such as Biovitroceramic, remain stable, whereas the surface–active glass ceramic Ceravital is subject to varying rates of degradation.

Ossicular prostheses fabricated from ionomeric cement, a hybrid bone replacement material, are distinguished by their compatibility, long–term stability, and excellent intraoperative workability.

Bibliography

Bellucci R J. Dual classification of tympanoplasty. Laryngoscope 1973; 83: 1754–8.

Fisch U. Tympanoplasty Mastoidectomy and Stapes Surgery. Stuttgart: Thieme; 1994.

Gerlach H. Die Stepp-Plastik zur Erhaltung der Trommelfellebene. Arch klin exp Ohr Nas u Kehlk-Heilkd 1972; 202: 662–6.

Geyer G. Implantate in der Mittelohrchirurgie. Eur Arch Oto-Rhino-Laryngol Suppl. 1992/I, 185–221.

Heermann J. Autograft tragal and conchal palisade cartilage and perichondrium in tympanomastoid reconstruction. ENT Journal 71 (1992)

Plester D, Hildmann H, Steinbach E. Atlas der Ohrchirurgie. Stuttgart: Kohlhammer; 1989.

Sadeé, J, Berco, E. Atelactais and secretory otitis media. Ann Otol Rhinol Laryngol 1976; 85 (suppl 25): 62–72.

Tos M. Manual of Middle Ear Surgery. Stuttgart: Thieme; 1993.

Wullstein H L, Wullstein S. Tympanoplasty: osteoplastic epitympanotomy. Stuttgart: Thieme, 1990.

Zöllner, F. Hörverbessernde Operationen bei entzündlich bedingten Mittelohrveränderungen. Arch Ohren Nasen Kehlkopfheilkd 1957; 171: 1–62.

5 Temporal Bone Trauma

Robert A. Jahrsdoerfer and Bechara Y. Ghorayeb

Surgery of External Canal Injuries

External auditory canal injuries may involve one or more of the tissues which form the canal. Canal skin lacerations are the most common. At times, cartilage is also involved and it is not uncommon to encounter a fracture of the bony canal. Treatment is aimed at restoring function and preventing complications which can range from infection to canal stenosis and even cholesteatoma formation.

Incidence

Isolated injuries of the external auditory canal are rare. Most often, the canal is involved by an adjacent injury such as a fracture of the glenoid fossa or a temporal bone fracture. Severe external canal lacerations are observed in one–third of temporal bone fractures.

Causes

Simple skin lacerations are most frequently self–inflicted by the introduction of a foreign object into the external auditory meatus. Ironically, the most common cause is from the use of a cotton–tipped applicator stick ordinarily used to clean the ear. Also included in this category are injuries inflicted by medical personnel while removing impacted cerumen. Avulsions and lacerations of the auricle may extend into the external canal causing complex injuries which involve the meatal cartilage. It is not uncommon to see a complete transection of the external canal from facial trauma which involves the auricle.

Fractures through the area of the glenoid fossa of the temporomandibular joint result in injuries of the anterior canal wall. Oblique (longitudinal) temporal bone fractures extend into the posterior or posterosuperior canal wall. Finally, penetrating trauma from handguns may severely disrupt the external auditory canal.

Diagnosis and Preoperative Evaluation

Physical Examination

The diagnosis of temporal bone trauma is established by inspection of the involved ear. The presence of blood in the concha and external auditory meatus may be mistaken for blood trickling from facial or scalp lacerations. It is therefore essential to perform an otoscopic examination to determine the source of bleeding. Sterile instruments and aseptic technique are used to aspirate the blood. Clots should never be lavaged. The examiner should be on the alert for cerebrospinal fluid. If the patient's condition allows, the tympanic membrane is inspected with the operating microscope.

Debris and cerumen are removed and the torn skin is carefully replaced over the bone. It is sometimes necessary to remove or reposition fragments which occlude the canal. In the absence of evidence of external ear injury, anterior canal lacerations or fractures are indicative of a glenoid fossa fracture. These fractures are also accompanied by trismus and tenderness over the temporomandibular joint. Posterior and posterosuperior lacerations and fractures of the canal occur in temporal bone fractures and are usually associated with a hemotympanum or a torn tympanic membrane. Profuse arterial hemorrhage may be temporarily controlled by packing the external canal. However, bleeding of this magnitude indicates injury to the internal carotid artery and should be investigated with carotid angiography.

Imaging

The most useful procedure is high resolution computed tomography (HRCT) of the temporal bones. This study shows the bony ear canal in its entirety and confirms the presence and course of a fracture. HRCT will be discussed later in this chapter under temporal bone fractures.

Audiometric Evaluation

In general, audiometry is not easy to perform when the external ear is acutely injured or in the presence of severe head trauma. This study may be postponed until the patient is stable.

Indications

Surgery is seldom indicated for acute injuries of the external auditory canal. Most soft tissue and bony fragments may be repositioned or removed during physical examination. A transected canal is usually stented during the primary repair of the auricular injury. Long–term sequelae of a canal transection are serious and deserve further discussion. These include canal stenosis and cholesteatoma formation.

Stenosis of External Canal

Traumatic external ear canal stenosis occurs as a result of displaced bone fragments which have become lined with canal skin. Stenosis can also result from circumferential scarring of soft tissue and is particularly common with the auricle has been amputated.

Cholesteatoma

When skin is trapped beneath bony fragments of behind soft tissue scarring a cholesteatoma may form.

Goal of the Operation

- Resection of soft tissue stenosis;
- Removal of bone fragments;
- Recontouring of ear canal.

Anesthesia

General

General endotracheal anesthesia may be preferable to local anesthesia, especially if an autogenous skin graft is required.

Local

Infiltration anesthesia using lidocaine 1 or 2% with epinephrine 1 : 100,000 may be used. This provides both anesthesia and hemostasis (see also Chapter 1).

Operative Technique

The patient is placed in the supine position with the affected ear up. The surgical approach is through the external ear canal (transcanal) or postauricular. The external auditory meatus is infiltrated with a local anesthetic agent.

Bony Stenosis, Removal of Bone Fragments

In acute injuries, bone fragments may be encountered within the lumen of the external canal. These fragments are usually mobile, but may be impacted in the fracture line. The lacerated canal skin is gently teased away from the bone fragments. The fragments are mobilized and extracted with a hook or a needle (Figs. 5.1 and 5.2). The skin is debrided and the ear canal lightly packed. Occasionally, a piece of temporalis fascia is interposed between the bone and canal skin to prevent the ingrowth of skin into the fracture line (Fig. 5.3).

Excision of Soft Tissue Stenosis and Bone Fragments—Recontouring of Ear Canal, Skin Grafting

When an injury has had time to heal, new skin may have grown over the bone fragments. These must be removed if they are large enough to occlude the ear canal, or if it is necessary to gain access to the tympanic membrane or middle ear. A tympanomeatal flap is elevated until the bony stenosis is reached. Skin is carefully elevated from the bony fragments which are then removed with a curette or a power drill. The tympanomeatal flap is replaced and the canal lightly packed.

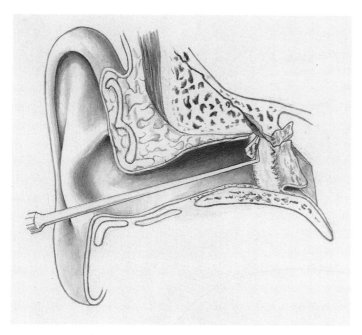

Fig. 5.**1**   Bony fragments extracted with a hook from fractured external auditory canal.

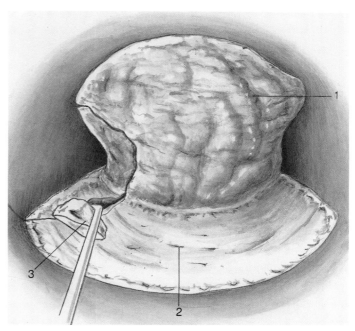

Fig. 5.**2**   Tympanomeatal flap elevated to allow extraction of bony fragments.
1   Tympanomeatal flap
2   Bony canal wall
3   Bony fragment

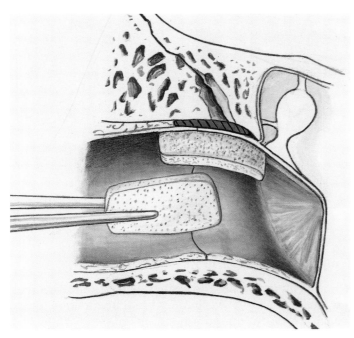

Fig. 5.**3**   Temporalis fascia interposed between skin and fracture line.

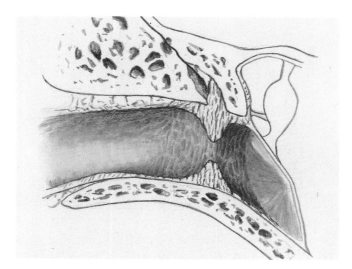

Fig. 5.**4**   Circumferential cicatricial stenosis.

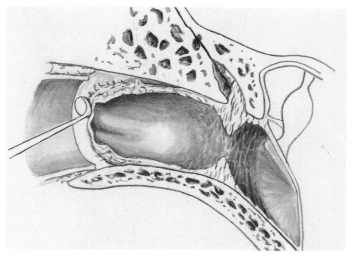

Fig. 5.**5**   Circumferential incision.

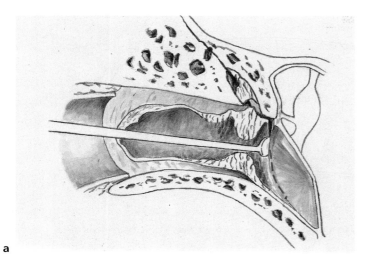

a

Fig. 5.**6**   Removal of stenotic segment.

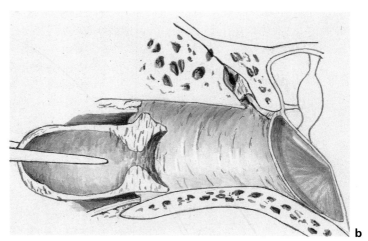

b

Severe soft–tissue scarring may result in a circumferential stenosis which occludes the ear canal lumen (Fig. 5.**4**). The stenotic segment needs to be excised and the bare bone covered with a split–thickness skin graft. A circumferential incision is made lateral to the area of stenosis (Fig. 5.**5**). The canal skin is elevated subperiosteally, incised medial to the stenosis, and removed (Fig. 5.**6 a** + **b**). Any displaced bone or bony projection is drilled away thus recontouring the ear canal.

A split–thickness skin graft 0.008 to 0.010 inches thick is harvested, trimmed to the size of the excised segment, and placed over the denuded bone of the ear canal (Fig. 5.**7**). The lateral edge of the skin graft is sutured to the meatus. The ear canal is lightly packed. (Details see p. 72)

Surgical Landmarks and Danger Points

Temporomandibular Joint

When drilling the anterior canal wall to remove bone fragments or a bony overhang, it is not uncommon to encroach upon the temporomandibular joint. While this does not usually pose a problem, the surgeon should recognize the whitish fibrous capsule of the joint and refrain from further drilling.

Canal Skin Trapped between Fragments can cause Cholesteatoma

Canal skin trapped between the bony fragments of a fracture, or beneath a skin graft, may cause a cholesteatoma. It is therefore imperative to remove any shreds of skin when recontouring the bony canal.

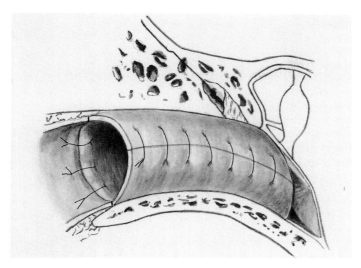

Fig. 5.**7**   Split–thickness skin graft placement.

Postoperative Care

Postoperative Broad–Spectrum Antibiotics

In acute injuries requiring surgery, the wound is cultured and broad–spectrum antibiotics are administered.

Removal of Packing

The ear is inspected a week after surgery and the packing is removed between the 7th and 15th postoperative days. Antibiotic–steroid ear drops are helpful in controlling infection.

Postoperative Complications

Infection

Postoperative infection is uncommon. If infection occurs, however, it may cause the skin graft to slough. Infection that progresses to auricular perichondritis requires aggressive treatment.

Temporomandibular Joint Dysfunction

If the temporomandibular joint is injured or surgically irritated, the patient may suffer from trismus or pain on mastication.

Recurrence of Soft–Tissue Stenosis

Circumferential stenosis from soft–tissue scarring is difficult to treat and may recur. Dilatation or merely stenting the stenosed segment may not be sufficient. Skin grafting will reduce the likelihood of restenosis.

Cholesteatoma

Cholesteatomas can arise from trapped skin fragments deep to the canal surface.

Surgery of Tympanic Membrane Injuries

Tympanic membrane injury is caused by forces applied directly through the external auditory canal, through the eustachian tube, or indirectly by forces transmitted through the skull as a result of head trauma.

Incidence

The overall incidence of traumatic tympanic membrane perforations is estimated to be 2% of all disorders of the ear. The exact incidence of each type of injury is unknown. In a study of 531 ruptured tympanic membranes, blast injuries accounted for 57% of the cases, penetrating injuries 15%, skull trauma 15%, and barotrauma 4% (Strohm, 1986).

Causes

Penetrating injuries are caused by the introduction of a foreign object into the external auditory canal. The most frequently reported objects include cotton–tipped applicators, hairpins, pencils, and match sticks. Also included in this category is ear drum rupture from irrigation for the removal of impacted cerumen, or during the removal of a foreign body from the ear of a restless child. A sudden increase in air pressure may also rupture the tympanic membrane. This may be caused by an open palm slap to the side of the face compressing the column of air trapped in the ear canal. Similarly, an explosion may produce a sudden increase in air pressure which may implode the tympanic membrane.

Barotrauma may, on occasion, cause pressure severe enough to rupture the tympanic membrane. There are anecdotal reports of tympanic membrane rupture from a Valsalva maneuver or eustachian tube insufflation.

In temporal bone fractures, one third of patients will exhibit a fresh tympanic membrane perforation. These perforations are more common in longitudinal fractures and are often associated with external canal skin lacerations.

Thermal burns of the tympanic membrane are an occupational hazard of welders. These are caused by hot slag fragments which enter the external ear canal. Lightning may cause an electrical burn of the tympanic membrane. Finally, chemical burns of the tympanic membrane are observed in patients who sustain acid or alkali facial burns.

Diagnosis and Preoperative Evaluation

Physical Examination

The appearance of the tympanic membrane often reflects the cause of injury. Most traumatic perforations have sharp, ragged edges with fresh blood in the ear canal or middle ear. Associated canal skin lacerations or ossicular injuries are often observed.

The examination is carried out with sterile instruments and preferably the use of a surgical microscope. Blood clots are carefully aspirated. Clear liquid may indicate a cerebrospinal fluid leak (see Chapter 9 in Vol. I /2). A dislocated or fractured footplate may also allow perilymph to leak into the middle ear although the small volume would not be grossly apparent. The surgeon should exercise caution when aspirating in the oval or round window niches. Burn injuries of the tympanic membrane have a tendency to become infected and are usually associated with purulent otorrhea. It is important to check the patient for nystagmus and facial paralysis.

Audiometry

Audiometric testing is performed as soon as the patient's condition allows. Large air–bone gaps raise the suspicion of ossicular chain disruption. Profound sensorineural loss is observed with labyrinthine window ruptures. Patients may experience severe labyrinthine symptoms and tinnitus which make the examination much more difficult. Auditory brainstem response testing may be necessary in comatose or uncooperative patients, and in children. Electronystagmography and other labyrinthine tests may also be indicated.

Indications

Most traumatic tympanic membrane perforations heal spontaneously and rapidly without visible scars. Even large perforations may heal completely without treatment (Bellucci, 1983). Surgery is reserved for the following conditions:
- Persistent tympanic membrane perforation,
- Persistent conductive hearing loss.

Goal of the Operation

- Closure of perforation—prevention of infection,
- Restoration of hearing.

Preparation for Surgery

Treatment of Infection

Patients are instructed to keep the affected ear dry. Swimming is contraindicated and it is best to plug the ear when taking a shower or shampooing the hair. Should the ear become infected, the discharge is cultured and proper antibiotic therapy is begun.

Anesthesia

- Local (see Chapter 1),
- General.

Operative Technique

Immediate Therapy

Traumatic perforations may be treated immediately at the time of the first physical examination. Otoscopy is performed using an aseptic technique. The external ear canal may be infiltrated with local anesthetic for anesthesia and hemostasis. This procedure is simple and may be performed as an outpatient procedure.

Elevation and Splinting of Drum Remnant

If the ragged edges of the perforation are inverted, they may be gently elevated with a small hook (Fig. 5.**8**) and splinted with Gelfilm or Gelfoam (Fig. 5.**9**).

Inspection of Middle Ear

The edges of the perforation may be gently retracted to visualize the ossicles.

Delayed Therapy

Surgery is indicated when a perforation has not healed within six weeks. Tympanoplasty is performed in the operating room using one of the following approaches:
- Transcanal,
- Postauricular.

Details of these surgical procedures are described elsewhere in this book (see pages 110–118).

Surgical Landmarks and Danger Points

In dealing with a traumatic perforation, the surgeon should be aware of some difficulties that may not be ordinarily encountered in a straightforward tympanoplasty.

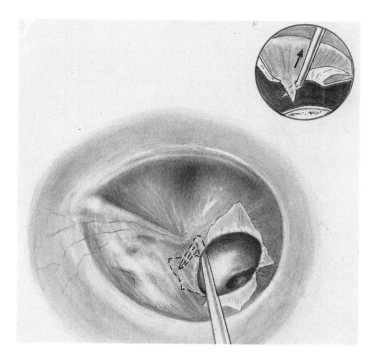

Fig. 5.**8**   Elevation of perforation edges.

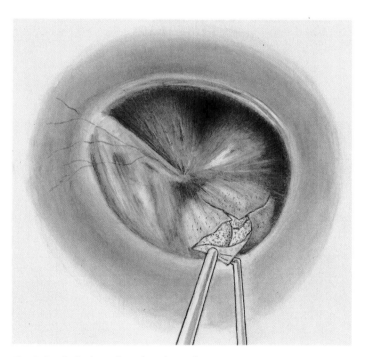

Fig. 5.**9**   Splinting of perforation edges.

Distorted Ear Canal Anatomy

Temporal bone fractures cause distortion of the bony canal wall, particularly in the posterior or posterosuperior portion where longitudinal fractures cross the external auditory canal. A bony step–off may occur along the fracture line which makes it difficult to raise a tympanomeatal flap and elevate the anulus.

Bleeding from Fracture Line

Bleeding along the fracture line may be heavy and compound the difficulties encountered in elevating the flap.

Associated Ossicular Chain Lesions

Traumatic perforations may also be associated with ossicular chain disruption or fracture which should be identified and repaired at the same time as the tympanic membrane. A massive dislocation of the incus is known to occur in longitudinal temporal bone fractures. The incus may be found lying in the fracture line or seen as an irregular mass beneath the skin of the external canal. A massive incus displacement of this sort is usually discovered at the time the tympanomeatal flap is elevated (Fig. 5.**10**).

Rules, Tips and Pitfalls

- Early surgery is unnecessary.
- Early surgery may introduce infection and cause meningitis.
- Always check ossicular chain.
- Be alert for facial nerve injury.
- Be alert for brain herniation.

Postoperative Care

Postoperative Antibiotics

Many surgeons do not routinely administer antibiotics for tympanoplasty, however, the repair of traumatic perforations is tedious and requires a longer period of time than ordinary tympanoplasty. Because of the prolonged exposure, broad–spectrum antibiotics may be necessary.

Postoperative Complications

Meningitis

Temporal bone fractures heal by fibrous union and it is not unusual to encounter a small cerebrospinal fluid leak from the attic during a middle ear exploration. This is a potential route of meningeal infection.

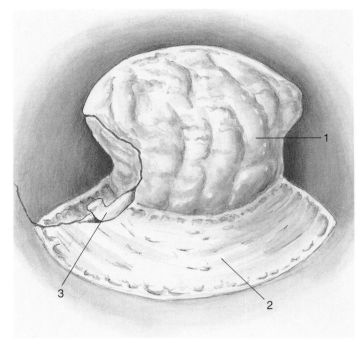

Fig. 5.**10**   Massively displaced incus in fracture line.
1   Elevated skin flap
2   Bony canal wall
3   Incus

CSF Otorrhea

If cerebrospinal fluid (CSF) otorrhea is present, or is surgically induced, the source should be identified and the leak repaired. Failing this, the CSF otorrhea may go unrecognized by draining down the eustachian tube. Persistant CSF may also retard healing of the grafted tympanic membrane and leak directly into the external ear canal (See Vol 1/II, pp. 576–577).

Facial Nerve Paralysis

The fallopian canal may be fractured. Bony fragments may impinge upon the facial nerve causing a paresis or paralysis.

Surgery of Ossicular Chain Injuries

(See also Chapter 4, pp. 119–129.)

Causes

Temporal bone fractures are the most frequent cause, followed by penetrating injuries.

Incidence

The incidence of ossicular chain injuries is unknown. Conductive hearing loss is observed in one–third of patients with temporal bone fractures and a mixed hearing loss occurs in one–half. In the majority of patients, the conductive loss resolves spontaneously in 4–6 weeks. About 12% of the patients will continue to have a conductive loss which is severe enough to require middle ear exploration. The most common finding at exploration is incudostapedial joint disruption, followed by incus dislocation. The malleus and the footplate of the stapes are relatively stable structures. The ligaments of the incus are fragile, facilitating dislocation even following minor trauma. Thus, the most vulnerable parts of the ossicular chain are the incus and adjacent incudostapedial and incudomallear joints. Fractures of the ossicles are less common than dislocations. A common fracture site are the stapes crura. The long process of the incus and the neck of the malleus may be fractured less commonly.

Diagnosis and Preoperative Evaluation

Otoscopy

In an acute injury, the ossicular chain may be difficult to inspect because of blood clots and soft–tissue injury. A perforated tympanic membrane may provide better exposure of the ossicles. In some patients with an intact tympanic membrane, the only physical finding is hemotympanum.

Audiometry

A persistent, large air–bone gap of 40 dB or more indicates an ossicular chain disruption. When behavioral audiometry is impossible in the severely head–injured patient, one should do auditory brainstem response testing.

Imaging

High resolution computed tomography of the temporal bones provides good visualization of the ossicles. It is particularly useful in the detection of incudomalleal dis-

articulation or massive incus dislocation. The incudomallear joint is easily seen and resembles an ice–cream cone in the axial view (Fig. 5.**11**). The incudostapedial joint is better demonstrated on coronal views, where the handle of the malleus and the long process of the incus form an image that looks like the letter "Y" (Fig. 5.**12**).

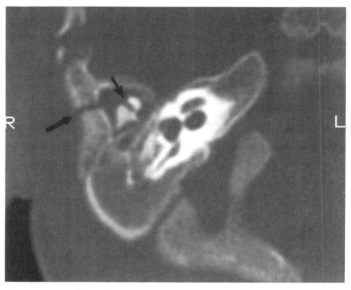

Fig. 5.**11**   High resolution CT scan, ice–cream cone appearance of incus and malleus on axial view.

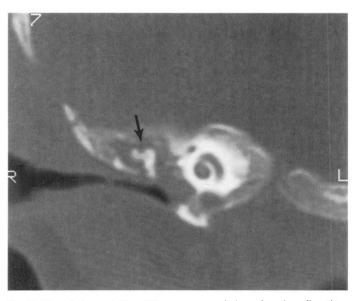

Fig. 5.**12**   High resolution CT scan, coronal view showing disarticulated ossicles: "Y" sign.

Indications

- Restoration of hearing,
- Closure of perilymphatic fistula.

Goal of the Operation

Reconstruction of Middle Ear Conductive Mechanism

The timing of surgery is determined by the general condition of the patient and the resolution of neurological and other life threatening injuries. Even if the patient is fit for surgery, ossicular reconstruction is postponed for about 6 weeks following the injury to allow the tympanic membrane time to heal spontaneously, and a hemotympanum, if present, to resolve. If the patient still has a persistent conductive hearing loss (Fig. 5.**13a**–**c**) after six weeks, the middle ear is explored and the ossicular chain inspected for the following:

- Incudostapedial disarticulation,
- Massive dislocation or fracture of incus,
- Fracture of stapedial superstructure,
- Fracture of footplate,
- Rupture of the round window membrane.

Closure or Perilymphatic Fistula

Perilymphatic fistulas occur when the stapes footplate is subluxed or fractured. This condition occurs most often from direct penetrating trauma and is usually associated with severe tinnitus, sensorineural hearing loss, and vertigo. Exploration may be deferred and the patient placed on complete bed rest.

Anesthesia

- Local (see Chapter 1)
- General

Operative Technique

Transcanal

Surgery is performed in the operating room. In a widely patent external auditory canal, it may be possible to perform the exploration via a transcanal approach. A tympanomeatal flap is elevated and the middle ear is entered. The ossicular chain is inspected and its integrity gently tested with a fine pick or needle.

Postauricular

When the external auditory canal is narrow or anatomically distorted by a fracture, a postauricular approach is preferable. This approach provides a better view of the

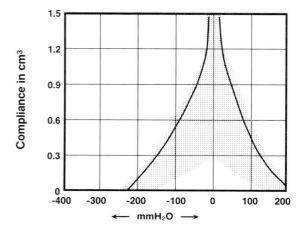

IMPEDANCE AUDIOMETRY

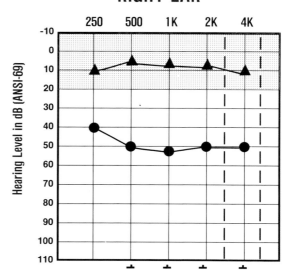

RIGHT EAR

Fig. 5.**13a**—**c**   Audiogram showing conductive hearing loss and type A$_D$ tympanogram.

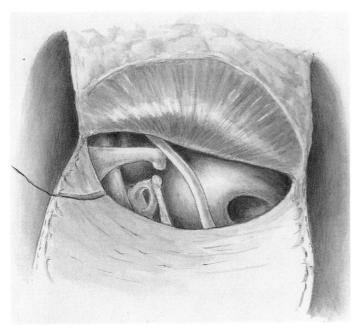

Fig. 5.**14**   Incudostapedial joint disarticulation in good alignment.

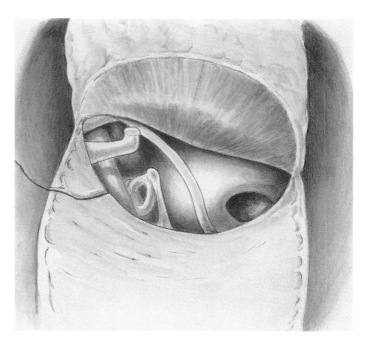

Fig. 5.**15**   Incus disarticulation and 180 degree rotation.

anterior tympanic sulcus and allows the harvesting of fascia or cortical bone for possible later use in grafting the drum or reconstructing the ossicular chain. The tympanomeatal flap may be initially outlined transcanal or incised and elevated after entering the lumen of the external auditory canal through a posterior canal skin incision.

Inspection of Ossicular Chain

The ossicular chain is inspected by challenging the malleus with a fine instrument and observing the movement of the incus and stapes. Excessive mobility of the ossicles suggests a dislocation. The incudostapedial joint should be inspected closely since it may be disrupted but still appear well aligned (Fig. 5.**14**). The incus may be massively dislocated and trapped between the edges of a bony ear canal fracture. The incus may also be rotated 180 degrees around its vertical axis or displaced into the aditus (Fig. 5.**15**). It may also be propelled laterally into the ear canal and lodged between the posterior canal skin and bone at the bony–cartilagenous junction (Cannon and Jahrsdoerfer, 1983).

Removal of Dislocated Incus

If found, the dislocated incus is removed. If it is impacted in the aditus or caught within the fracture line, it may be difficult to extract. In this situation, it is best left alone. However, it can be curetted or drilled if it obscures the stapes or impairs the reconstruction (Fig. 5.**16**).

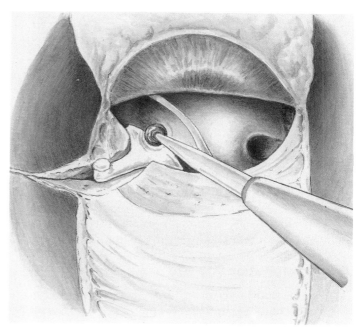

Fig. 5.**16**   Drilling of dislocated incus.

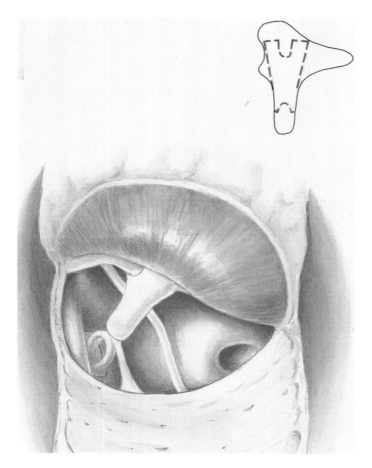

Fig. 5.**17**   Sculptured incus interposition.

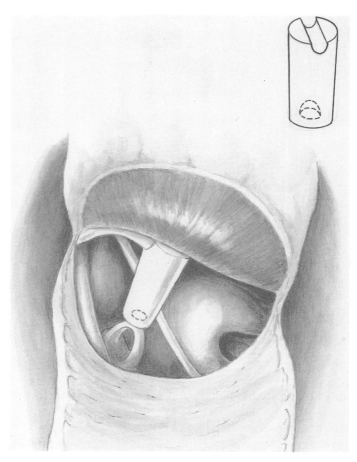

Fig. 5.**18**   Reconstruction with pre–sculptured incus homograft.

Stapes Intact and Incus Dislocated

If the malleus and stapes are intact, reconstruction is achieved by one of the following techniques.

Incus Interposition

The dislocated incus is sculptured and interposed between the malleus and stapes (Fig. 5.**17**).

Incus Homograft

An incus homograft or banked incus is used (Fig. 5.**18**).

Partial Ossicular Replacement Prosthesis

Partial ossicular replacement prostheses may also be used. These are particularly useful in instances where the malleus and stapes head lie at an unfavorable angle (Fig. 5.**19**).

Incus Intact and Stapes Fractured

Stapedectomy

When the malleus and incus are intact but the stapes is fractured or dislocated, a stapedectomy should be performed (Fig. 5.**20**). This is recommended for healed injuries only, i. e. six weeks must have elapsed since time of injury. A stapedectomy should not be performed electively in an acute injury.

Incus and Stapes are Fractured/Dislocated

Total Ossicular Replacement Prosthesis

A total ossicular replacement prosthesis is useful in those cases in which both the incus and stapes are involved. Total ossicular replacement prostheses may be placed over an intact footplate. If the oval window is open, a tissue graft is interposed between the labyrinth and the medial end of the prosthesis (Fig. 5.**21**).

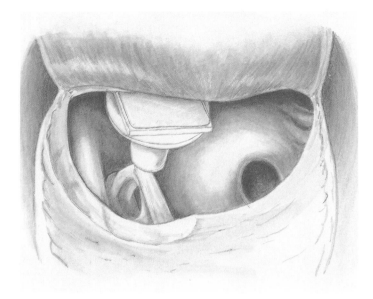

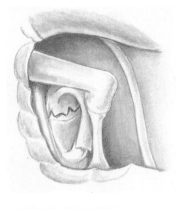

Fig. 5.**19** Partial ossicular replacement prosthesis.

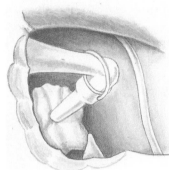

Fig. 5.**20** Stapedectomy.

◁ Fig. 5.**21** Total ossicular replacement prosthesis.

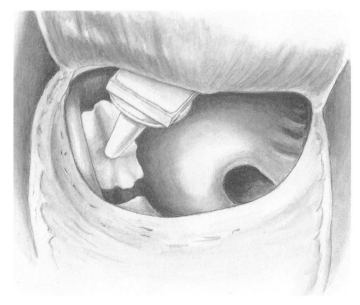

Other

Various other prostheses (hydroxylapatite, metal, bioglass, Teflon, etc.) are available and are equally effective in reconstructing the ossicular chain.

Perilymphatic Fistula Closure

A small subluxation of the stapes may be treated by gently replacing the stapes in its normal position and covering the stapedial anulus with a tissue graft to block the flow of perilymph. Fractures of the footplate, or a gaping subluxation of the stapediovestibular joint, are better managed by performing a stapedectomy, placing a tissue graft over the oval window, and inserting a stapes prosthesis.

Surgical Landmarks and Danger Points

- Bleeding from fracture line, difficult elevation of canal skin, distorted anatomy.
- Massive incus dislocation associated with sensorineural loss.
- Incus may not be easily found since it is either displaced into attic, or lodged between fracture fragments.
- Distorted facial nerve anatomy.
- Brain herniation.

Postoperative Care

Postoperative antibiotics are given.

Postoperative complications

- Sensorineural hearing loss—partial or complete.
- Meningitis.
- Facial paralysis.

Surgery of Facial Nerve Injuries

Facial nerve paralysis is a common manifestation of temporal bone fractures. It usually occurs at the time of injury, but can also develop several days later. See also Vol. 1/II, Chapter 16.

Incidence

The incidence of traumatic facial nerve paralysis varies tremendously in the otolaryngologic literature. In a series of 123 temporal bone fractures proven by high resolution computed tomography, one–half had immediate facial nerve paralysis and one–tenth developed delayed paralysis (Ghorayeb and Rafie, 1989).

Etiology

Temporal Bone Fractures

Temporal bone fractures occur in 4% of blunt head injuries. They are unilateral in 90% of cases and three times more frequent in males than in females. They are more common in adults, but have also been observed in infants. The majority are caused by automobile accidents (63%). Other causes include falls, assaults, and fire arm injuries (Ghorayeb and Rafie, 1989).

Pathology

Classically, temporal bone fractures are grouped according to the course of the fracture line in relation to the longitudinal axis of the petrous pyramid. Fractures that run parallel to the longitudinal axis are called longitudinal fractures (Fig. 5.22), those that cross this axis are transverse (5.23) and the irregular ones are mixed. Most authors agree that the classification should not be based solely on the direction of the fracture, as much as it should on symptomatology. Transverse fractures produce mostly inner ear symptoms, while longitudinal fractures mostly affect the middle ear. Facial nerve paralysis accompanies 20% of longitudinal fractures and 40% of transverse fractures. The incidence of each type of fracture seems to vary: 70% to 90% of all temporal bone fractures are longitudinal, 10% to 30% are transverse. Mixed fractures account for approximately 10%.

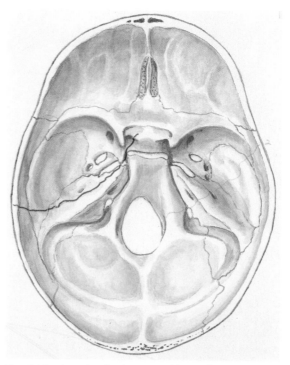

Fig. 5.**22**   Longitudinal temporal bone fracture.

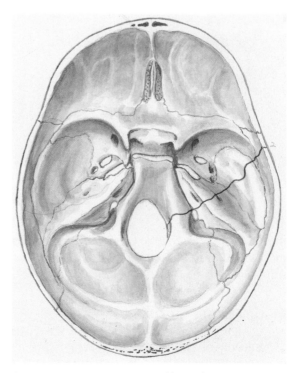

Fig. 5.**23**   Transverse temporal bone fracture.

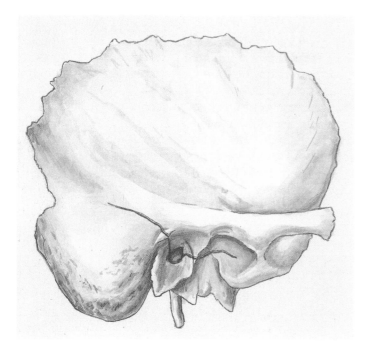

Fig. 5.**24** Oblique temporal bone fracture.

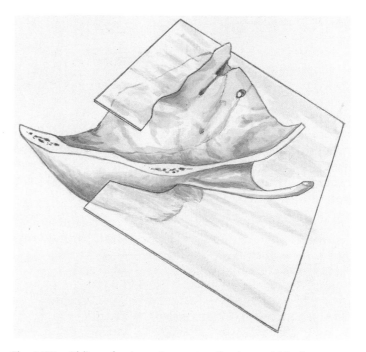

Fig. 5.**25** Oblique fracture plane extending into middle fossa.

Many fractures are neither transverse nor longitudinal but oblique. They run in an inclined plane which crosses the mastoid laterally at the level of Henle's spine, enters the external auditory meatus and slants anteriorly toward the glenoid fossa and petrotympanic fissure (Fig. 5.**24**). Medially, this plane slants upward to involve the lateral wall of the attic. The plane then projects to the geniculate ganglion area where the facial nerve is injured. Superomedially, the plane continues into the floor of the middle cranial fossa, Meckel's cave, and the posterior clinoid (Figs. 5.**25** and 5.**26**), (Ghorayeb and Rafie, 1989).

Diagnosis and Preoperative Evaluation

Physical Examination

Physical examination should be thorough and must include all of the cranial nerves. When the patient is conscious and cooperative, facial movements are examined carefully, comparing the affected side to the normal side. This is difficult in patients who suffer from bilateral facial nerve paralysis. The eyes should be carefully checked for Bell's phenomenon, keratitis, pupil size, nystagmus and movement of the extraocular muscles. Periorbital chemosis (raccoon sign) alerts the examiner to a skull base fracture.

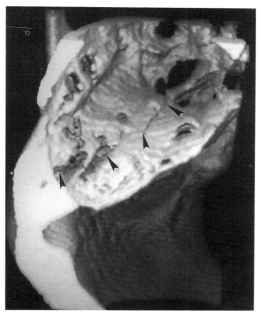

Fig. 5.**26** Three–dimensional reconstruction of high resolution CT scan showing oblique fracture plane.

Classification

- Complete
- Incomplete
- Immediate
- Delayed

Facial paralysis may not be apparent in the presence of severe head injury and coma. When discovered, facial paralysis may be complete or incomplete. Patients with incomplete paralysis should be watched carefully in order to detect, at the earliest possible time, a progression to complete paralysis. As long as the paralysis remains incomplete, a good prognosis is assured (Lambert and Brackmann, 1984).

In the majority of patients, paralysis is immediate. However, in one–tenth, delayed facial paralysis appears 24 to 36 hours following trauma. Delayed paralysis also has a good prognosis.

Grading

The assessment of facial function is very subjective and may vary between individual examiners. In order to avoid confusion, a 6–point grading system has been proposed by J. W. House (1983):

Grade I   Normal
Grade II   Mild dysfunction
Grade III   Moderate dysfunction
Grade IV   Moderately severe dysfunction
Grade V   Severe dysfunction
Grade VI   Total paralysis

An alternative scheme has been proposed by Stennert (1977 and 1979) involving the following two questionnaires.

Index for Paresis according to Stennert (1977):

Resting tone				
Eyelid slit difference	< 3 mm		3 mm or more	
Ectropion	no		yes	
Nasolabial groove lapsed (provided that it is present on the healthy side)	no		yes	
Depression of labial commissure	< 3 mm		3 mm or more	
Motility				
Frowning (formation of skin creases or, resp., elevation of eyebrows) [> 50%]	possible		not possible	
Residual lid slit — in sleeping position	no		yes	
Residual lid slit — at max. innervation	no		yes	
Exposure of teeth — upper and lower canines	visible		not visible	
Exposure of teeth — full width of second upper incisor	visible		not visible	
Apices of mouth (reduced separation between philtrum and angle of mouth as compared to healthy side)	50% or more		< 50%	
			Index for Paresis	☐

Index for Defective Healing according to Stennert (1979):

Hyperacusis		yes ☐		no ☐
Disorder of taste		yes ☐		no ☐
Synkinesia between:	☐ forehead ☐ eyes ☐ nasolabial crease ☐ angle of mouth ☐ chin		no	yes
	more than 3 regions			
Generalized blinking ("sec. spasm")				
Contractures				
Lacrimal secretion	less than 70%			
Lacrimal secretion	less than 70% with residual lip slit			
Lacrimal secretion	0%			
Crocodile tears				
Index for Defective Healing				☐

Imaging

High resolution computed tomography (HRCT) of the temporal bones provides in excellent view of the facial nerve canal. Fracture planes are also clearly seen as they cross the temporal bone. HRCT is performed by obtaining 25 to 30 pretargetted axial slices, 1.5 mm thick at 1 mm increments, from the base of skull to the tegmen. Direct coronal pretargetted 1.5 mm sections are performed when possible. Multiplanar reconstruction is achieved using a special algorithm to process data in sagittal, coronal or other planes (Aguilar et al., 1985).

Magnetic resonance imaging, with or without gadolinium enhancement, does not appear to be useful in demonstrating facial nerve lesions in temporal bone fractures (Millen et al., 1990).

Audiologic Testing

Audiology is performed as soon as the patient's condition allows. In addition to the hearing loss associated with temporal bone fractures, the stapedius muscle reflex must be assessed.

Topodiagnosis

It is important to determine the site of injury along the path of the facial nerve. Several topodiagnostic tests have been devised, ranging from electrogustometry and submaxillary salivary flow tests to the stapedius reflex and Schirmer's test. Schirmer's test and the stapedius reflex are still used, while the others have been abandoned.

Schirmer's Test

Since the surgical approach to the facial nerve depends mainly on whether the injury is proximal or distal to the geniculate ganglion, Schirmer's test is the most useful topodiagnostic study. The result is considered positive if lacrimation is reduced unilaterally by more than 30% of the total lacrimation secretion, or when the total amount of lacrimation is less than 25 mm (Fisch, 1980).

Stapedius Reflex

When present, the stapedius reflex indicates that the injury to the facial nerve is distal to the stapedius muscle.

Electrodiagnostic Tests

These tests are used to determine the extent of nerve degeneration and to assist the otolaryngologist in deciding on a further course of action.

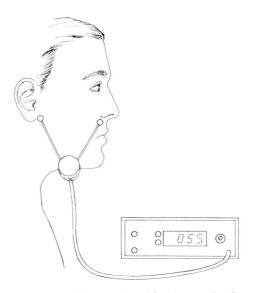

Fig. 5.**27**   Nerve excitability testing with a nerve stimulator.

Nerve Excitability Test

Nerve excitability testing determines the lowest electric current necessary to produce a facial twitch in the affected side of the face and compares this threshold value to the normal side. This test is performed with a nerve stimulator (Fig. 5.**27**) and a difference of 3.5 mA or greater suggests a poor prognosis.

Maximal Stimulation Test

In the maximal stimulation test, the stimulator is initially set at 5 mA and increased to the level of the patient's tolerance. The responses of the affected side are compared with those of the normal side. Patients tested within 10 days of the onset have a 92% chance of complete recovery when the responses are equal on both sides. Markedly decreased responses indicate a 73% chance of incomplete recovery, while those with no response always have an imcomplete recovery. This test is more accurate than the nerve excitability test because it recruits both large and small nerve fibers (Blumenthal and May, 1986).

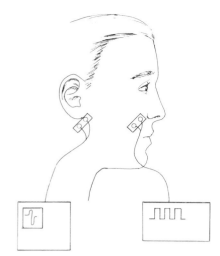

Fig. 5.**28**   Electroneuronography.

Electroneuronography (ENoG)

This test measures electrically evoked facial muscle compound action potentials. It utilizes bipolar surface electrodes for both stimulation and recording (Fig. 5.**28**). A supramaximal stimulus is used to obtain a smooth biphasic compound action potential. Response amplitude is compared to the contralateral side and a percent reduction is calculated. This reduction correlates well with axonal degeneration. An amplitude reduction of 90% or more is associated with a 91% chance of incomplete recovery. Electroneuronography has the greatest prognostic accuracy of all electrodiagnostic tests (Kartush and Prass, 1988).

Electromyography

This test uses intramuscular needle electrodes to measure electrical responses at rest and during volitional movement. If degeneration sets in, fibrillation potentials start appearing 14 to 21 days after the onset of paralysis. Electromyography is beneficial in detecting early regeneration (Kartush and Prass, 1988).

Indications

Surgery is indicated in patients who show no response or show a barely discernible response upon 10 mA of stimulation with the nerve stimulator. With electroneuronography, exploration is indicated if there is degeneration of 90% or more of motor nerve fibers within six days of the onset of the paralysis.

- Transected nerve.
- Immediate, complete paralysis
  — no response or markedly reduced response to 10 mA maximal stimulation from 48 hours to 10 days after injury,

  — or 90% degeneration on ENoG within 6 days after onset of paralysis.
- Patient seen one month after onset
  — no regeneration potentials by EMG 4 to 6 months after onset of paralysis.

Goal of the Operation

- Exploration of facial nerve from labyrinthine portion to stylomastoid foramen.
- Removal of bony fragments compressing nerve.
- Reanastomosing or grafting transected nerve.

The initial surgical approach for all patients, even those with a positive Schirmer's test, is a transmastoid–facial recess exploration of the tympanic and mastoid portions of the nerve. Patients with a positive Schirmer's test should then undergo inspection of the geniculate ganglion and distal portion of the labyrinthine segment of the nerve. This can be achieved either via the middle fossa approach or through the transmastoid–extralabyrinthine–subtemporal approach (Fisch, 1980). The type of approach used to explore the labyrinthine portion of the facial nerve is a subject of personal preference. May, who originally described the transmastoid–extralabyrinthine–subtemporal approach, is able to explore the geniculate ganglion and distal portion of the nerve without disturbing the hearing in all cases and without having to resort to the middle fossa approach (May, 1983). Other authors have found this technique useful in the majority of cases, but have had to resort to the middle fossa approach in 7% of their cases (Zini et al., 1985). Lambert and Brackmann used this technique in 20% of their cases (Lambert and Brackmann, 1984) and Ghorayeb and Rafie in 18% (Ghorayeb and Rafie 1989).

In longitudinal fractures, the site of facial nerve injury is in the perigeniculate area (1—2 mm distal and proximal to the ganglion) in approximately 80% of cases (Lambert and Brackmann, 1984; Zini et al., 1985; Fisch, 1980). The most common finding at exploration is the presence of bony spicules impinging on the nerve at the fracture site (Lambert and Brackmann, 1984). Fisch (1980) describes bony fragments in 20% only, while complete section of the nerve distal to the genu was observed in 30% and intraneural hematoma in 50% of longitudinal fractures.

The results of surgery are encouraging with facial movement returning in 80% to 92% of the cases. The timing of surgery is still an unresolved issue. While most authors advocate early facial nerve exploration if electrodiagnostic tests show evidence of degeneration within 48 hours to 6 days post–injury, others have decompressed facial nerves 3 to 14 months after the injury with good recovery of facial function within 6 months of the surgery (Lambert and Brackmann, 1984; Brodsky et al., 1983).

When the nerve is transected, every effort should be made to reapproximate the segments. If this cannot be achieved without tension, a greater auricular nerve cable graft is interposed between the distal and proximal segments.

Preparation for Surgery

Neurological Status

Because a number of patients with temporal bone fractures have other interrelated neurological problems, it is essential that the patient be cleared from a neurosurgical standpoint before being submitted to prolonged surgery.

Permission for Middle Fossa Exploration

Although in most cases a transmastoid–extralabyrinthine approach is adequate to explore the facial nerve from the labyrinthine portion to the stylomastoid foramen, it may sometimes be necessary to resort to a middle fossa approach. It is therefore necessary to obtain permission for a middle fossa approach and to enlist the aid of a neurosurgeon, if needed.

Head Shaving

In preparing the patient for surgery, it is important to have the temple adequately shaved in case a middle fossa approach is used.

Anesthesia

- General

Operative Technique

Transmastoid–Extralabyrinthine

The ear and neck are prepared and draped in such a way as to allow access to the neck in case a greater auricular nerve graft is needed.

A postauricular incision is performed and carried medially through soft tissue to the mastoid cortex where the fracture line may be readily apparent (Fig. 5.**29**). The periosteum is incised and elevated to expose the external auditory canal anteriorly. Self retaining retractors are applied and a simple mastoidectomy is performed. The lateral semicircular canal is identified in the floor of the mastoid antrum. The cavity is enlarged

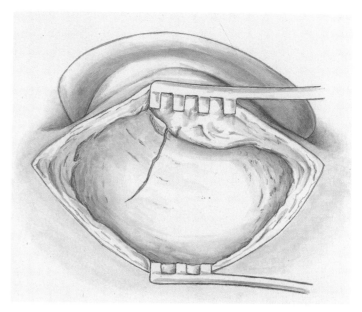

Fig. 5.**29** Oblique fracture line involving mastoid cortex and Henle's spine.

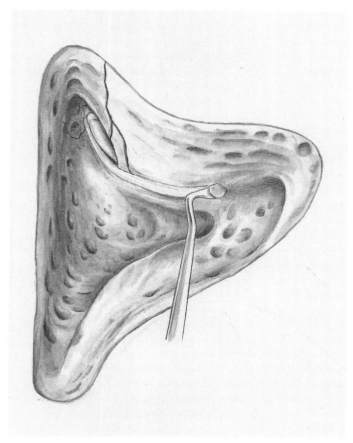

Fig. 5.**30**   Transmastoid extralabyrinthine facial nerve exploration.

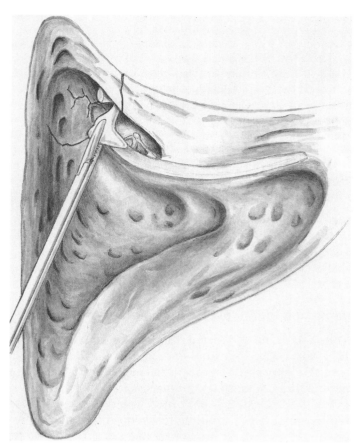

Fig. 5.**31**   Dislocation and rotation of incus to expose facial nerve.

to expose the tegmen superiorly, the sigmoid sinus pos-teriorly, and the digastric ridge inferiorly. The sinodural angle is opened and the sigmoid sinus skeletonized. The posterior and superior bony canal walls are thinned and the incus is identified in the aditus. The facial recess is opened between the fossa incudis superiorly, the chorda tympani inferiorly, and the descending facial nerve medially. This dissection is performed by care-fully thinning the posterior canal wall with a small dia-mond burr, until the ossicles are seen in the middle ear. Continuous irrigation should be used when drilling near the facial nerve to prevent thermal injury. The fa-cial nerve is identified from the cochleariform process to the stylomastoid foramen. Its canal is unroofed with the drill or a fine curette. The horizontal facial canal is very thin and does not require drilling. It is easily un-roofed with a curette. The descending portion is better skeletonized with the drill until a fine shell of bone re-mains. This is removed with a curette or a dental excava-tor. With this dissection, the facial nerve can be exposed from the processus cochleariformis to the stylomastoid foramen without disturbing the ossicles (Fig. 5.**30**).

When the labyrinthine portion of the facial nerve needs to be explored, it becomes impossible to follow

the nerve proximally without disturbing the ossicular chain. At this point, many surgeons opt for the middle fossa approach in the belief that this is a safer pro-cedure. On the other hand, May, who developed the transmastoid–extralabyrinthine approach, believes that the distal 3 mm of the labyrinthine portion can be reached through the mastoid approach by working under the dura and just above the ampullated ends of the horizontal and superior semicircular canals. This usually requires dislocation and rotation of the incus. May also believes that this approach can be performed safely and with less morbidity than the middle fossa ap-proach (Brackmann, 1986). Zini et al. describe a pro-cedure which is identical to that of May's, however, they routinely remove the incus. The ossicular chain is then reconstructed at the end of the procedure (Zini, 1985).

If the surgeon chooses to continue through the mas-toid, the incudostapedial joint is disarticulated. The bridge over the fossa incudis is shaved with the drill, so that the entire body of the incus is exposed. The incus is then separated from the malleus and rotated toward the aditus. This maneuver allows exploration proximal to the cochleariform process (Fig. 5.**31**). The incus is

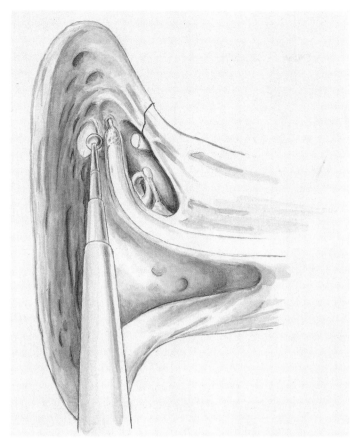

Fig. 5.**32** Drilling a hole in the tegmen facilitates identification of facial nerve in the middle fossa.

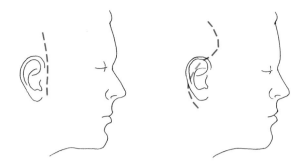

Fig. 5.**33** Incisions for middle fossa approach.

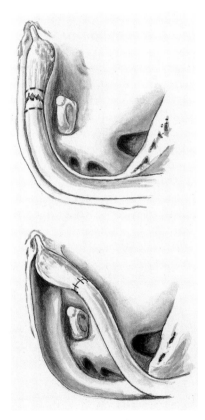

Fig. 5.**34** Rerouting of the facial nerve.

then replaced in its anatomical position (May et al., 1986).

Middle Fossa Exploration

If one chooses to continue exploration of the labyrinthine segment via a middle fossa approach, it is worthwhile to drill the tegmen tympani at the level of the geniculate ganglion (i.e. at the level of the cochleariform process) until the middle fossa dura is exposed (Fig. 5.**32**). This window in the tegmen facilitates the middle fossa procedure by making the geniculate ganglion readily visible from above.

The postauricular incision may be extended superiorly and anteriorly in a "lazy S" to reach the temple. The upper extremity of the incision should reach 5—6 cm above the top of the auricle. If a separate incision is preferred, it is usually placed 0.5 cm anterior to the tragus and curved gently posterosuperiorly (Fig. 5.**33**).

The details of the middle fossa operation are discussed in detail elsewhere in this book (see page 313).

Anastomosis

For small defects, every attempt should be made to anastomose a severed facial nerve by approximating the distal and proximal segments without tension. In order to gain a few millimeters, the nerve is removed from its bony canal and rerouted (Fig. 5.**34**). The ends of the severed nerve are freshened with a blade, approximated and covered with a piece of temporalis fascia.

Grafting with Greater Auricular Nerve

For larger defects, or in situations where rerouting and end–to–end anastomosis have failed, cable grafting with a segment of greater auricular nerve is an alternative. The greater auricular nerve has roughly the same diameter as the facial nerve and is readily available for harvesting as it crosses the lateral surface of the upper third of the sternocleidomastoid muscle (Fig. 5.**35**). The graft is interposed between the freshened ends of the facial nerve and covered with a piece of temporalis fascia (Fig. 5.**36**).

Surgical Landmarks and Danger Points

- *Digastric ridge, lateral semicircular canal, fossa incudis:* In a fractured temporal bone, the anatomy may be distorted and one should proceed carefully while drilling the mastoid in search of the facial nerve. The landmarks are the same as in any other mastoid operation. They include the digastric ridge and the lateral semicircular canal. If the incus cannot be found, the fossa incudis is still a good landmark. The cochleariform process and tensor tympani tendon should also be identified in order to locate the geniculate ganglion.
- *Bleeding from fracture line:* Bleeding from the fracture line can be annoying. One way of controlling this constant ooze of blood is by applying bone wax to the source of bleeding.
- *Distorted anatomy.*
- *Vibratory trauma to inner ear:* When the ossicular chain is intact, the incudostapedial joint may be disconnected to avoid the transmission of vibrations from the drill to the inner ear.
- *Brain herniation, CSF leak:* Defects in the tegmen around fracture lines may be associated with brain herniation and cerebrospinal fluid leak or both. Sometimes, vigorous dissection may detach or disturb the fibrous union of bony fragments precipitating a leak. Small defects are plugged with a piece of temporalis muscle. Larger defects may require a craniotomy.
- *Bleeding from fractured sigmoid sinus:* Fortunately, fractures of the sigmoid sinus are rare because fracture lines tend to run anterior and parallel to the sigmoid sinus. Bleeding from the sigmoid sinus tamponnades quickly, but may resume at surgery if the blood clot, or granulation tissue, are disturbed. The sinus is packed extraluminally with oxidized regenerated cellulose (Surgicel) to control hemorrhage.

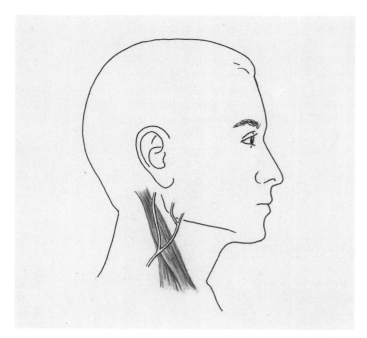

Fig. 5.**35**   Greater auricular nerve crossing sternocleidomastoid.

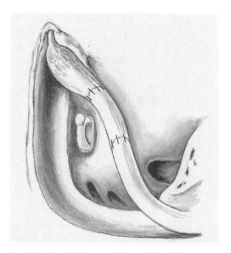

Fig. 5.**36**   Cable grafting of facial nerve.

Rules, Tips, and Pitfalls

● Associated brain injuries.

Postoperative Care

Exposure keratitis should be avoided. This is achieved by one or more of the following methods:
● Artificial tears,
● Patching of eye,
● Tarsorrhaphy,
● Gold lid weight.

Postoperative Complications

● Meningitis.
● Seizures.
● Hearing loss and tinnitus.

Sequelae

● Incomplete recovery.
● Mass movements.
The majority of patients in whom facial nerve continuity is preserved will recover facial function. The earlier recovery begins, the better the results will be. Patients who start recovering three to six weeks postoperatively will have a satisfactory recovery. Those who start recovering three to six months postoperatively will have an incomplete recovery with synkinesis and spasm. Finally, those who do not show return of function until a year postoperatively rarely recover useful function (Brackmann, 1986; Editor's note).

Alternative Techniques

● Hypoglossofacial anastomosis.
● Spinal accessory to facial anastomosis.
Patients who do not recover facial function or show very little function a year after surgery are candidates for a hypoglossofacial anastomosis (Fig. 5.**37**). This procedure is usually performed two years following injury. Recovery is unusual if the procedure is performed after four years (Brackmann, 1986; Editor's note). Some surgeons prefer a spinal accessory to facial nerve anastomosis.

See also Vol. 1/II, Chapter 16.

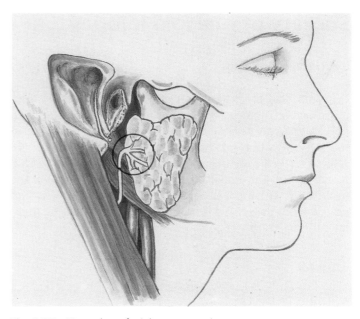

Fig. 5.**37**   Hypoglossofacial anastomosis.

Surgery of Mastoid Injuries

Incidence

Pure mastoid fractures are rare. In a series of 147 temporal bone fractures, Strohm found only one longitudinal fracture traversing the mastoid and terminating in the labyrinth behind the lateral semicircular canal. He also describes four other cases with atypical horizontal fractures of the mastoid which did not involve the middle ear. In one of these cases the mastoid tip was separated from the rest of temporal bone exposing the jugular bulb (Strohm, 1986).

Causes

- Blunt trauma.
- Gunshot wounds.

The majority of mastoid fractures are caused by blunt trauma. A smaller group result from gunshot wounds. In civilian population studies, the incidence of gunshot wounds varies greatly. Duncan et al. (1984) reported 22 cases from three major medical centers in 10 years. Ghorayeb and Rafie (1989) described 10 cases over a period of 4 years.

Diagnosis and Preoperative Evaluation

Physical Examination

Battle's Sign

This sign is not specific for mastoid fractures. It is an external sign of a temporal bone fracture, in particular, a fracture involving the base of the skull and mastoid bone. In essence, it is an ecchymosis of the postauricular skin which results from the extravasation of blood along the path of the posterior auricular artery.

Griesinger's Sign

Patients who develop sigmoid sinus thrombosis may present with an edematous swelling behind the mastoid bone, at the site of emergence of the mastoid emissary vein. This is the result of thrombosis of the emissary vein itself as the thrombus extends laterally.

Imaging

High Resolution CT

Fractures involving the mastoid bone are well demonstrated on high resolution computed tomography of the temporal bone. Usually, the mastoid air cells are

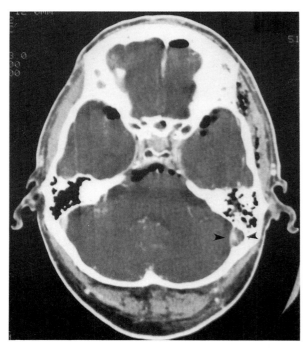

Fig. 5.**38**   High resolution CT showing sigmoid sinus thrombosis and central liquefaction of the thrombus.

clouded from blood and one may see an occasional air–fluid level. The sigmoid sinus may be involved by the fracture and show evidence of thrombosis, i. e., the lumen of the sinus is occluded with a soft tissue density. A liquified thrombus (Fig. 5.**38**) may show a central lucency inside the density (Ghorayeb et al., 1987). Sigmoid sinus thrombosis may also be diagnosed by magnetic resonance scanning with gadolinium.

Indications

Surgery for mastoid injury is indicated in the following situations:
- CSF otorrhea
- Brain herniation
- Cholesteatoma
- Sigmoid sinus thrombosis

Goal of the Operation

- Stop CSF leak
- Prevent meningitis
- Remove cholesteatoma
- Prevent intrasinus abscess formation

The sinus is usually explored as part of the facial nerve exploration. Should a sigmoid sinus thrombus become infected, an abscess may form inside the lumen and thrombophlebitis could extend to other sinuses. This is a dangerous situation requiring rapid surgical intervention. See also Chapter 9.

Preparation for Surgery

- Shaving
- Permission to ligate internal jugular vein
- Permission to obtain abdominal fat
- Typing and cross–matching blood

Generous head shaving is recommended for surgical exploration of the mastoid. The neck is also scrubbed and draped in case it is necessary to ligate the internal jugular vein.

Permission to harvest abdominal fat should be obtained. Fat is particularly useful to obliterate large defects through which brain may herniate into the mastoid. Fat is also a good seal for major cerebrospinal fluid leaks.

A thrombus (or in the case of a gunshot wound, the bullet, or its fragments) may become dislodged and embolize to the heart. To prevent this it is recommended to ligate the internal jugular vein on the side of the injury.

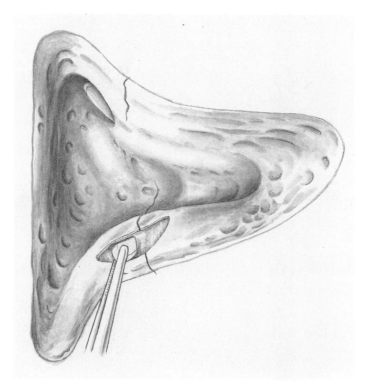

Fig. 5.**39**   Packing of sigmoid sinus.

Anesthesia

- General
- Mannitol and hyperventilation

In dealing with brain herniation, it is sometimes useful to give mannitol or ask the anesthesiologist to increase the ventilation rate, thus reducing brain swelling. This greatly facilitates the repair of defects from a mastoid approach.

Operative Technique

- Simple mastoidectomy
- Uncovering of sigmoid sinus
    — Packing sigmoid sinus
    — removal of thrombus
- Exposure of tegmen
    — Identification of CSF leak
    — Excision of herniated brain
    — Closure of tegmen defect
        — temporalis muscle flap
        — abdominal fat

A simple mastoidectomy is performed and the sigmoid sinus is skeletonized. The edges of the fracture are inspected and gently lifted away from the sinus. If the lumen of the sinus is open or if it is about to be surgically explored, it is safer to ligate the internal jugular vein in the neck. This is done through a separate neck in-

cision over the sternocleidomastoid. The posterior margin of the sternocleidomastoid is elevated to expose the internal jugular vein. The vein is identified inside the carotid sheath and ligated. The surgeon may now proceed with the removal of the thrombus or bullet fragment from within the lumen of the sigmoid sinus. The superior portion of the sinus may be packed with Gelfoam and muscle (Fig. 5.**39**) or may be closed with a suture ligature (Fig. 5.**40**).

Brain which has herniated into the mastoid is usually covered with a thick layer of glial tissue. The herniated brain is shaved at the level of the tegmen and packed into the middle fossa with a piece of temporalis muscle or fascia. Larger defects require a temporalis muscle rotation flap (Fig. 5.**41**) or abdominal fat grafting, or may need to be repaired through a craniotomy.

Surgical Landmarks and Danger Points

- Bleeding and distorted anatomy.
- Hemorrhage from sigmoid sinus.
- Dislodging thrombus.

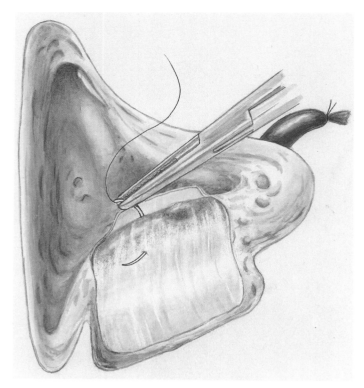

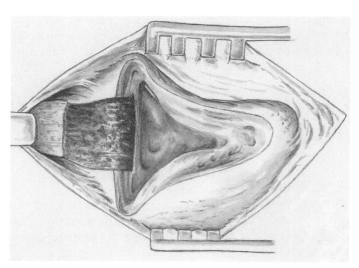

Fig. 5.**41**   Rotation of temporalis muscle flap into mastoid.

Fig. 5.**40**   Suture ligature around sigmoid sinus.

Postoperative Care

- Check for meningitis.
- Antibiotics.

Postoperative Complications

- Meningitis.

Bibliography

Aguilar EA, Ghorayeb BY, Hauser M, Yeakley JW, et al. High resolution CT scan of temporal bone fractures. XIII World Congress of Otolaryngology Abstracts, Vol. 1:36, 1985.

Bellucci RJ. Traumatic injuries of the middle ear. Otolaryngologic Clin North Am 633-50, 1983, 16(3).

Blumenthal F, May M. Electrodiagnosis. In: The Facial Nerve (May M, Ed.), Chapter 12, pp 241-263, New York: Thieme, 1986.

Brackmann DE. Otoneurosurgical procedures. In: The Facial Nerve (May M, Ed.), Chapter 33, pp 589-613, New York: Thieme, 1986.

Brodsky L, Evitar A, Daniler A. Post-traumatic facial nerve paralysis: three cases of delayed temporal bone exploration with recovery. Laryngoscope 1983; 93:1560-5.

Cannon CR, Jahrsdoerfer RA. Temporal bone fractures, review of 90 cases. Arch of Otolaryngol 1983; 109(5):285-8.

Duncan NO, Coker NJ, Jenkins HA, Canalis RF. Gunshot injuries to the temporal bone. Otolaryngol Head Neck Surg 1986; 94(1):47-55.

Fisch U. Management of infratemporal facial nerve injuries. J Laryngol Otol 1980; 94(1):129-34.

Ghorayeb BY, Rafie JJ. Fractures du rocher, bilan de 123 cas. Ann. Oto-Laryng. (Paris) 1989; 106:294-301.

Ghorayeb BY, Yeakley JW, Hall JW, Jones E. Unusual complications of temporal bone fractures. Arch Otolaryngol Head Neck Surg 1987; 113(7):749-53.

House JW. Facial nerve grading systems. Laryngoscope 1983; 93(8):1056-69.

Jahrsdoerfer RA, Hall JW. Congenital malformations of the ear. Am J Otol 1986; 7(4):267-9.

Kartush JM, Prass RL. Facial Nerve testing: Electroneuronography and intraoperative monitoring. Instructional courses, Volume 1, Chapter 21, pp 231-247; Johnson, Blitzer, Ossof, and Thomas, Eds, St. Louis: C. V. Mosby, 1988.

Lambert PR, Brackmann DE. Facial paralysis in longitudinal temporal bone fractures: a review of 26 cases. Laryngoscope 1984; 94(8):1022-6.

May M. Trauma to the facial nerve. Otolaryngol Clin North Am 1983; 16(3):661-70.

May M, Blumenthal F, Klein SR. Acute Bell's palsy: prognostic value of evoked electromyography, maximal stimulation and other electrical tests. Am J Otol 1983; 5:1.

May M, Prodvinec M, Ulrich J, Peiterson E, Klein S. Idiopathic (Bell's) palsy, herpes zoster cephalicus and other facial nerve disorders of viral origin. In: The Facial Nerve (May M, Ed.), Chapter 18, pp 365-399, New York: Thieme, 1986.

Millen SJ, Daniels D, Meyer G. Gadolinium-enhanced magnetic resonance imaging in facial nerve lesions. Otolaryngol Head Neck Surg 1990; 102(1):26-33.

Schubiger O, Valavanis A, Stuckmann G, Antonucci F. Temporal bone fractures and their complications, examination with high resolution CT. Neuroradiology 1986; 28(1):93-9.

Stennert E, Limburg CH, Frentrup KP. Parese- und Defektheilungs-Index. HNO 1977; 25:238-45.

Strohm M. Tympanic membrane lesions. Advances in Oto-Rhino-Laryngology. 1986; 35:6-71.

Zini C, Sanna M, Jemmi G, Gandolfi A. Transmastoid-extralabyrinthine approach in traumatic facial palsy. Am J Otolarnyngol 1985; 6(3):216-21.

6 Surgery for Tumors of the Middle Ear and Lateral Skull Base

Jan Helms

Surgery for Tumors of the Auditory Canal

Benign Tumors

Exostosis is the most common benign tumor occurring in the external auditory canal. The treatment of exostoses is described in Chapter 6.

Malignant Tumors

Malignant Tumors Outside the Tympanic Membrane

Preoperative Diagnostic Studies

A histologically confirmed malignant tumor of the external auditory canal requires a general tumor staging workup in addition to CT evaluation to detect possible infiltration of the petrous pyramid.

Indications

All malignant tumors that are confined to the external auditory canal should be managed by surgical extirpation.

Principle of the Operation

The tumor is extirpated with a margin of healthy tissue.

Preoperative Preparations

The patient is positioned as for a tympanoplasty (see page 81).

Anesthesia

The resection of tumors confined to the external auditory canal is usually performed under local anesthesia. General anesthesia may be appropriate for highly anxious or apprehensive patients.

Operative Technique

The ear is opened with a postauricular incision, and the meatal orifice is circumcized close to the conchal cavity. The tragal cartilage is also divided. The soft–tissue dissection is carried inferiorly to the stylomastoid foramen outside the petrous bone, and the facial nerve is exposed at that level (see Fig. 6.**1**).

Next the mastoid is opened, and the facial nerve is exposed from the lateral semicircular canal to the stylomastoid foramen (Fig. 6.**2**).

The posterior canal wall is thinned with a burr close to the tympanic anulus. The meatal skin is divided just outside the tympanic membrane. The tympanic bone is drilled open circumferentially around the tympanic anulus, taking care to leave the tympanic ring anchored in the bone. The meatal skin and the attached soft tissues in front of the tympanic bone and outside the tragus are progressively divided.

Finally the specimen, consisting of the tumor and the complete external auditory canal, is removed in one piece (Fig. 6.**3**).

The mastoidectomy cavity is closed with an inferiorly based, postauricular soft–tissue flap (Figs. 6.**4** and 6.**5**). If necessary, a cartilage autograft from the external ear can be implanted to keep the aditus patent and reconstruct the bridge. Skin grafts and prolonged packing are needed to achieve epithelialization and stabilization of the anterior canal wall.

Modifications

With a malignant tumor located so close to the tympanic membrane that clear margins cannot be confidently established on that side of the neoplasm, the tympanic membrane should be included in the resection (see page 112).

Landmarks and Pitfalls

The facial nerve should be preserved, so it should be identified at the stylomastoid foramen, as in a parotidectomy, and along its mastoid segment, as in any type of mastoid surgery, before extensive dissection or drilling are carried out.

Rules, Hints, and Common Errors

An en bloc resection should be attempted for all tumors of the external ear canal, including malignancies, and the margins of the specimen should consist entirely of noninfiltrated tissue. This strategy requires sufficiently

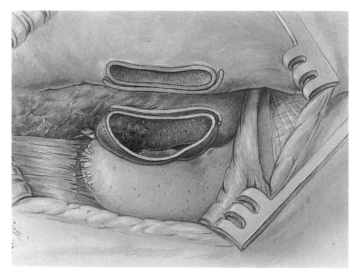

Fig. 6.**1**

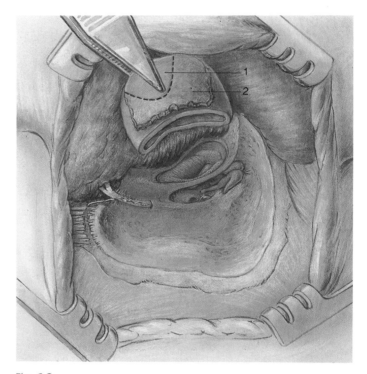

Fig. 6.**2**
1: Tumor is inside
2: Bony posterior canal wall

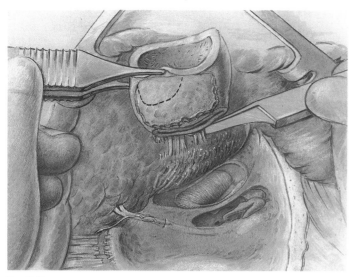

Fig. 6.**3**

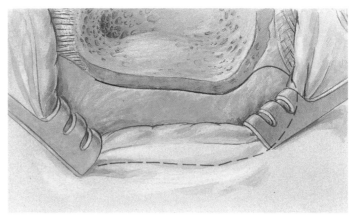

Fig. 6.**4**

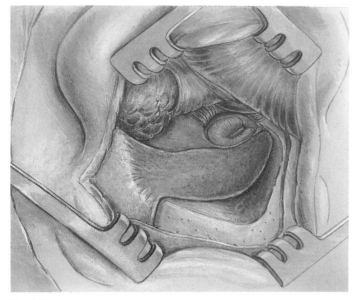

Fig. 6.**5**

broad dissection of the tissues surrounding the neoplasm, and this is facilitated by adequate mastoidectomy. A common error is inadequate dissection of the healthy tissues surrounding the tumor.

Postoperative Care

At the end of the operation, the external ear is lined with silicone sheeting and packed. The packing is removed at three weeks, as after a tympanoplasty, and may be replaced as often as required. Further postoperative measures are like those described for otologic surgery (see pages 101–102).

Postoperative Complications

An artery below the ear that was inadequately secured at operation can lead to profuse postoperative bleeding, necessitating surgical exposure and definitive control of the site. Rarely, perichondritis may develop following the routine perioperative use of prophylactic antibiotics.

Postoperative stenosis of the external ear canal is best avoided by leaving the meatal packing in place for a sufficient length of time. Re–epithelialization from the tympanic membrane should occur below the silicone lining. If this does not occur, thin split–thickness skin grafts are inserted in a subsequent operation.

Functional Sequelae

If meatal stenosis develops, it will generally result in conductive hearing loss. Dermatitis may develop as well as a cholesteatoma.

Alternative Methods

Local tumor excision and postoperative irradiation may be considered as an option in elderly patients with multiple morbidity.

Malignant Tumors of the External Auditory Canal with Involvement of the Tympanic Membrane

Preoperative Diagnostic Studies

Computed tomography can establish whether the tumor is an ear canal malignancy involving the tympanic membrane, or whether it is a carcinoma of the middle ear that has invaded the petrous bone. General tumor staging is also indicated.

Indications

The treatment of choice is surgical resection.

Principle of the Operation

The principle is to surgically encompass the tumor with an adequate margin of uninvolved tissue.

Preoperative Preparations

The preparations are the same as for a tympanoplasty (see page 80).

Anesthesia

General anesthesia is indicated due to the extent of the resection.

Operative Technique

Mastoidectomy is carried out, producing a funnel–shaped cavity with a wide inlet. For this purpose the soft tissues are widely dissected from the mastoid cortex (Fig. 6.**6**), and the auditory canal is opened (Fig. 6.**7**).

The external auditory canal is closed just below the conchal cavity. The anterior canal wall, with the tragal cartilage and the adjacent tympanic bone, is separated from the soft tissues.

A suture technique that everts the keratinizing squamous epithelium is used (Figs. 6.**8** and 6.**9**).

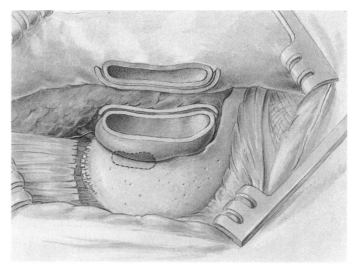

Fig. 6.**6**

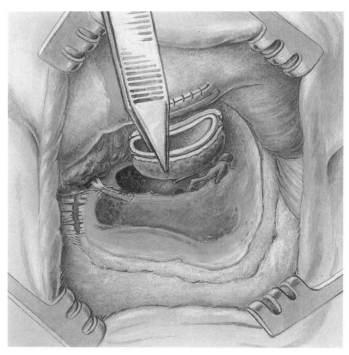

Fig. 6.**7**

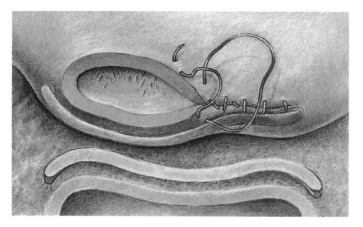

Fig. 6.**8**

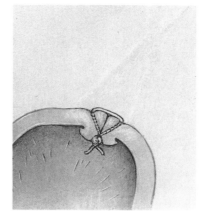

Fig. 6.**9**

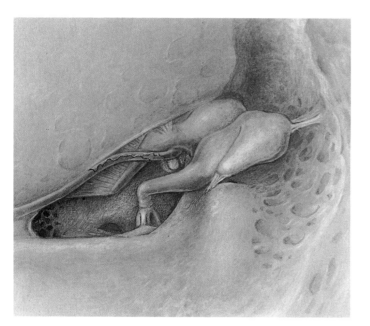

Fig. 6.**10**

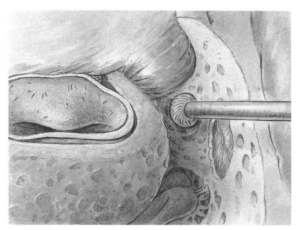

Fig. 6.**11**

The mastoid segment of the facial nerve is exposed until much of the promontory is visible through the chordofacial angle (Fig. 6.**10**). The posterior and inferior circumference of the tympanic anulus are identified. At this stage the floor of the auditory canal and the hypotympanum are clearly visible.

While retracting the surrounding soft tissues, the surgeon drills through tympanic bone between the epitympanum and the temporomandibular joint so that the posterior bony wall of the joint can be resected into the anterior part of the middle ear space (Fig. 6.**11**). This bone work can be accomplished more broadly and with better vision in an extensively pneumatized rather than in a small, dense petrous bone.

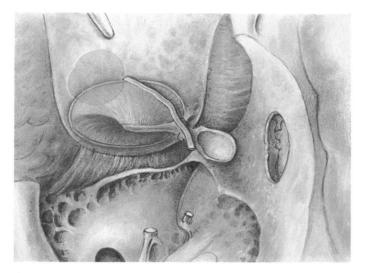

Fig. 6.**12**

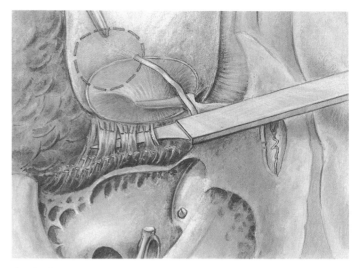

Fig. 6.**13**

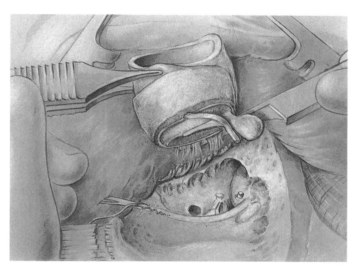

Fig. 6.**14**

The posterior wall of the temporomandibular joint is exposed above the auditory canal from the middle ear space, without opening the middle cranial fossa. Finally the tumor specimen is removed in continuity with the auditory canal and tympanic membrane (Figs. 6.**12**, 6.**13**, and 6.**14**). (The red area indicates the tumor in the external canal. The incus was removed, the tendon of the tensor tympani muscle transsected.)

Since all the walls of the external ear canal and tympanic membrane have been removed, there is little chance for the restoration of hearing. Generally, therefore, it is better to close the ear securely than attempt to restore hearing. A large, inferiorly based muscle and soft–tissue flap is transposed to seal off the ear canal.

Modifications

Local resection and postoperative irradiation (e. g., afterloading therapy) are a possible alternative to the above procedure. This option should be limited to patients with multiple morbidity who would be poor candidates for more extensive surgery.

Landmarks and Pitfalls

The facial nerve should remain intact throughout the procedure; it should not be traumatized. This is aided by identifying the tympanic portion of the nerve in the middle ear early in the operation and by exposing the nerve at the stylomastoid foramen, as would be done in the initial phase of a parotidectomy. The surgeon can safeguard the temporomandibular joint most effectively by staying very close to the cartilage and bone while dissecting the soft tissues from the anterior wall of the ear canal.

Rules, Hints, and Common Errors

The facial nerve should be positively identified before any extensive dissections are performed close to the nerve.

Closure of the external auditory canal should be done first, immediately after the opening phase, since this is far more difficult to accomplish later. The soft tissues about the auditory canal undergo considerable distortion during the operation, and the residual effects of these manipulations can make it difficult to close the external ear canal at a later stage in the procedure.

A common problem is to discover that preoperative CT images did not delineate the full extent of the tumor, i. e., failed to demonstrate invasion of the middle ear. Informed consent is generally inadequate in these cases, since the surgeon must proceed without regard for facial nerve function and conservation of hearing.

Postoperative Care

The wound area is inspected daily so that problems such as bleeding and infection can be detected early and managed appropriately.

Postoperative Complications

One potential complication is the development of a fistula in the sealed auditory canal. This usually results from deficient primary closure of the canal. Prolonged curettage or even reoperation may be required.

Functional Sequelae

Conductive hearing loss must be accepted as a functional sequel to this type of surgery.

Alternative Methods

Besides the modifications noted above, radiotherapy without surgery may be considered as an alternative. Radiotherapy alone, however, is less effective than surgery, which may be followed by radiotherapy as an adjunct.

Surgery for Tumors of the Middle Ear and its Surroundings

Subtotal Petrosectomy with Preservation of the Labyrinth

Preoperative Diagnostic Studies

A pulsatile "tumor" in the middle ear is routinely investigated by means of high–resolution computed tomography and angiography.

Preoperative Investigation of a Suspected Tumor

If a richly vascularized tumor is found in the middle ear space, therapeutic embolization should be attempted during preoperative angiography. Surgery is performed two to four days after preoperative embolization.

Preoperative Investigation of a Suspected Vascular Anomaly

If CT scans do not show the typical features of a glomus tumor but instead show continuity between the soft tissues of the middle ear and the internal carotid artery or jugular bulb, and if angiograms demonstrate a large vessel but no tumor, then embolization would not be indicated. The consulting neuroradiologist would proceed no farther than diagnostic angiography.

Indications

The procedure is indicated for benign tumors in the middle ear space and mastoid and for vascular anomalies (e. g., glomus tympanicum tumor, facial nerve neuroma, arachnoid cyst, ceruminoma, high jugular bulb, anomalous course of the internal carotid artery with involvement of the middle ear space).

While tumors in the middle ear almost invariably require operative treatment, vascular anomalies require surgery only if there is a significant mass effect caused by a hernia–like protrusion of the jugular bulb or an aneurysm in a large vessel. These are manifested by increasing subjective complaints and noticeable enlargement on CT scans taken at about three–month intervals.

Principles of the Operation

A tumor resection should include the complete removal of all neoplastic tissue.

The treatment of vascular anomalies involves the reduction of ectatic segments with the creation of new, pressure–resistant walls for the vascular bed.

Preoperative Preparations

The patient is positioned as for otologic surgery (see page 81).

Anesthesia

The operation is performed under general anesthesia.

Operative Technique

For the removal of a *glomus tympanicum tumor,* the ear is entered through a postauricular approach. The meatal skin is incised to permit exposure of the canal floor; it is dissected as far as the tympanic anulus (Fig. 6.**15**). The anulus is freed from its bony bed gradually, proceeding in small steps, since the lateral aspect of the tumor may be encountered at any moment. The surgeon should avoid opening the tumor if at all possible. Bleeding may obscure the field at this stage, and bipolar coagulation is used as needed. The meatal flap, including the inferior portions of the tympanic membrane, is resected and removed to provide free access for bone removal in the auditory canal.

The floor of the auditory canal is excavated with a cutting burr until the lower portions of the tumor can be seen (Fig. 6.**16**). Feeding vessels are either occluded with bipolar cautery or sealed off by drilling with a low–speed diamond burr (Figs. 6.**17** and 6.**18**). Care is taken to keep instruments from touching the intact ossicular chain and round window. The frequently large vessels that course to the eustachian tube in the mucosa (anterior tympanic artery) can be coagulated with bipolar forceps. If the petrous bone is extensively pneumatized, additional bone is removed between the basal turn of the cochlea in the anterior part of the promontory and the floor of the tubal entrance, if necessary, exposing the lateral wall of the internal carotid artery to permit the removal of tumor remnants in that area.

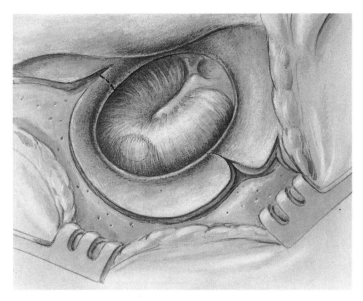

Fig. 6.**15**

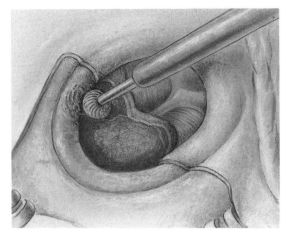

Fig. 6.**16**

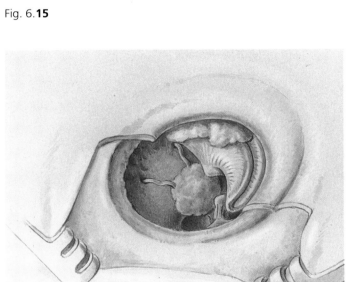

Fig. 6.**17**

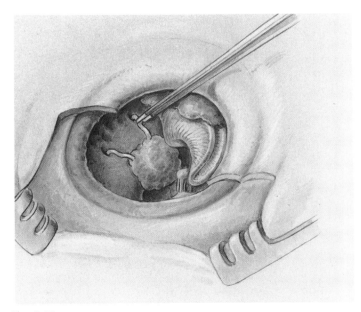

Fig. 6.**18**

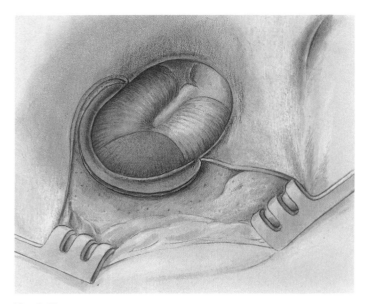

Fig. 6.**19**

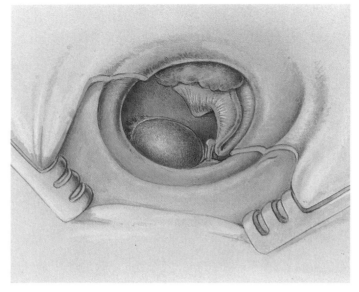

Fig. 6.**20**

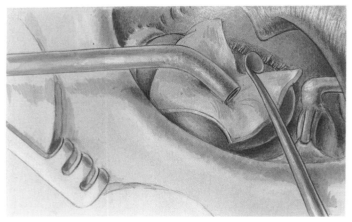

Fig. 6.**21**

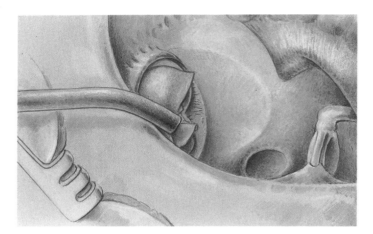

Fig. 6.**22**

In cases where an *ectatic jugular bulb* has produced pulsatile tinnitus or conductive hearing loss (Fig. 6.**19**), the ear is entered using the same technique as for a small glomus tumor. Again, the floor of the ear canal is burred down at its junction with the middle ear without opening the jugular bulb (Fig. 6.**20**). A piece of banked dura is placed on top of the high–riding bulb so that pressure can be applied broadly to the bulb without opening it (Figs. 6.**21** and 6.**22**). Adhesions bordering the bed of the jugular bulb are progressively freed from the bone by sharp dissection so that the bulb can gradually be displaced inferiorly to a normal level.

A wafer of bone cement, prehardened to a doughy texture, is placed over the fixed dura protecting the top of the bulb and is pushed down to the level of the hypotympanum. Over the next few minutes the cement will harden, protecting the jugular bulb and permanently separating it from the middle ear (Fig. 6.**23**).

Very rarely, the vascular anomaly will involve an aneurysmal dilatation of the *internal carotid artery* secondary to partial aplasia of the vessel. In this case the technique for exposing the carotid is like that described previously for small glomus tumors or the reduction of an ectatic jugular bulb. The exposed carotid artery is encased with bone cement to construct a new, stable canal for the vessel (Figs. 6.**24** and 6.**25**).

Smaller *facial nerve neuromas* confined to the middle ear and mastoid present a tumor–like contour behind the tympanic membrane. The absence of pulsations in the pale red lesion distinguishes it from a glomus tumor or aberrant blood vessel.

Operative treatment involves extensive excavation of the mastoid, antrum, and epitympanum without altering the external auditory canal or tympanic membrane.

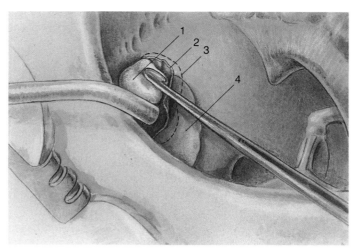

Fig. 6.23
1: Viscous bone cement
2: Margin of dural onlay
3: Bony margin that will support cement
4: Bed of the high jugular bulb at the start of the operation

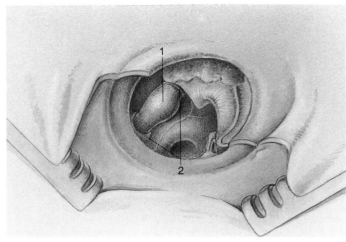

Fig. 6.24
1: Aneurysm
2: Vascular canal

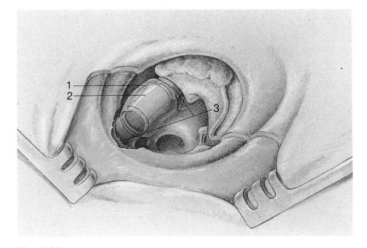

Fig. 6.25
1: Cement sheath
2: Preserved dura
3: Ends of bony vascular canal

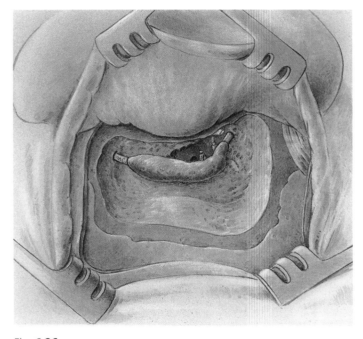

Fig. 6.26

The tumor is approached by the postauricular route (see page 60). Tumor exposure with preservation of the labyrinth is achieved by clearing the surrounding mastoid cells until the tumor can be lifted from its bony bed (Fig. 6.**26**). The resection should extend far enough toward the stylomastoid foramen and geniculate ganglion to encompass healthy nerve tissue. Occasional tumors are associated with some degree of ossicular erosion or even erosion of the lateral semicircular canal. These defects are managed accordingly (see page 119 and page 98).

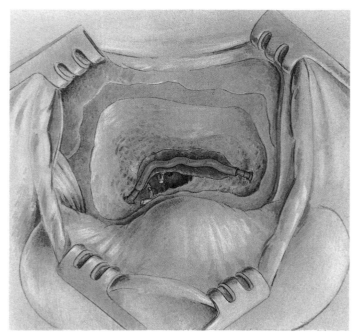

Fig. 6.**27**

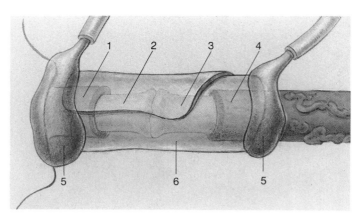

Fig. 6.**28**
1: Epineurium
2: Axonal tissue
3: Axonal tissue of the graft
4: Graft epineurium
5: Fibrin glue
6: Collagen film

About 2—3 mm of epineurium is removed from the central and peripheral nerve stumps. An adequate length of nerve autograft, similarly prepared and preferably taken from the great auricular nerve, is interposed. The fresh cut ends of the nerves are fully and evenly approximated (Fig. 6.**27**).

It is advantageous to wrap the anastomotic sites with pieces of thin collagen film to prevent any premature ingrowth of connective tissue from around the anastomosis. The collagen film can be secured with fibrin glue (Fig. 6.**28**).

If neuroma has grown past the stylomastoid foramen into the parotid gland, the exposure must be extended until healthy nerve tissue, perhaps even past the main division of the facial nerve, can be seen within the parotid gland. A transaxonal anastomosis is performed in the soft tissue at that level using simple interrupted sutures. The essential mechanical stability of the nerve is restored by encasing it in collagen film secured with fibrin glue.

If tumor has spread to the geniculate ganglion or farther toward the internal auditory canal or even the posterior cranial fossa while hearing is still intact, the operation must be extended to a transtemporal procedure (see page 223). At the intracranial level as well, the central nerve stump is fixed using simple interrupted sutures reinforced with a collagen sheath and fibrin glue. If the nerve suture proves too difficult, a graft can be interposed using collagen and fibrin glue without sutures. Adhesive can even be used to attach a cable graft directly at the site of emergence of the facial nerve from the brainstem. For mechanical stability about 1 cm of the graft is glued to the brain surface, and the graft is passed without tension through the petrous bone and anatomosed peripherally.

Modifications

The procedure described above for benign tumors or vascular anomalies can be modified only by using different materials to reconstruct a stable vascular channel. The implantation of solid prefabricated ceramic half–shells is a possible option, but the use of individually sculpted bone cement has proven very effective.

Landmarks and Pitfalls

The same middle ear structures that figure in the surgery of inflammatory diseases (tympanoplasty) constitute the principal landmarks and hazards. One pitfall is the inadequate primary diagnostic workup of an apparently small glomus tumor, especially the failure to obtain an angiogram. Unexpected intraoperative findings may compel the surgeon to discontinue the procedure pending a more complete workup and new informed consent.

Rules, Hints, and Common Errors

Angiography should routinely precede the treatment of glomus tumors or vascular anomalies in the middle ear. This reduces the likelihood of diagnostic error (glomus tumor vs. a large vessel). Tumor removal is facilitated by exposing the lateral aspect of the tumor as broadly as possible before removal is begun. A common error is failure to follow all of the tumor below the basal turn of the cochlea. Tumor remnants left in that area can lead to a "recurrence."

Postoperative Care

The postoperative regimen is the same as that following tympanoplasty (see page 101). Patients who have undergone the excision of a facial nerve neuroma should be advised that much time will be needed for nerve regeneration to occur. At least six months will pass before there is any evidence of reinnervation, and that may be detectable only by myography. In approximately 80% of cases the definitive result in mobility of the face is achieved by about one year.

Therapeutic electrical stimulation starting, say, four months after surgery will not delay the return of nerve function at about six months but neither will it accelerate that process, even though the physician and (grateful) patient may mistakenly regard electrostimulation as a valuable adjunct. Training of facial movements in front of a mirror may be helpful.

Postoperative Complications

The persistence of conductive hearing loss is a potential complication that may follow the above procedures. Sensorineural hearing loss can result from extensive bone work at the promontory, destruction of the round window, or a labyrinthine fistula.

Functional Sequelae

Occasionally a degree of hearing loss must be accepted. The often distressful preoperative pulsatile tinnitus is consistently improved by the surgery.

Alternative Methods

Glomus tumors are occasionally treated with irradiation, but this therapy is inadequate, especially for smaller tumors. There are no alternatives to the techniques described above for the surgical treatment of vascular anomalies and facial nerve neuromas.

Supralabyrinthine Subtotal Petrosectomy with Preservation of the Labyrinth or with Labyrinthectomy

This technique is indicated for benign tumors in the middle ear, mastoid, and those medial and superior to the labyrinth.

Preoperative Diagnostic Studies

Besides function tests (audiometry, electrophysiologic facial nerve testing), the preoperative workup should include imaging of the lesion by high–resolution computed tomography. Magnetic resonance imaging is also indicated in select cases to evaluate for intracranial extension.

Indications

A true *cholesteatoma* (epidermoid), *meningioma*, or *facial nerve neuroma* involving the medial portion of the petrous bone should be managed by surgical removal. A true *petrous apex cholesteatoma* located medial to the labyrinth can be resected by the transtemporal route. The procedure in this case corresponds to that used for a small acoustic neuroma (see page 313). Many of these tumors extend from the middle ear to the petrous apex at the time of diagnosis, necessitating translabyrinthine removal. Preservation of the cochlea may be feasible in these cases owing to the presence of connective tissue separating the cholesteatoma from the perilymphatic space.

In patients with multiple morbidity, it is acceptable to monitor the growth of the mass in the pyramid by obtaining follow–up films at six months. The anesthetic risk and postoperative balance disturbance justify a "wait–and–scan" approach in these patients.

Principle of the Operation

Surgery aims at the complete removal of the neoplasm, if possible, with conservation of hearing and facial nerve function. If the labyrinth (vestibular organ and cochlea) is resected due, for example, to the ingrowth of cholesteatoma into the perilymphatic space, a translabyrinthine or transotic (Fisch) approach is used. The facial nerve can be transposed without serious loss of function, permitting, for example, the removal of tumor matrix from all aspects of the facial nerve epineurium. The internal auditory canal is opened in these cases to access the matrix in the fundal portion of the canal. The extensive mastoidectomy cavity is then obliterated.

The tympanic orifice of the eustachian tube can also be closed to prevent ascending infection.

An alternative concept involves sealing off the internal auditory canal and establishing drainage of the petrous cell mucosa through the eustachian tube to the nasopharynx. The advantage of this method is that it prevents the formation of a mucocele or cholesterol granuloma, which can occur following inadequate mastoidectomy and closure of the eustachian tube.

Preoperative Preparations

The patient is positioned as for other types of otologic surgery (see page 81). Only the transtemporal approach requires special positioning (see page 223).

Anesthesia

The operation is performed under general anesthesia.

Operative Technique

The mastoid and middle ear space are widely opened through a postauricular incision. The mastoidectomy leaves a thin layer of bone covering the middle fossa dura superiorly and the sigmoid sinus posteriorly. The posterior wall of the auditory canal is thinned to about 1 mm. The facial nerve canal below the lateral semicircular canal is burred down until the nerve is clearly identified, leaving a thin bony layer covering the epineurium. Cholesteatoma extensions into the antrum and epitympanum are removed (Fig. 6.29).

The semicircular canals are progressively burred down until the inferior portions of the cholesteatoma can be seen and the matrix can be elevated. If the cholesteatoma is not too large, it may be possible to preserve hearing despite destruction of the semicircular canal system and remove all matrix from the petrous apex medial to the superior semicircular canal.

Leaving matrix behind will of course lead to residual cholesteatoma and is incompatible with hearing conservation. If the cholesteatoma has infiltrated large portions of the cochlea or has spread forward below the labyrinthine segment of the facial nerve, a corresponding cochlear resection is required. The matrix is completely exposed and removed along with adherent vestibular nerves, for example (Fig. 6.30). This creates a cerebrospinal fluid (CSF) fistula in the fundus of the internal auditory canal.

When all matrix has been removed, this dural opening below and behind the facial nerve is repaired by covering it with a free muscle flap and then preserved

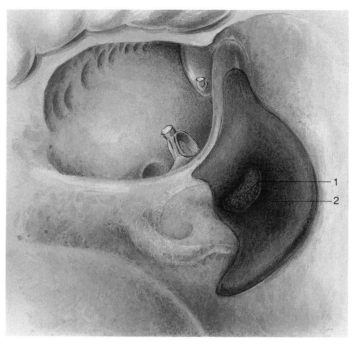

Fig. 6.**29**
1: Debris
2: Matrix

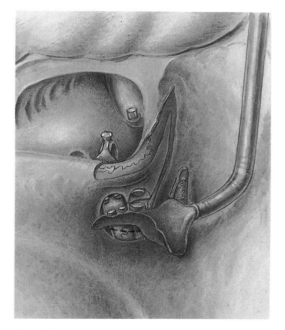

Fig. 6.**30**

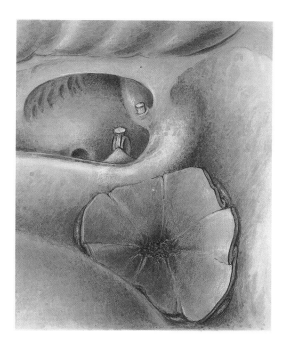

Fig. 6.**31**

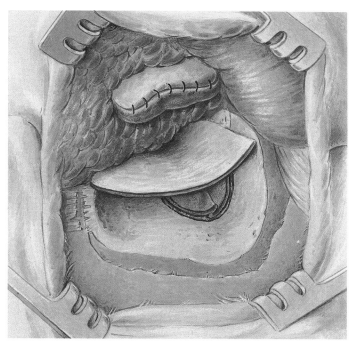

Fig. 6.**32**

dura, both attached with tissue adhesive (Fig. 6.**31**). To avoid subsequent CSF leak, the funnel–shaped cavity in the petrous apex should be packed with autogenous soft tissue, such as abdominal fat, or sealed off with a hard material like bone cement. The entire mastoid also may be obliterated (e. g., with abdominal fat) after clearing all the mastoid cells and occluding the tympanic tubal orifice.

If the posterior canal wall has been partially or completely removed to follow an anterior extension of cholesteatoma, or if the tympanic membrane has been removed to access, say, the region of the anterior hypotympanum and the area about the internal carotid artery, cartilage can be implanted to separate the middle ear and mastoid spaces from the external ear canal (Fig. 6.**32**), or the ear canal can be closed below the level of the concha (see Fig. 6.**8**). The latter procedure requires the previous clearing of all mastoid and pyramidal cells and the resection of all keratinizing squamous epithelium from the tympanic membrane and external canal in the area of the closure. This is necessary to prevent the formation of a cholesteatoma, mucocele, or cholesterol granuloma (Fig. 6.**24**).

Preoperative imaging studies do not demonstrate the extent of a petrous apex cholesteatoma with complete precision. Consequently, the matrix must be systematically exposed and identified during the operation and progressively elevated from underlying structures. Sometimes very thin matrix shells that have formed in small, preformed spaces may overlie more extensive

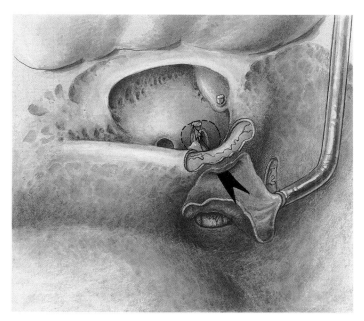

Fig. 6.**33**

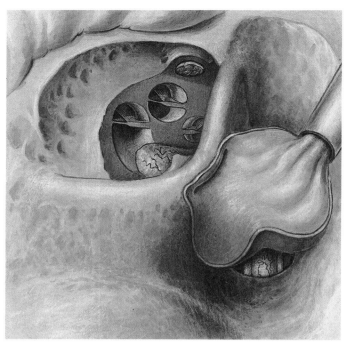

Fig. 6.**34**

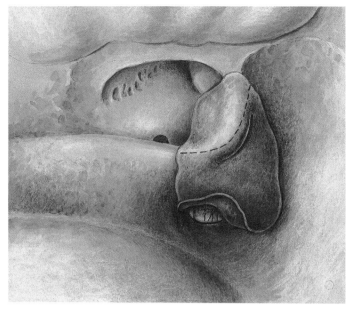

Fig. 6.**35**

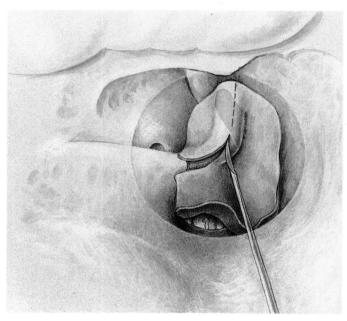

Fig. 6.**36**

zones of cholesteatoma growth involving, say, the cochlea or the internal auditory canal (Fig. 6.**33**). The surrounding bone, including overhangs, should be taken down in these cases to allow complete matrix removal from all turns of the cochlea and from the internal auditory canal (Fig. 6.**34**).

With a very delicate matrix, it is difficult to distinguish the final keratin layer of the cholesteatoma sac from the matrix tissue that has to be removed. The matrix is always located on a subepithelial layer of connective tissue that is traversed by blood vessels. In doubtful cases this vascularized, often transparent layer should be elevated from the substrate along with the matrix and removed.

If the cholesteatoma has invaded the internal auditory canal, Scarpa's ganglion should also be removed to minimize postoperative vertigo (see Fig. 6.**30**).

Matrix that encases the facial nerve is incised along the lateral wall of the mastoid segment of the facial nerve and is dissected medially around the nerve establish a plane of separation (Figs. 6.**35** and 6.**36**). The greater petrosal nerve is divided at the geniculate ganglion to permit upward mobilization of the facial nerve (Fig. 6.**37**).

By repeated superior and lateral displacement of the facial nerve, it should be possible to dissect all of the matrix from the nerve. These manipulations must not compromise the continuity of the nerve.

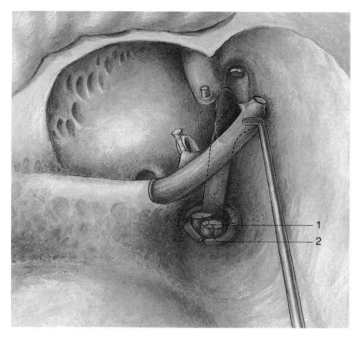

Fig. 6.**37**
1: Vestibular nerve
2: Cochlear nerve

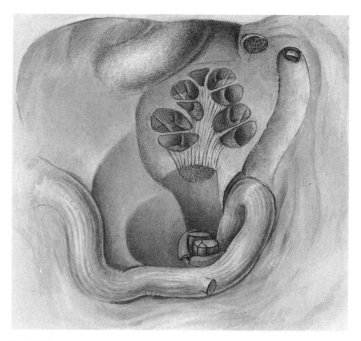

Fig. 6.**38**

Extensive cholesteatomas may additionally require exposure of the internal carotid artery so that matrix can be elevated along the vessel in its course toward the foramen lacerum (Fig. 6.**38**). With very extensive disease, the jugular bulb also will be visible at the base of the operative field (Fig. 6.**39**).

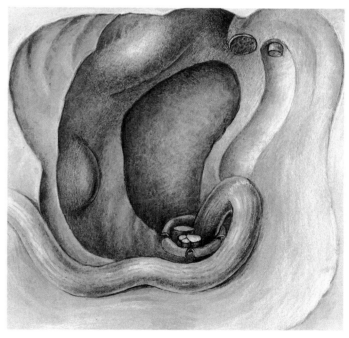

Fig. 6.**39**

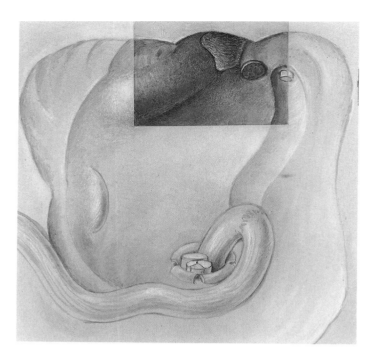

Fig. 6.**40**

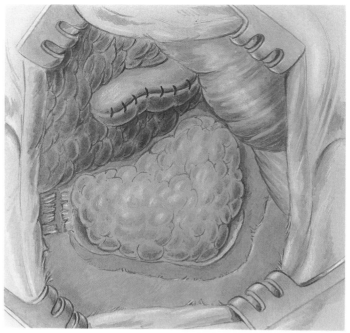

Fig. 6.**41**

Following resections of this extent, which generally leave very thin areas of dura, the eustachian tube is occluded, e. g., by burring the orifice and sealing it with bone cement or bone dust mixed with fibrin glue (Fig. 6.**40**).

The surgical cavity is obliterated with abdominal fat (Fig. 6.**41**) after the dural openings have been repaired with banked dura and fibrin glue. The external meatus is sutured as previously described (Fig. 6.**8**).

Modifications

The transmastoid–translabyrinthine approach can be modified by varying the extent of the resection of aerated mastoid and pyramidal cells. With a relatively small cholesteatoma and very extensive pneumatization, it may be preferable to seal off the petrous apex (e. g., with bone cement) rather than obliterate the entire mastoid.

Landmarks and Pitfalls

Intraoperative facial nerve damage is a significant hazard in patients who have normal preoperative facial nerve function and a relatively small cholesteatoma or other benign tumor. Consequently, the surgeon should positively identify the facial nerve at operation and minimize mechanical trauma to the nerve by dissecting slowly and using low-intensity suction.

Of course, dissections about the internal carotid artery or jugular bulb should also proceed slowly and deliberately, avoiding excessive traction that might tear the vessel and cause heavy bleeding.

Even if a CSF leak stops spontaneously during the operation, it should still be securely and definitively repaired; otherwise the leak might reoccur with the postoperative rise in CSF pressure.

Rules, Hints, and Common Errors

Before obliteration and closure of the external auditory canal, the surgeon must remove all keratinizing squamous epithelium from the medial portion of the petrous bone and tympanic membrane to prevent cholesteatoma formation. Also, the surgeon must remove all matrix tissue and must carefully follow the matrix to ensure that none is left behind. The extraction of a "matrix remnant" from a small, preformed cavity may result in overlooking larger matrix collections located distal to the apparent remnant.

Postoperative Care

No further antibiotics are necessary besides the perioperative prophylactic dose. If vestibular function was intact prior to surgery, a potent antivertiginous agent should be administered for 3—4 days postoperatively to relieve dizziness following labyrinthectomy.

Postoperative Complications

CSF leakage and facial nerve palsy are typical post-operative complications. Before additional surgery is done to repair a CSF fistula, a lumbar CSF drain should be inserted with the help of a neurosurgeon. If it is certain that the continuity of the facial nerve has been preserved during the operation, a wait–and–see approach is warranted owing to the favorable prognosis associated with an intact facial nerve.

Functional Sequelae

Balance disturbance occurs only in cases where vestibular nerve function was intact prior to surgery. Vestibular nerve integrity cannot be reliably established by preoperative studies, however, so the patient should understand that vertiginous symptoms may be experienced after the operation. Deafness most commonly occurs after removal of the semicircular canal system for petrous apex cholesteatoma, but it will not necessarily occur if the surgeon is able to preserve the membranous containment of the cochlea while removing the matrix.

Alternative Methods

Simply debulking a petrous apex cholesteatoma without resecting the matrix is not a valid alternative to the procedure described and is useful only for temporary palliation. Revision surgery is always necessary in these cases and should be performed by a highly proficient surgeon.

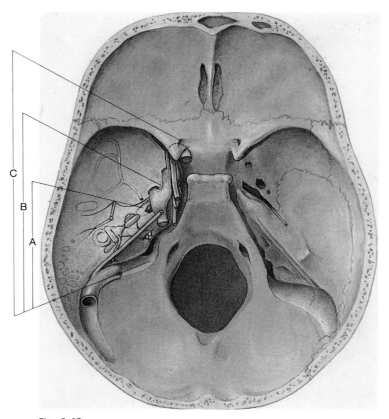

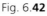

Fig. 6.**42**

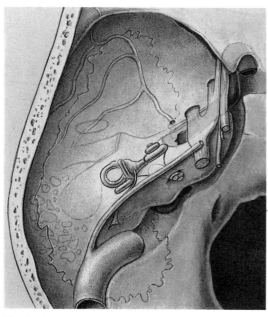

Fig. 6.**43**

Subtotal or Total Petrosectomy, with Facial Nerve Transposition or Resection, and Transposition of the Internal Carotid Artery

This technique is used in surgery for extensive tumors in the middle ear and mastoid, those medial and inferior to the labyrinth, and in the petrous apex (e. g. glomus jugulare tumors).

Preoperative Diagnosis

The internationally accepted Fisch classification defines surgical approaches of variable extent for varying degrees of tumor involvement of the temporal bone and skull base (Figs. 6.**42** and 6.**43**). The Fisch classification of the location and extent of tumor involvement is internationally recognized for its practical value in preoperative evaluation and planning.

Class A tumors (Fig. 6.**44**) arise from the tympanic plexus. They derive most of their blood supply from the tympanic artery, with some contribution from the caroticotympanic arteries.

Class B tumors (Fig. 6.**45**) arise from the tympanic canal above the jugular bulb. The bony roof of the jugular bulb is intact.

Class C tumors (Fig. 6.**46**) originate in the glomus jugulare and erode the bony covering of the jugular bulb. There is variable extension to the internal carotid artery, which may be encased by tumor.

Class D tumors (Fig. 6.**47**) are marked by intracranial extension. These tumors are further classified as extradural (*De*) or intradural (*Di*). De1 tumors displace the posterior fossa dura by less than 2 cm, while De2 tumors displace it by more than 2 cm.

Intradural tumors (Fig. 6.**48**) are subclassified as *Di1*, *Di2*, or *Di3* according to their extent. Di1 tumors are smaller than 2 cm, Di2 tumors are larger than 2 cm, and Di3 signifies multifocal intracranial metastasis.

Indications

Surgical treatment is indicated in all cases where the prognosis for quality of life without surgery appears less favorable than the prognosis with surgery. Smaller tumors are almost always managed by surgical re-

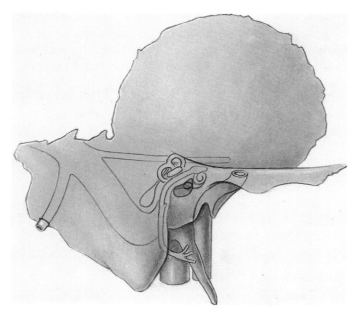

Fig. 6.**44**

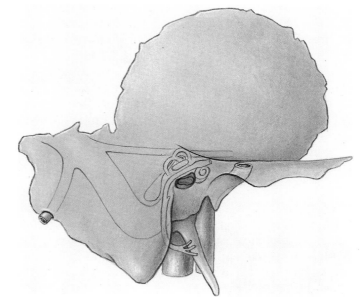

Fig. 6.**45**

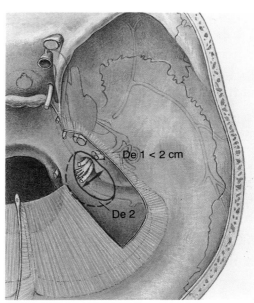

Fig. 6.**46**

C4

C3

C1 C2

De 1 < 2 cm

De 2

Fig. 6.**47**

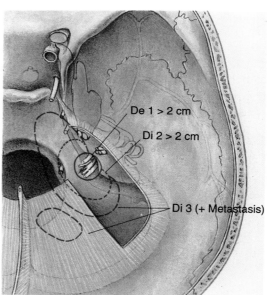

De 1 > 2 cm

Di 2 > 2 cm

Di 3 (+ Metastasis)

Fig. 6.**48**

moval. With extensive tumors, extirpative surgery can degrade the quality of life by damaging structures such as the cochleovestibular, facial and lower cranial nerves, which cannot always be preserved at the jugular foramen during this type of operation. Frequently, however, lower cranial nerve deficits are already present on the affected side, and it is unlikely that surgery will cause much additional trauma. Of course the risks of intracranial extension include the possibility of spontaneous tumor hemorrhage, which can have devastating consequences.

Because glomus tumors grow very slowly, radiation therapy should be considered in patients with multiple morbidity. Irradiation can provide a long–term reduction in tumor size. Occasionally this may be supplemented by arterial embolization of the tumor. Recanalization and revascularization develop slowly following successful tumor embolization.

Principles of the Operations

This chapter follows largely the techniques described by Fisch.

Resection of the Jugular Bulb without Transposing the Internal Carotid Artery

This type of surgery for smaller tumors involves identifying the major neurovascular structures in the neck, ligating or occluding the upper part of the sigmoid sinus, opening the jugular foramen, and removing the tumor with the jugular bulb. Generally the facial nerve is left alone. The Janssen–Grunert technique is used (see page 275).

Resection of the Jugular Bulb and Transposing the Internal Carotid Artery and Facial Nerve

For more extensive tumors that extend to the lateral genu of the internal carotid artery in the petrous bone but do not reach the foramen lacerum, it is additionally necessary to burr open the carotid canal. This requires opening the temporomandibular joint. The mandible may be displaced forward, or the posterior portion of the mandible, including the condyle, may be resected. It is generally necessary to mobilize the facial nerve from its tympanic and mastoid canal and transpose it anteriorly over the eustachian tube into the parotid region.

Resection of the Jugular Bulb, Transposing the Internal Carotid Artery and the Entire Facial Nerve, or Dividing the Facial Nerve

Very extensive glomus tumors may infiltrate the wall of the internal carotid artery, necessitating its resection. This precondition should be established prior to surgery.

Pre– or intraoperative neuroradiologic balloon occlusion is used as required. With pronounced tumor growth into the petrous apex, it may also be necessary to mobilize the labyrinthine segment of the facial nerve after sectioning the greater petrosal nerve and transpose the facial nerve inferiorly to facilitate the dissection of tumor components medial to the internal auditory canal.

Tumors with Intracranial or Intradural Extension

Neurosurgical consultation is advised for the resection of these lesions to ensure correct surgical handling of the vessels and brain surface in the posterior cranial fossa, especially when intradural extension is present.

Preoperative Preparations

In patients with large tumors, preoperative angiography with embolization may have to be supplemented by occlusion of the internal carotid artery with balloons positioned proximal and distal to the tumor site. Preparations include providing a sufficient volume of banked blood or a system for the retransfusion of blood lost at operation. The standard position for otologic surgery may be used, or the patient may be placed in a sitting position with the head immobilized in a clamp, as for a neurosurgical suboccipital exposure.

Anesthesia

The operation is performed under general endotracheal anesthesia. Mild controlled hypotension is desirable. The use of intraoperative hypothermia should be discussed with the anesthesiologist.

Operative Techniques

Resection of the Tumor and Jugular Bulb without Labyrinthectomy (Fisch C1 and C2 Tumors)

A curved incision (red) starting above the ear and passing behind the auricle to the anterior border of the sternocleidomastoid muscle (Fig. 6.49) (alternative in black) provides exposure of the major vessels and nerve in the neck and the facial nerve below the stylomastoid foramen (Fig. 6.50). The sigmoid sinus is widely exposed by extensive mastoidectomy. An area of bone 3–4 cm long and a full 1 cm wide parallel to the sigmoid sinus is removed from over the posterior fossa dura (Fig. 6.51). Then the sigmoid sinus is ligated, if necessary with neurosurgical assistance (Figs. 6.52 and 6.53). A tagged neurosurgical cottonoid is placed on the cerebellar surface below the ligature. If considerably less bone has been removed, the sinus can be com-

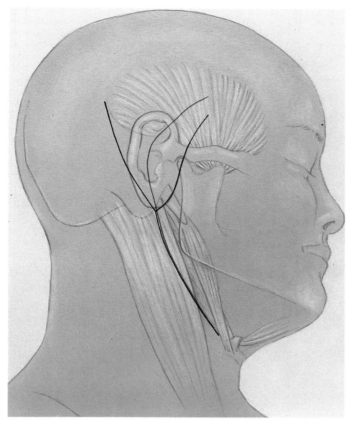

Fig. 6.**49**

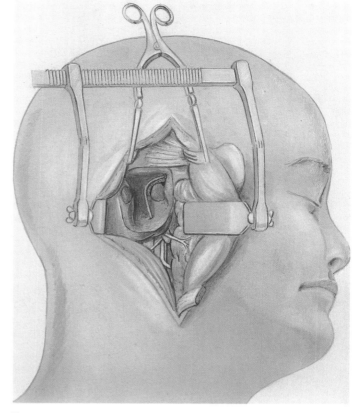

Fig. 6.**50**

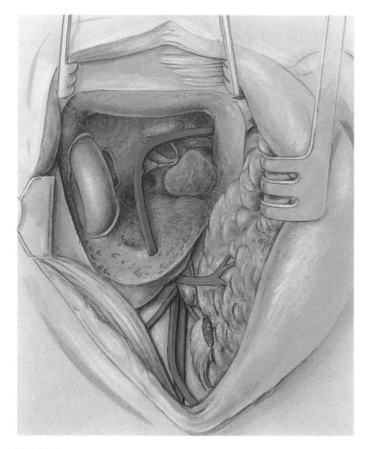

Fig. 6.**51**

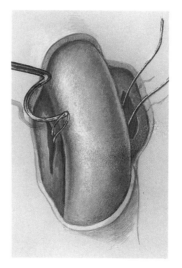

Fig. 6.**52**

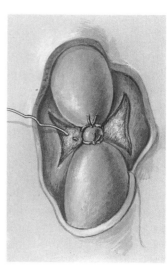

Fig. 6.**53**

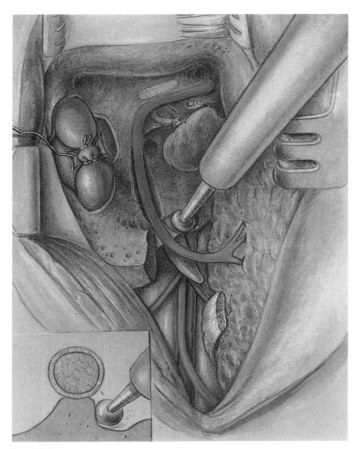

Fig. 6.**54**

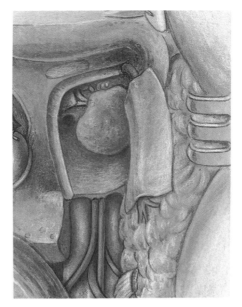

Fig. 6.**55**

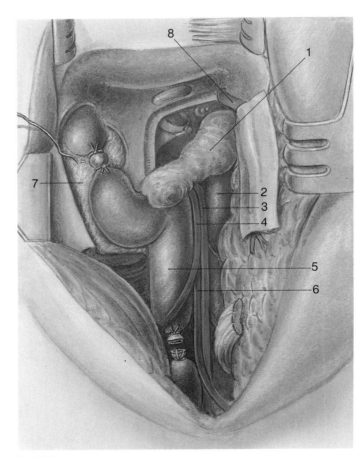

Fig. 6.**56**
1: Tumor
2: Internal carotid artery
3: Vagus nerve
4: Accessory nerve
5: Internal jugular vein
6: Hypoglossal nerve
7: Cotton on cerebellum
8: Transposed facial nerve

pressed in its bony canal from the lateral side and completely occluded by packing in Tabotamp or other material (see also Chapter 9).

Topographic constraints may make it necessary to mobilize and transpose anteriorly the tympanic and mastoid portions of the facial nerve. This involves opening the fallopian canal and burring down its sidewalls to a level below the nerve (Fig. 6.**54**). At that point the surgeon should be able to lift the facial nerve from its bony bed with epineurium intact, displace it anteriorly from the area of the geniculate ganglion, and lay it on the parotid or adjacent soft tissues without subjecting it to undue pressure or tension. A piece of banked dura is glued over the nerve at that site to protect it (Fig. 6.**55**). This follows previous closure of the external auditory canal below the concha and removal of the tympanic membrane and tympanic bone (see Figs. 6.**8** and 6.**12**).

The lateral aspect of the tumor is exposed by dissecting from the sigmoid sinus and upward along the jugular vein (Fig. 6.**56**).

Ideally the tumor is removed in one piece. Often this is not feasible, however, and bits of tumor have to be resected piecemeal from the jugular bulb. The sigmoid

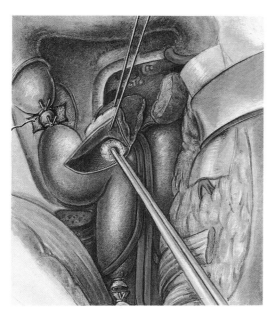

Fig. 6.**57**

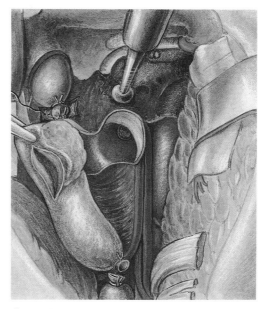

Fig. 6.**58**

sinus and jugular bulb are opened. Profuse bleeding from the inferior petrosal sinus is common at this stage and is managed by packing the sinus orifice with Tabotamp or other hemostatic material (Fig. 6.**57**). If the previous packing and ligature of the sigmoid sinus prove inadequate, Tabotamp can be packed up into the residual lumen through the incision in the sinus wall. It is helpful to impregnate the hemostatic pack with fibrin glue before insertion. The infiltrated portions of the jugular bulb are resected under direct vision (Fig. 6.**58**). A thin, partially transparent layer of connective tissue is left covering the lower cranial nerves in the pars nervosa of the jugular foramen (see Fig. 6.**60**).

If the tumor extends to the internal carotid artery, the ascending ramus of the mandible is either displaced forward or tangentially resected, with a condylectomy, so that the course of the internal carotid artery can be adequately visualized. The tympanic bone and other portions of the petrous bone medial to the mandibular fossa and lateral to the carotid foramen are removed until the anterior margin of the tumor can be seen. The eustachian tube is retracted from the skull base with the soft tissue (Fig. 6.**59**).

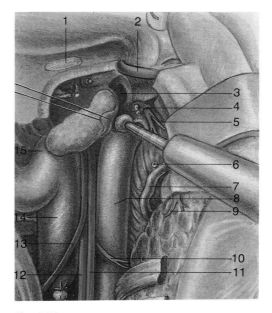

Fig. 6.**59**
 1: Lateral semicircular canal
 2: Transposed facial nerve
 3: Eustachian tube
 4: Middle meningeal artery
 5: Mandibular nerve
 6: Middle meningeal artery
 7: Maxillary artery
 8: Internal carotid artery
 9: Facial nerve
10: Glossopharyngeal nerve
11: Vagus nerve
12: Hypoglossal nerve
13: Accessory nerve
14: Jugular vein
15: Jugular bulb

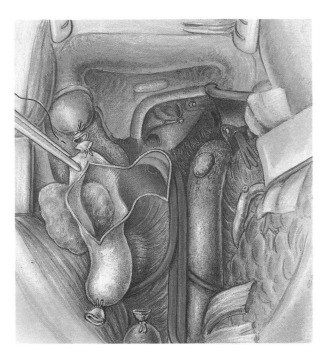

Fig. 6.**60**

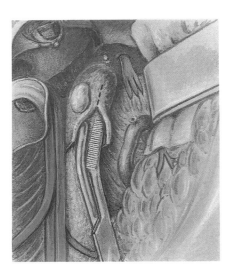

Fig. 6.**61**

The tumor is progressively dissected from the internal carotid artery, taking with it the arterial adventitia and the underlying fine venous plexus (Figs. 6.**60** and 6.**61**). Bleeding points are controlled with bipolar cautery, taking care to avoid coagulating over a large area of the artery. In this way tumor can be freed from the carotid artery as far as its horizontal segment lateral to the foramen lacerum.

Resection of the Jugular Bulb, Transposition of the Infraganglionic Facial Nerve Segment, Transposition of the Internal Carotid Artery in the Lower Part of the Petrous Bone, if Necessary, with Labyrinthectomy (Fisch C3 and C3 Tumors)

If the tumor not only reaches the carotid artery but also partially or completely encases it, it is necessary to transpose the vessel so that the tumor can be removed from its medial aspect. For this purpose the vessel is snared with a vascular tape and slowly elevated. The superficial layers of the encasing mass are divided and displaced to one side with the tumor as the carotid artery is progressively freed from the neoplasm. The eustachian tube is retracted forward and laterally to permit dissection of the horizontal carotid segment. The middle meningeal artery and maxillary nerve are sectioned. Small, briskly bleeding tumor–feeding vessels are coagulated as the dissection proceeds (Fig. 6.**62**).

If tumor infiltration extends beyond the adventitia to involve the deeper layers of the carotid artery wall, the affected portion of the vessel can be resected after balloon occlusion so that complete tumor clearance can be

achieved. Shekar (1993) notes that the vascular defect in these cases can be bridged with a saphenous vein graft, or the wall of the carotid artery can be partially reconstructed in its petrous segment.

With tumor extension into the foramen lacerum, the operation becomes considerably more difficult. The surgical cavity is deep, and it is also quite narrow at the petrous apex. Inferior displacement or tangential resection of the mandible is inadequate to improve tumor exposure, and the root of the zygoma has to be resected in order to demonstrate the region of the foramen lacerum (Fig. 6.**63**).

After retraction of the soft tissues from the skull base, bony ridges and prominences below the foramen spinosum and foramen ovale are burred down until the dura is visible through the bone. The posterior border of the pterygoid process is also taken down, especially near the base. The pharyngeal muscles are progressively released from their attachments to the skull base. Finally there is only a very thin boundary layer of connective tissue at the foramen lacerum separating the wall of the cavernous sinus, the trochlear nerve, and the maxillary nerve (Fig. 6.**64**).

Bleeding from the cavernous sinus and the entrance of the superior and inferior petrosal sinuses into the cavernous sinus is controlled by compression with Tabotamp, which may be applied in conjunction with fibrin glue.

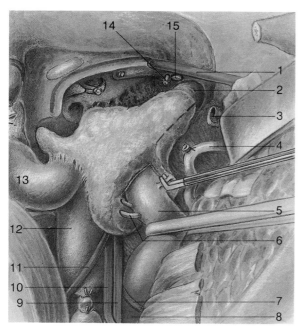

Fig. 6.**62**
 1: Anteriorly transposed facial nerve
 2: Internal carotid artery
 3: Eustachian tube
 4: Maxillary artery
 5: Internal carotid artery
 6: Tumor–feeding artery
 7: Glossopharyngeal nerve
 8: Internal carotid artery
 9: Vagus nerve
10: Hypoglossal nerve
11: Accessory nerve
12: Jugular vein
13: Sigmoid sinus
14: Middle meningeal artery
15: Mandibular nerve

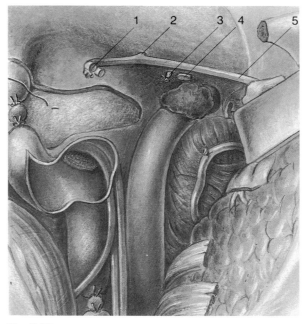

Fig. 6.**63**
 1: Fundus of the internal auditory canal after labyrinthectomy
 2: Greater petrosal nerve
 3: Middle meningeal artery
 4: Mandibular nerve
 5: Facial nerve

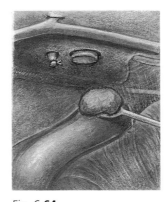

Fig. 6.**64**

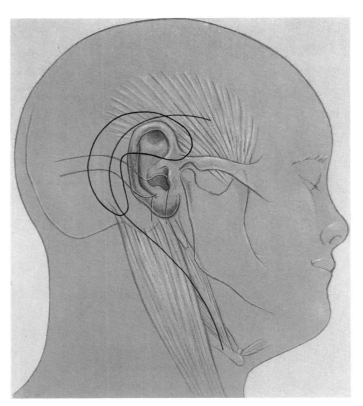

Fig. 6.**65**

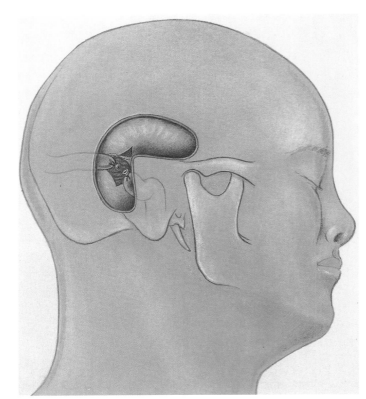

Fig. 6.**66**

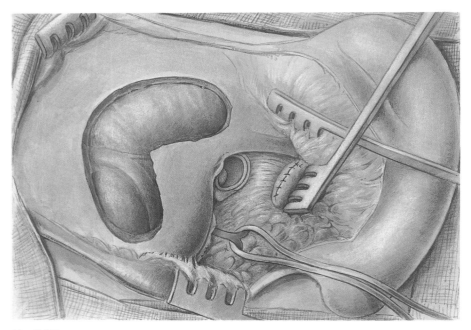

Fig. 6.**67**

Resection of the Jugular Bulb, Transposition of the Entire Facial Nerve and Internal Carotid Artery, Labyrinthectomy, and Intradural Tumor Removal

Principle

For glomus tumors that have extended into the posterior cranial fossa (Fisch De and Di neoplasms) and also for tumors of the petrous apex and clivus, broad access to the medial portions of the posterior fossa can be ob-

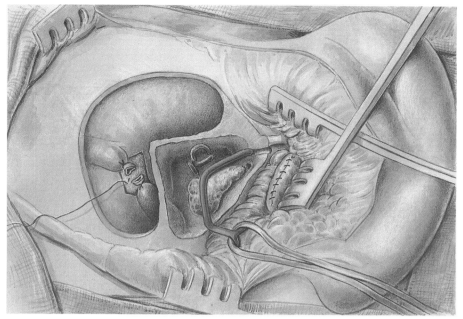

Fig. 6.**68**

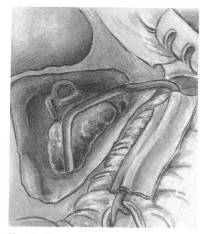

Fig. 6.**69**

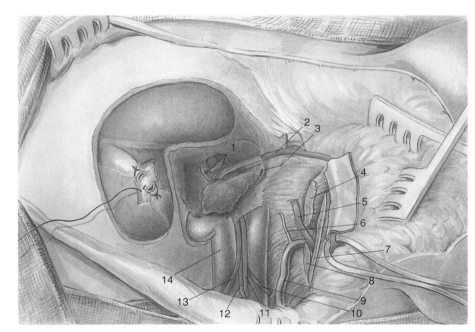

Fig. 6.**70**
 1: Semicircular canals
 2: Transposed facial nerve
 3: Eustachian tube
 4: Lateral pterygoid muscle
 5: Mandibular nerve
 6: Middle meningeal artery
 7: Mandibular border after resection
 8: Medial pterygoid muscle
 9: Maxillary artery
10: Glossopharyngeal nerve
11: Vagus nerve
12: Hypoglossal nerve
13: Accessory nerve
14: Jugular vein

tained without excessive cerebellar retraction by resecting most of the petrous bone. This extensive resection is particularly appropriate in cases where the patient does not possess serviceable hearing on the affected side. The approach requires considerable transposition of the facial nerve. First the nerve is displaced anteriorly as shown in Fig. 6.**55**. The lower part of the pyramid and the jugular bulb are resected. Then the internal carotid artery is transposed. After division of the superior petrosal nerve at the geniculate ganglion and labyrinthectomy, the facial nerve can be transposed inferiorly to gain access to the petrous apex (Schürman and Helms, 1979).

Technique

The first step is neurosurgical as the middle and posterior cranial fossae are opened by craniectomy (red line: skin incision) (Figs. 6.**65** and 6.**66**). The sigmoid sinus is divided just below the superior petrosal sinus. Opening the posterior and middle fossa dura above and below the transverse sinus permits the surgeon to view the tentorium from above and from below (Fig. 6.**66**). The lateral margins of the floor of the middle fossa and the posterior wall of the mastoid lateral to the sigmoid sinus are initially left intact to facilitate the petrosectomy (Figs. 6.**67** and 6.**68**).

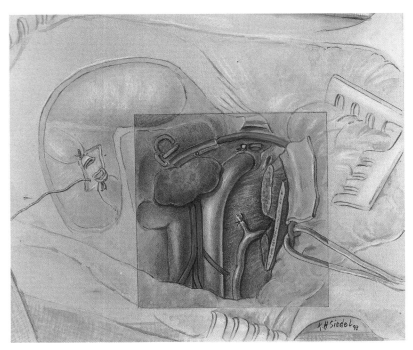

Fig. 6.**71**

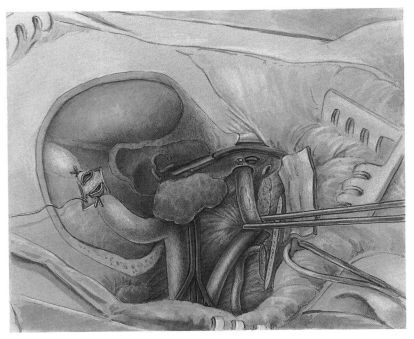

Fig. 6.**72**

The petrous bone is progressively excavated with a burr while the facial nerve is displaced from the area of the geniculate ganglion over the tympanic tubal orifice and placed upon the posterior aspect of the parotid. There it is covered with preserved dura and fibrin glue to protect it from additional trauma (Fig. 6.**69**). If the lesion involves the horizontal segment of the internal carotid artery, the temporomandibular joint should be opened and the mandible displaced forward or, if necessary, tangentially resected (Fig. 6.**70**).

Next, the lateral portions of the petrous bone are burred down over the carotid canal until the carotid artery and jugular bulb are exposed (Fig. 6.**71**). The carotid artery is snared with a tape and retracted forward (Fig. 6.**72**).

Tumor components in the lower petrous bone are removed with the jugular bulb, and the inferior petrosal sinus is packed (Fig. 6.**73**). As the dissection is carried superiorly, the labyrinth is resected. The lateral wall of

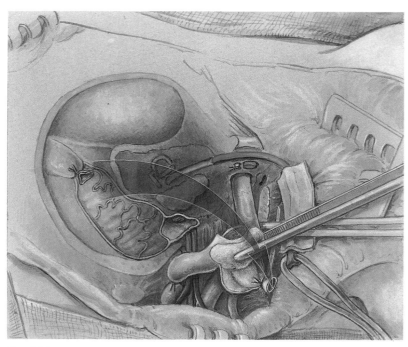

Fig. 6.**73**

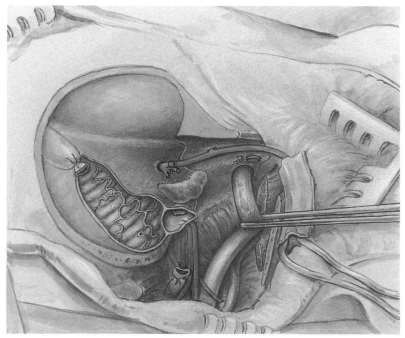

Fig. 6.**74**

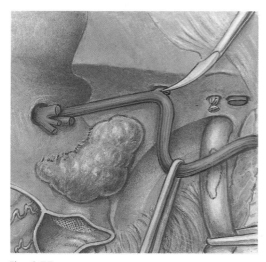

Fig. 6.**75**

the labyrinthine fallopian canal is thinned down until the very thin connective tissue covering the facial nerve is broadly exposed. In this way the fundus of the internal auditory canal is opened by the translabyrinthine route. Cerebrospinal fluid is noted (Fig. 6.**74**).

The facial nerve is dissected by further bone removal above and below its initial segment between the internal auditory canal fundus and the geniculate ganglion (Fig. 6.**75**). The greater petrosal nerve is dissected at the

geniculate ganglion toward the facial nerve hiatus and is divided. Bleeding points at the peripheral stump of the nerve are controlled with bipolar coagulation.

Next the entire facial nerve is transposed inferiorly from the internal acoustic porus and internal auditory canal. The nerve can be transposed downward for a considerable distance, especially after incision of the dura of the posterior pyramidal wall below the porus acousticus. Freed from its temporary placement on the poste-

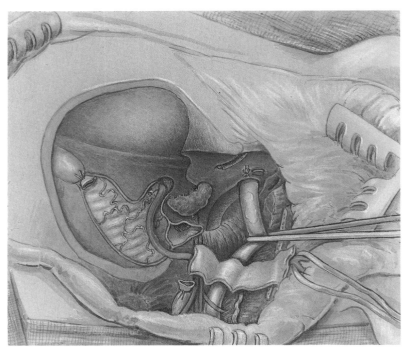

Fig. 6.**76**

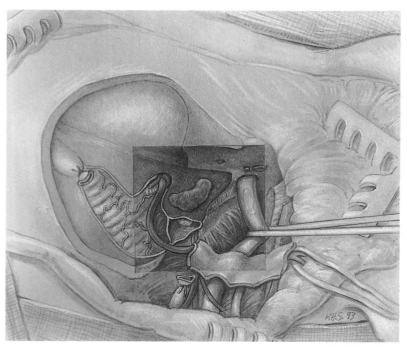

Fig. 6.**77**

rior aspect of the parotid gland and over the eustachian tube, the nerve is transposed to the lower part of the operative field, where it is again protected by covering it with a piece of preserved dura (Fig. 6.**76**).

Further dissection in the upper part of the pyramid can now be carried along the internal carotid artery without further danger to the facial nerve (Fig. 6.**77**). A thin plate of bone is left covering the middle fossa dura

to prevent premature sagging of the dura into the operative field. The bony posterior wall of the pyramid (if not already eroded by tumor) is thinned, leaving only a thin bony covering medial to the internal acoustic porus.

With the help of a neurosurgeon, the arachnoid is slowly elevated from the intradural tumor surface (Fig. 6.**78**). Vessels entering the tumor are coagulated, and the tumor is progressively dissected from the facial

Fig. 6.**78**
  1: Greater petrosal nerve (sectioned)
  2: Middle meningeal artery
  3: Mandibular nerve
  4: Internal carotid artery
  5: Lateral pterygoid muscle
  6: Mandibular ramus
  7: Maxillary artery
  8: Glossopharyngeal nerve
  9: Internal carotid artery
10: Vagus nerve
11: Hypoglossal nerve
12: Accessory nerve
13: Jugular vein
14: Facial nerve, transposed inferiorly
15: Jugular bulb with intact pars nervosa
      and packed inferior petrosal sinus
16: Stump of cochlear nerve
17: Sigmoid sinus
18: Arachnoid adhesions
19: Superior petrosal sinus
20: Dura at posterior pyramidal surface

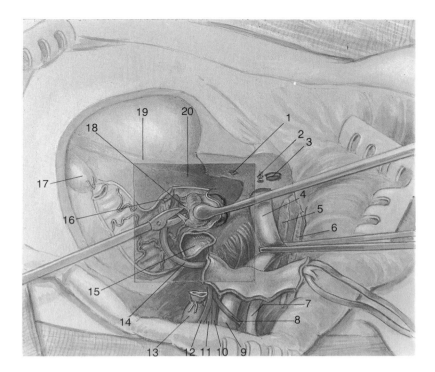

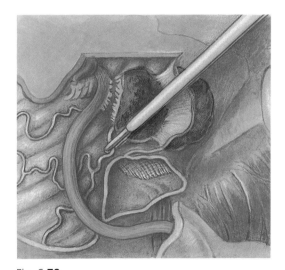

Fig. 6.**79**

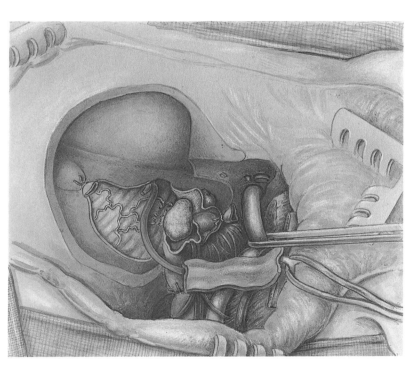

Fig. 6.**80**

nerve, trigeminal nerve, etc. The cochlear and vestibular nerves are sectioned just lateral to the brainstem (Fig. 6.**79**).

Extensive tumors may develop some firm adhesions with arterial loops in the posterior fossa. These adhesions can be separated from the tumor along with the arachnoid. While the arteries themselves should be preserved, small branches entering the tumor are coagulated. In this way the tumor is progressively freed from its intracranial contacts and, with the lower part of the sigmoid sinus and jugular bulb, reflected downward. At this point the lower cranial nerves are visible in the pars nervosa of the jugular foramen (Fig. 6.**80**).

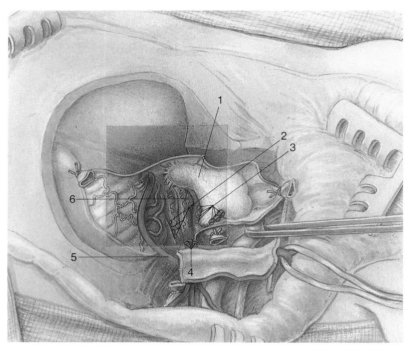

Fig. 6.**81**

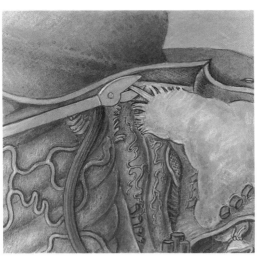

Fig. 6.**82**

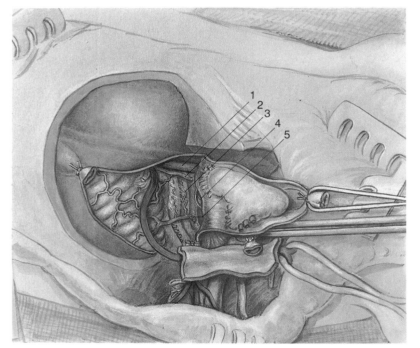

Fig. 6.**83**

Fig. 6.**81**
1: Tumor with infiltrated dura and sigmoid sinus
2: Central stumps of the lower cranial nerves
3: Lower cranial nerves in the tumor
4: Peripheral stumps of the lower cranial nerves
5: Facial nerve
6: Packed inferior petrosal sinus

Fig. 6.**83**
1: Trigeminal nerve
2: Anterior inferior cerebellar artery
3: Basilar artery
4: Packed inferior petrosal sinus
5: Posterior inferior cerebellar artery

If these nerves are infiltrated by tumor and no intact nerve bundles can be isolated, cranial nerves IX, X and XI should be divided intradurally before their entry into the jugular foramen (Fig. 6.**81**).

In this way the tumor can be fully mobilized and rolled into the petrous bone (Fig. 6.**82**).

The medial tumor margins in the petrous apex or on the clivus are similarly dissected and progressively separated from surrounding tissues. The abducens nerve and tentorial incisure come into view as the dissection proceeds, along with the oculomotor nerve and occasionally a short segment of the basilar artery and its branches (Fig. 6.**83**).

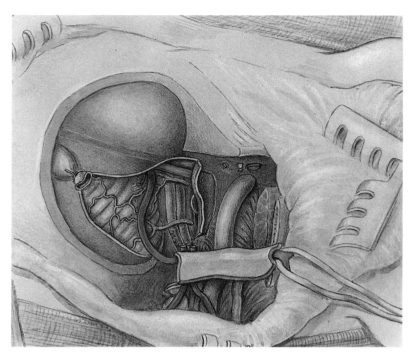

Fig. 6.**84**

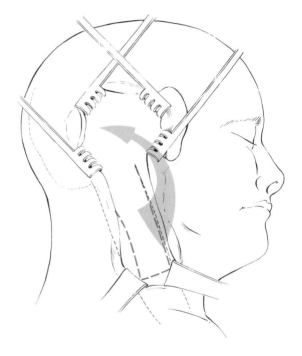

Fig. 6.**85**

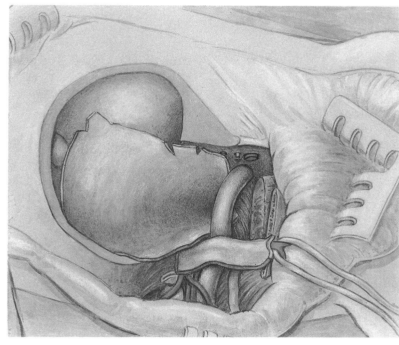

Fig. 6.**86**

After all tumor components have been removed, the operative field is bounded anteriorly by the internal carotid artery and medially by the clivus, cranial nerves III and IV, and the basilar artery. The abducens nerve and trigeminal nerve are found laterally, and still farther laterally is the inferiorly transposed facial nerve (Fig. 6.**84**).

The operative field may be obliterated with a large free graft of abdominal fat or by transposing a sterno-cleidomastoid muscle flap of sufficient length based on the postauricular skin (Fig. 6.**85**). Before the abdominal fat or muscle flap is implanted, the large dural defect on the posterior aspect of the pyramid is securely covered with banked dura and fibrin glue (Fig. 6.**86**).

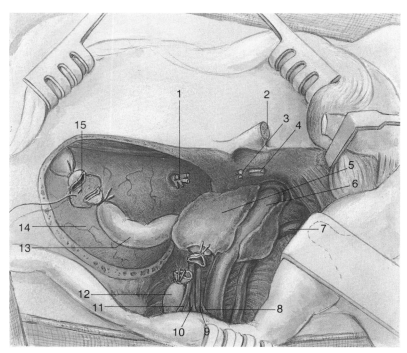

Fig. 6.**87**

Fig. 6.**87**
1: Nerves VII and VIII, sectioned in the internal auditory canal
2: Zygomatic arch, sectioned
3: Middle meningeal artery
4: Mandibular nerve
5: Tumor with jugular bulb
6: Internal carotid artery
7: Maxillary artery
8: Glossopharyngeal nerve
9: Vagus nerve
10: Hypoglossal nerve
11: Abducens nerve
12: Jugular vein
13: Sigmoid sinus
14: Dura at posterior pyramidal surface
15: Cottonoid on the cerebellum

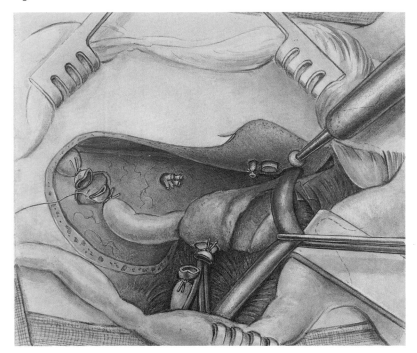

Fig. 6.**88**

Modifications

The Fisch modification of this procedure affords a somewhat more anterior exposure of the pyramid without extensive craniectomy of the middle and posterior fossae. In this technique the mandible is displaced farther anteroinferiorly, and the base of the zygomatic arch is resected. As in the exposure of the foramen lacerum described earlier (see Figs. 6.**63** and 6.**64**), the entire posterior surface of the pyramid is accessible below the internal auditory canal as far as the jugular bulb and inferior petrosal sinus (Fig. 6.**87**).

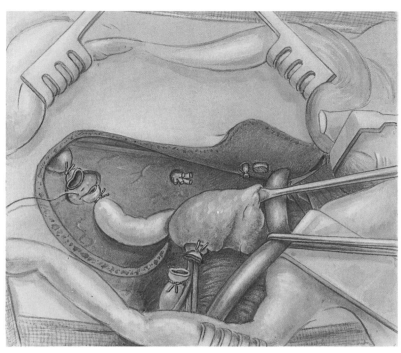

Fig. 6.**89**

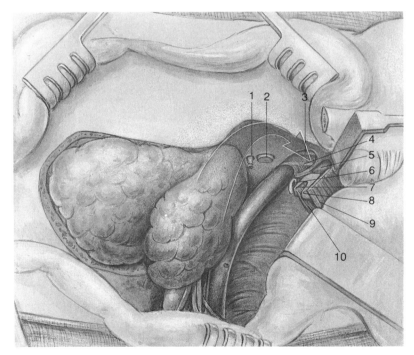

Fig. 6.**90**

Fig. 6.**90**
1: Middle meningeal artery
2: Mandibular nerve
3: Abducens nerve in cavernous sinus
4: Trochlear nerve in cavernous sinus
5: Pterygopalatine fossa
6: Cartilaginous eustachian tube
7: Medial plate with medial pterygoid muscle
8: Lateral plate with lateral pterygoid muscle
9: Lateral pterygoid muscle, partially resected
10: Medial pterygoid muscle

Following dissection and resection of the tumor from the posterior fossa as described above, this approach likewise provides a clear view of the posterior fossa. The tumor is progressively separated from the internal carotid artery aided by extensive bone removal below the middle fossa (Figs. 6.**88** and 6.**89**). The lateral wall of the cavernous sinus is exposed, and the abducens and trochlear nerves are seen. The field is obliterated with abdominal fat (Fig. 6.**90**).

Landmarks and Pitfalls

Attention should be given to bleeding sites outside the tumor itself: the sigmoid sinus, the inferior and superior petrosal sinuses, and cerebellar veins that enter the superior petrosal sinus above the internal acoustic porus (petrosal veins). Bleeding from brain arteries whose branches enter the tumor also must be controlled. Manipulations on the cerebellar surface and especially the flocculus, which may well be in contact with tumor tissue, should be performed slowly using tagged, moist cottonoids to protect the cerebellar surface.

Rules, Hints, and Common Errors

Preoperative embolization of the tumor is advantageous. If the tumor has infiltrated the internal carotid artery, preoperative balloon occlusion should be considered. Since the sigmoid sinus will have to be ligated, venous return from the intracranial space should be evaluated prior to surgery. Also, neuroradiologic techniques should be used to define the inferior extent of the tumor, since it can be difficult to identify the demarcation between the tumor and the soft tissues below the skull base at operation.

Postoperative Care

Postoperative medical treatment in the intensive care unit is planned in consultation with the neurosurgeon, if one is attending, and with the anesthesiologist. Routine measures include several hours of ventilatory support, treatment with corticosteroids, and monitoring of coagulation status.

Postoperative Complications

Besides the complications noted above, surgery of this extent is occasionally followed by the formation of CSF collections outside the subdural space. Treatment consists of lumbar CSF drainage and the application of a local, light pressure dressing, which can be made, for example, from the thick, sterile foam slabs used in packing materials.

In some cases reoperation may be necessary to locate and control bleeding sites within the operative field.

Functional Sequelae

The operation will destroy any hearing that was present prior to surgery. If the vestibular organ was partially intact, the patient may experience balance disturbances for several months postoperatively. If the lower cranial nerves (IX, X, and XI) were also damaged, which usually cannot be avoided, patients with normal preoperative laryngeal function may experience hoarseness and severe swallowing difficulties that may necessitate a corrective deglutition operation like that described by Denecke.

Alternative Methods

Alternatives include radiation therapy, embolization, or a combination of both. These options should be discussed only if the patient is considered an unacceptable surgical risk due to pre–existing multiple morbidity, or if it appears that surgery would significantly degrade the patient's quality of life. This would be the case with bilateral tumors, for example, where surgery on one side has left the patient with only one internal carotid artery.

Malignant Tumors of the Middle Ear

Preoperative Diagnostic Studies

Besides the preoperative studies used to evaluate benign tumors, general tumor staging must be carried out in patients with malignancies of the lateral skull base (petrous pyramid).

Indications

Complete tumor resection with a margin of healthy tissue is not the only rationale for the surgical treatment of a middle ear malignancy. Surgery can also increase the efficacy of postoperative radiation therapy by reducing the bulk of malignant tissue. A radical tumor resection should be performed if it appears to be possible without causing additional, unacceptable functional deficits. In many cases a partial resection is all that can be accomplished.

Principles of the Operation

If a complete tumor removal is planned, the dissection must completely encompass the tumor with a margin of healthy tissue. If at all possible, the tumor is removed in one piece.

Preoperative Preparations

The patient is positioned as for the removal of a benign tumor (see page 81).

Fig. 6.**91**
  1: Bone edges after resection of zygomatic arch
  2: Lateral pterygoid muscle
  3: Pterygopalatine fossa
  4: Internal carotid artery
  5: Cartilaginous eustachian tube
  6: Mandibular condyle
  7: Inferiorly displaced zygomatic arch
  8: Parotid gland
  9: Sternocleidomastoid muscle
 10: Facial nerve
 11: Jugular vein
 12: Styloid process
 13: Middle meningeal artery
 14: Mandibular nerve

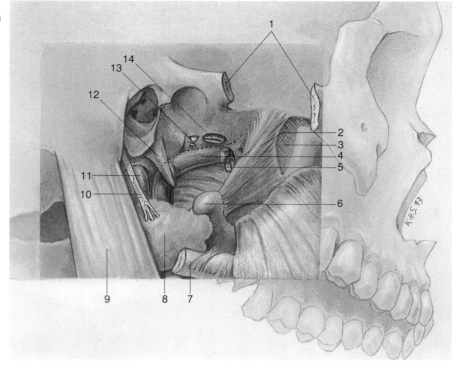

Fig. 6.**91**

Anesthesia

The operation is performed under general anesthesia.

Operative Technique

The approach most commonly used and most familiar to otosurgically trained head and neck surgeons is the Fisch type C infratemporal fossa approach (Figs. 6.**91** and 6.**92**).

Fisch summarizes the key steps in the operation as follows:

— Large postauricular and temporal skin incision.
— The frontal branch of the facial nerve is exposed.
— The zygomatic arch is reflected downward on the temporalis muscle, and a subtotal petrosectomy is performed.
— The middle meningeal artery and the mandibular branch of the trigeminal nerve are sectioned. The ascending ramus of the mandible is displaced inferiorly.
— The pterygoid process and the surrounding bone at the skull base are taken down with a burr.
— The maxillary branch of the trigeminal nerve is divided.
— The internal carotid artery is exposed from the carotid foramen to the foramen lacerum at the cavernous sinus.

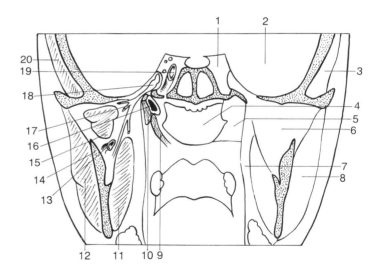

Fig. 6.**92**
  1: Cavernous sinus
  2: Middle cranial fossa
  3: Temporal fossa
  4: Nasopharynx
  5: Peritubal space
  6: Infratemporal fossa
  7: Parapharyngeal space
  8: Masseter space
  9: Levator veli palatini muscle
 10: Tensor veli palatini muscle
 11: Medial pterygoid muscle
 12: Masseter muscle
 13: Maxillary artery
 14: Mandible
 15: Lateral pterygoid muscle
 16: Eustachian tube
 17: Mandibular nerve
 18: Trigeminal nerve
 19: Internal carotid artery
 20: Temporalis muscle

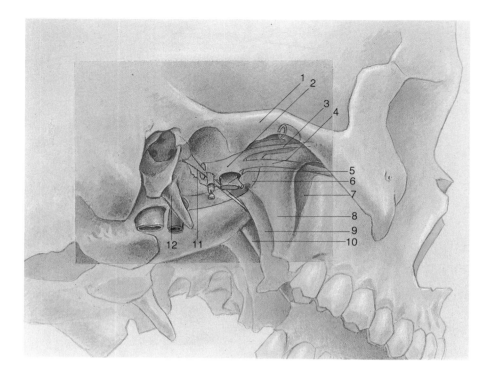

Fig. 6.**93**
1: Zygomatic arch
2: Gasserian ganglion
3: First division of trigeminal nerve
4: Second division of trigeminal nerve
5: Third division of trigeminal nerve
6: Internal carotid artery
7: Pterygopalatine fossa
8: Lateral plate of pterygoid process
9: Medial plate of pterygoid process
10: Posterior margin of vomer
11: Eustachian tube
12: Styloid process

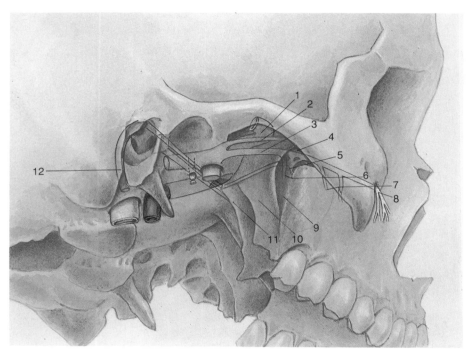

Fig. 6.**94**
1: Internal carotid artery
2: First division of trigeminal nerve
3: Second division of trigeminal nerve
4: Inferior orbital fissure
5: Sphenopalatine ganglion
6: Palatine nerves
7: Alveolar nerves
8: Infraorbital nerve
9: Pterygopalatine fossa
10: Lateral plate of pterygoid process
11: Medial plate of pterygoid process
12: Facial nerve

— The above steps provide exposure of the entire in-fratemporal fossa, the pterygopalatine fossa, the pa-rasellar region, and the nasopharynx for removal of the tumor.
— The zygomatic arch is returned to its original posi-tion and reattached (e. g., with transosseous wires).
— The surgical cavity is obliterated with pedicled soft-tissue flaps from the temporalis, postauricular re-gion, or sternocleidomastoid muscle.

This approach is made on a transverse plane at a some-what lower level than in the operations previously de-scribed. Hence the approach requires greater inferior displacement of the disarticulated mandible. The essen-tial anatomic landmarks for the procedure are shown in Figs. 6.**93** to 6.**100**, after Fisch.

Fig. 6.**95**
1: Internal carotid artery
2: Optic nerve
3: Ophthalmic artery
4: Superior orbital fissure
5: Oculomotor nerve
6: First division of trigeminal nerve
7: Abducens nerve
8: Second division of trigeminal nerve
9: Vidian nerve
10: Superficial petrosal nerve
11: Pterygoid process
12: Foramen ovale
13: Third division of trigeminal nerve
14: Middle meningeal artery
15: Superficial petrosal nerve
16: Geniculate ganglion
17: Posterior margin of vomer
18: Opened sphenoid sinus
19: Sella

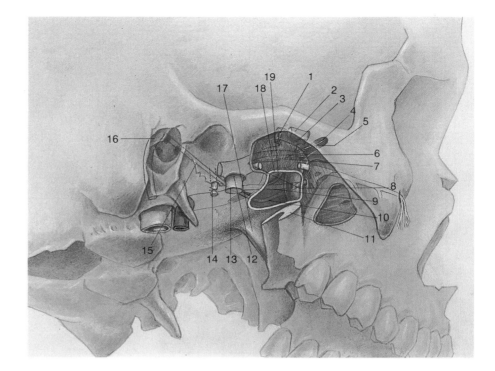

Fig. 6.**96**
1: Lateral pterygoid muscle
2: Medial pterygoid muscle

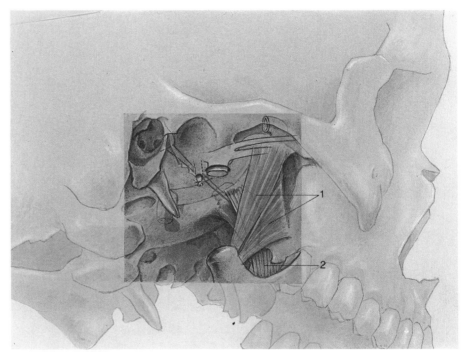

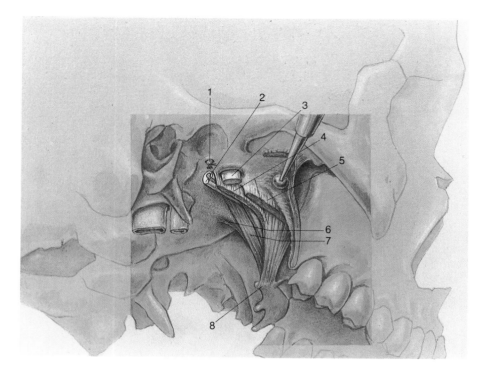

Fig. 6.**97**
1: Middle meningeal artery
2: Cartilaginous eustachian tube
3: Third division of trigeminal nerve
4: Tensor veli palatini muscle
5: Medial pterygoid muscle
6: Posterior margin of vomer
7: Levator veli palatini muscle
8: Hamulus

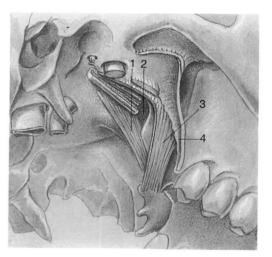

Fig. 6.**98**

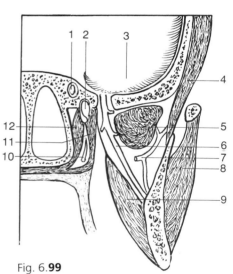

Fig. 6.**99**

Fig. 6.**98**
1: Opened nasopharynx
2: Levator veli palatini muscle
3: Tensor veli palatini muscle
4: Pterygoid process (burred down)

Fig. 6.**99**
1: Internal carotid artery
2: Eustachian tube
3: Middle cranial fossa
4: Temporalis muscle
5: Lateral pterygoid muscle
6: Mandibular nerve
7: Maxillary artery
8: Masseter muscle
9: Medial pterygoid muscle
10: Pterygoid process
11: Tensor veli palatini muscle
12: Levator veli palatini muscle

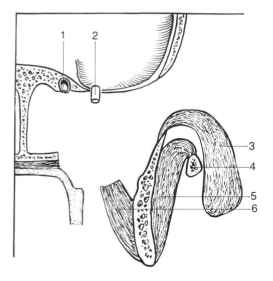

Fig. 6.**100**
1: Internal carotid artery
2: Mandibular nerve
3: Temporalis muscle
4: Displaced zygomatic arch
5: Masseter muscle
6: Medial pterygoid muscle

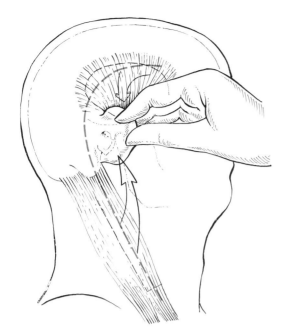

Fig. 6.**101**

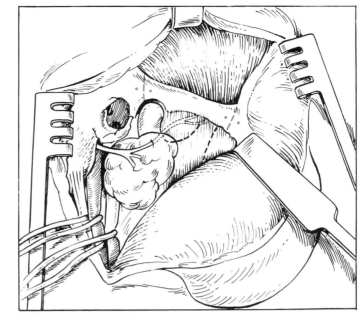

Fig. 6.**102**

After the skin incision (**red**), which has a greater frontal extent than previous incisions (Fig. 6.**101**), the skin is dissected anteriorly, and the superficial soft tissues are reflected anteroinferiorly. The zygomatic arch is divided and mobilized inferiorly, sparing the frontal branch of the facial nerve. Before the arch is mobilized, drill holes can be made on each side of the osteotomy cuts to permit later reattachment with interosseous wires (Fig. 6.**102**). Next a subtotal petrosectomy is performed as described earlier, except that the tympanic and mastoid segments of the facial nerve are not mobilized, and there is greater exposure of the infratemporal fossa anteriorly and medially (Fig. 6.**103**).

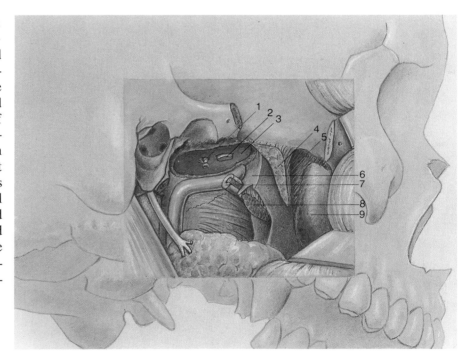

Fig. 6.**103**
1: Middle meningeal artery
2: Mandibular nerve
3: Middle fossa dura
4: Remnant of lateral pterygoid muscle
5: Pterygopalatina fossa
6: Root of pterygoid process
7: Eustachian tube
8: Remnant of medial pterygoid muscle
9: Posterior wall of maxillary sinus

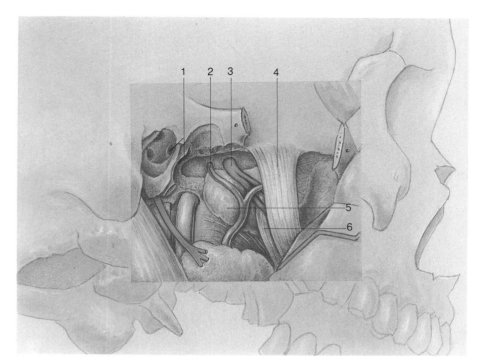

Fig. 6.**104**
1: Bony eustachian tube
2: Middle meningeal artery
3: Mandibular nerve
4: Lateral pterygoid muscle
5: Tumor
6: Medial pterygoid muscle

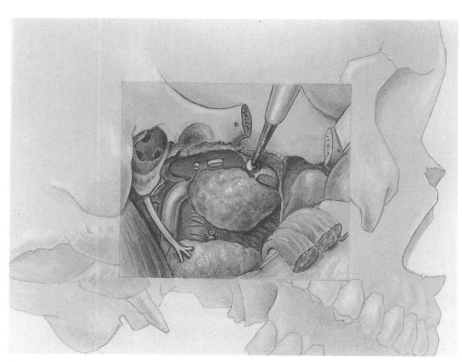

Fig. 6.**105**

The temporomandibular joint is opened to permit adequate inferior mobilization of the mandible. The dissection is progressively deepened, and the middle meningeal artery and mandibular nerve are identified and sectioned. As the dissection continues, the eustachian tube is included in the resection. Most of the pterygoid process is removed with a burr (Figs. 6.**104** and 6.**105**).

Proceeding from below upward, the medial aspect of the tumor is excised from the lateral wall of the choana and epipharynx (Fig. 6.**106**). This provides a clear view into the epipharynx (Fig. 6.**107**).

The dissection can also be carried downward to separate the tumor from more inferior soft tissues. The internal maxillary artery is ligated (Fig. 6.**108**).

Fig. 6.**106**
1: Middle meningeal artery
2: Mandibular nerve
3: Posterior margin of vomer
4: Choana
5: Eustachian tube in tumor
6: Reflected pterygoids

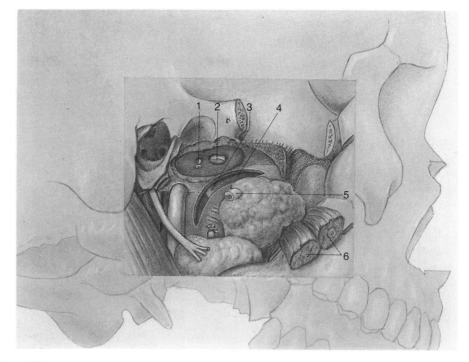

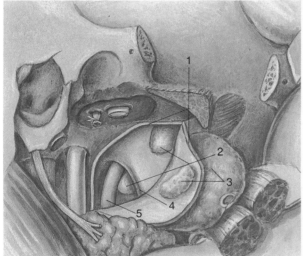

Fig. 6.**107**
1: Edge of incision for opening nasopharynx
2: Tails of turbinates
3: Tumor
4: Posterior margin of vomer
5: Feeding tube

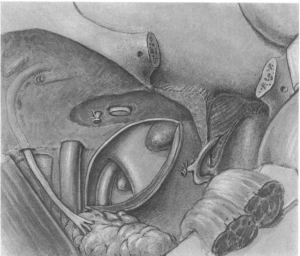

Fig. 6.**108**

For wound closure, the temporalis muscle is transposed into the infratemporal fossa (area within the black broken line in Fig. 6.**101**), and the zygomatic arch is reattached at the orbital margin. The mastoid tip and the bone behind the sigmoid sinus are burred down to form a shallow cavity after subtotal petrosectomy that can be obliterated with surrounding soft tissues (Fig. 6.**109**). The skin is closed in layers over a suction drain.

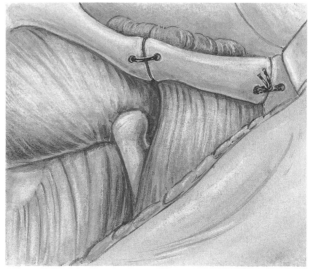

Fig. 6.**109**

Modifications

The infratemporal fossa can be widely explored through a more cranial approach that avoids extensive mandibular displacement but requires neurosurgical skills. Tumor removal is basically the same as described above. A large parietal craniectomy is performed to permit elevation of the temporal lobe of the brain. The floor of the middle fossa (the roof of the infratemporal fossa) is removed, and the tumor is followed down into the temporal fossa and if necessary into the epipharynx.

Tumor that has invaded the maxillary sinus and ethmoid region may necessitate additional transmaxillary surgery in both the Fisch and neurosurgical approaches. With malignant tumors, surgery is routinely followed by adjunctive radiotherapy with the goal of providing complete tumor clearance.

Landmarks and Pitfalls

Essential landmarks for orientation are the mandibular branch of the trigeminal nerve in the foramen ovale and the pterygoid process, which restrict access to the lateral pharyngeal wall unless most of it is removed with a burr. Of course, close attention should be given to the internal carotid artery at the back of the operative field to avoid inadvertent injury.

Rules, Hints, and Common Errors

Fisch (pp. 388, 398) emphasizes the following points:

- The working space required for the type C approach is obtained by removing as much bone as possible at the base of the middle cranial fossa.
- If the condylar process of the mandible is preserved, the mandible can be displaced inferiorly by no more than about 4 cm. Thus, the infratemporal fossa approach requires a full mastery of microsurgical techniques.
- If the eustachian tube is not infiltrated, it may be possible to preserve the eustachian tube to provide for subsequent aeration of the middle ear.
- If the infratemporal vertical segment of the carotid artery is surrounded by tumor, the artery should be identified in the neck below the carotid foramen.
- In this approach bone should be left covering the mastoid and tympanic portions of the facial nerve to protect it from inadvertent injury.
- The facial nerve trunk between the stylomastoid foramen and parotid gland should not be needlessly exposed. It is better to leave it protected by surrounding connective tissues.

- Care should be taken that the shafts of retractors and other instruments do not push against the facial nerve trunk while the surgeon's attention is deep in the infratemporal fossa.
- Removal of the mandibular fossa and articular disc will not cause significant masticatory dysfunction if the mandibular condyle is preserved.
- The medial plate of the pterygoid process is the lateral wall of the choana.
- Inferior displacement of the mandibular condyle is much easier after section of the middle meningeal artery and mandibular nerve.
- The "foramen ovale" and "foramen spinosum" are actually 5–mm–long canals, which are thinned at the base of the middle fossa.
- Section of the mandibular nerve does not cause permanent loss of sensory function of the tongue and chin. Some functional recovery will occur over 6 to 12 months.
- Well–encapsulated portions of a juvenile nasopharyngeal angiofibroma can be removed from the lower infratemporal fossa by traction and gentle mobilization of the tumor margins.
- If a tumor obscures important landmarks in the infratemporal fossa, its size should be reduced by intracapsular debulking.
- Branches from the maxillary artery in the infratemporal fossa should be coagulated before they are sectioned. Otherwise they will retract into the soft tissues, and bleeding from them will be far more difficult to control.
- Tumors medial to the internal carotid artery can displace the vessel laterally and can make it difficult to separate the artery from the cartilaginous eustachian tube.
- The vidian nerve is found inferior and anterior to the maxillary nerve within the pterygopalatine fossa.
- In the infratemporal type C approach, the nasal cavity is entered anterior to the medial plate of the pterygoid process to remain as far away from the tumor as possible.
- If a malignant tumor grows lower down in the pharynx, a retromandibular fossa approach must be added to the procedure.
- A temporalis muscle flap is most suitable for reconstructing the pharyngeal defect.
- Tumor extending into the middle fossa and parasellar region should not be resected en bloc. It is better to remove the tumor from the middle fossa first and then proceed with the parasellar dissection.
- The abducens nerve lies directly below the medial portion of a tumor compressing the cavernous sinus, where it is highly susceptible to injury.
- The pituitary gland may be exposed if tumor has invaded the sphenoid sinus.

- Exposure of the parasellar region requires extradural elevation of the temporal lobe to obtain an adequate view. Bleeding from the cavernous sinus is easily controlled by compression with free muscle grafts. This is difficult only if the sphenoid sinus has been partially removed in previous surgery. Balloon occlusion of the internal carotid artery can be used whenever there is massive tumor infiltration of the foramen lacerum and cavernous sinus.
- Large intracranial tumor extensions from the infratemporal fossa are best removed in a second-stage neurosurgical procedure. This will reduce the risk of CSF leaks and ascending meningitis.
- Malignant tumors that have infiltrated the cavernous sinus are treated by irradiation.
- An intraoperative suction drain should be placed only if the eustachian tube has been securely closed.

Postoperative Care

Postoperative care consists of standard surveillance in the intensive care unit. The nasopharyngeal packing is removed at about three to five days.

Postoperative Complications

Bleeding, CSF leakage, and infection should be recognized early and managed appropriately.

Functional Sequelae

The subtotal petrosectomy leaves a slight depression in the temporal area. Initial sensory deficits should improve with time.

Adverse functional sequelae are relatively minor considering the extent of the resection.

Alternative Methods

Radiotherapy alone or combined radiotherapy/chemotherapy may be considered as alternatives for the treatment of malignant disease.

Bibliography

Denecke H J. Operative Korrektur des Schluckaktes. In: Die oto-rhino-laryngologischen Operationen im Mund- und Halsbereich, Operationslehre V/3 (Denecke H J. ed), 678-690, Heidelberg: Springer; 1980.

Fisch U, Mattox D. Microsurgery of the Skull Base. Stuttgart: Thieme; 1988.

Helms J, Geyer G. Surgery of Cranial Base Tumors (Sekhar L, Janecka J. eds), 461–469, New York: Raven Press; 1993.

Helms J, Schürmann K. Interdisciplinary approach to benign tumors of the lateral skull base. In: Tumors of the skull base (Scheunemann H, Schürmann K, Helms J. eds), 227–229, Berlin: De Gruyler; 1986.

Lang J. Clinical Anatomy of the Posterior Cranial Fossa. Stuttgart: Thieme; 1991.

Lang J. Klinische Anatomie des Ohres. Heidelberg: Springer; 1992.

Poch Broto J, Traserra J, Garcia Ibánez E, Clarós P, Avellaneda R. Cirugia de la Base del Craneo. In: Ponencia Oficial del XV Congreso Nacional, Madrid: Editorial Garsi; 1993.

Samii M, Draf W. Surgery of the Skull Base. Heidelberg: Springer; 1989.

Sekhar L, Janecka J (eds). Surgery of Cranial Base Tumors. New York: Raven Press; 1993.

7 Surgery of the Intracranial Facial Nerve Proximal to the Stylomastoid Foramen

Wolfgang Draf

The cause of peripheral facial nerve paralysis must be established before surgical treatment is planned. This may be a simple matter, as in the case of malformations and trauma, but an etiologic diagnosis can also be quite difficult, as in patients with latent inflammatory disease, "idiopathic" facial paralysis, or occult tumors. A diagnosis of Bell's palsy should be made only after all other potential causes of facial paralysis of acute onset have been excluded. It is often helpful to elicit the prior history and obtain appropriate laboratory tests.

In any case, the disfigurement associated with significant facial nerve paralysis is very distressful to patients and can seriously hamper their ability to communicate effectively in their personal and vocational environments.

Diagnosis

Clinical Findings

It is important to distinguish *supranuclear (central) lesions* of the facial nerve (cortex and internal capsule, operculum, extrapyramidal pathways, midbrain, pons) from *infranuclear (peripheral) lesions* (cerebellopontine angle, skull base, internal auditory canal, geniculate ganglion and tympanomastoid segment, extracranial, extratemporal; Fig. 7.1). Central paralysis is generally a spastic form of paralysis, so that the face appears symmetrical at rest. Normal forehead movements are frequently preserved by the crossed supranuclear fibers. Lesions involving the facial nucleus or more distal nerve segments are characterized by flaccid paralysis in which there is conspicuous facial asymmetry even at rest.

We use Stennert's paresis score and residual defect score (Stennert, 1977) as parameters for evaluating the degree of facial paralysis and for monitoring the

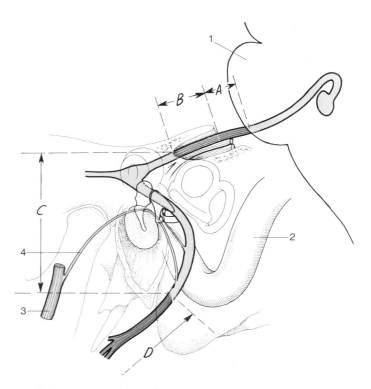

Fig. 7.**1**   Segments of the facial nerve.
A   Cerebellopontine angle segment
B   Meatal segment
C   Fallopian canal
D   Extratemporal segment
1   Pons
2   Sigmoid sinus
3   Lingual nerve
4   Chorda tympani

patient's progress. Other schemes have also been proposed for the documentation of facial nerve deficits and recovery (see May, 1986 for details). The House-Brackmann grading system for facial paralysis is a valuable alternative.

Site-of-Lesion Determination

Besides the type of nerve lesion present, the *site of the lesion* is a key factor in treatment planning. It is determined by a differentiated neurologic examination, vestibular function testing, and detailed audiometric tests that include brainstem audiometry and stapedius reflex testing. These tests may be supplemented by Schirmer's lacrimal secretion test, taste testing, and salivation tests. These latter tests provide limited diagnostic information, however.

Plain and contrast–enhanced magnetic resonance imaging (MRI) has gained increasing importance in recent years for the precise localization of facial nerve lesions.

Electrical Testing

Electrodiagnostic testing is of great value in determining the extent of nerve damage in patients with idiopathic facial paralysis, malformations, trauma, inflammation, and tumors, for determining prognosis in idiopathic facial paralysis, and for selecting patients for facial nerve decompression. These tests require costly equipment, and the examiner must have a detailed knowledge of neuroelectrophysiology in order to interpret the tests correctly. Cooperation with a neuroradiologist is advised.

The current mainstays of electrodiagnostic testing are the maximal stimulation test (MST; May, Harvey, Morovitz, et al., 1971), electroneurography (Fisch and Esslen, 1972), more correctly termed evoked electromyography (EEMG; Blumenthal and May, 1986), and electromyography (EMG).

MST and EEMG can differentiate between neurapraxia and the axonal degeneration of peripheral motor neurons. Serial testing can be done to monitor the progression of paralysis and recovery. EMG can detect recovery of nerve function before any such signs can be observed clinically. One disadvantage is that MST and EEMG are unable to document detectable changes until an average of 72 h after the onset of facial paralysis. In EMG, abnormal fibrillation potentials do not occur until at least eight days after significant nerve injury has occurred. Another limiting factor is the broad range of variation in normal facial nerve responses to electrical stimulation. Side–to–side comparisons are of critical importance.

Radiologic Studies

Conventional Radiography and Tomography

Conventional radiographic views of the petrous bone (e.g., Schüller, Stenvers, Wullstein, Meyer, etc.) can do no more than provide a basic diagnostic impression. The radiation exposure is justified only if more modern diagnostic methods are unavailable and help is needed in deciding whether to refer the patient to a better equipped center. Conventional tomography can provide more accurate information on the site of a facial nerve lesion, e.g., secondary to malformation, trauma, inflammation, or tumor (Mündnich and Frey, 1959; Reisner and Gosepath, 1973; Valvassori and Buckingham, 1975), but the attainable image quality still falls short of the currently accepted standard.

Computed Tomography and Magnetic Resonance Imaging

High–resolution, thin–section computed tomography (CT) using a 2–4 mm slice thickness is the current standard for providing detailed views of the intratemporal course of the facial nerve. Multiplanar reconstruction can be used to document all the facial nerve segments and surrounding bone and to demonstrate abnormalities (Haas and Kahle, 1988; Valvassori and Buckingham, 1975). CT also provides positive identification of intracranial mass lesions, especially in contrast–enhanced scans.

Magnetic resonance imaging (MRI) can provide high–definition views of even small neoplastic lesions (e.g., intrameatal acoustic and facial neuromas) unobscured by superimposed bone, especially when paramagnetic contrast enhancement is used. MRI is superior to CT in this regard. Not infrequently, both modalities must be applied as complementary studies. Osseous structures are portrayed more clearly on CT scans. The capabilities of MRI for facial nerve evaluation have not yet been fully explored (Valvassori et al., 1988; Traxter et al., 1989), and further important developments are expected. MRI is becoming increasingly important for site–of–lesion determinations. Cooperation and close consultation with a neuroradiologist is advised.

Informed Consent

Informed consent is often a key element in current medicolegal proceedings. Physicians are well advised to accede to the wishes of most patients to receive adequate information and, when various treatment options are available, to have some decision–making power based on a reasonable knowledge of specific problems and issues.

The patient information process should be thorough and unemotional. This is possible only if the surgeon masters the full spectrum of procedures that may be applied in the treatment of facial paralysis.

We have found it helpful to use an anatomic diagram when explaining the etiology, pathogenesis, and location of the facial nerve lesion and the related problems of surgical treatment. Preoperative consultation can be difficult in patients who already have iatrogenic morbidity following a previous operation. The consulting physician should help the patient understand the specific pathoanatomic situation that led to the facial nerve injury by a different surgeon or by the consulting physician himself. Disparaging remarks about the previous surgeon do not benefit the latter, the patient, or the surgeon to whom the patient has entrusted the task of facial nerve rehabilitation. In the discussion of the surgical procedure itself, the patient, who usually has high expectations for the operation and is pressing for it, should be given very explicit information on the rationale for the procedure and the chances of success. The indications for facial nerve decompression surgery (see. pp. 216 ff.) are especially problematic. The patient can appreciate the fact that the degree of residual dysfunction can be reduced in selected cases by an experienced surgeon. The chance for a successful end–to–end anastomosis or free nerve graft by current microsurgical standards is approximately 80% in terms of achieving a satisfying clinical result. A complete functional recovery is not possible following nerve reconstruction, and a residual degree of involuntary spastic twitching and synkinesis must be accepted. More centrally located lesions are associated with a greater degree of synkinesis.

The patient should also be made aware of the usually mild sensory deficits that will follow the removal of donor nerves (e.g., cervical plexus, sural nerve).

The definitive outcome of a nerve reconstruction cannot be assessed until about 1–2 years postoperatively. The patient may not notice initial signs of regeneration until about three months, depending on the proximity of the defect to the facial muscles. The rate of regeneration does not depend significantly upon age. Postoperative radiotherapy has no lasting adverse effects on nerve regeneration.

We make an effort during the preoperative consultation to motivate the patient for the active facial exercises that will follow surgery. There is no point in initiating facial exercises until clinical evidence of regeneration has been observed (motor twitches and incipient voluntary movement). We have had good results with the use of a special exercise instruction sheet. The rationale and benefits of electrotherapy are controversial, but such therapy should not be withheld from patients who expressly desire it.

Multiple video documentation, which is superior to static photographic documentation, is useful for reminding patients of their preoperative condition and motivating them to perform their exercises at home. Video documentation of the nerve reconstruction can be a valuable document in the event of a medicolegal dispute.

Indications

Detailed diagnostic studies are essential in selecting patients for facial nerve surgery. Early and late paralysis cannot be differentiated in the unconscious trauma patient, but it is safe to wait until the patient regains consciousness before assessing the extent of the facial nerve injury. In doubtful cases it is best to proceed with atraumatic microsurgical exploration of the nerve.

Absolute Indications

Immediate Posttraumatic Paralysis

For combined injuries of the petrous bone and facial soft tissues, we feel that immediate nerve exploration in the face is warranted if there are deep lacerations in the region of the parotid gland. Restraint is advised in patients with more superficial and more peripherally located lacerations and abrasions, as in these cases the numerous facial anastomoses can often compensate satisfactorily for the transection of individual facial nerve branches. Surgical measures should not aggravate the severity of existing traumatic lesions (see also Surgery of the Extratemporal Facial Nerve, Vol. 1, Chapter 16).

Confirmed Intraoperative Nerve Injury

This type of injury includes inadvertent lesions caused by dissection close to the facial nerve as well as unavoidable transection of the nerve necessitated by tumor removal, for example. Any nerve irritation that would prevent a complete, spontaneous recovery should be precisely analyzed and, if necessary, corrected by reconstructive measures. The latter should be performed by a surgeon experienced in facial nerve surgery.

Postoperative Facial Paralysis

Any postoperative facial nerve paralysis that is not obviously referable to temporary swelling and is not promptly improved by measures to reduce swelling should be surgically explored to advance the diagnosis and avoid medicolegal consequences. If necessary, the original surgeon should not hesitate to refer the patient to a surgeon considered to be more competent.

Facial Paralysis Secondary to Otitis Media

Decompression of the middle ear cleft by myringotomy and tube insertion is often sufficient in patients with acute otitis media. In cases complicated by mastoiditis, more extensive decompressive measures must be undertaken by performing a mastoidectomy and exploring the middle ear space.

With chronic otitis media (usually cholesteatoma), the surgeon should expose the facial nerve while clearing the middle ear of disease. Delays could allow irreversible axonotmesis or neurotmesis to develop, resulting in incomplete recovery.

Relative Indications

Late Posttraumatic Palsy

Surgical exploration of the facial nerve is appropriate in cases where electrodiagnostic tests confirm a severe injury and there is no clinical evidence of spontaneous improvement. CT evidence of discontinuities in the bony canal will facilitate the decision to expose the nerve and locate the site of the lesion. In many cases the lesion can be directly visualized with MRI.

Idiopathic Facial Paralysis

Surgical decompression is appropriate for idiopathic facial paralysis only in the rare cases where there is complete paralysis showing no tendency to improve, and electrophysiologic tests show marked signs of degeneration and objectively confirm the absence of voluntary innervation. Follow–up examinations should be scheduled following the decompression.

Irreversible Partial Paralysis

The decision to operate is always difficult in this population. The reasonably attainable degree of improvement should be explained to the patient and weighed carefully against the possibility that surgery may cause additional damage. In principle, simple exposure and epineural neurolysis of the facial nerve by an experienced surgeon should carry an acceptable degree of risk.

Surgical Options for Lesions of the Intracranial and Intratemporal Portions of the Facial Nerve

Several basic options exist for the surgical rehabilitation of facial nerve palsy, depending on the site of the lesion and the interval between the occurrence of the lesion and operative treatment:

1) Decompression,
2) Direct anastomosis,
3) Indirect anastomosis,
4) Secondary plastic reconstruction.

Some cases require a combined approach involving the use of both direct and indirect anastomoses ["diversification" concept of Stennert (1979)], or it may be advantageous to combine a direct or indirect anastomosis with secondary plastic reconstruction. Again, there are some patients who will benefit from just one of these methods (cf. Volume 1, Chapter 16), while others will require a comprehensive rehabilitative approach involving all three. The decision in a given case will depend on which of the methods, alone or in combination, is likely to produce the most favorable result with the fewest disadvantages.

The timing of facial nerve surgery can be simple or quite difficult. This is because it is not always easy to determine the extent of a posttraumatic or postoperative lesion and accurately predict the capacity for spontaneous regeneration.

Serial electrophysiologic testing and especially clinical observation are appropriate when the extent of the nerve lesion cannot be clearly ascertained. This is often the case after tumor excisions and with intractable facial palsy that is secondary to inflammatory disease and persists after the cause has been eliminated. There is still controversy regarding the interval after the onset of significant facial palsy during which surgical therapy is still feasible. As a general rule of thumb, the prospects for successful surgical therapy are unfavorable after more than one year has passed, and they are definitely poor after more than two years. On a shorter time scale, there is no appreciable difference in functional outcome between performing immediate surgery for a nerve defect and deferring the surgery for six to eight weeks after the injury. We personally favor the definitive primary repair of nerve transection injuries, assuming that satisfactory technical facilities and personnel are available. This is especially true if the extratemporal facial nerve has sustained damage. If several weeks have passed since the injury, it can be more difficult to locate and identify the nerve stumps in the buccal soft tissues than it is to carry out the repair itself.

If the paralysis patient seeks facial rehabilitation after a period of months or even years, then the history of the causative injury and the results of electrophysiologic testing will determine whether it is worthwhile to undertake surgery to restore nerve conduction to the still-functional musculature, or whether it is better from the outset to plan a secondary plastic reconstruction. We know from experimental and clinical experience that collateral innervation in patients with a unilateral facial nerve transection can provide some degree of innervation to the palsied muscles from the opposite side, even if the patient appears clinically to have total paralysis. It would be appropriate in such cases to attempt a direct or indirect anastomosis to take advantage of the fact that functional muscles are still present (Samii and Draf, 1989).

Surgical Procedures

Basic Methods

Surgical Segmental Anatomy of the Facial Nerve

The thickness of the connective tissue sheath surrounding the facial nerve increases from the center toward the periphery, so the peripheral portions of the nerve are less sensitive to mechanical irritation than its more central segments. This variation in mechanical sensitivity, along with site–to–site variations in the recipient bed and the diversity of surgical approaches, provide a basis for subdividing the facial nerve into four main segments (fig. 7.**1**):

1) The cerebellopontine angle segment,
2) The meatal segment (within the internal auditory canal),
3) The intratemporal segment (within the fallopian canal),
4) The extratemporal portion.

As the facial nerve emerges from the brain stem, about the first 2 mm of the nerve is covered only by central glial cells. Past that point the nerve is accompanied by Schwann cells (Lang, 1989). The epineural and perineural connective–tissue sheath investing the nerve becomes thicker within the fallopian canal and extratemporally, providing effective protection from mechanical irritation. As it traverses the cerebellopontine angle and the internal auditory canal, the facial nerve is exposed to rhythmic movements of the recipient bed within the CSF, a circumstance that must be considered in the creation of anastomoses. The segment traversing the fallopian canal is the most favorable in terms of graft placement and nutrition. The recipient bed is immobile, and in many cases an interpositional graft can be stably positioned without sutures. The extratemporal region is also very favorable for graft nutrition, but the graft length should be sufficient to allow for nerve motion. There is some degree of overlap among the surgical approaches to the various facial nerve segments: the cerebellopontine angle segment and the meatal segment in the internal auditory canal are both accessible through the lateral suboccipital approach or the transtemporal extradural approach; the translabyrinthine route can be used in patients with total hearing loss. The initial, labyrinthine portion of the fallopian canal about the geniculate ganglion is also accessible by the transtemporal approach, or it can be reached by the transmastoid route. If the bone is poorly pneumatized, it may occasionally be necessary to disrupt the ossicular chain in order to gain access to the geniculate ganglion following mastoidectomy. If the dura occupies a low position, it may not be possible to reach the geniculate ganglion by the transmastoid route or through the external auditory canal (see pp. 216 ff.). The extratemporal facial nerve can be approached through existing soft–tissue injuries or through an incision like that used for parotidectomy (see p. 226).

Obtaining Graft Material for Nerve Reconstruction

Grafts used in restoring facial nerve continuity must match the anatomic caliber of the facial nerve following removal of the epineurium (Fig. 7.**2** and 7.**3**). Also, it must be possible to harvest a sufficient length of the graft material. A branched graft is often desirable for reconstructing the extratemporal portion of the nerve. Finally, the harvesting of the graft should produce minimal functional and cosmetic deficits for the patient.

Branches of the cervical plexus are excellent in terms of matching the facial nerve caliber. The great auricular nerve and sural nerve are particularly well suited, and branched grafts can be obtained if desired. Another advantage is the proximity of the cervical plexus to the operative site (Fig. 7.**4**). In terms of length, however, 10 cm is about the maximum graft length than can be obtained from the cervical plexus. Following malignant tumor surgery, the graft should be taken from the plexus that is contralateral to the side where the tumor was removed. With proper suture technique, the extra neck incision should not be conspicuous. Experience has shown that the resulting sensory disturbances in the neck and auricle do not cause significant discomfort.

The sural nerve can provide a branched or unbranched graft up to 40 cm long whose caliber closely matches that of the facial nerve. Removal of the sural nerve creates relatively minor sensory deficits on the lateral side of the foot (Figs. 7.**5** and 7.**6**). A certain amount of experience is needed for harvesting the graft. The advantages and disadvantages of the remoteness of the donor area from the recipient bed tend to balance out.

One advantage is that the operating time can be shortened by having two teams simultaneously prepare the recipient site and harvest the graft. Potential contamination of the donor site with malignant cells is not a concern. On the negative side, extra sterile draping of the donor site would be necessary in cases where the need for the graft was not appreciated before the operation.

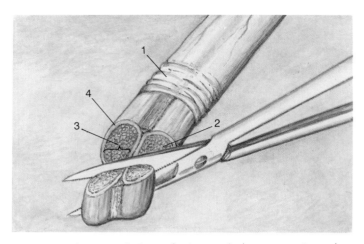

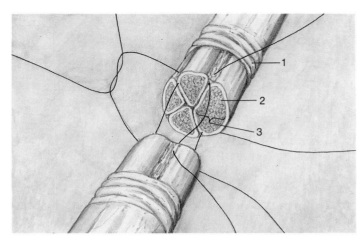

Figs. 7.**2** and 7.**3** Technique of microsurgical nerve anastomosis.

Fig. 7.**2** Several millimeters of the epineurium are resected. The fascicles are freshened with serrated microscissors.
1 Epineurium
2 Axon bundles
3 Fascicles
4 Perineurium

Fig. 7.**3** Perineural–fascicular sutures.
1 Epineurium
2 Perineurium
3 Fascicle

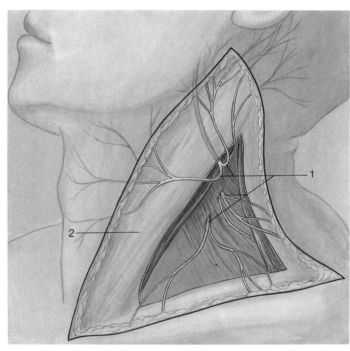

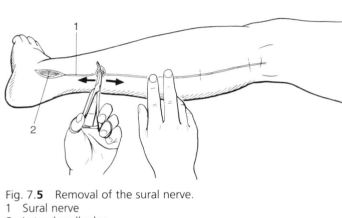

Fig. 7.**5** Removal of the sural nerve.
1 Sural nerve
2 Lateral malleolus

Fig. 7.**4** Sensory branches of the cervical plexus that are available as branched or unbranched nerve graft material.
1 Cervical plexus
2 Sternocleidomastoid muscle

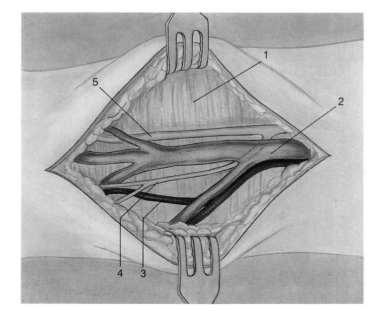

Fig. 7.**6** Topographic anatomy dorsal to the lateral malleolus (left side).   ▷
1 Lateral malleolus
2 Short saphenous vein
3 Peroneal artery
4 Branch of sural nerve
5 Sural nerve

Obtaining a Graft from the Cervical Plexus
(Figs. 7.**4**)

In most laterobasal extracranial surgical procedures, a graft can be harvested through the main surgical incision. If necessary, the incision can be extended inferiorly along the posterior border of the sternocleidomastoid muscle. A retroauricular incision from the superior root of the auricle to the mastoid tip should suffice if only a short graft is needed. The great auricular nerve is exposed just below the skin and can be followed as far as Erb's point at the junction of the middle and upper thirds of the posterior border of the sternocleidomastoid muscle, depending on the graft length required. A branched graft can be obtained by identifying a large-caliber branch of C2, transecting it as centrally as possible, and removing it along with its peripheral branches including the great auricular nerve.

Harvesting the Sural Nerve
(Figs. 7.**5** and 7.**6**)

The patient may be placed in a supine or prone position. The dissection is somewhat easier in the prone position, but moving the patient from the supine to the prone position can be time-consuming. We prefer the supine position, therefore. Starting at the junction of the middle and anterior thirds of an imaginary line connecting the tip of the calcaneus with the lateral malleolus, an anteriorly concave skin incision is made parallel to the posterior circumference of the calcaneus. The main trunk of the sural nerve is generally located slightly anterior and medial to the short saphenous vein (Fig. 7.**6**). Care is taken not to mistake branches of the main nerve trunk for the trunk itself, which may be located somewhat more centrally. The nerve is bluntly exposed in the area of the incision, and a mosquito forceps is passed underneath it. The surgeon identifies the cranial course of the nerve by pulling gently on the nerve with the forceps while palpating lateral to the posterior midline of the lower leg 10 to 15 cm above the lateral malleolus. A second incision, preferably horizontal, is made at that level. The nerve is again bluntly exposed and elevated on a forceps, and traction is applied with the lower forceps to confirm its identity. The longitudinal fibers visible through the epineurium serve to distinguish the nerve from the short saphenous vein. The nerve can be exposed at one or two additional levels, depending on the required graft length, as far as the division of the two muscle bellies of the gastrocnemius. At that level the nerve passes deeply in front of the gastrocnemius muscle and generally cannot be followed further. The nerve is sectioned at the desired level and extracted from its bed with the mosquito forceps. In some cases large central branches will tether the sural nerve to its bed; these branches have to be exposed and sectioned through additional horizontal incisions so that they will not seriously damage the main trunk of the graft during the extraction. Afterward all the skin incisions are closed in layers, and a compressive elastic dressing is applied to the lower leg.

Technique of Nerve Anastomosis

Three main factors account for the superiority of the microsurgical technique over naked-eye neurorhaphy (Samii, 1975):

1) The ability to evaluate the precise extent of the nerve lesion,
2) Optimum coaptation of the nerve ends,
3) Reduced surgical trauma owing to the use of microsurgical instruments and extremely fine suture material (10—0).

Before the advent of microsurgical nerve anastomosis, interrupted epineural sutures were used in the attempt to achieve optimum coaptation of the nerve stumps. Although precise coaptation can be obtained with this technique, the overriding, kinking, and shifting of individual fascicles can significantly reduce the number of functioning axons in the periphery (Fig. 7.**7**). Another factor to be considered is that the facial nerve does not contain well-defined connective-tissue sheaths producing a fascicular architecture like that observed in the peripheral nerves. Consequently, the classic fascicular suture described by Milesi is not strictly applicable to the facial nerve, especially its intratemporal portion (Milesi, 1969). The surgeon must attempt, rather, to adapt the multifascicular nerve graft optimally to the monofascicular structure of the central facial nerve stump.

Operative Technique

The first 1–2 mm of epineurium, if present, is resected from the nerve stump and from the graft with a serrated microscissors (Figs. 7.**2** and 7.**3**). Next a smooth interface is prepared at each nerve end by resecting the nerve bundles protruding from the perineural sheaths. The axon bundles will tend to extrude from the interface again, so suturing should be performed without delay. The cross-sectional architecture of the facial nerve varies from site to site. The sparse amount of investing connective tissue in the cerebellopontine angle gives that segment of the facial nerve a monofascicular structure. By the time it reaches the stylomastoid foramen, the nerve has acquired a markedly thicker epineural sheath, but its perineural segmentation generally produces no more than two or at most three units that are identifiable as fascicular substructures under the microscope. Our suture material of first choice is nonabsorbable 10—0 monofilament. During suturing

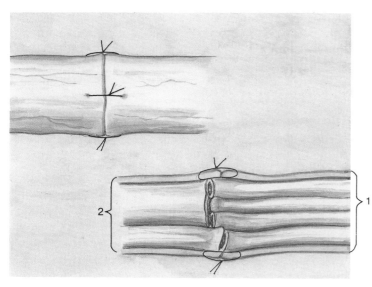

Fig. 7.**7**   A pure epineural suture may allow shifting or overriding of the fascicles, inhibiting the growth of central nerve fibers into the peripheral part of the nerve.
1   Nerve graft
2   Facial nerve

the needle is passed through the connective–tissue sheath surrounding the fascicular bundles. The peripheral part of the facial nerve is anastomosed with perineural and interfascicular sutures, while the meatal and cerebellopontine angle portions are sutured without removing the epineurium. Besides accurate coaptation of the nerve ends, a successful functional result depends on a completely tension–free suture line. In doubtful cases it is better to interpose an autogenous nerve graft, producing two anastomotic sites, than perform an end–to–end anastomosis that is under tension (Samii, 1975).

Special Methods

The techniques of direct anastomosis are of primary interest in the intracranial and intratemporal portions of the facial nerve. They produce the best results in terms of voluntary motor function *and* emotional expression. Techniques of indirect facial nerve repair are generally applied distal to the stylomastoid foramen, so they are outside the scope of this chapter. They are considered second–line techniques in terms of their functional and aesthetic outcomes, while secondary plastic reconstructions (see Volume 1, Chapter 16) are considered third–line techniques. It should be added that the different methods in each group can vary considerably in terms of the functional result and the surgery–related disadvantages for the patient.

Techniques of practical importance for exposing the cerebellopontine angle and intratemporal portions of the facial nerve, and their capabilities, are discussed in the sections below. The emphasis is on the treatment of the facial nerve itself rather than the surgical approach. Technical details on the various routes of approach can be found in the chapters dealing with surgery of the mastoid process, middle ear, internal auditory canal, and cerebellopontine angle.

Simple Nerve Exploration

Indications

Simple exposure of the facial nerve is an option in post-traumatic and postsurgical cases where unexpected facial nerve palsy develops that (1) is not explained by the trauma mechanism or radiologic findings and (2) is so severe according to electrophysiologic tests (see above) that exposure of the nerve to relieve pressure, remove a bone fragment, etc. could positively influence the quality and the rate of facial nerve recovery.

Principle of the Operation

The surgery involves selective exposure of the facial nerve in the presumed area of irritation. Bone splinters are removed as required, and the degree of damage is assessed. In many cases this simple exploration will lead to more extensive measures such as decompression or nerve repair, so it should always be performed by a surgeon experienced in facial nerve surgery so that unnecessary second and third operations can be avoided.

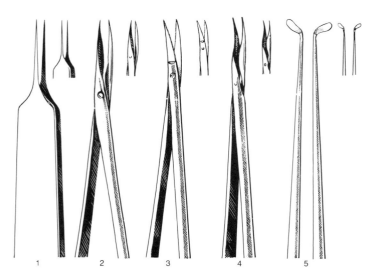

Fig. 7.**8** Assortment of microsurgical instruments used for nerve anastomosis and exposure.
1 Watchmaker's forceps
2 Nerve grasping forceps
3 Serrated scissors (Samii design)
4 Needle holder
5 Nerve excavators (right and left)

Special Instruments

The micro–otosurgical instrument set (Fig. 7.**8**) includes cutting and diamond burrs, facial nerve excavators, and microneurosurgical instrumentation with micro–grasping forceps, serrated and nonserrated microscissors, watchmaker's forceps, and micro–needle holders.

Suture material: We use 10—0 nonabsorbable or slowly absorbing monofilament. Fibrin glue may be used in selected cases.

The above instruments are necessary for all the techniques described below. Neural stimulators are not required, since anatomic landmarks are sufficient for identifying the facial nerve in its intracranial and intratemporal course.

Anesthesia

Although local anesthesia is adequate for exposing the tympanic and mastoid segments of the facial nerve, most of these operations are performed under general anesthesia (neuroleptanalgesia) augmented by the local infiltration of an anesthetic/vasoconstrictor solution. This is done because most patients desire it, because the surgeon may have to extend the field toward the internal auditory canal, and because it may be necessary to harvest a nerve graft. The systolic blood pressure should range from 80 to 100 mm Hg to help clear the field of blood. Topostasin solution (Schobel) is an ef-

fective local hemostatic agent and can obviate the potential side effects of the direct injection of epinephrine solution.

Operative Technique

The simple exposure of a selected portion of the facial nerve is one aspect of the procedures described below, so the technique will be described within the context of those procedures.

Facial Nerve Decompression and Neurolysis

Decompression of the facial nerve is indicated after trauma, in rare cases of Bell's palsy, in patients with a severe inflammatory process in the petrous bone such as acute otitis media or a specific form of chronic otitis media, cholesteatoma, necrotizing otitis externa, facial nerve compression by tumor, and finally for hemifacial spasm secondary to vascular compression at the brain stem. Even with modern diagnostic studies, it cannot always be predicted whether exposure of the facial nerve will be adequate in a given case, or whether a repair or reconstruction will be required.

Classic Transmastoid Facial Nerve Decompression (Bonnel, 1927; Wullstein, 1958)

Indications

See above (pp. 209–210).

Principle of the Operation

The surgery involves complete exposure of the mastoid and tympanic segments of the facial nerve as far as the geniculate ganglion, with incision of the epineurium.

Position: The patient is positioned as for a tympanoplasty with mastoidectomy. The head and upper body are slightly elevated, and the head is hyperextended and turned to the opposite side.

Operative Technique

(Figs. 7.**9** and 7.**10**)

The operation starts with a wide mastoidectomy (see p. 80) with cortex removal to the level of the middle cranial fossa dura and posterolaterally to the sigmoid sinus. After exposure of the aditus, incus, and lateral semicircular canal, the bony layer covering the mastoid segment of the facial nerve is first identified below the

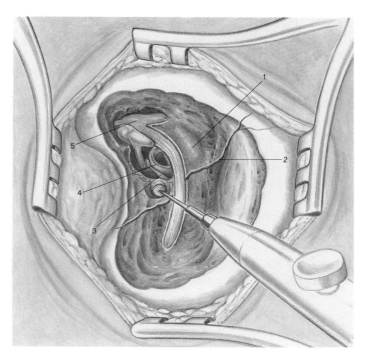

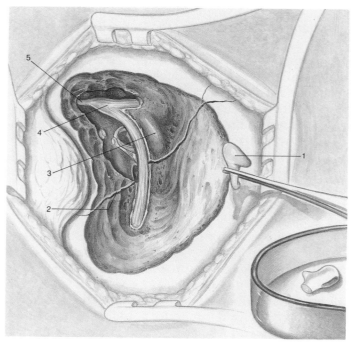

Figs. 7.**9** and 7.**10**   Transmastoid facial nerve decompression with preservation of the ossicular chain.

Fig. 7.**9**   The facial nerve is exposed to the geniculate ganglion in well–pneumatized bone, preserving the ossicular chain. An extensive mastoidectomy is performed. The fracture line runs below the semicircular canal. The dura is high, allowing somewhat more extensive bone removal about the stylomastoid foramen. The geniculate ganglion lies in front of the anterior stapes crus by a distance roughly equal to the distance between the crura.
1   Lateral semicircular canal
2   Fracture
3   Stapedius tendon
4   Stapes
5   Geniculate ganglion

Fig. 7.**10**   The facial nerve after dismantling of the ossicular chain, exposed as far as the geniculate ganglion. The petrous bone is poorly pneumatized. The malleus head and incus are removed and reconstructed by a type III tympanoplasty.
1   Incus
2   Fracture
3   Lateral semicircular canal
4   Geniculate ganglion
5   Greater petrosal nerve

tip of the short process (crus) of the incus. The more heavily the bone is pneumatized, the thinner the bony plate covering the facial nerve. Occasionally the facial canal may be dehiscent due to the presence of a "Pogany cell*." As the burr aproaches the actual facial canal, the pale nerve sheath can be seen shimmering through the bone when viewed under the microscope. A relatively large arterial vessel can be seen on the sheath, following the course of the nerve. As bone removal is carried close to the thin bony layer covering the facial nerve, the surgeon's experience will dictate whether it is best to use a round–cutting burr or a diamond burr. In any case, a constant up–and–down motion of the burr should be maintained while gentle pressure and continuous irrigation are applied to avoid overheating close to the nerve. The surgeon should keep in mind that the facial nerve may occasionally follow an

atypical course (Helms, 1981). The bony shell covering the facial nerve is exposed as far as the stylomastoid foramen, which generally is located at the anterior end of a ridge that is formed by the start of the digastric muscle and projects into the mastoid. At that point the bone around the stylomastoid foramen is excavated somewhat more broadly. Then, using the diamond burr, the surgeon thins the bony layer in front of, over, and behind the facial nerve, leaving an eggshell thickness that can easily be elevated at a later time. After the mastoid portion of the facial canal has been exposed, the chordofacial angle between the chorda tympani and the facial nerve is excavated until the incudostapedial joint, stapes, and tympanic facial nerve segment can be identified. The surgical cavity should closely approach the geniculate ganglion medial to the long process of the incus. If access to the geniculate ganglion is required, as in patients with idiopathic facial nerve palsy and many types of laterobasal fracture, this can be accomplished in well–pneumatized bone by dissecting along the bone

* A Pogany cell is a large cell located over the mastoidal part of the facial nerve.

covering the middle fossa dura and approaching the ganglion from above (Fig. 7.**9**). This preserves the continuity of the ossicular chain. With moderate pneumatization and a low position of the dura, the ossicular chain will have to be disarticulated at the incudostapedial joint, the incus extracted, and the malleus head removed with a nipper to gain access to the geniculate ganglion. The procedure concludes with a type III tympanoplasty in which generally the body of the incus is interposed between the stapes and malleus remnant to reestablish continuity (Fig. 7.**10**). These are the two options available for exposing the geniculate ganglion, which is located anterior to the anterior stapedial crus by a distance approximately equal to the distance separating the stapedial crura. After also thinning the bony plate covering the tympanic facial nerve segment (where spontaneous dehiscences may again be encountered), the surgeon progressively elevates the bony shell from all portions of the facial nerve using a knife–elevator, House curette, and excavators. Indriven bone fragments may have to be removed in patients with fractures. At the conclusion of the operation, the nerve sheath is incised with the sickle knife, a sharp microscissors, or a micro–razor blade. At this time, the relatively thick connective–tissue ring around the stylomastoid foramen should be divided until the nerve fascicles can be seen. Suction trauma to the nerve bundles can be avoided by applying the suction tip over cottonoid strips covering the nerves. If heavy intraoperative bleeding has occurred, it is a good precaution to insert a silicone drainage tube for several days; usually this is unnecessary, however. The periosteum covering the mastoidal corticalis is sutured to the meatal skin to prevent stenosis of the meatal entrance, and the wound is closed in layers using subcutaneous interrupted sutures and a simple running suture in the skin.

In patients with irreversible hearing loss due to a laterobasal fracture, for example, the mastoidectomy can be extended to a labyrinthectomy so that the facial nerve can be followed into the cerebellopontine angle (p. 224). A standard pressure dressing is applied over the ear.

Postoperative Care

The ear dressing is removed on the second postoperative day. If a drain has been inserted, it is removed three days postoperatively. Active facial exercises should be initiated as soon as clinical signs indicate a return of nerve function. As noted on page 209, electrotherapy is controversial, but we feel it should be offered to patients who request it.

Errors, Pitfalls, and Hints

The short process (crus) of the incus points to the facial nerve canal! The semicircular canal lies posterosuperiorly and should not be violated. The gray line exposed by thinning its bony covering should alert the surgeon to drill no farther. Drilling around the nerve itself requires continuous, copious irrigation to prevent overheating. In all trauma patients, the tympanic and mastoid segments of the facial nerve should be completely exposed. If no abnormalities are found, the labyrinthine segment and geniculate ganglion should be decompressed through the transtemporal–extradural route in patients with good hearing or by the translabyrinthine route in patients with total hearing loss on the affected side. Intraoperative findings will dictate whether nerve decompression is sufficient, or whether reconstructive measures are required.

Decompression of the Geniculate Ganglion through the External Auditory Canal

Indications

Selective decompression of the geniculate ganglion is appropriate in the rare cases of idiopathic facial paralysis that meet the clinical and electrophysiologic criteria for operability (see p. 210). The bony canal of the facial nerve is narrowest at the geniculate ganglion, so swelling at that level can lead very rapidly to neurapraxia and axonotmesis (Fowler, 1956; Helms, 1976).

Principle of the Operation

The area of the geniculate ganglion, considered critical in the pathogenesis of idiopathic facial palsy, is selectively decompressed through a limited surgical approach.

Position: The patient is positioned supine with the head turned to the opposite side. As in operations for otosclerosis, the head is not hyperextended.

Anesthesia

The procedure is performed under local anesthesia with sedation. General anesthesia supplemented by local infiltration is used only if the patient requests it.

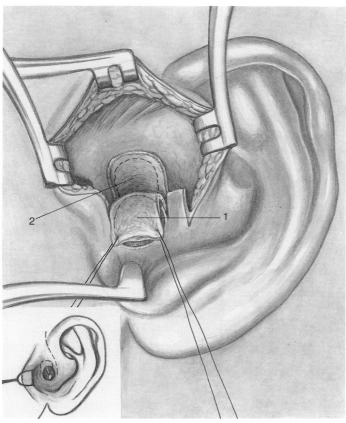

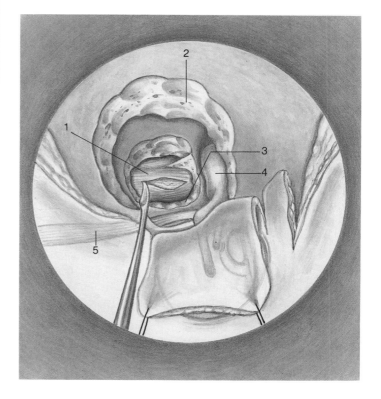

7.**11**   7.**12**

Figs. 7.**11** to 7.**13** Decompression of the geniculate ganglion through the external auditory canal (Helms, 1976).

Fig. 7.**11** Incision (overview).

Fig. 7.**12** Endaural auxiliary incision with a superior tympanomeatal flap. The area of bone removal is marked by a red dotted line.
1 Superior tympanomeatal flap
2 Bone removal

Fig. 7.**13** Geniculate ganglion exposed anterior to the malleus handle.
1 Geniculate ganglion
2 Lateral attic wall
3 Bony tympanic facial canal
4 Malleus head
5 Tensor tympani muscle

Operative Technique

(Figs. 7.**11**, 7.**12**, and 7.**13**)

An endaural auxiliary incision is made (Fig. 7.**11**), and a superior tympanomeatal flap based on the tympanic membrane is developed in the superior portion of the auditory canal (Fig. 7.**12**). The malleus head is exposed, the anterior part of the bony anulus is burred away from 12 to 3 o'clock, and the lateral bony layer covering the geniculate ganglion is progressively thinned anterior to the malleus head. Several smaller cells will have to be opened first if the bone is well pneumatized. The geniculate ganglion is positively identified by exposing the origin of the greater petrosal nerve anteriorly and the start of the tympanic facial nerve segment posteriorly (Fig. 7.**13**). The surgical cavity is bounded posteriorly by the malleus head, inferiorly by the anterior liga-ment of the malleus, superiorly by the bone covering the middle fossa dura, and anteriorly by the anterior wall of the tympanic cavity.

The nerve sheath surrounding the geniculate ganglion is incised. At the conclusion of the operation the tympanomeatal flap is replaced and supported with two silicone strips, the external auditory canal is packed with sponge packing, the endaural auxiliary incision is closed, and the ear dressing is applied.

Postoperative Care

The ear dressing is removed on the second postoperative day. The sponge packing and silicone strips can be removed on the sixth postoperative day.

Errors, Pitfalls, and Hints

The surgeon should review the CT scans preoperatively to determine whether the dura is sufficiently high to allow access to the geniculate ganglion from the lateral side. The tympanomeatal flap should be broadly based on the tympanic membrane between nine and three o'clock. If tearing of the tympanic membrane cannot be avoided, the tear can be repaired by backing it with a small piece of fascia, and the sponge packing is left in place for three weeks postoperatively. The surgeon should avoid touching the malleus head with the diamond burr to avoid inner ear trauma. The diamond burr should be "as large as possible and as small as necessary" in order to reduce the risk of iatrogenic injury.

Advantages and Disadvantages

Our own experience is consistent with that of Helms (1976). The operation is relatively simple for the experienced surgeon compared with the classic transmastoid facial nerve decompression. It is also associated with less morbidity and provides safer access to the geniculate ganglion, especially in terms of preserving the ossicular chain. One disadvantage is that the less experienced surgeon may find it difficult at first to become oriented in the region anterior to the malleus head.

Alternative Procedures

Classic transmastoid facial nerve decompression.

Complete Meatolabyrinthine–Tympanomastoid Exposure of the Facial Nerve (Fisch, 1973; 1979)

Principle and Indications

This procedure involves exposure of the facial nerve in the internal auditory canal and the labyrinthine portion of the fallopian canal through the middle cranial fossa by the extradural, transtemporal route combined with exposure of the tympanic and mastoid facial nerve segments through a mastoidectomy in the same sitting. Its main indication is for extensive petrous bone fractures in patients with intact preoperative hearing.

For Bell's palsy, Fisch exposes the facial nerve in the internal auditory canal and the labyrinthine portion of the fallopian canal. If intraoperative neuronography localizes the lesion to this area, the procedure concludes with incision of the epineurium at the geniculate ganglion. Fisch reports that this is not the case in 6% of patients, who will require transmastoid exposure of the facial nerve in the same sitting. He states further that transtemporal exposure is adequate in patients with zoster oticus.

Operative Technique

This procedure combines the transtemporal–extradural approach to the lateral central skull base (see p. 223) with transmastoid facial nerve decompression (see p. 216), so the description does not need to be repeated here.

Vascular Decompression of the Facial Nerve in the Cerebellopontine Angle (Jannetta, 1967; 1970)

Campbell and Keedy (1947) and Gardner (1962) made early references to vasogenic compression of the facial nerve in the cerebellopontine angle as having causal significance in facial nerve spasm. With the advent of the operating microscope, Jannetta was able to perform a systematic microsurgical exploration of the cerebellopontine angle with vascular decompression of cranial nerve VII. His excellent results have since been duplicated and confirmed by numerous authors.

Hemifacial spasm is now considered an established indication for microsurgical exploration of the cerebellopontine angle with vascular decompression of the nerve. Unlike other common surgical treatments for hemifacial spasm, this procedure is both nondestructive and causal, as it eliminates the cause of facial twitching by removing vascular pressure from the nerve near its site of emergence from the brain stem. Jannetta et al. (1978) also achieved good results in six patients with "Ménière-like" vestibulocochlear dysfunction by performing vascular decompression of cranial nerve VIII in the cerebellopontine angle. These results have not yet been confirmed by other authors (see Samii and Draf, 1989 for a detailed discussion and further references).

Principle of the Operation

The operation involves exposing the facial nerve at its origin from the brain stem and identifying the impinging vascular segments, most commonly the posterior and anterior inferior cerebellar arteries. These vessels are isolated, and a muscle graft is interposed between them and the facial nerve. The cerebellopontine angle segment of the facial nerve can be exposed through the extended transtemporal extradural approach (Wigand et al., 1982), or, more commonly, by the lateral suboccipital route.

Facial Nerve Surgery from the Cerebellopontine Angle to the Stylomastoid Foramen

End–to–End Anastomosis in the Cerebellopontine Angle

An end–to–end anastomosis of the facial nerve in the cerebellopontine angle may be necessary in cases where the facial nerve has been severely stretched and thinned by a large cerebellopontine angle tumor, and its continuity cannot be preserved at tumor removal despite meticulous dissection through the suboccipital approach. The stretched, elongated condition of the nerve allows an end–to–end anastomosis to be performed following tumor removal, provided the anatomy is clear enough to allow positive identification of the proximal and distal stumps (Fig. 7.**14**). If this cannot be done, intraoperative stimulation of the questionable peripheral stump is of little help due to the various anastomoses among the nerves in the internal auditory canal, so that eliciting a facial twitch does not establish the identity of the nerve. It remains to be seen whether contemporary stimulators such as the Brackmann device (Brackmann EMG System) will help to resolve this uncertainty (Leonetti et al., 1989).

Owing to the elongated condition of the facial nerve, it is still possible to accomplish an end–to–end repair after about a 1– to 1.5 cm segment of the nerve has been sacrificed at tumor removal. The results of direct facial nerve repairs in the cerebellopontine angle are satisfactory (Samii, 1981). A direct repair is worth attempting, as it is superior to other reconstructive techniques.

After the nerve ends have been freshened, it is generally sufficient to use one or at most two sutures for performing the anastomosis. Due to the pulsations in the cerebellopontine angle, it is advantageous to position the anastomosis against the brain stem or porus acousticus if possible, or to support the repair temporarily by backing it with sponge packing.

For larger defects in the cerebellopontine angle, a nerve graft can be interposed once the central and peripheral nerve stumps have been positively identified (Fig. 7.**15**).

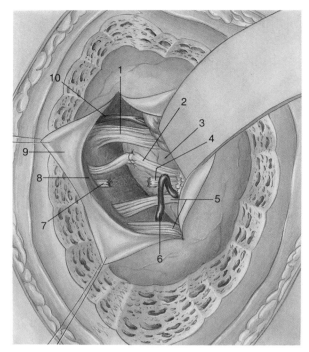

Fig. 7.**14**   End–to–end anastomosis of the facial nerve in the cerebellopontine angle.
1 Trigeminal nerve
2 Facial nerve
3 Pons
4 Stump of vestibulocochlear nerve
5 Lower cranial nerves
6 Anterior inferior cerebellar artery
7 Stump of vestibulocochlear nerve
8 Porus acousticus
9 Dura
10 Petrosal vein

Intracranial–Intratemporal Anastomosis

In an effort to maintain emphasis on preserving or restoring facial nerve continuity following the advent of the operating microscope, neurosurgeons and otosurgeons have collaborated since 1975 to develop the technique of the intracranial–intratemporal anastomosis for cases that cannot be managed by a direct repair (Samii, 1977; Draf, 1980; Draf and Samii, 1982). It represents a simplification of Dott's intracranial–extratemporal repair (Dott, 1958) and is appropriate when the peripheral facial nerve stump cannot be positively identified before its entry into the internal auditory canal.

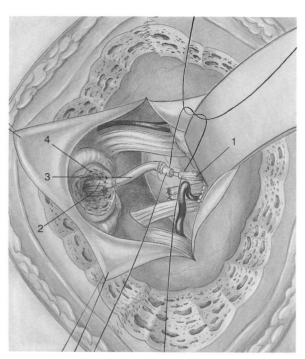

Fig. 7.**15**   Facial nerve reconstruction with a free nerve graft in the cerebellopontine angle.
1   Central stump of facial nerve
2   Peripheral stump of facial nerve
3   Graft
4   Internal auditory canal

Operative Technique

(Fig. 7.**16**)

Usually it is possible to isolate an adequate central facial nerve stump about 1–1.5 cm long at the brain stem even during the removal of a large acoustic neuroma. Once this has been accomplished, an autogenous free nerve graft about 5 cm long (see p. 212) is taken from the sural nerve and anastomosed to the central facial nerve stump at the brain stem using one or two sutures (Fig. 7.**16**). An area measuring about 1 cm^2 has previously been burred from the posterior surface of the petrous bone in the sinodural angle so that the graft can be delivered into the mastoid from the suboccipital approach through an oblique incision in the dura. This site can be sealed from the intracranial side by covering it with small pieces of muscle secured with fibrin glue. Without moving the patient, the otosurgeon performs a broad mastoidectomy through a separate postauricular incision. The mastoid segment of the facial nerve is exposed as far as the stylomastoid foramen, transected below the lateral semicircular canal, and transposed posteriorly toward the sinodural angle by routing it through a newly–created bony groove. The nerve graft previously delivered into the mastoid through the dural incision is pulled farther through while the anastomosis

in the cerebellopontine angle is observed. Sufficient slack should be left intracranially so that the anastomosis can be positioned against the brain stem, and the graft is joined to the peripheral facial nerve trunk with one or two microsurgical sutures (Fig. 7.**16**). The site where the graft pierces the dura can also be sealed from the mastoid side with small pieces of muscle or fat as an added safeguard against CSF leakage. The operation concludes with closure of the dura, the soft tissues over the craniotomy, and the mastoid opening. With proper organization, this procedure should prolong the basic operation for acoustic neuroma removal by no more than one hour. Considering its excellent results, this additional investment is worthwhile.

Facial Nerve Reconstruction in the Internal Auditory Canal

In cases where the facial nerve is stretched and severed following the transtemporal or translabyrinthine exposure of a basal skull fracture or the removal of a tumor, continuity can be restored by a simple end–to–end anastomosis in the internal auditory canal. If up to 1 cm of the facial nerve substance has been lost, sufficient length for an end–to–end repair can be gained by utilizing the natural curvature of the nerve and "rerouting" it so that the ends can be approximated without tension (Bonnel, 1927; Fisch, 1969; 1970). Another option in this situation is the interposition of a nerve graft. Regardless of which technique is used, it is essential to obtain a tension–free anastomosis. The functional results of an end–to–end anastomosis and interpositional free nerve graft are the same when proper technique is employed.

Transtemporal Extradural Approach

Operative Technique

The technique for performing an end–to–end anastomosis in the internal auditory canal is basically similar to that used in the cerebellopontine angle. At this site as well, the facial nerve has an extremely thin connective–tissue investment.

Here the rerouting technique involves exposing the central nerve stump from above, mobilizing it from the labyrinthine portion of the fallopian canal, exposing and mobilizing the tympanic facial nerve segment, drilling a new bony canal to gain length, and suturing the nerve ends together (Fig. 7.**17**). On occasion, simple apposition of the nerve ends may provide a sufficiently strong anastomosis through the adhesive action of the interfacial fibrin.

Fig. 7.**16** Intracranial–intratemporal anastomosis of the facial nerve. The cerebellopontine angle and mastoid fields are shown.
1 Sural nerve graft
2 Central stump of facial nerve
3 Anterior inferior cerebellar artery
4 Lower cranial nerves
5 Fat grafts
6 Mastoid facial nerve segment
7 Anastomosis
8 Internal auditory canal
9 Petrosal vein
10 Trigeminal nerve

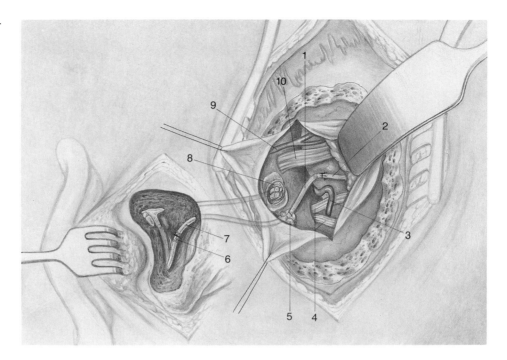

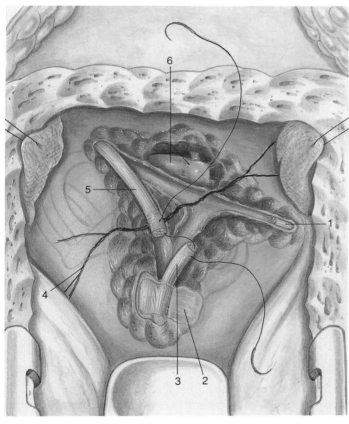

Fig. 7.**17**

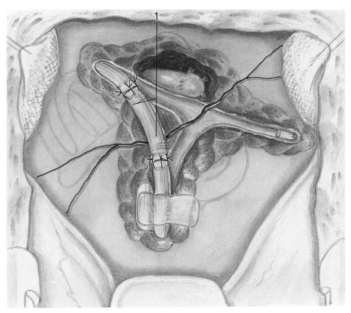

Fig. 7.**18**

Figs. 7.**17** and 7.**18**   Facial nerve reconstruction in the internal auditory canal through the transtemporal extradural approach.

Fig. 7.**17**   Rerouting.
1 Greater petrosal nerve
2 Dura, internal auditory canal
3 Facial nerve, labyrinthine segment
4 Fracture
5 Facial nerve, tympanic segment
6 Malleus and incus

Fig. 7.**18**   Interpositional free nerve graft.
1 Auricular nerve graft

If the defect cannot be bridged by rerouting, an autogenous nerve graft is interposed (Fig. 7.**18**).

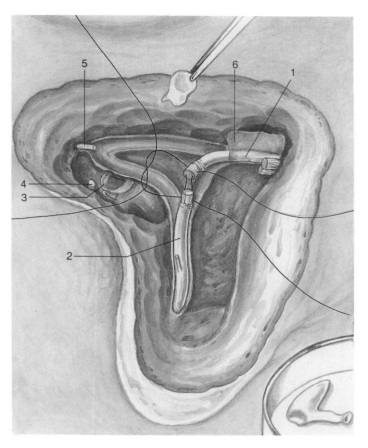
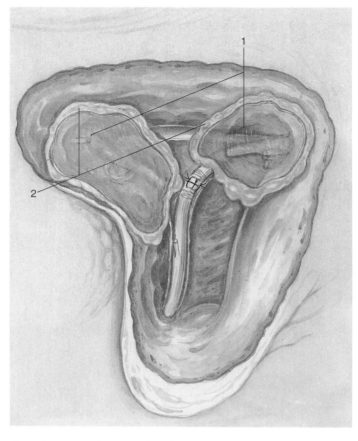

Figs. 7.**19** and 7.**20**   Facial nerve reconstruction in the internal auditory canal through the translabyrinthine approach.

Fig. 7.**19**   Rerouting, initial step.
1   Central facial nerve
2   Facial nerve, mastoid segment
3   Stapes
4   Malleus handle
5   Greater petrosal nerve
6   Dura, internal auditory canal

Fig. 7.**20**   Rerouting completed.
1   Preserved dura
2   Fibrin glue

Translabyrinthine Approach

Operative Technique

A basically similar technique is used in cases where the internal auditory canal has been entered by the translabyrinthine route (see p. 313). The essential problem is to distinguish the central stump of the facial nerve from the stumps of the superior and inferior vestibular nerves and cochlear nerve. By incising the posterior fossa dura backward and laterally from the posterior lip of the porus acousticus to a point just short of the sigmoid sinus, the surgeon can see into the cerebellopontine angle well enough to identify the facial nerve emerging from the brain stem in front of the vestibulocochlear nerve so that he can anastomose the correct stump. After the greater petrosal nerve has been

divided at the geniculate ganglion, the peripheral stump of the facial nerve can be transposed posteriorly with the exposed tympanic and mastoid segments and anastomosed to the central stump in the internal acoustic meatus by rerouting it posteriorly and obliquely through a newly constructed bony facial canal (Figs. 7.**19** and 7.**20**).

Mobilization of the peripheral part of the nerve is facilitated by dismantling the ossicular chain, leaving the stapes in place.

If rerouting is not possible, a free nerve graft of adequate length, usually obtained from the cervical plexus, is interposed to restore continuity. Sutures must be used to attach the proximal end of the graft to the mobile central facial nerve stump in the internal auditory canal. At the distal anastomosis, simple apposition of the graft and nerve ends is often sufficient within the

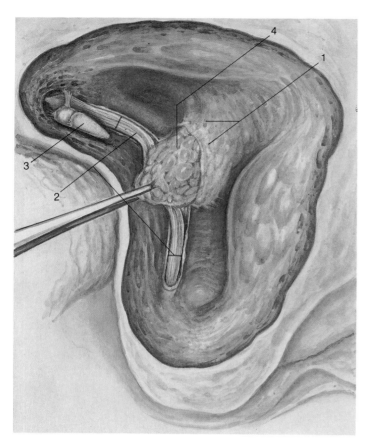 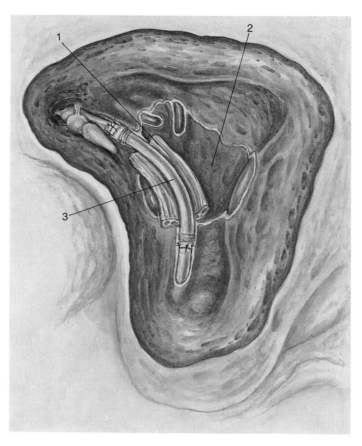

Figs. 7.**21** and 7.**22**   Tympanomastoid reconstruction of the facial nerve.

Fig. 7.**21**   Facial neuroma is removed. Resulting defect is shown.
1   Neuroma capsule
2   Facial nerve section
3   Incus
4   Abdominal fat graft

Fig. 7.**22**   Autogenous nerve graft has been interposed.
1   Muscle graft
2   Posterior fossa, dura
3   Great auricular nerve graft

stable bony graft bed. The internal auditory canal must be well sealed off from the mastoid by means of fascia or banked dura applied with adhesive. The mastoid, completely freed of mucosa, is then obliterated with abdominal fat grafts secured with adhesive to prevent CSF leakage through the eustachian tube with risk of ascending intracranial infection.

Tympanomastoid Reconstruction

(Figs. 7.**21** and 7.**22**)

Large facial nerve defects can result from laterobasal fractures or the removal of a tumor such as facial neuroma (Figs. 7.**21** and 7.**22**) involving the tympanomastoid portion of the nerve. Ossicular chain disruption is common in trauma patients, and a dural defect is frequently present. Besides reconstruction of the ossicu-

lar chain and repair of the dural defect, the operation must include the interposition of a free nerve graft between the central, tympanic end of the nerve and its peripheral, mastoid end. The graft may be positioned within the existing bony canal, or the canal may have to be reconstructed. Two drops of blood are sufficient to bond the nerve and graft ends together through the adhesive action of endogenous fibrin.

Intratemporal–Extratemporal Reconstruction

Reconstruction of the main trunk of the facial nerve can be difficult if the lesion extends into the stylomastoid foramen from the mastoid or extratemporal side. This is especially true if the surgeon is unfamiliar with the intramastoid and extratemporal topography of the facial nerve. Interdisciplinary cooperation is recommended in these cases. The passage of the nerve through the stylomastoid foramen should never be the cause of a faulty anastomosis in cases where the surgeon is unable to obtain normal–appearing proximal and distal facial nerve ends.

Operative Technique

(Figs. 7.**23**, 7.**24**, and 7.**25**)

If the main lesion in the facial nerve trunk is extratemporal following trauma or a tumor excision (as in the illustrations), that region is exposed first. The skin incision can be placed in existing scars, or an incision can be made like that used for parotidectomy. In this case, the incision extends from the superior margin of the tragus along the auricle to the root of the earlobe. There it turns sharply downward and first runs along the anterior border of the sternocleidomastoid muscle, then turns forward and terminates in a skin crease. Our preferred landmarks for identifying the extratemporal facial nerve trunk are the anterior attachment of the sternocleidomastoid muscle, the origin of the posterior digastric muscle belly on the mastoid, and the apex of the cartilaginous auditory canal [the "pointer" of Conley (1975)]. The facial nerve trunk is located just cranial to these muscle attachments, medial to the posterior belly of the digastric muscle, and about 10 mm medial to the apex of the cartilaginous auditory canal when the auricle is pulled upward. Broad dissection with separation of the connective tissue fibers passing from the cartilaginous auditory canal to the parotid capsule provides good visibility (Fig. 7.**23**). Once the main trunk of the facial nerve has been exposed, it is isolated as far as its branches and if necessary beyond, in which case the superficial parotid lobe is also dissected free. The nerve is now inspected under the microscope. If it is found that a deficient or pathologically altered portion of the nerve extends into the stylomastoid foramen, two options present themselves. The first is to follow the facial nerve trunk farther cephalad from the stylomastoid foramen by the progressive excavation of bone (Fig. 7.**24**). This may prove difficult due to the dense ring of connective tissue surrounding the stylomastoid foramen. In this case, it is better to perform a standard mastoidectomy through a postauricular incision, like that used for facial nerve decompression (see p. 216).

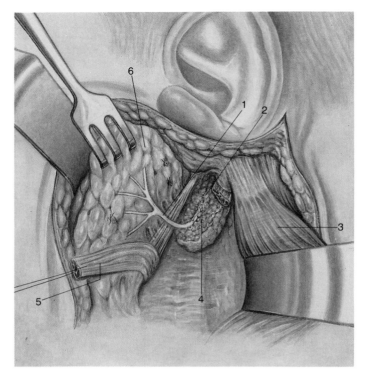

Figs. 7.**23** to 7.**25**   Intratemporal–extratemporal reconstruction of the facial nerve.

Fig. 7.**23**   Facial nerve trunk with glomus tumor, exposed extratemporally as far as the stylomastoid foramen.
1   Main trunk of facial nerve
2   Glomus tumor involving the facial nerve
3   Sternocleidomastoid muscle
4   Glomus tumor
5   Posterior belly of digastric muscle
6   Parotid gland

The mastoid segment of the facial nerve is exposed, and its junction with the extratemporal portion is isolated by broad bone removal about the stylomastoid foramen. This requires dividing the thick connective–tissue ring in the stylomastoid foramen. After the abnormal part of the facial nerve has been resected and healthy central and peripheral stumps have been obtained, a nerve graft is interposed between the mastoid and extratemporal trunks and secured with sutures (Fig. 7.**25**). Tumor infiltration of the facial nerve requires a microscopically guided resection with frozen–section evaluation.

The mastoid is closed in layers in standard fashion. An easy-flow drain (capillary drain without suction) is placed in the extratemporal part of the field, and a head dressing is worn for five days.

Fig. 7.**24** The mastoid tip is removed, and the facial nerve is exposed within the mastoid.
1   Mastoid cavity

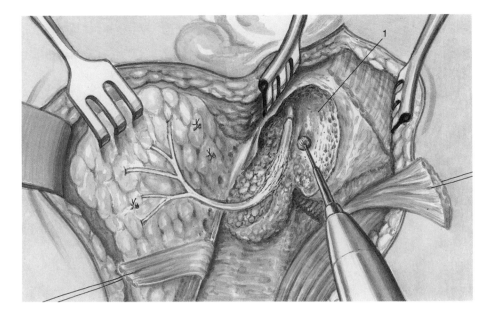

Fig. 7.**25** A free nerve graft has been interposed.
1   Sural nerve graft

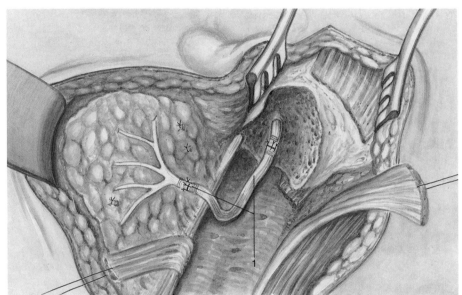

Concluding Remarks

We have considered all segments of the facial nerve from its origin at the brain stem to the stylomastoid foramen as well as the transitional area between the intra– and extratemporal segments, and we have reviewed the options available for decompression, repair, and reconstruction in an effort to promote interdisciplinary understanding and stimulate cooperation. Patients are grateful when their complex facial nerve problem can be solved at one time, rather than in multiple stages, through the collaborative efforts of multiple specialties. Another advantage of this approach is that it tends to yield better functional and aesthetic results.

Bibliography

Blumenthal F, May M. Electrodiagnosis Chapter 12. In: May M (ed): The Facial Nerve, New York: Thieme Inc., 1986.

Draf W. Zur Beurteilung des Transplantatlagers bei der autogenen Nerventransplantation im HNO-Bereich. In: Hierholzer G, Zilch H (eds): Transplantatlager und Implantatlager bei verschiedenen Operationsverfahren. p. 147 ff, Berlin, Heidelberg, New York: Springer, 1980.

Draf W. Intracranial–intratemporal Anastomosis of the Facial Nerve after Cerebellopontine Angle Tumor Surgery. In: Graham MD, House WF (eds): Disorders of the Facial Nerve. pp. 441–9, New York: Raven, 1982.

Draf W. (1995) Rehabilitation of the Paralyzed Face. In: Tardy ME, Kastenbauer ER, Naumann HH (eds): Head and Neck Surgery, 2nd edn, Vol. I/II, Chapter 16, Stuttgart, New York: Thieme, 1995.

Fisch U. Transtemporal Surgery of the Internal Auditory Canal. Report of 92 Cases, Techniques, Indications and Results. Adv Otorhinolaryngol 1970; 17: 203.

Haas JP, Kahle G. Wie kann heute das Felsenbein am besten radiologisch dargestellt werden? HNO 1988; 36: 89–101.

Helms J. The Transmeatal Approach to the Geniculate Ganglion Acta Otorhinolaryng Belg 1976; 30: 84–9.

Helms J. Variations of the Course of the Facial Nerve in the Middle Ear and Mastoid. In: Samii M, Jannetta P (eds): The Cranial Nerves. p. 391, Berlin, Heidelberg, New York: Springer, 1981.

Jannetta PJ. Microsurgical Exploration and Decompression of the Facial Nerve in Hemifacial Spasm. Curr Top Surg Res 1970; 2: 217–20.

Lang J. Surgical Anatomy of the Skull Base. In: Samii M, Draf W (eds): Surgery of the Skull Base. p. 82, Springer, 1989.

May M. The Facial Nerve. New York: Thieme Inc., 1986.

Millesi H. Wiederherstellung durchtrennter peripherer Nerven und Nerventransplantation. Münch Med Wschr 1969; 52: 2669–74.

Samii M. Modern Aspects of Peripheral and Cranial Nerve Surgery. In: Krayenbühl H (ed): Advances and Technical Standards in Neurosurgery. Vol 2, Vienna, New York: Springer, 1975.

Samii M. Panel Discussion Management of Facial Nerve in Intracranial Tumors. In: Fisch U (ed): Facial Nerve Surgery. p. 475, Amstelveen: Kugler, and Birmingham: Aesculapius, 1977.

Samii M. Preservation and Reconstruction of the Facial Nerve in the Cerebellopontine Angle. In: Samii M, Jannetta P (eds): The Cranial Nerves. Berlin, Heidelberg, New York: Springer, 1981.

Samii M, Draf W. Surgery of the Skull Base. Chapt. Facial Nerve and Skull Base Surgery. Springer, 1989.

Stennert E. Combined Approach in Extratemporal Facial Nerve Reconstruction. Clin Plast Surg 1979; 6: 481–6.

Traxler M, Gritzmann N, Kramer J, Grasl MCh, Hajek PCH. Der intratemporale Verlauf des N. facialis in der Magnetic Resonance – (MR) Darstellung. HNO 1989; 37: 19–22.

Wigand ME, Haid T, Berg M, Rettinger G. The Enlarged Transtemporal Approach to the Cerebellopontine Angle. Technique and Indications. Acta Otorhinolaryngol Ital 1982; 2: 571–82.

8 Operations for Stapedial Ankylosis

Hans H. Naumann and Eberhard Wilmes

Otosclerosis is the most common cause of stapedial ankylosis. Although its cause is still unknown, the resulting conductive deafness can be relieved surgically in a very high proportion of patients. This *symptomatic* treatment is likely to succeed if the disease is confined to the sound conducting apparatus, and if the labyrinthine windows and the inner ear function are preserved.

Two *different surgical principles* can be used:

- Reconstruction of normal function of the ossicular chain and labyrinthine windows, for example by stapedectomy.
- Bypassing of the ossicular chain and oval windows by creation of a new route for access of sound to the inner ear, for example by fenestration either of the horizontal semicircular canal (see page 254) or of the promontory (see page 126). This technique is rarely used.

The principle of both the stapedial operation (Kessel, 1878; Miot, 1890) and of fenestration (Passow, 1897) was appreciated as early as the end of the last century. These procedures did not become established at that time because the important prerequisites for lasting success such as antibiotics, microscopes, and instruments, were not available.

The fenestration operation was developed as a routine procedure by the work of Lempert who, in turn, built on the earlier work of Holmgren, Sourdille, and others.

The fenestration remained the operation of choice for fixation of the stapes by otosclerosis for about 20 years, but it then began to be displaced by a direct attack on the fixed stapes and its footplate (Rosen's indirect and direct mobilization or stapediolysis), and finally by the partial or total replacement of the stapes and/or the footplate (Shea, Heermann, Schuknecht, and others).

Today, the *stapes operation* is the method of choice. Initially, *complete removal* of the stapes was preferred by most surgeons, but in recent years *partial removal* has become increasingly popular. The latter procedure is less traumatic for the inner ear, and the function of the inner ear after a *partial stapedectomy* is better than that after *complete removal* of the stapes (McGee, 1981). Moreover, reclosure of the oval window after partial stapedectomy is no more common than after complete removal. However, complete removal of the stapes may be necessary for pathological or anatomical reasons.

Different authors use a variety of terms for *partial stapedectomy* such as stapedotomy, stapes replacement, piston procedure, small fenestra technique, etc. The following nomenclature will be used in this chapter:

- *Partial stapedectomy* will be used for the currently most popular technique of removal of part of the stapedial structures (the posterior crus and part of the footplate) followed by their replacement.
- *Complete stapedectomy* will be used for classic complete removal of the stapes together with the entire footplate, and replacement by appropriate materials.

Both techniques will be described. The classical technique of *fenestration* is still occasionally needed, for example for congenital anomalies, and will be described in brief.

Stapedectomy

Preoperative Diagnostic Procedures

A careful *history* should also include a family history. The otoscopic findings are recorded, and generalized bone diseases looked for, such as osteogenesis imperfecta, van der Hoeve-de Kleyn syndrome, Paget's disease, acromegaly, etc. The *patency of the eustachian tube* is tested.

The *differential diagnosis* includes middle ear effusion, ankylosis of the head of the malleus, subluxation of the ossicular chain or fracture of the ossicles due to trauma, adhesions, congenital anomalies of the ossicular chain or windows, and disorders of aeration of the eustachian tube.

Accurate *audiological investigation* should include tuning fork tests, pure tone and speech audiograms, impedance audiometry, and measurement of the stapedial reflex. Satisfactory masking must be used where appropriate.

Radiological investigation includes Schueller's plain view and high resolution CT scan to assess the chain, the oval window (in congenital anomalies), and to demonstrate cochlear otosclerosis.

Nasal disease should be excluded, and the patient's *fitness for anesthesia* should be assessed.

Before the operation, the prognosis of the procedure in general and for the specific situation should be explained to the patient. For example, the patient must be told that the hearing may become worse in 1% of patients (and a considerably higher percentage in revision operations), but that serious postoperative symptoms are to be expected in fewer than 1% of operations. The patient must also be told of the possibility of persistence or even development of tinnitus and of unilateral disorders of taste, usually temporary, due to division of the chorda tympani.

Indications

- Typical otosclerosis of the oval window with fixation of the stapes to a varying extent.
- Otosclerosis or fixation of the annular ligament of the oval window in chronic otitis media, as a staged procedure (see Chapter 4).
- Osteogenesis imperfecta.
- Certain congenital anomalies (see Chapter 3).
- Tympanosclerosis in which removal of the stapes is indicated, usually as a staged operation.

Other criteria which may influence the decision include:

- The *patient's age:* a stapedectomy may be carried out in patients as young as 12 years. There are no upper age limits provided that the operation is not contraindicated for other reasons.

Audiological criteria:

- The extent of the conductive deafness. The operation is indicated for conductive deafness with a negative Rinne at 500 and 1000 Hz, and even more so if the conductive deafness exceeds 20 dB.
- Rapid deterioration of the conductive component.
- In *unilateral otosclerosis,* stapedectomy is only carried out if a useful gain in hearing is to be expected. However, unilateral otosclerosis is usually an indication for surgery to improve directional and stereophonic hearing.
- The extent of sensorineural deafness: an operation may be useful even if hearing in the operated ear does not return to normal after the operation but allows a hearing aid to be used more efficiently, and improves discrimination;
- Carhart's notch causing an apparent perceptive deafness disappears with the creation of new sound access. The average values for bone conduction loss before operation in stapedial ankylosis are: 5 dB at 512 Hz, 10 dB at 1024 Hz, 15 dB at 2048 Hz, and 5 dB at 4096 Hz.
- Choice of side: in bilateral otosclerosis it is usual to operate on the worse ear first, or on the ear with the greatest loss of discrimination if there is a prospect of a useful increase in hearing.
- The second ear should not be operated on for at least six months after the first procedure.
- If the patient experiences a marked inner ear response or dizziness to the first operation, the operation on the second ear should be postponed for at least twelve months, and the most atraumatic procedure possible such as the partial removal of the footplate or stapedotomy (see page 238) should be chosen. Operation on the second ear may indeed be completely contraindicated.
- Marked tinnitus: it is not possible to predict whether noises in the ear will disappear after the operation, and the chance of improvement is at the most 50%.
- Particular care is needed for the patient with total hearing loss in one ear. Such patients need very careful explanation of the possibility of total deafness in the operated ear. An operation on the sole hearing ear must always be considered carefully, and sometimes it is safer to rely on a hearing aid. In the U.S.A. a stapedectomy *is not performed* in cases of unilateral total deafness under any circumstances.

- *Revision operations:* reoperation may be indicated for an atypical response of the inner ear immediately after the operation, shown by persistent dizziness, hearing loss, or for recurrence of the conductive deafness. Revision surgery may also be indicated for persistent dizziness due to a fistula or for a stapes prosthesis which is too long (see also page 250).
- Revision for unsatisfactory improvement of hearing should not be carried out for at least 6 months after the first operation.

Contraindications

- Very poor inner ear function or rapid loss of inner ear function.
- Otosclerosis combined with Ménière's disease.
- Hemophilia which has not been treated by substitution therapy.
- Marked perceptive deafness after a previous stapedial operation.
- Acute inflammatory diseases of the external or middle ear.
- A perforated tympanic membrane should be closed first, and a stapedectomy delayed for six months or longer until the conditions in the closed middle ear have returned to normal.

Principles of the Operation

Partial Stapedectomy

The middle ear is opened, the superstructure (both crura and the head of the stapes) of the fixed stapes identified and removed from the oval window. An opening is created in the posterior part of the footplate and a stapedial prosthesis introduced. The vestibule is covered and the middle ear closed.

Alternatives include simple perforation of the footplate with the removal of the stapes superstructure (stapedotomy). The opening of the footplate is only slightly larger than the piston of the teflon prosthesis.

Complete Stapedectomy

The middle ear is opened and the entire fixed stapes is isolated and removed from the oval window. The open vestibule is covered by connective tissue and a suitable interposition is placed between the long process of the incus and the vestibular covering.

Preoperative Preparation

On the day before operation: The meatus is cleaned carefully, and hairs in the meatus are clipped, but no local or general antibiotics or chemical preparation are necessary. *Premedication* depends on the type of anesthesia planned (see Chapter 1).

On the day of operation: In the operating room the external ear is washed with colorless antiseptic solution [for example phenylmercuric borate (Merfen), Dibromol, 1:1000 thiomersal (Merthiolate), or 70% alcohol]. The hair around the ear is turned back, fixed, and covered with strips of plaster or Op-site.

Local anesthetic is injected even if the operation is to be carried out under general anesthesia, because of its vasoconstrictor action. The technique of injection is described on pages 1 ff, and is shown in Figure 8.3. A strip of gauze soaked in antibiotic solution is introduced into the external meatus, and the auricle and surrounding area washed again with antiseptic solution. Finally the surgical field is draped.

Special instruments include: an operating microscope, drill, bipolar electric coagulation and a selection of microsurgical instruments.

The following are particularly useful for stapedial surgery:
- small self–retaining retractors or small endaural retractors for endaural operations
- bony curette
- angled and straight incision knife
- mucosal curettes
- sickle knife
- microperforator
- curved dissecting needle
- several long 45° hooks, 0.3, 0.6, and 1 mm long
  several long fine 90° hooks, 0.3, 0.6, 1, and 2 mm long
- fine and very fine aspirators with hand–controlled pressure adjustment
- very fine cup forceps
- fine smooth jawed alligator forceps for introduction of a wire prosthesis
- very fine diamond burr with a commercial handpiece, 0.5 mm, 1 mm, and 2 mm diameter head
- House pattern prefabricated stapedial prosthesis of tantalum wire or stainless steel in various sizes, 4 mm, 4.5 mm, 5 mm, 5.5 mm, and 6 mm long (Fig. 8.**1a**)
- platinum wire-Teflon prosthesis in 0.4, 0.6, or 0.8 mm diameter depending on individual anatomical situations and the technique used. The usual length is 4.5 mm (Fig. 8.**1b**)
- McGee wire closing forceps for the wire prosthesis (Fig. 8.**1c**)
- measuring rod for determining the distance between the long process of the incus and the level of the oval window (Fig. 8.**2**).

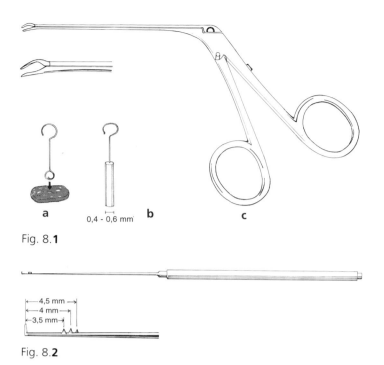

Fig. 8.**1**

4,5 mm
4 mm
3,5 mm

Fig. 8.**2**

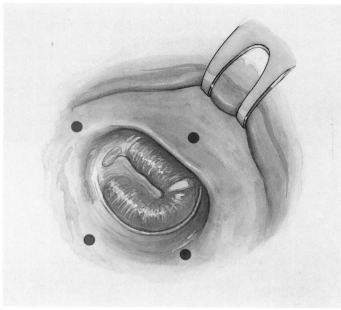

Fig. 8.**3**

Anesthesia

The stapedectomy may be carried out either under local anesthesia with sedation, or under general endotracheal anesthesia.

Bleeding in either technique can be kept to a minimum by the use of hypotensive anesthesia combined with endotracheal intubation, and/or by placing a few drops of 1:100000 adrenaline on the mucosa of the middle ear.

Local Anesthesia

An important prerequisite is thorough sedation by premedication which can be deepened or prolonged if necessary.

The local anesthesia should be injected *before* draping for maximal effect. Suitable agents include 2% lidocaine with adrenaline, or 1% ultracaine with adrenaline, 1:200000.

Technique

A depot of 0.2–0.5 ml of anesthetic solution is introduced with a fine short bevelled and angled needle at 4 points in the external meatus as shown in red in Figure 8.**3**. It is important to hold the bevel of the needle parallel to the bony surface of the meatus to ensure that the fluid is injected under the meatal skin, to prevent its leaking into the lumen of the meatus, and to prevent a hematoma. If too much anesthetic is injected the resultant swelling narrows the meatal lumen.

General Anesthesia

Depots of local anaesthesia are also introduced in smaller amounts to reduce the bleeding, even if intubation anesthesia is to be used. The details of the technique of anesthesia are given in Chapter 1, Vol. I.

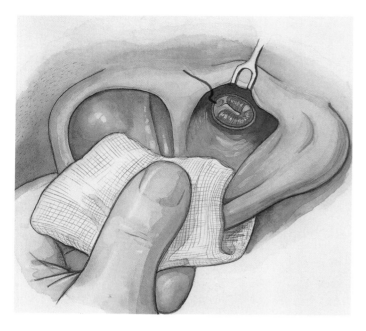

Fig. 8.**4**

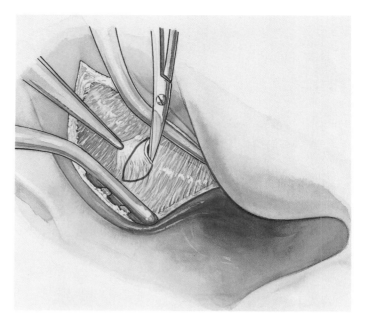

Fig. 8.**5**

Surgical Technique

A Heermann skin incision (Figs. 8.**4** and 8.**5**) serves both to widen the entrance to the meatus, and to allow removal of loose connective tissue to be used later to close the oval window (Figs. 8.**22**, 8.**34**, and 8.**35**). The piece of connective tissue is stored in Ringer's solution until it is needed.

Bleeding points are grasped with a fine forceps and coagulated.

The cartilage of the external ear must on no account be exposed or damaged by the incision.

If the meatus is narrow the incision can be extended further into it. A *tympanomeatal flap* is now developed separately from the incision, using a sharp moderate sized incision knife to create an incision shown by the broken line in Figure 8.**6**.

The knife is carried through the skin down to the bone of the meatus. The resulting curved incision should lie at most 5–8 mm from the tympanic membrane to ensure that sufficient skin remains to close off the middle ear if a large amount of bone is removed from the posterior meatal wall to gain access to the oval window.

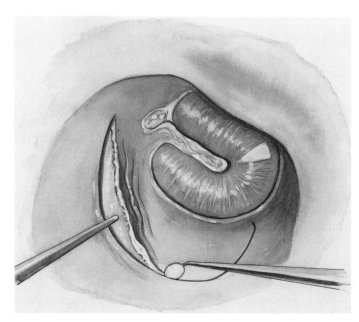

Fig. 8.**6**

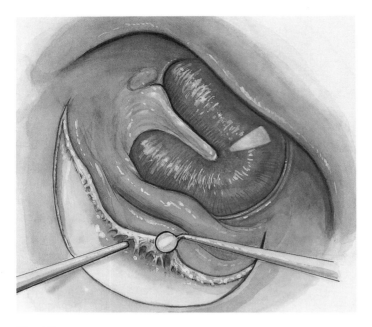

Fig. 8.**7**

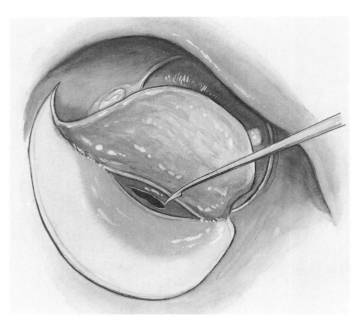

Fig. 8.**8**

The meatal skin is carefully elevated from the bone towards the fibrocartilaginous anulus of the tympanic membrane using an angled incision knife (Fig. 8.**7**). It is important that neither the skin flap nor the tympanic membrane is torn during this procedure. An incision knife or elevator is used to probe carefully through the tympanic sulcus by freeing the fibrocartilaginous anulus at this point.

There now usually follows a bony area, 1–2 mm wide, before the middle ear mucosa appears as a delicate, tense, transparent membrane. This membrane is divided with a sickle knife parellel to the fibrocartilaginous anulus, and the middle ear is thus opened (Fig. 8.**8**).

An elevator is introduced into the resulting defect, and the tympanic membrane is elevated carefully above and below out of the tympanic sulcus. The freeing of the tympanic membrane is carried far enough to provide good access to the oval window, and a view of the round window (Fig. 8.**9**).*

The resulting tympanomeatal flap is turned anteriorly (Fig. 8.**10**), and usually remains in the position without further fixation. If the tympanic membrane has not been mobilized widely enough, or if the tympanomeatal flap is particularly stiff, the tympanic membrane must be freed further, and it may be necessary to

* In Figure 8.**9** and the following views, the tympanic membrane has been elevated liberally below to provide a better view.

fix the tympanomeatal flap in the desired position by a small piece of moist gelatine sponge.

The chorda tympani may lie close to the fibrocartilaginous anulus, but it may also be hidden behind the bone of the posterior meatal wall or run free through the middle ear. It is easily identified by dissection with a sickle knife or a dissecting needle. It should be preserved if possible, and this can be achieved in 90% of cases. Depending on the local anatomy, it is usually possible to displace the chorda in the direction of the handle of the malleus, or if it does not otherwise give sufficient access to the oval window to stretch it a little with an elevator towards the handle of the malleus (Fig. 8.**10**). The chorda should seldom be divided, and then only when the anatomy is very unfavorable.

It is usually necessary to remove bone from the posterosuperior meatal wall to provide satisfactory access to the stapes and oval window. The individual anatomy determines the amount of bone to be removed. A fine rigid curette can be used, but a fine diamond burr is more elegant and no more time consuming (Fig. 8.**10**).

The following points require attention during removal of bone with the diamond burr:

- The burr must be irrigated sufficiently to prevent heating of the bone leading to necrosis.
- The tympanic ostium of the tube should be closed temporarily by a gelatine sponge.
- The bone dust must be carefully removed by suction.

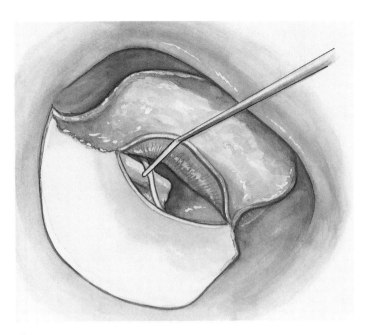

Fig. 8.**9**

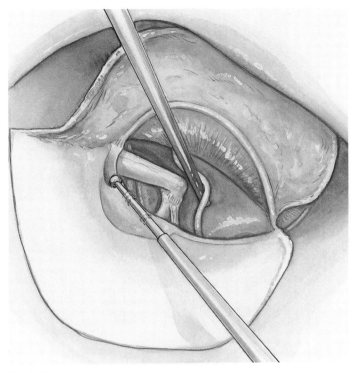

Fig. 8.**10**

- The head of the burr should be small enough to en-sure that the underlying long process of the incus and the chorda tympani are not disturbed. It may be suitable to begin with a small burr, and then to pro-gress to a larger one.
- The tympanomeatal flap and the chorda tympani must be kept away from the burr using a fine aspira-tion cannula (Fig. 8.**10**).
- The chorda tympani demands particular attention when removing bone in an inferior direction.

Removal of bone is sufficient once the following struc-tures can be seen (Fig. 8.**11**):

1) The tendon of the stapedius muscle and the pyra-midal process.
2) The canal of the facial nerve, the long process of the incus and the incudostapedial joint.
3) The posterior crus of the stapes and its junction with the footplate.

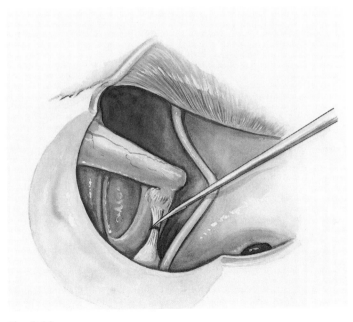

Fig. 8.**11**

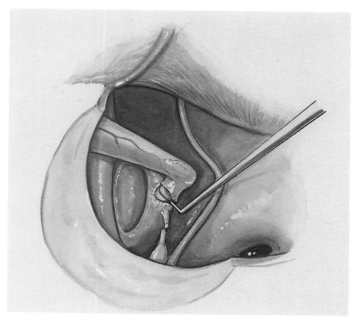

Fig. 8.**12**

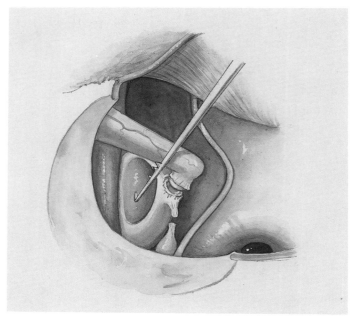

Fig. 8.**13**

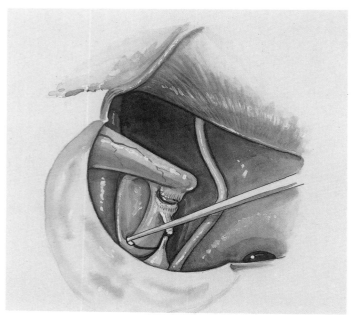

Fig. 8.**14**

Inspection of the Ossicular Chain

Fixation of the stapes is confirmed by a slight lateral movement of the long process of the incus. This step also allows the mobility of the ossicular chain in the epitympanum to be checked, and fixation of the head of the malleus to be excluded.

The tendon of the stapedius muscle is now divided with a sickle knife (Fig. 8.**11**).

If the pyramidal process obscures the oval window, it and the origin of the tendon can be removed with a diamond burr.

At this point 1–2 drops of 1:100000 adrenaline are injected into the oval window niche with a blunt cannula, and any excess fluid removed by suction. This step ensures that there will be little or no bleeding during the later removal of the mucosa from the niche.

Next the incudostapedial joint is divided carefully with a 90° hook, a fine sickle knife or a small angled incision knife (Fig. 8.**12**).

The distance between the long process of the incus and the footplate is measured (Fig. 8.**13** and 8.**2**) and a suitable prosthesis chosen. The piston of the prosthesis should project about 0.2–0.3 mm into the vestibule, whereas the connective tissue wire prosthesis should reach the level of the footplate precisely.

The next step is division of the stapes superstructure from the stapedial footplate. A fine incision knife is applied from the side of the facial nerve, that is immediately above the footplate (Fig. 8.**14**), to the base of the posterior crus of the stapes, and the stapedial crus is fractured by cutting or tilting movements towards the promontory. This step must be carried out carefully to prevent the footplate from being mobilized at this time. If a large focus of otosclerosis is present on the posterior crus, with a normal anterior stapedial crus, division of the superstructure may begin on the anterior crus: unfortunately the view may be obstructed by the stapedial arch.

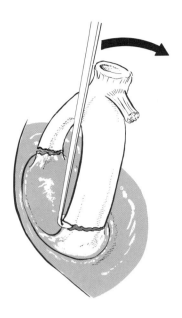

Fig. 8.**15**

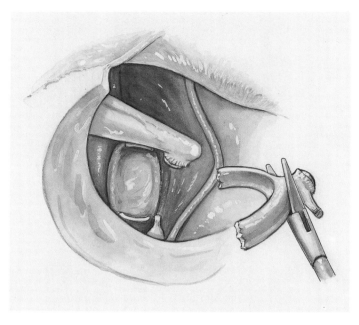

Fig. 8.**16**

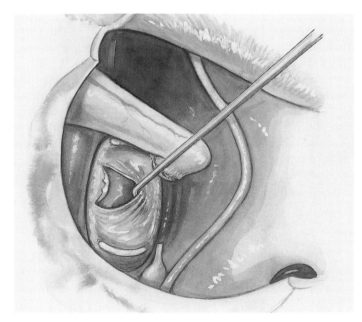

Fig. 8.**17**

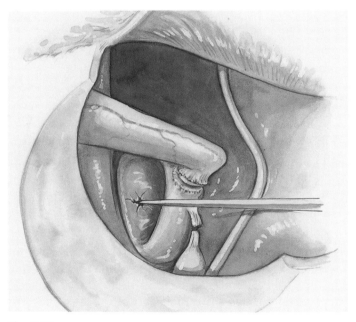

Fig. 8.**18**

After one of the crura has been divided, it usually suffices to push the stapedial arch towards the promontory using an incision knife to break the second crus at an appropriate point. Alternatively, a 90° hook can also be used (Fig. 8.**15**).

The now isolated superstructure of the stapes can be removed with a hook, a forceps or an aspirator (Fig. 8.**16**).

The niche of the oval window is usually now easily visible, and a free view can be obtained of the stapes footplate (Fig. 8.**16**).

Next, the mucosa covering the footplate is removed, using magnification for this and subsequent steps.

The mucosa is removed from the window using a fine 45° hook: the mucosa over the footplate is torn and pushed towards the edge of the footplate or the wall of the niche (Fig. 8.**17**). If the mucosa is thick it is first mobilized as far as the wall of the niche (Fig. 8.**18**) and then removed with a fine forceps. However, if the mucosa is very delicate it may be simply pushed off the footplate. Bleeding after removal of the mucosa is dealt with by placing a piece of gelatine sponge soaked in 1:100 000

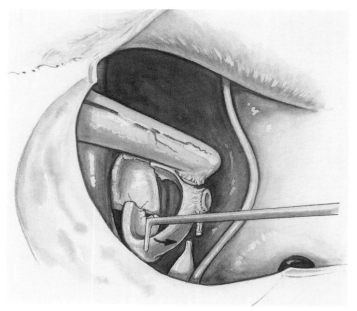

Fig. 8.**19**

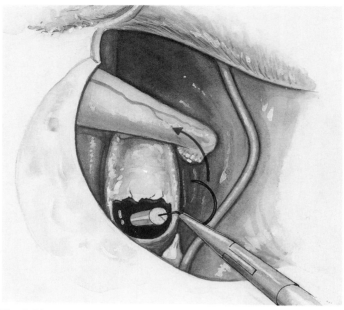

Fig. 8.**20**

adrenaline in the oval niche. If the footplate is already mobile the adrenaline should be omitted.

From this point on the technique of *partial* and *complete* stapedectomy differ.

Partial Stapedectomy

A) Removal of the Posterior Third of the Footplate

The footplate is perforated with a perforator or needle at the junction between the posterior and middle thirds of the footplate, producing one or more fracture lines (Fig. 8.**18**).

The mobile posterior third of the footplate is removed in one or more fragments. To prevent splintering of the footplate, it is preferable to use a fine Plester's footplate elevator rather than a hook because this instrument has a broader working surface that distributes the tractive force over the entire fragment of the footplate (Fig. 8.**19**). The piece of footplate is immediately pushed away from the window and then removed with a fine grasping instrument.

Many surgeons perforate the footplate *before* removing the stapes superstructure. The stapes superstructure is then removed as described above, lifting the posterior third or quarter of the footplate out of the oval niche together with the posterior crus. Separate removal of the footplate is then unnecessary.

The prosthesis is grasped with alligator forceps, in such a way that the forceps and the long axis of the prosthesis form an obtuse angle (Fig. 8.**20**). The prosthesis is now introduced into the open vestibule.

McGee's wire closing forceps (Fig. 8.**1c**) are introduced so that both jaws grip the open loop of the prosthesis exactly. The other hand is used to elevate and stabilize the long process of the incus using a 90° hook while the McGee forceps closes around the loop of the prosthesis which concentrically grasps the long process of the incus (Fig. 8.**21**). This step must be carried out directly with no force or tilting because of the danger of fracture (Fig. 8.**21**). Pressure on the long process of the incus must be avoided at all costs because of the danger of necrosis, but on the other hand it must lie tightly enough against the bone to avoid a dead space.

The vestibule is now closed with a piece of connective tissue taken at the start of the procedure (Fig. 8.**22**).

If the *entire footplate* becomes *mobile* before it is removed (floating footplate), extreme care is needed to prevent the mobile footplate sinking into the vestibule. Occasionally it suffices to grasp the stump of one of the stapedial crura with a fine alligator forceps or hook to allow the footplate to be manipulated out of the oval window (Fig. 8.**23**). If this is not possible, a small window is created in the vestibule on the promontory side of the oval window using a fine diamond burr (Fig. 8.**24**); a 90° hook can be introduced through this window under the footplate (Fig. 8.**25**). The footplate can then usually be lifted out of the window in this manner (Fig. 8.**26**).

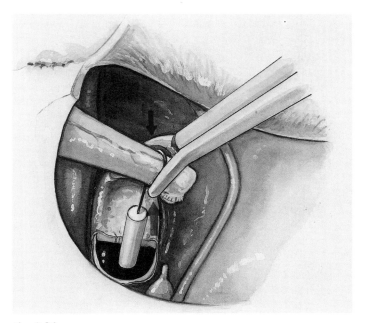

Fig. 8.**21**

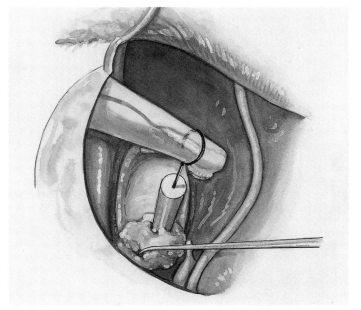

Fig. 8.**22**

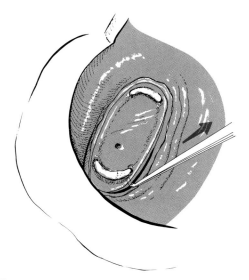

Fig. 8.**23**

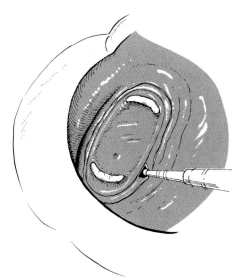

Fig. 8.**24**

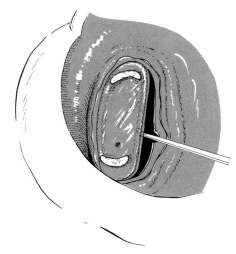

Fig. 8.**25**

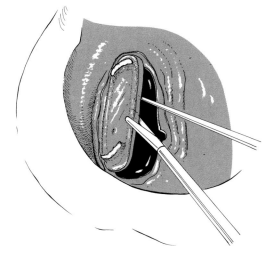

Fig. 8.**26**

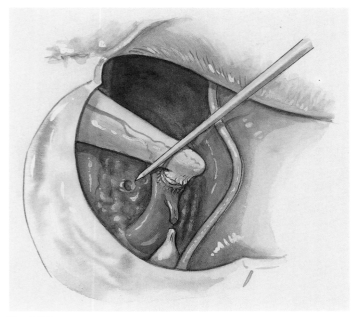

Fig. 8.**27**

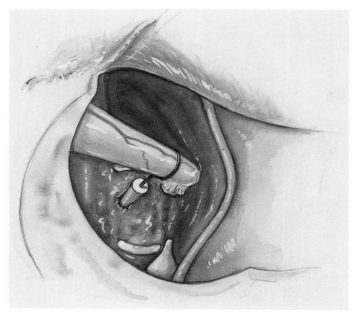

Fig. 8.**28**

B) Stapedotomy

In order to minimize the trauma to the inner ear during creation of a new portal for sound access, Shea in 1963 described a technique in which a hole is created in the footplate. A Teflon piston attached to the long process of the incus (Fig. 8.**1b**) then transmits the to–and–fro movements of the sound waves to the inner ear fluids through this defect. Other surgeons (Guilford, Schuknecht, Fisch a. o.) have adopted this principle, modified the material, the shape of the piston and the method, and have also recorded very good long–term results. This technique is suitable for extremely thick footplates.

Technique: The early phases of this operation are exactly the same as the steps described above. However, partial removal of the footplate is replaced by simple perforation without removal of any part of the footplate. The vestibule is usually opened *before* removal of the stapes structure by a perforation (Fig. 8.**27**). A Teflon piston with a diameter of 0.4 mm must be able to vibrate freely in the opening (Fig. 8.**28**). A suitable piston is placed in the opening in the footplate and its wire loop is fixed to the crura of the incus as described in detail on page 239. Loose connective tissue is placed around the piston and the footplate to close off the perforation.

Complete Stapedectomy

Principles: The entire footplate of the fixed stapes is removed from the oval window niche, the open vestibule is closed with connective tissue, and the stapes is replaced by a suitable prosthesis.

Technique: The stapedial superstructure and the mucosa covering the footplate are removed as described above. The fixed footplate is then divided transversely at its thinnest point, that is usually in the middle, using a needle, or preferably a straight fine footplate knife. Usually the two parts of the footplate are then so mobile that they can be removed with a fine 90° hook (Figs. 8.**29** to 8.**31**).

If small parts of the footplate remain attached to the annular ligament a 90° hook is placed carefully beneath them, they are tilted out of the window and removed (Fig. 8.**32**).

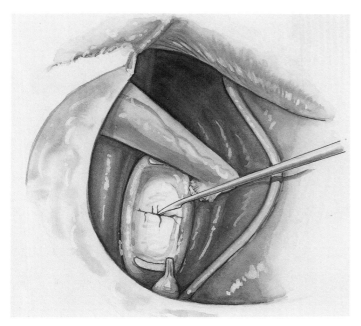

Fig. 8.**29**

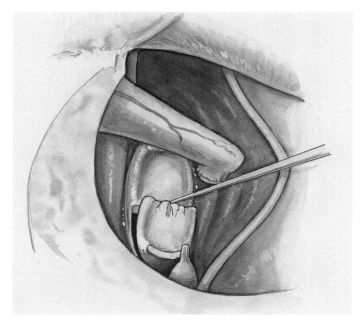

Fig. 8.**30**

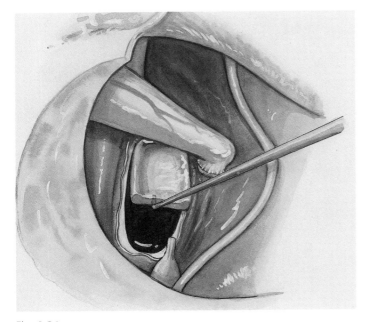

Fig. 8.**31**

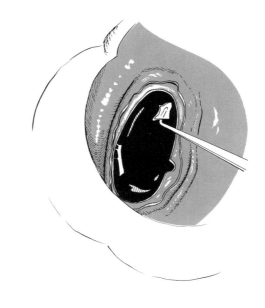

Fig. 8.**32**

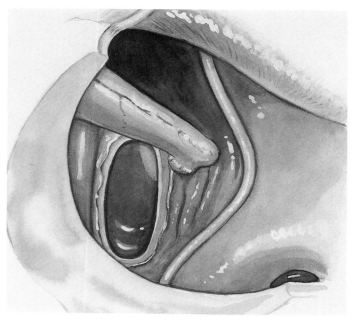

Fig. 8.**33**

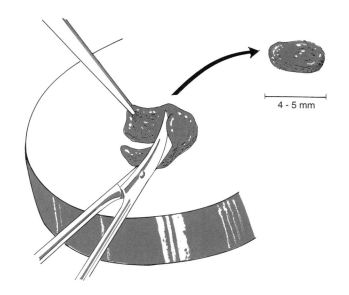

Fig. 8.**34**

The oval window is now completely open with smooth walls, and the vestibule filled with perilymph can be seen through it as shown in Figure 8.**33**. This figure also shows the clear macula of the saccule lying deeply in the anterior part of the window.

As soon as the footplate has been removed, the oval window is closed as quickly as possible with a piece of connective tissue which has already been prepared before the vestibule was opened (Fig. 8.**34**). It is introduced with a dissecting needle and a very small incision knife so that it overlaps the oval window and seals it securely (Fig. 8.**35**).

The distance to be bridged is assessed with a measuring rod. A wire prosthesis of suitable length is chosen and fixed to the long process of the incus (Figs. 8.**36** to 8.**38**), then pushed as far as possible towards the free end of the long process of the incus.

If the foot of the prosthesis should become displaced, for example during closure of the loop, its position is corrected with two 90° hooks as shown in Figure 8.**39**.

The remainder of the procedure is now practically the same in both partial and complete stapedectomy.

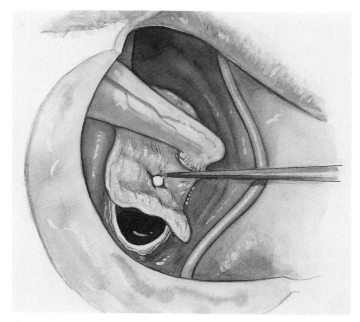

Fig. 8.**35**

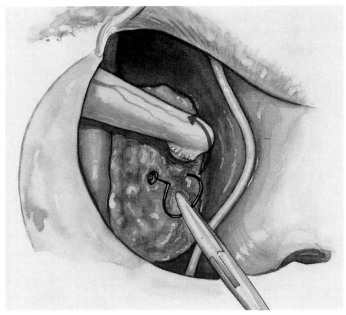

Fig. 8.**36**

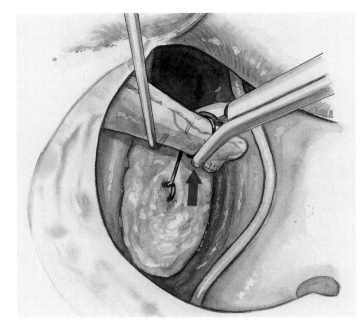

Fig. 8.**37**

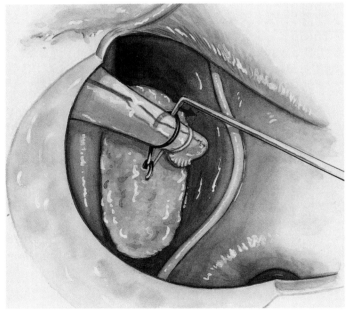

Fig. 8.**38**

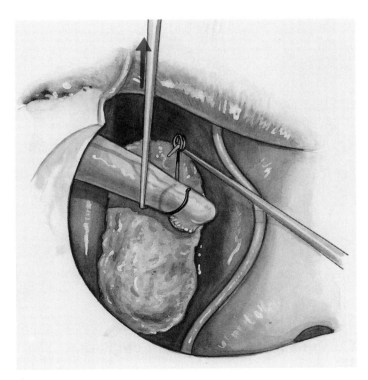

Fig. 8.**39**

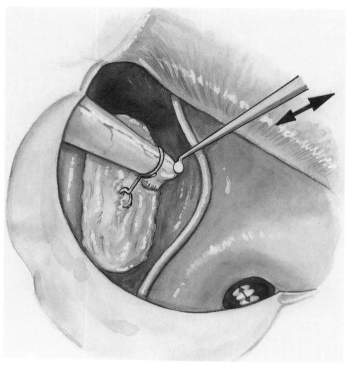

Fig. 8.**40**

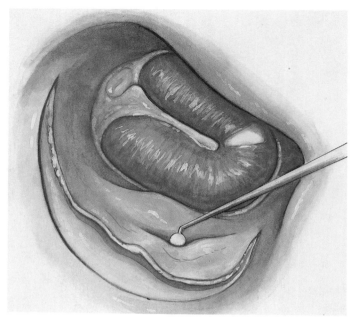

Fig. 8.**41**

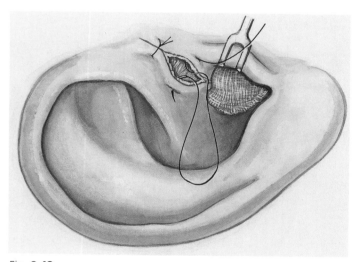

Fig. 8.**42**

Closing Stages of Partial or Complete Stapedectomy

The incus is now moved gently and carefully with a curette, and the round window niche is observed to test that the round window reflex is positive (Fig. 8.**40**). If the test is negative the cause of failure of transmission of vibrations must be sought in the ossicular chain and be eliminated, provided that the round window niche is free.

After careful suction of blood clots, bone fragments, etc. from the middle ear cavity, a tympanomeatal flap is replaced to close the middle ear (Fig. 8.**41**).

The flap is adjusted with the aspirator and the curette in such a way that the tympanic membrane has no folds, and the attached meatal skin lies on the bony wall of the meatus and covers the bone defect securely.

The meatus is now packed from the tympanic membrane to the junction of the inner and middle thirds of the meatus using pieces of gelatine foam soaked in antibiotic solution. The packing is continued with the introduction of small pieces of gauze soaked in antibiotic ointment about 1 cm^2 in size as far as the inner end of the incision. The incision is now closed by two or three fine skin sutures (Fig. 8.**42**), and the remaining part of the meatus is then filled with a continuous strip of gauze soaked in ointment which also covers the incision (Fig. 8.**43**).

Finally the ear is bandaged (Fig. 8.**44**).

Modifications and Alternative Procedures

Apart from the two techniques *partial* and *complete stapedectomy* described in detail above, numerous other modifications of the technique for stapedial ankylosis have been described so far. They have not become generally established, and will therefore not be considered further. Several special techniques which may be used in particular problem situations will be briefly described.

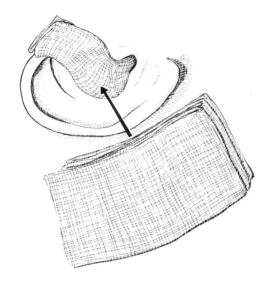

Fig. 8.**43**

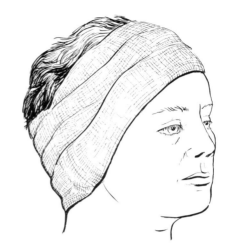

Fig. 8.**44**

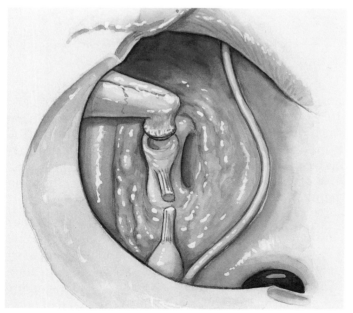

Fig. 8.**45**

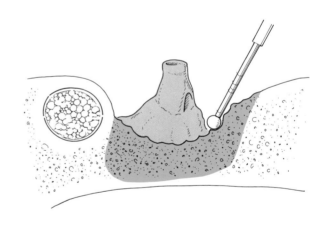

Fig. 8.**46**

1. Procedure for a Thick Footplate or an Obliterated Oval Window Niche

There are two methods for this situation. The first using a piston is described in greater detail on page 239 ff (see stapedotomy). The alternative procedure consists of careful removal of excess otosclerotic bone from the niche and footplate area until the level of the footplate and the original shape of the niche are restored.

Technique: The initial situation is illustrated in Figure 8.**45**. The otosclerotic osteophyte is removed gradually and carefully using a fine diamond burr to recreate the original contours of the oval window niche (Fig. 8.**46**).

Once the suspected original level of the footplate has been reached the entire footplate area is drilled down using continuous suction and irrigation under higher magnification until the blueness of this bony area is seen (Fig. 8.**46**). Premature opening of the vestibule should be avoided as this allows bone dust to reach the perilymph.

The following points are important during removal of bone with the drill:

• The finest diamond burr should be used for exact concentric dissection, that is without making strokes with the drill. The diameter of the head of the burr should be between 0.5 and 1.0 mm.
• Dissection should be on the surface without boring deeply.
• Drilling at a very low rate of revolutions.
• Drilling only finishes when a normally shaped, homogenous, blue–tinted footplate has been created.

The footplate area is now incised with a footplate knife as shown in Figure 8.**29**, both vertically and across the footplate, and is fractured (Fig. 8.**29**) as in the standard procedure (page 241). After the fragments of the footplate have been mobilized they are carefully removed. Despite previous mobilization this step may be difficult because in these cases the fragments of the footplate often adhere firmly to the bony edges of the window. The further procedure is described on page 242.

This method demands a steady hand and much experience. The two *specific complications* of this procedure are as follows:

a) If the drill is used in the region of the footplate it can produce sensorineural hearing loss even if the drill is used with extreme care and at the lowest possible rate of revolutions.
b) If an active focus of otosclerosis is dissected with the drill, and nothing of the annular ligament remains there is an increased probability of subsequent bony reclosure of the oval window.

2. Procedure for a Narrow Oval Window Niche

The normal anatomical variants include wide and narrow niches. In addition there are abnormal causes of narrowing of the entrance to the niche through an overhanging facial nerve or a very marked projection of the wall of the promontory.

Technique: A *projecting facial nerve canal* (Fig. 8.**47**) is the more difficult problem. Without doubt the part of the bony wall of the facial canal facing the oval window niche can be removed with a diamond burr. However, the bone in this area is very thin so that not much further space can be created, especially as the nerve bulges through the resulting bony defect. Furthermore, the facial nerve sometimes does not have a bony cover in this area, and there is then nothing which can be removed. In order to ensure successful sound transmis-

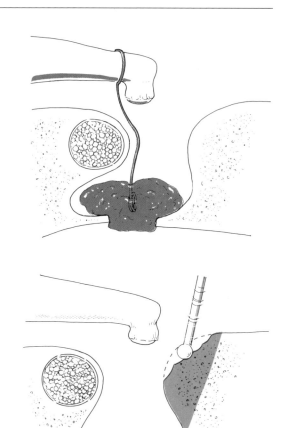

Fig. 8.**47**

Fig. 8.**48**

sion, a rather longer wire prosthesis should be inserted after opening and covering the oval window, a step which may be difficult if the niche is very narrow. The prosthesis should be so curved that it avoids the projecting facial canal without touching it or the other structures of the wall of the niche. The principle is shown in Figure 8.**47**.

An *overhanging wall of the promontory* on the other hand can be smoothed flat with a diamond burr turning at low revolutions, either before or after the stapedial superstructure has been removed, but *before* beginning work on the footplate (Fig. 8.**48**). The scala tympani of the cochlea must not be opened during removal of bone from the promontory.

3. Otosclerosis Around the Round Window

Very occasionally, access to the round window is impeded by a focus of otosclerosis, either combined with fixation of the stapes or independently. For cases with stapedial fixation a stapedectomy is first carried out, and then the round window reflex is elicited. A positive result will be obtained if even only a narrow slit of the niche remains patent. In such a case dissection in the round window should be avoided.

On the other hand if the round window niche is completely obstructed by an osteophyte — a very rare finding — with or without otosclerosis of the oval window, the wall of the promontory of this area should be removed very carefully with a diamond drill. The surgeon must constantly bear in mind that the membrane of the round window is very thin and its relation to the promontory can also vary widely. For example, it can lie at almost the same level as the wall of the promontory, but may also lie deep within the niche. Should the membrane be damaged the round window must be immediately covered with loose connective tissue or middle ear mucosa.

4. Fixation of the Ossicular Chain at Several Points

Fixation of the ossicular chain by otosclerosis at sites other than the oval window is very rare. However, otosclerosis may be combined with chronic otitis media and its sequelae, or with a congenital anomaly of the middle ear. Thus combinations of fixation of the footplate by otosclerosis with adhesions, tympanosclerosis, or bony bridges obstructing the function of the ossicular chain in the attic may occasionally be found behind an intact tympanic membrane. It is important to test the mobility of the malleus and the incus as well as the round window reflex by slight pressure on the handle of the malleus before finishing a stapedectomy so as not to overlook these anomalies. Usually the surgeon will notice immediately after dividing the incudostapedial joint that the mobility of the long process of the incus is limited if there is multiple fixation of the chain. Such rigidity of the long process of the incus almost certainly indicates additional points of fixation around the tympanic membrane and the articular process of the long process of the incus usually in the attic. In such cases the entire ossicular chain must be inspected beginning with a limited atticotomy.

If investigation shows additional mechanical obstruction, and this cannot be overcome by manipulation of the chain with a dissecting needle for example, a stapedectomy is first carried out with cover of the opened oval window by fascia or connective tissue and the fixed chain is now bypassed by a *malleovestibuloplasty*.

Technique: The tympanic membrane is further mobilized above until the neck of the malleus is accessible.

Small parts of the lateral attic wall can be removed to allow inspection of the tympanic recess. The neck of the malleus is now divided either with a malleus head punch or a conical diamond burr. The incus and the head of the malleus are then removed from the epitympanum.

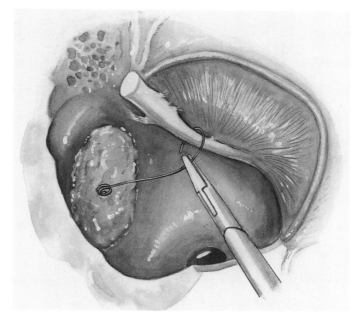

Fig. 8.**49**

The handle of the malleus is now separated carefully from the tympanic membrane from its lateral process to the umbo. Figure 8.**49** shows the situation after release of the tympanic membrane.

The distance between the handle of the malleus and the layer of connective tissue closing the oval window is measured, and if a prosthesis of suitable length is not available an appropriate steel wire prosthesis is fashioned. The end of the prosthesis intended to clasp the handle of the malleus is shaped in the form of a long loop that is longer than that for the incus (Fig. 8.**49**). This prosthesis must usually be longer (5.5–6.5 mm) than one which is fastened to the incus.

The end of the prosthesis is now attached to the isolated handle of the malleus (Fig. 8.**49**). The wire loop is closed and then pushed as far superior as possible in the direction of the lateral process of the malleus (Fig. 8.**50**).

The foot of the prosthesis is now placed on the center of the connective tissue pad over the oval window, and the stability of the conducting mechanism from the tympanic membrane to the oval window is confirmed. The operation then proceeds as described under the standard technique on page 244).

A caveat should be mentioned concerning the wire prosthesis to the malleus handle: these have been known to migrate laterally, transect the malleus handle, and extrude through the tympanic membrane. An alternate prosthesis would be one wherein the "crutch" end of the prosthesis would accommodate the malleus neck or handle and the shaft of the prosthesis would contact the oval window graft. The prosthesis may be hydroxylapatite, homograft bone, Teflon, etc.

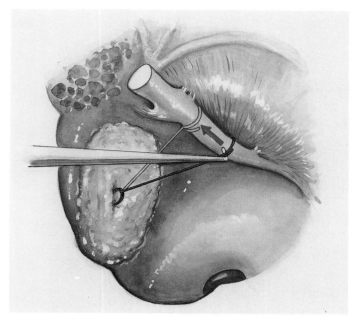

Fig. 8.**50**

Table 8.**1**   Complications after stapedial operations (from Plester, Hildmann, Steinbach; 1989).

Complication	Number of Patients	Percent
1. Loose prosthesis due to inadequate fixation or partial necrosis of the long process of the incus	208	20.00
2. Loose prosthesis due to complete necrosis of the long process of the incus	57	5.48
3. Adhesions in the oval window changing the position of the prosthesis	217	20.86
4. Reduced mobility of the tympanic membrane due to adhesions in the middle ear	115	11.06
5. Fistula at the oval window	52	5.00
6. Bony reclosure of the oval window	101	9.71
7. Prosthesis too short	94	9.04
8. Prosthesis too long	76	7.31
9. Previous partial stapedectomy or mobilization, recurrent fixation	60	5.77
10. Granulations at the oval window	28	2.69
11. Fixation of the head of the malleus	13	1.25
12. Closure of the round window	9	0.87
13. Cholesteatoma	6	0.58
14. Ruptured wire prosthesis	4	0.38
Total	1040	100.00

An alternative procedure is to fenestrate the promontory (see Chapter 4, page 126).

5. Ossified Tendon of the Stapedius Muscle

Occasionally the tendon of the stapedius muscle is ossified, either with or without fixation of the footplate. For patients with simultaneous stapedial ankylosis the above technique requires no modification since the tendon of the stapedius is divided in any case. On the other hand, if fixation of the stapes is due solely to ossification of the tendon of the stapedius it suffices to divide the tendon with a fine diamond drill. In these cases stapedectomy is obviously not necessary, although it may be appropriate to drill down the pyramidal eminence.

Congenital Anomalies of the Ossicular Chain

Occasionally stapedial ankylosis is combined with anomalies of the ossicular chain, and in these cases otosclerosis *can* play an additional role. The procedure to be adopted is determined by the condition of the oval window, the ossicular chain, the tympanic membrane, and the middle ear (see Chapters 3 and 4). A stapedotomy, possibly combined with a malleovestibulopexy, often suffices for anomalies confined to the ossicular chain. However, if the oval window is completely absent a fenestration of the lateral semi-

circular canal may be considered as a less traumatic alternative, provided that the round window is still functioning.

7. Intraoperative Complications

The intraoperative complications include *floating footplate* (see page 239) and a *perilymph fistula.*

In the latter, a profuse escape of fluid follows opening of the oval window. The fluid includes not only perilymph but also cerebrospinal fluid. It is thought that this phenomenon arises in patients with an abnormally wide cochlear aqueduct *(oozers)*, and in congenital anomalies where the defect lies in the internal acoustic meatus *(gushers)* (Schuknecht and Reisser, 1988). Such cases are treated during the operation by elevating the patient's head and waiting for the flow of CSF to cease. The oval window is then closed with a large piece of connective tissue fixed with adequate pressure in the oval window niche.

Revision Surgery

Although more than 90% of patients have a good long-term result after stapedectomy, a few patients develop a considerable conductive deafness either in the immediate postoperative healing phase or some weeks, months or years later.

Indications for revision surgery include:

- Sudden marked tinnitus.
- A suspected early granuloma.
- Increasing or fluctuating conductive or sensori-neural deafness.
- Persistent or intermittent dizziness.

The most frequent causes of failure after stapes surgery are shown in Table 8.**1**, summarized from Plester et al.

Revision surgery should not be carried out *before three to six months* after the first operation, with the exception of an early granuloma (see below).

The danger of damage to the inner ear at a revision operation is obviously higher than at the first operation. Shea reports complete deafness in 10% of patients after revision operation for disease around the oval window.

Early Granuloma

An early granuloma is to be feared because it endangers the inner ear. The clinical picture includes the symptoms of vestibular irritation and a rapid loss of inner ear function between 5 and 17 days after the operation. Weber's test is lateralized to the unoperated ear. Dizziness and severe tinnitus may develop suddenly.

Steroids and antibiotics are urgently indicated: if this treatment is not successful within 24 hours immediate reoperation is indicated. Typically, massive granulations are found in the oval window.

Histological examination in such cases of early granuloma shows a foreign body reaction at the oval window niche.

Facial Paralysis

Facial paralysis is a very unusual complication during or after stapedectomy. Immediate paralysis that persists after the effect of the local anesthetic has worn off is probably due to injury to the nerve. It demands *immediate* exploration of the course of the nerve.

A facial paralysis coming on a few days after the operation has a much better prognosis. It is probably due to a transient edema around the nerve, and requires no further treatment.

Subluxation of the Ossicular Chain

A malleovestibulopexy is indicated (see also page 247) for subluxation of the ossicular chain shown by abnormal mobility of the incus. Loss of continuity of the ossicular chain may be due to rough dissection at the first operation.

Loose Prosthesis

The phenomenon is expressed as a considerable improvement of hearing after aeration of the middle ear by the Valsalva maneuver. The hearing deteriorates again after swallowing *(fluctuating hearing)*. This fluctuating hearing is caused by a loose prosthesis due to inadequate fixation or erosion of the long process of the incus.

The tympanic membrane and the long process of the incus move laterally as a result of the Valsalva maneuver, gaining close contact with the prosthesis, causing a temporary improvement in hearing.

Reoperation and adequate fixation of the prosthesis leads to a stable improvement in hearing.

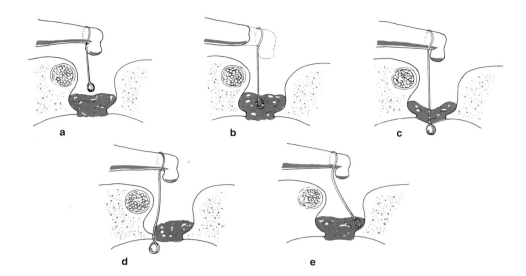

Fig. 8.**51**

Occasionally it may be found that the peripheral part of the long process of the incus is atrophic or converted into connective tissue, causing loss of continuity between the ossicular chain and the stapedial prosthesis (Fig. 8.**51b**). Fixation of the loop of the existing prosthesis to the stump of the long process of the incus may restore a solid union. In other cases the prosthesis must be completely removed (see below) and be replaced by a new, longer and individually–shaped prosthesis to create good contact with the remnant of the incus. If this is impossible a malleovestibulopexy must be carried out. Incudal necrosis was more common in the early years of stapes surgery when relatively plump polyethylene prostheses were used rather than the wire prosthesis.

Incorrect Position of the Prosthesis

Incorrect position of the prosthesis after partial stapedectomy using a platinum wire–Teflon piston is extremely unusual. Displacement of a connective tissue–wire prosthesis, particularly after complete stapedectomy, is more common. The end of the prosthesis sits on the edge of the oval window (Figure 8.**51e**) causing a moderate or high grade conductive deafness.

The most common cause of deafness persisting after the operation is a short prosthesis (Fig. 8.**51a**). The prosthesis is removed at a further operation and replaced by a new one of the correct length.

The removal of a piston prosthesis usually does not endanger the function of the inner ear. However there is a danger that the connective tissue of a connective tissue–wire prosthesis can adhere to the inner ear structures. In this case the prosthesis must on no account be simply removed from the oval window. The old prosthesis must be divided. The covering of the oval window remains in one piece. The new prosthesis (for example, a piston prosthesis) is then introduced after creating a small opening in the connective tissue covering, if possible in the posterior quarter of the oval window. This step also confirms that the oval window has not suffered bony reclosure under the connective tissue covering.

Long Prosthesis

The distance from the long process of the incus and the footplate varies from 3.9 to 5.0 mm. In most patients with otosclerosis a prosthesis 4.5 mm long will be suitable. A prosthesis which is too long can impinge upon the saccule or the utricle causing persistent dizziness and tinnitus (Fig. 8.**51c, d**).

Recurrent Closure of the Oval Window

If the *oval window* has been *completely closed by bone* under the soft tissue, the membrane is released stepwise from the underlying bone. The new osteophyte is now removed with a fine diamond burr until the outline of the former footplate with a blue appearance shines through. The further steps of the procedure are described on pages 240 and 245.

Perilymph Fistula

The main symptoms are fluctuating hearing in the operated ear, and mild temporary vestibular symptoms. A fistula may become manifest immediately after the operation or several months later. It appears to be determined by the technique used, and by the materials used for closing the oval window, and making the stapedial prosthesis.

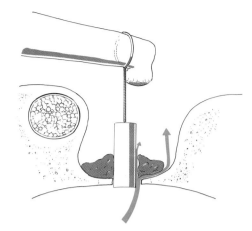

Fig. 8.**52**

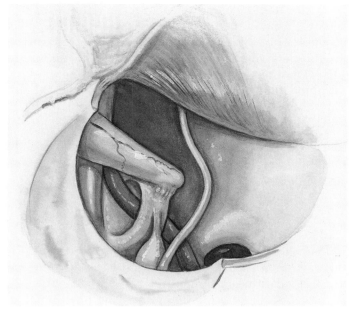

Fig. 8.**53**

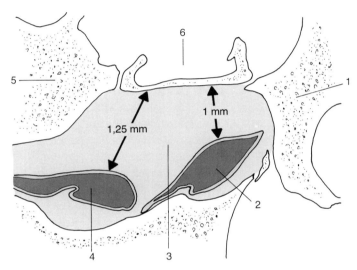

Fig. 8.**54**
1 Ventral wall of the oval window (promontory)
2 Saccule
3 Vestibule
4 Utricle
5 Dorsal wall of the oval window
6 Stapes

If a perilymph fistula is suspected the oval window niche and all the edges of the cover should be checked (Fig. 8.**52**). If a leak is confirmed, the covering of the site of the leak is freshened, and supplemented by further connective tissue. In unfavorable cases, that is a very large, gaping fistula, the entire connective tissue covering of the oval window must be removed (see above) and be replaced by a new reliable overlapping layer of connective tissue.

Landmarks and Danger Points

- The site of exit of the *chorda tympani* from the bony posterior meatal wall.
- A *persistent stapedial artery* is unusual. The typical course of this vessel is shown in Figure 8.**53** which shows that the persistent artery usually rises out of the hypotympanum, runs superiorly along the promontory and between the crura of the stapes to the canal of the facial nerve. A stapedectomy should be abandoned in favor of a fenestration in the presence of a persistent stapedial artery (see page 254). In some cases it may be possible to work around the persistent stapedial artery and perform a stapedectomy/stapedotomy. If the artery is not large, it may be electrocoagulated and the operation completed in the usual manner.

Important data

In adults the footplate is on average 3 mm long and 1.5 mm wide. The distance from the long process of the incus to the footplate is on average 4 mm, but it can vary within relatively wide limits. It is usually less in women than in men.

The distance between the handle of the malleus and the footplate is on average 1–1.5 mm longer than that between the long process of the incus and the footplate. The relations of the membranous labyrinth to the oval window are of surgical relevance in stapedectomy (see Fig. 8.**54**).

Part of the saccule projects into the anterior half of the oval window, and the utricle is related to the posterior border of the oval window. The saccule and utricle are thus in danger during operations on the stapes footplate. Prostheses should be placed in the free part of the vestibule, that is the posteroinferior part, since the distance from the utricle is greatest at this point.

The distance between the stapedial footplate and the saccule is 1 mm. The distance between the stapes footplate and the utricle is 1.25 mm (Anson and Donaldson).

Rules, Hints, and Typical Mistakes

1) As in most operations in the head and neck, it is very useful and saves time if the surgeon has trained himself to use all the instruments with equal facility with either hand. The hand must always be supported and instruments, especially drills, must be protected from sudden unexpected movement.
2) Instruments, particularly the drill, should never be worked towards the facial nerve, but always in the opposite direction.
3) It is appropriate to change the magnification during individual phases of stapedectomy. Low power is used for all phases of the operation up to dissection on the footplate and after the oval window has been covered. Dissection under higher power increases safety during work on the footplate and the oval window.
4) Force should never be applied with the instruments, particularly around the ossicular chain and the oval window niche, because of the danger of subluxation from a fracture.
5) The round window reflex should only be tested once or twice during the entire procedure, and it must always be done as carefully as possible.
6) Great care is necessary during identification and freeing of the fibrocartilaginous anulus during creation of the tympanomeatal flap to prevent tearing of the tympanic membrane.
7) The tympanic membrane must be elevated sufficiently to ensure a good view into the middle ear. Dissection through an inadequate slit is not only more difficult but also more dangerous. Instillation of one or two drops of 1:100000 adrenaline solution into the oval window niche immediately after the tympanic membrane has been turned back facilitates the ensuing phases of the procedure. Excess fluid should be suctioned out immediately.
8) The chorda tympani can be retracted to one side but should not be severely stretched because of abnormalities, usually temporary, of taste after the operation.

9) The operation can be continued after accidental subluxation of the malleoincudal joint with minimal dislocation of the long process of the incus. Minimal damage of the joint is usually followed by normal healing. However, if the entire incus is dislocated from its normal position it must be removed, and a malleovestibulopexy carried out.
10) A malleovestibulopexy is also indicated for a fracture of the long process of the incus if the remnant of the long process is no longer adequate to ensure reliable fixation of the wire prosthesis.
11) The oval window should not be opened until absolute hemostasis has been achieved. Even then bleeding may occur after the footplate has been opened from vessels lying at its edge or from a focus of otosclerosis. In such cases a blood clot should be allowed to form over the vestibule, and it is then removed carefully by suction or a 90° hook; the latter must not be inserted deeper than the level of the footplate. Slight bleeding can often be managed satisfactorily by covering the open vestibule as quickly as possible with a previously prepared piece of connective tissue.
12) Before the oval window is opened the suction tubing must be fitted on a very fine suction cannula consisting of a handpiece with a finger plate and an on/off valve, and the suction pump should be turned low.
13) While the oval window is open the aspirator should never be allowed to lie in the window itself. If fluid must be sucked out, the tip of a very fine suction tube aspirator should be placed in the hypotympanum at some distance from the oval window.
14) The plug of connective tissue prepared before the operation, to cover the oval window after complete stapedectomy, should be neither too thick nor too thin. An inexperienced surgeon should shape the connective tissue *before* removing the footplate. It is also dangerous to make a connective tissue plug too small because it then sinks into the vestibule allowing escape of perilymph.
15) Removal of the entire stapes with the intact footplate should be avoided because this procedure exerts excessive hydraulic pressure on the inner ear.
16) The hooks used for removing adherent parts of the footplate from the oval window must be manipulated very delicately, otherwise the hook can break and the fragment sink into the vestibule. If this happens no attempt should be made to remove the piece of metal from the vestibule.
17) No attempt should be made to manipulate a floating footplate out of the vestibule with instruments. The surgeon should wait until the vestibule is full to the brim with perilymph, and then introduce a drop of blood on the open oval window, wait until this has clotted, and finally suck out the clot carefully.

Sometimes the loose footplate then adheres to the clot. If this step is not successful the footplate should be left in the vestibule, and the operation should be completed in the normal fashion. The patient may complain of dizziness for some time, but this symptom gradually resolves during the ensuing months.

18) Small individual fragments of the footplate which cannot be removed safely from the edge of the window with a 90° hook are better left alone rather than risking bleeding or damage to the inner ear caused by rough manipulations within the window.

19) If the footplate is very thick it is important that the canal created for a Teflon piston lie exactly in the axis of vibration of the piston. If necessary, the position of the piston can be corrected by bending the wire part of the prosthesis slightly.

20) If the tympanomeatal flap is too short to close the middle ear because more bone than expected has been removed, the defect is bridged by a piece of fascia lying under the tympanomeatal flap and upon the posterior meatal wall.

21) A perforation of the tympanic membrane is closed by an underlay of a piece of loose connective tissue or fascia, and the tympanic membrane is then returned to its correct position (see Chapter 4).

Postoperative Course

- If the patient feels well he can get out of bed on the day after operation. However, he should remain in bed if there are symptoms or signs of irritation of the labyrinth such as nystagmus due to bleeding into the vestibule and manipulations in the oval window niche, etc., and should not get up until these symptoms subside.

- For the first 8 days the patient should not blow his nose and if possible should not sneeze.

- The dressing is changed for the first time on the fifth or sixth day after operation. The meatus is treated with ointment alone after removal of the dressing.

- In the first few days after operation nystagmus should be looked for and Weber's test should be done using 512 and 1024 Hz tuning forks. If there is any suspect adverse response from the inner ear a bone conduction audiogram should be done daily.

- Labyrinthine irritation or reduction of bone conduction, indicating labyrinthitis or foreign body reaction, should be treated by low molecular weight dextrans, antibiotics, and steroids. Antivertiginous drug also help to reduce the symptoms.

- A stapedectomy/stapedotomy operation is usually done on an outpatient basis, or requires an overnight stay, especially if the patient's home is far away. Patients with poststapedectomy complications, i. e., vertigo, may require a longer hospital stay.

- The rate of improvement varies widely, being quicker with the piston technique or partial stapedectomy and longer after complete stapedectomy. A conductive deafness of 10 dB can be due to hemotympanum. Slight high tone loss of bone conduction is found occasionally, but this usually improves within the ensuing months.

- The patient must be told that the hearing can vary in the first few weeks and only stabilizes about 6 or 8 weeks after operation. The Tullio phenomenon often annoys the patient but usually resolves within 6 to 8 weeks. The patient must also be warned that this effect may make him unsteady, for example in city traffic.

- Washing the hair, swimming, etc. can be resumed after 14 days if healing is normal.

Functional Results

A sudden perceptive deafness may arise months or years after the operation, precipitated by sudden variations in atmospheric pressure, diving, intensive sunlight, chilling, or similar external insults. However, the mechanism is not always obvious, particularly as the pathogenesis of such deafness is often unclear.

A revision operation should be considered if conductive deafness recurs.

Tinnitus present before the operation will improve or disappear in about half the cases.

Vestibular symptoms are not normally to be expected after the operation, but some patients may feel dizzy in the few days immediately after the operation. Patients with a perilymph fistula may also experience dizziness.

It is impossible to predict with certainty whether the function of the inner ear will remain stable after a stapedectomy or whether it will decline with the course of time, for example in a patient with cochlear otosclerosis.

Clinical experience shows that the otosclerotic process can be halted or slowed by surgery.

Excess stretching or cutting of the chorda tympani can lead to a partial loss or change of taste of the anterior quadrant of the same side of the tongue, and to dryness of the mouth due to interference with the innervation of the salivary glands. However, even complete division of both chorda tympani seldom causes severe long–standing symptoms which are to be expected in fewer than 10% of all cases.

Fenestration

Although the fenestration is nowadays seldom carried out there are still situations in which it is appropriate such as *congenital anomalies of the middle ear.* The operative technique will therefore be described briefly.

Preoperative Diagnostic Procedures

The current, special indications for fenestration demand a detailed history of previous operations on the ear, vestibular tests, and detailed radiological investigation of the middle ear by high resolution CT, etc.

Indications

Fenestration, in either one or two stages, may be used as a last resort in the following circumstances.

- After previous, possibly repeated, unsuccessful operations on the oval window.
- In "malignant" juvenile obliterating otosclerosis of the oval window niche.
- For severe tympanosclerosis.
- For severe congenital middle ear anomalies if it is not possible to achieve improvement in the hearing using both windows.
- If the oval window is completely obstructed by the facial nerve.
- For a persistent stapedial artery (see page 251).

Contraindications

- Conductive deafness with less than a 40 dB hearing loss.
- Patients with occupations which make particular demands on the balance mechanism.
- Infection of the external or middle ear.

Principle of the Operation

A "new oval window" (Lempert) is created in the lateral semicircular canal because sound can no longer enter the inner ear through the oval window for one of the reasons named above.

Preoperative Preparation

See page 231.

Special Instruments

These include an operating microscope, a drill, electrocoagulation, and the usual set of microsurgical instruments. The following instruments are useful for creating the fenestration in the semicircular canal:

— short and long angled excavators, right and left (Fig. 8.**55**)
— suction–irrigation
— malleus head punch
— special self retaining retractors for the right and left side (Fig. 8.**56**)

Anesthesia

Although fenestration can be carried out under local anesthesia with adequate premedication, it is preferably done under general intubation anesthesia.

Operative Technique

One–Stage Endaural Procedure (Lempert, Shambaugh)

Shambaugh's incision begins at the origin of the auricle above, then runs inferiorly between the helix and tragus, passes around the posterior circumference of the meatal introitus, and ends in front of the sulcus between the tragus and the antitragus (Fig. 8.**57**).

A large *tympanomeatal flap* (Sourdille) that will cover the window in the semicircular canal securely is now created. A straight incision knife is used to create an incision in the skin of the meatal floor, between 6 and 7 o'clock in the right ear, beginning just in front of the tympanic membrane and running externally. The incision is carried right down to the bone, and ends externally at the end of the bony meatus where it meets the lower end of the initial incision (Fig. 8.**58**).

The second meatal incision begins immediately in front of the tympanic membrane, but lying between 3 and 4 o'clock for the right ear. This incision is also carried down to the bone externally and then to the initial incision shown in Figure 8.**57**.

The skin–periosteal flap which is defined by these incisions is now carefully freed with a fine elevator from the underlying bone ending just in front of the edge of, the tympanic membrane (Fig. 8.**59**). The outer part is usually relatively thick and stiff. It should be immedi-

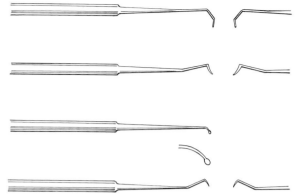

Fig. 8.**55**

Fig. 8.**56**

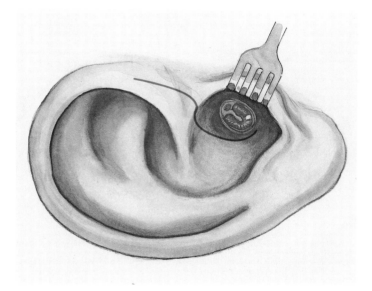

Fig. 8.**57**

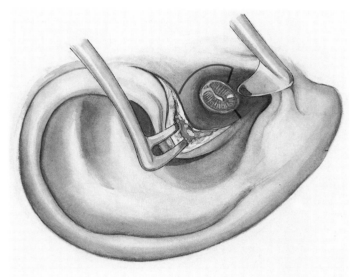

Fig. 8.**58**

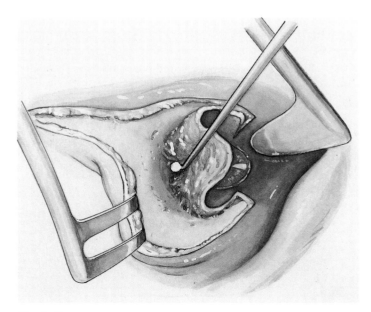

Fig. 8.**59**

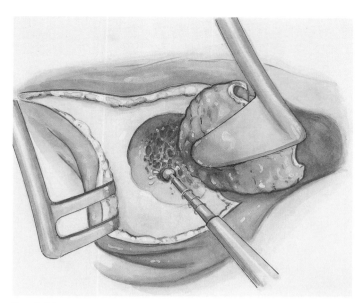

Fig. 8.**60**

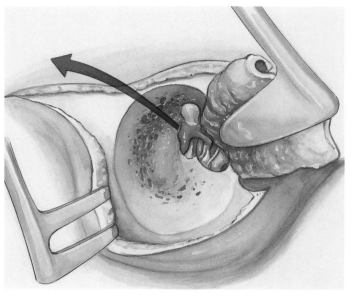

Fig. 8.**61**

ately thinned carefully with a fine scissors so that it can be later fitted easily over the fenestration or into the mastoid cavity, without being perforated. The posterior bony meatal wall in the region of the antrum is removed with a drill (Fig. 8.**60**) to create better access to the middle ear and antrum. The fibrocartilaginous anulus of the tympanic membrane to which the meatal flap is attached is now carefully freed from the tympanic sulcus so that the tympanic membrane together with the attached meatal flap can be turned forward as one tympanomeatal flap. The flap turns around the handle of the malleus, so that the neck of the malleus is exposed (Fig. 8.**61**).

The tympanomeatal flap is held forwards with a special retractor until it is needed to cover the new window (Fig. 8.**61**). The cell system of the mastoid process is now dissected out with the drill, beginning at the exposed bone of the posterior meatal wall until the antrum and the region of the lateral semicircular canal is easily visible and accessible.

The next step is the removal of the lateral attic wall and of the bridge, down to the level of the floor of the meatus. The attic with the malleus and incus, the chorda tympani and the bony block containing the lateral semicircular canal are now exposed (Fig. 8.**61**).

The incudomalleolar joint is divided with a dissecting needle or a sickle knife from the incus which is removed (Fig. 8.**61**). The neck of the malleus is divided with a malleus head punch or a conical fine diamond burr, and the head of the malleus is also removed (Fig. 8.**62**).

Sufficient space has now been created to provide a good view for dissection of the semicircular canal and

to allow the tympanomeatal flap to be spread out over the semicircular canal easily once the fenestration has been created. At this point in the operation it is wise to ensure that the tympanomeatal flap fits well: if it is under tension or forms folds, the base of the flap on the tympanic membrane should be mobilized further. After being tried for size, the flap should again be turned anteriorly and held by the retractor.

So far the operation has been carried out under low—power magnification, but it is now advisable to change to higher power.

The cells surrounding the compact bone of the lateral semicircular canal are now removed with a small cutting drill, watching out for the facial nerve, until the labyrinthine block projects from its surroundings as an arched white bony complex (Fig. 8.**63**). Enchondralization (Shambaugh) of the horizontal semicircular canal is now carried out using diamond burrs of various sizes. Initially a large diamond burr (2–3 mm diameter) is used under continuous and copious irrigation to burr down the bone of the labyrinthine capsule over the semicircular canal in a flat and gradually deepening plane (Fig. 8.**64**) (the diagrams of enchondralization in Figure 8.**64** et seq. are taken from Wullstein).

Figure 8.**64** shows the extent of the area to be drilled down. The flat plane is gradually and carefully deepened until a fine grey line shines through the bone (Fig. 8.**65**). This line marks the lumen of the bony semicircular canal which must not be opened at this stage.

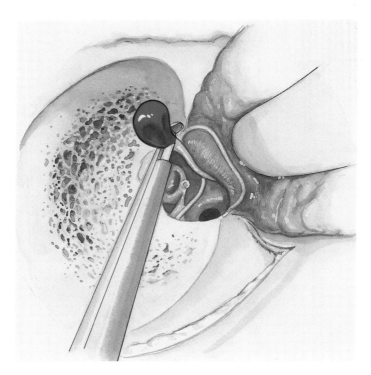

Fig. 8.**62**

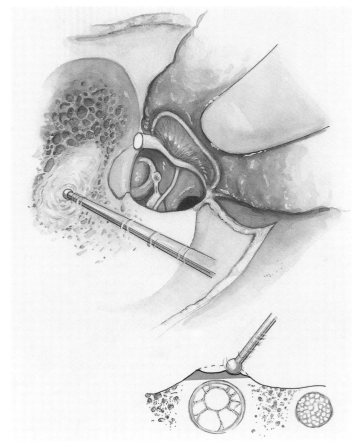

Fig. 8.**63**

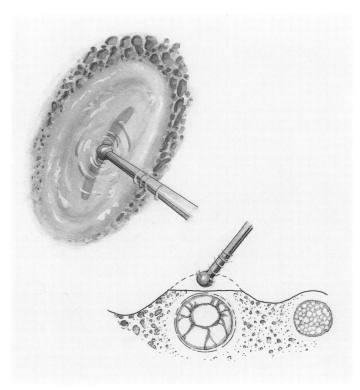

Fig. 8.**64**

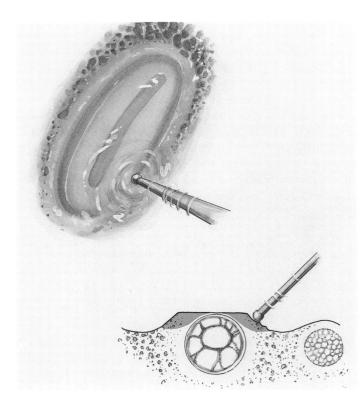

Fig. 8.**65**

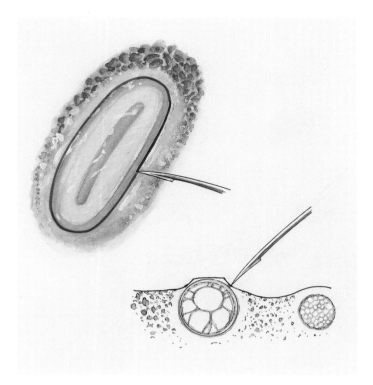

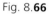

Fig. 8.**66**

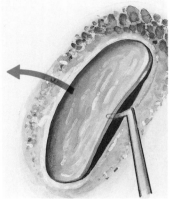

Fig. 8.**67**

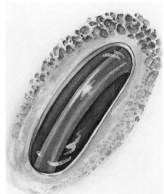

Fig. 8.**68**

A cupola is now defined in the labyrinthine block (Fig. 8.**66**) using a fine diamond burr 1 mm in diameter under higher optical magnification and continuous irrigation. This fine diamond burr is used to encircle the lumen of the bony semicircular canal at some distance from the grey line, thus gradually forming a bony groove surrounding the lumen of the semicircular canal (Fig. 8.**66**). In this way an arched cupola forming a lid for the labyrinthine lumen is created (Lempert). At the same time the lateral wall of the semicircular canal is thinned more and more so that finally the lumen of the labyrinth is accompanied by two parallel intense grey lines.

The grey line which first appears *above* the labyrinthine lumen should only be visible weakly but the two deeper lying grey lines lying parallel to the *edge* of the lumen of the semicircular canal are darker if they have been created properly (Fig. 8.**66**) (double blue line technique).

Finally, the two parallel dark grey lines are each joined by a transverse groove, both over the ampulla (that is close to the facial nerve) and also at the posterior end of the future fenestration (Fig. 8.**66**). The grey lines should not lie too close together as the cupola would then be too flat, but they must also not be too far

apart: the cupola should not take up more than half the circumference of the bony semicircular canal.

Absolute hemostasis must now be achieved using the diamond burr to deal with any bleeding points in the bone.

The wound is cleaned again carefully of bone dust by thorough irrigation. Irrigation should not be used during the remaining part of the operation (Lempert's dry fenestration technique).

Once the grey line has been completely and uniformly defined all around, the bone is slit carefully with a sickle knife (Fig. 8.**66**).

A suitable excavator is now introduced into the resulting fissure from the facial nerve side and the entire cupola is levered off in one piece (Fig. 8.**67**).

The delicate grey band of the endolymphatic space can now be seen lying in the newly created window (Fig. 8.**68**). The fenestration should be between 4 and 6 mm long and 0.9–1 mm wide in the region of the ampulla (Wullstein). The endolymphatic space must not protrude above the edges of the fenestration, but its summit should lie at the level of the edges of the fenestration (Fig. 8.**68**).

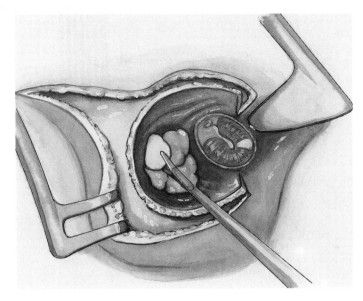

Fig. 8.**70**

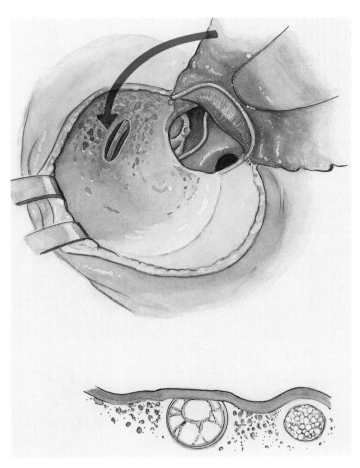

Fig. 8.**69**

Bony splinters adhering to the edges can be removed carefully with dissecting needles or fine hooks, but extensive manipulation within the open labyrinthine lumen must be avoided.

The already prepared tympanomeatal flap is now turned over the semicircular canal to close the fenestration securely (Fig. 8.**69**).

The flap is then secured with a layer of gelatine sponge soaked in antibiotic (Fig. 8.**70**) followed by a continuous packing with gauze soaked in ointment which is somewhat invaginated over the open window. The rest of the mastoid cavity is covered with fascia and/ or skin as necessary and then it and the external meatus are packed loosely with gauze.

The incision in the meatus is now sutured and packing of the meatus and the concha completed.

The auricle is covered with a padded dressing, and an ear bandage is applied.

Landmarks and Danger Points

The facial nerve lies close to the semicircular canal. It is in danger during creation of the cupola if its course has not been first identified.

Brisk bleeding during drilling of the bone close to the course of the facial nerve indicates the proximity of the nerve sheath. The bone over the lumen of the semicircular canal is on average 2 mm thick.

Rules, Hints, and Typical Mistakes

1. Creation of a Standard Fenestration

A tympanomeatal flap that is too narrow or too short does not cover the fenestration securely.

If the tympanomeatal flap is acccidently torn it can be used as a free graft. In this case it is laid over the edge of the tympanic membrane which should be first de–epithelialized: gelatine sponge soaked in antibiotic is laid under the part of the tympanic membrane which is now no longer fixed in the cartilaginous annulus.

The inner layer of the tympanomeatal flap must be absolutely clean and free from bone dust; the latter can cause new bone formation, particularly around the new window (Shambaugh).

An inadvertent perforation of the tympanic membrane part of the tympanomeatal flap is treated by an underlay of fascia. A perforation lying in the part which will later cover the mastoid bone can be ignored.

However, if the perforation lies in the part of the flap which is to cover the fistula, the tympanomeatal flap must either be used as a free graft which is rotated as necessary, or the defect must be lined with fascia to ensure secure closure of the open fenestration.

The niches of the oval and round windows must be checked carefully before creation of the fenestration.

The patency of the eustachian tube must be tested carefully in patients with previous chronic otitis media, including those who have been subjected to tympanoplasty.

The tympanic membrane may be damaged during removal of the head of the malleus by the levering action.

The round window niche and the ostium of the eustachian tube must be thoroughly cleaned of bone dust and blood clots before creation of the fenestration.

Procedures for injury to the facial nerve are described in Chapter 7, for injury to the dura in Chapter 5, and for injury to the sigmoid sinus in Chapter 9.

2. Dissection of the Semicircular Canal and Creation of the New Window

Drilling must be carried out under continuous irrigation to prevent the development of heat. Thinning of the semicircular canal and the creation of a cupola must be carried out under a fluid level. The fluid should leave the irrigation tube at body temperature, particularly if the operation is being done under local anesthetic. Ringer's or Locke's solution is suitable for irrigation. Irrigation should cease as soon as the cupola is ready to be pried off.

Drilling of the semicircular canal and the creation of the cupola should be carried out flat. Drilling begins with a relatively wide burr to be followed by one of finer caliber (1 mm in diameter) for creation of the oval grey contour. Diamond burrs are suitable for drilling the labyrinthine block. A "hatching" movement transverse to the long axis of the semicircular canal until the first grey line appears has proved most useful for drilling down the bone of the canal. *After* the grey line appears the drilling should be carried out parallel to the axis of the semicircular canal.

The course of the facial nerve requires particular care during drilling of the labyrinthine bone between the lumen of the canal and the facial nerve.

The drill should always be worked parallel to the course of the facial nerve in the region of the oval window, and never at right angles to it.

If the facial nerve runs very close to the semicircular canal the fenestration may be created further posteriorly.

The period when the fenestration is open should be as short as possible: the flap should lie ready so that the fenestration can be covered immediately after the cupola has been pried off.

Instruments must not be introduced into the perilymphatic space, and certainly must not touch the endolymphatic space. Small splinters of bone adhering solely to the edge of the fenestration can be removed by an instrument, provided that the instrument does not enter the perilymphatic space to any extent.

The summit of the endolymphatic space should lie in the plane of the fenestration so that it adheres to the overlying skin flap and prevents reossification.

The fenestration must be as long and as wide as possible to prevent reclosure.

Slight bleeding from the bony edge of the fenestration can be allowed to cease spontaneously.

Electrocoagulation should not be used close to the semicircular canal or the facial nerve.

3. Mastoid Cavity

If a mastoid cavity must be created, it should be so shaped that all parts of the cavity can be inspected from the meatus.

The facial spur should be removed down to the meatal floor during creation of the mastoid cavity. Edges or steps in this area and other parts of the cavity must be avoided.

Fascia or periosteum is suitable for covering the mastoid cavity in an incompletely dissected cell system. Full-thickness skin is also reliable, but split skin less so.

The gelatine sponge used for packing the cavity, particularly that used for fixing the flap over the fenestration, should not be too moist. After it has been immersed in antibiotic solution it should be pressed out well, so that it is again capable of being shaped and absorbant.

The surgical field around the fenestration and antrum must not be too narrow, and a balloon– or pear-shaped space must be created in which the tympanomeatal flap, or a graft, can be fitted at all points.

Aftercare

- Antibiotic cover is given for 5 days.
- The patient must remain in bed for 3 days with the head fixed by two lateral sandbags. If the patient develops marked symptoms of vestibular irritation he must remain in bed until they resolve completely.
- The patient usually remains in the hospital for a week.

- The packing in the cavity and the meatus may be left undisturbed for 2 weeks and is then carefully removed. However, if desired, the first dressing may be carried out after 8 days, but it must then be ensured that adequate expert daily care of the wound is available for the following 14 days.
- A large mastoid cavity requires expert supervision and cleaning for many months, especially to prevent dermatitis.
- The patient should not blow his nose for the first 8 days, and should avoid sneezing if possible.
- During the first few days after operation Weber's test should be done daily and nystagmus looked for.
- The eustachian tube can be inflated at low pressure after 10 days.
- Marked dizziness is treated with drugs such as dimenhydrinate (Dramamine, Vomex), haloperidol, diazepam (Valium), triflupromazine (Psyquil), etc.
- Facial paralysis presenting immediately after the operation must be treated by immediate decompression of the nerve. However, facial paralysis presenting after an interval of a few days requires no active treatment.

Functional Results and Postoperative Complications

Symptoms of vestibular irritation are much more common after fenestration than after stapedectomy, and can persist for several days or even weeks.

After fenestration the patient still has a conductive deafness of about 25 dB in normal cases, because the ossicular chain is not used for transmission of sound to the new fenestration.

However, reversal of Carhart's notch (page 230) contributes to improvement in hearing by elevating bone conduction in certain frequencies.

The Tullio phenomenon, e. g. dizziness in response to loud sound, as observed after stapedectomy, is also noticeable immediately after a fenestration. Furthermore, the patient may complain of persistent sensitivity to noise.

Patients with a fenestration should usually not work in a noisy environment and should not dive because of caloric stimulation of the peri- and endolymphatic system which is now covered solely by skin.

Bibliography

Anson B J, Donaldson J A. Surgical anatomy of the temporal bone and ear. 2nd edn, Philadelphia: Saunders, 1973.
Bailey H A T, Pappas J J, Graham S S. Small fenestra stapedectomy. A preliminary report. The Laryngoscope 1981; 91: 1308–21.
Baron S H. Persistent stapedial artery, necrosis of the incus and other problems which have influenced the choice of technique in stapes replacement surgery in otosclerosis. Laryngoscope (St. Louis) 1963; 73: 769.
Beck C, Bader J. Ein Beitrag zur feineren Anatomie des menschlichen Innenohres.. Arch Ohr-, Nas- u Kehlk-Heilk 1963; 181: 245.
Beickert P. Otosklerose. In: Hals-Nasen-Ohren-Heilkunde, Vol. III/1, Eds J. Berendes, R. Link, F. Zöllner, Stuttgart: Thieme, 1965.
Bellucci R J. Trends and profiles in stapes surgery. Ann. Otol. 1979; 88: 708–13.
Causse J, Causse J-B. Surgeon's workshop. Eighteen-year report on stapedectomy. II. postoperative therapy. Clin. Otolaryngol. 1980; 5: 329–37.
Derlacki E L. Revision stapes surgery. Laryngoscope 1985; 95: 1047.
Farrior B, Rophie S S. Fenestration of the horizontal semicircular canal in congenital conductive deafness. Laryngoscope 1985; 95: 1025.
Fisch U. Stapedektomie oder Stapedotomie? HNO 1979; 27: 361–7.
Fisch U, Dillier N. Technik und Spätresultate der Stapedotomie HNO 1987; 35: 252–4.
Fisch U, Dillier N. Stapedotomie: Technik und Langzeitresultate. ORL 10, Bern: Huber, 1987.
Gristwood R E. The surgical concept for otosclerosis. Adv Otorhinolaryngol 1988; 39: 52.
House H P. Early and late complications of stapes surgery. Otology 1963; 78: 606–13.
Kessel J. Über das Mobilisieren des Steigbügels durch Ausschneiden des Trommelfelles, Hammers und Ambosses bei Undurchgängigkeit der Tube. Arch Ohrenheilk 1878; 13: 69.
Krmpotić-Nemanić J, Draf W, Helms J. Chirurgische Anatomie des Kopf-Hals-Bereiches. Berlin: Springer-Verlag 1985.
Lempert J. Fenestra nov-ovalis: A new oval window for the improvement of hearing in cases of otosclerosis. Arch Otolaryng 1941; 34: 880.
Mc Gee, T M. Comparison of small fenestra and total stapedectomy. Michigan: Panel on stapes surgery, 1981.
Miglets A W, Paparella M M, Saunders W H. Atlas of Ear Surgery. St. Louis: C. V. Mosby, 1986.
Nager F R, Meyer M. Die Erkrankungen des Knochensystems und ihre Erscheinungen an der Innenohrkapsel des Menschen. Berlin: Karger, 1932.
Passow H. Diskussion zu R. Panse. Verh dtsch Otol Ges 1897; 6: 143.
Pedersen C B. The use of a small fenestra technique with the Fisch piston in the surgical treatment of otosclerosis. The Journal of Laryngology and Otology 1987; 101: 542–7.
Plester D, Cousins V C. Otosclerosis: its modern surgical management. The British Journal of Clinical Practice 1986; 40: 401.
Plester D, Hildmann H, Steinbach E. Atlas der Ohrchirurgie. Stuttgart: Kohlhammer, 1989.
Rosen S. Mobilization of the stapes to restore hearing in otosclerosis. N Y J Med 1953; 53: 2650.
Schuknecht H F. Stapedectomy. Boston: Little, Brown & Co., 1971.
Schuknecht H F, Reisser C. The morphologic basis for perilymphatic Gushers and Oozers. Adv Oto-Rhino-Laryng. 1988; 39: 1–12.
Shambaugh G E, Glasscock M E. Surgery of the ear, 3rd edn, Philadelphia: Saunders, 1980.
Shea J J. The Teflon piston operation for otosclerosis. Laryngoscope (St. Louis) 1963; 73: 508.
Shea J J. Thirty years of stapes surgery. J Laryngol Otol 1988; 102: 14.
Smith M F, Hopp M L. 1984 Santa Barbara state-of-the-art symposium on otosclerosis. Ann Otol Rhinol Laryngol 1986; 95: 1.
Wullstein H L. Operationen zur Verbesserung des Gehörs. Stuttgart: Thieme, 1968.
Yanagisawa E, Gardner G. The Surgical Atlas of Otology and Neuro-otology. New York: Grune & Stratton, 1983.

9 Surgical Management of Otogenic Intracranial Complications

Konrad Fleischer

Otogenic Extradural Abscess and Otogenic Meningitis

Causes and Routes of Extension

Bacterial destruction involving the peridural cells of the temporal bone, e. g. mastoiditis, petrositis, or a bacterially infected cholesteatoma in that area can cause a collection of pus to form between the dura mater and bone, producing an *extradural abscess* (external pachymeningitis). The abscess may overlie the dura of the middle or posterior cranial fossa and may directly overlie the lateral sinus (episinus abscess). Generally, the abscess is easy to detect owing to destruction of the overlying bone (internal table), but occasionally there is only a narrow tract passing through the inner table to the purulent focus, which then is easily overlooked. Dural granulations are usually present. Further intracranial complications such as meningitis, sinus thrombosis, subdural empyema, and brain abscess can develop from an extradural abscess at any time.

In otogenic *meningitis* (leptomeningitis), the leptomeninges have become broadly involved by bacterial infection. The principal otogenic causes and routes of extension (Fig. 9.**1**) are given below.

- Meningitis may arise early in the course of an acute bacterial otitis media (early meningitis). The organisms can spread from the middle ear mucosa to the meninges along connecting vessels or through sites of bone dehiscence — especially a temporal bone fracture, which may have been sustained years before. Repeated bouts of infection can occur by this mechanism.
- Mastoiditis or petrositis: Spread occurs through a focus of liquefaction that has penetrated to the dura, often with an epidural abscess as an intermediate stage. Osteitic processes in the paralabyrinthine cells and pyramidal apex contribute to the pathogenesis (Fig. 9.**1**).

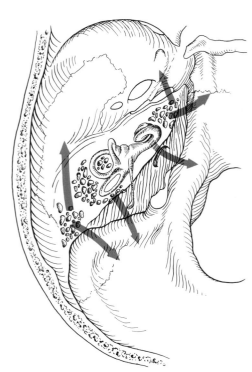

Fig. 9.**1** Potential routes for the development of meningitis from the air cells of the temporal bone and from the labyrinth. The middle cranial fossa is above, the posterior fossa below.

- A bacterially contaminated middle–ear cholesteatoma that has penetrated to the dura.
- Purulent labyrinthitis, which usually is secondary to an acute otitis media or chronic otitis media with bone destruction. The internal acoustic meatus or endolymphatic sac forms a pathway for spread from the labyrinth to the meninges. This *labyrinthogenic meningitis* is associated with total loss of labyrinthine function. It may commence within hours after

bacterial invasion of the labyrinth or, less commonly, may occur as a late complication following bone necrosis due to the labyrinthine disease.

Experience has shown that chronic suppuration of the middle ear mucosa (characterized by a central perforation of the tympanic membrane) is not significant as a precursor of meningitis, unless it is based on a masked mastoiditis.

Preoperative Diagnostic Procedures

Before the advent of MRI, an *extradural abscess* was very seldom diagnosed prior to surgery. It may be suspected in patients with mastoiditis or a middle–ear cholesteatoma who complain of a pounding ipsilateral headache. Because the typical tympanic membrane features of temporal bone involvement provide a definite indication for surgery, there appears to be no need for a more detailed workup (high–resolution CT). A pulsatile discharge of pus from the opened temporal bone is typically encountered at operation.

The diagnosis of *meningitis,* whose clinical symptoms are well known (headache, vomiting, fever, cranial tenderness to percussion, nuchal rigidity, positive Kernig and Brudzinski signs, opisthotonus), is established by examination of the cerebrospinal fluid (CSF). (The technique and hazards of CSF sampling are discussed in Volume 1, Chapter 10.) Otogenic meningitis, which is always bacterial, is characterized by cloudy CSF, an elevated CSF pressure, and usually a marked pleocytosis ranging from several hundred to many thousands of cells per mm^3. Granulocytes are predominant, Pandy's test is positive, and the total protein level is markedly elevated.

An attempt should always be made to isolate the causative organisms from the CSF and determine their sensitivities so that appropriate antibiotic therapy can be initiated. The CSF may be sterile in meningitis patients who have already been treated with antibiotics.

Meningitis should be classified as otogenic whenever any of the foregoing predisposing diseases are present in the temporal bone. It should be noted that the otoscopic and imaging features of a mastoiditis or petrositis may be obscured by previous antibiotic therapy, and that the initial otitis may have developed months before in neglected cases. The diagnosis of labyrinthogenic meningitis is based on deafness with a complete loss of vestibular nerve function as well as on the otologic history and corresponding tympanic membrane findings.

Differentiation from *viral meningitis* is notoriously difficult. This condition is not otogenic but represents one manifestation of a systemic viral illness. The inflammation typically involves the respiratory mucosa, and concomitant involvement of the middle ear mucosa is not unusual. This can mislead the examiner into believing that the meningitis is secondary to an acute bacterial otitis. At the same time, a secondary bacterial infection may supervene on a viral (e. g., influenzal) otitis. Viral meningitis is usually characterized by a low cell count in the CSF with a predominance of lymphocytes. A nonbacterial, superimposed viral otitis does not lead to tympanic membrane perforation, is usually bilateral, and does not yield pus on paracentesis.

Diagnostic problems also arise when a non–otogenic pneumococcal meningitis and a pneumococcal otitis coexist as parallel entities. Finally, a herpes zoster infection causing tympanic membrane eruptions and meningeal irritation is apt to be mistaken for otogenic meningitis.

Indications for Surgical Treatment

Despite the impressive response of otogenic bacterial meningitis to antibiotics given in proper dosage and matched to pathogen sensitivity, surgical eradication of the primary focus in the temporal bone is a mandatory part of treatment. This applies to cholesteatoma, of course, and to purulent foci of mastoiditis or petrositis that are insufficiently vascularized for reliable antibiotic penetration. Withholding surgery would carry the risk of continued bacterial seeding to the cranial cavity, quite apart from the potential risks to the middle and inner ear. Neither is medical treatment alone appropriate for early meningitis, as it is important to identify routes of extension (e. g., a fracture line) and prevent a later recurrence. Thus, a meningitis established as being otogenic constitutes a definite indication for otologic surgery. Admittedly, this principle is sometimes violated and, except for cholesteatoma, good results can be achieved with medical treatment alone. The residual risk in these cases, however, mandates close, long–term observation of the patient. The decision to operate for definitive cure is made easier by the fact that this surgery no longer poses a significant hazard to patients when proper technique is employed.

If the patient's condition permits, the surgery should be performed immediately upon completion of necessary preoperative studies. If the otologist is consulted only after the meningitis has been successfully controlled with antibiotics, he should urge that curative surgery be carried out even if there are only minimal signs of a persistent, potentially masked inflammatory disease in the temporal bone.

Principle of the Operation

The goal of the operation is to identify and remove all accessible purulent foci or cholesteatomatous tissue and thereby prevent further bacterial incursion into the cranial cavity. This is achieved by opening and exenterating the infected portions of the temporal bone and by obtaining broad exposure of the dura in the presumed area of spread to the middle or posterior cranial fossa. This should disclose any undetected sites of epidural suppuration still covered by the bone of the internal table.

Preoperative Preparations

Preparation of the patient (position, draping, etc.) is like that for any ablative procedure on the temporal bone (see Chapter 4). Special supplementary instruments are not required.

Anesthesia

General endotracheal anesthesia is most suitable. Given adequate muscular relaxation, this method permits a light plane of general anesthesia and provides access for ventilation if meningitis–related respiratory problems arise. Local anesthesia is acceptable in principle, but in restless patients it can compound the difficulty of the surgery, prolong the operating time, and increase the overall risk.

Premedicants and anesthetic agents that cause respiratory depression (barbiturates, morphine) should be withheld or used only in very selected cases with the approval of the anesthesiologist.

Operative Technique

The procedure used to eliminate the primary bacterial focus in the temporal bone depends on the findings and may consist of a simple mastoidectomy, a radical mastoid operation, or an operation on the petrous pyramid. With labyrinthogenic meningitis, the nonfunctioning labyrinth should always be opened and exenterated. The techniques for all these procedures are discussed in Chapter 4.

The following principles apply to otologic surgery carried out because of an intracranial complication.

- The retroauricular approach should be used. No other approach can ensure sufficient access in cases where involvement is extensive or the sites of involvement are more difficult to reach than anticipated.

- Eradication of the primary focus by surgery on the mastoid, pyramid, or labyrinth should be completed before dealing with the complication (for example, inspection and revision of the dura).

- Tympanoplastic measures that might prolong the operation are contraindicated or should be deferred until a second operation after the complication has resolved. Meanwhile, elements that might be useful for later surgery to improve auditory function (ossicular remnants, tympanic membrane tissue, middle ear mucosa) should be preserved whenever possible.

- The operating microscope, though essential for precision work in critical phases (dura, perilabyrinthine area), need not necessarily be used throughout the operation as it may limit the overall view of the diseased temporal bone and significantly prolong the operating time.

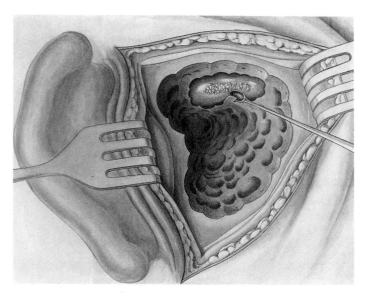

Fig. 9.**2**   Exposure of the dura. Note the dural granulations.

Extradural Abscess

The primary focus having been eradicated, attention is turned to the dura, which usually is already exposed and covered with granulations. Remaining portions of the internal table around the abscess (the "dural plate") are thinned with a burr, undermined with a small bone curette (with its convexity toward the dura) or elevator, and removed in small fragments until a margin of healthy dura about 5 mm wide has been exposed all around the abscess (Fig. 9.2). This eliminates the danger of leaving extensions of the abscess beneath intact portions of the dural plate.

Now the granulation tissue on the dura is closely scrutinized. If inspection reveals no fistulous tract, no trace of infection, no discharge of pus, and no dark, necrotic dura suggestive of subdural suppuration or brain abscess, the granulations may be left alone to preserve containment of the inflammation. Otherwise, the rest of the procedure is like that for a brain abscess (see p. 267).

Before closing, a gauze strip soaked in antibiotic solution is laid into the bony cavity and brought out through the lower part of the wound (a rubber drain may also be placed). In a radical operation, it is brought out through the external auditory meatus. In the absence of other complications, the retroauricular wound may be closed.

Meningitis

If the portal for the dural infection has been positively identified during the previous ablative surgery (granulating osteitis extending to the dura, epidural abscess, infected cholesteatoma with exposed dura), further surgery may be limited to exposing the affected region with a margin of healthy dura as described above. But if the site of the dural infection cannot be ascertained, approximately fingernail–sized areas of dura should be exposed in the middle and posterior fossae to disclose hidden purulent foci. This is done with particular care in the perilabyrinthine area and in the angle between the sinus and labyrinthine block (Trautmann's triangle).

The bone covering the dura is thinned with a burr and removed piecemeal with a small bone curette as described above. Fine bone forceps also may be used. On no account should bone fragments be left between the dura and bony plate. A fine elevator is used to separate the posterior and middle fossa dura from the bone of the labyrinthine block to check for epidural pus near the perilabyrinthine cells and endolymphatic sac. Finally, the bony cavity is loosely packed with a gauze strip as described, and the wound is closed.

Errors

- The dura may not be adequately exposed, infectious tracts may be left unopened, and all epidural purulent foci may not be detected. A labyrinthogenic meningitis may be overlooked, and the labyrinth may not be completely cleared of suppuration.
- The dura may be damaged during its exposure by removal of overlying bone. If the lesion is minor, and a CSF leak is either absent or very scant, it is sufficient to cover the defect with pieces of antibiotic–impregnated Gelfoam and pack the cavity with a gauze strip. The CSF leak should subside within a few days. Only large dural openings require suture closure or repair with a piece of fascia inserted beneath the bone edges.
- The meningitis may be superimposed on a brain abscess or subdural empyema that is missed. Corresponding symptoms may not become apparent until after meningitis–related impairment of consciousness has resolved.

Postoperative Care

- A drainage strip left in the surgical cavity can be removed on the 2nd or 3rd postoperative day if the meningitis regresses and the wound is healing satisfactorily. Otherwise the gauze strip should be changed.

- The patient should be nursed in an intensive care setting with monitoring of respiration, circulation, and renal function.
- Antibiotic therapy is of critical importance and should be matched to pathogen sensitivity whenever possible. Most antibiotics will penetrate the blood–CSF barrier when administered in the proper dosage.

- Lumbar puncture should be repeated every few days according to the severity of the meningitis and the cellularity of the CSF.
- Following the regression of meningitic symptoms and an improvement in the level of consciousness, the patient should be observed for signs of brain abscess (neurologic findings, optic fundus; CT or MRI also may be useful).

Otogenic Brain Abscess

Pathogenesis, Causes, and Location

Approximately 30% of all brain abscesses are otogenic or rhinogenic. Unlike abscesses having a metastatic, embolic, or traumatic etiology, otogenic abscesses tend to develop by the contiguous spread of bacterial infection from the temporal bone through the dura to the brain. This circumstance, important for the interpretation of operative findings, explains why dural change is almost always seen intraoperatively at the site of entry, and why otogenic brain abscesses tend to form near the dura. Frequently there is a coexisting epidural abscess.

Due to the nature of the blood supply to different brain regions, most of these abscesses develop just below the cortex in the white matter following initial local encephalitis (Fig. 9.**3**). The size and shape are variable (globular, tubular, cleft, or finger–shaped). Multiple and loculated abscesses are not uncommon. Older abscesses are enclosed by a capsule. With a fresh abscess, the accompanying encephalitis and brain edema are the main determinants of symptoms and prognosis. A purulent collection confined to a walled–off segment of the subdural space is termed a *subdural empyema.* This lesion may displace the brain substance but may also involve it (cortical abscess). It is difficult to distinguish between the two entities.

There are various possible sources of infection:

- Chronic otitis with cholesteatoma (most common).
- Mastoiditis or petrositis (less common).
- Purulent labyrinthitis.

An otogenic brain abscess may form in the temporal lobe or in the cerebellum. Abscesses of the *temporal lobe* most commonly involve the second and third gyri adjacent to the temporal bone. Large abscesses may continue to expand and break through into the inferior horn of the lateral ventricle. An otogenic *cerebellar ab-*

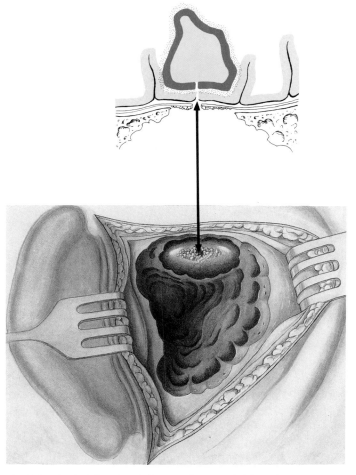

Fig. 9.**3** A draining tract from a temporal lobe abscess passes through the granulated dura. The schematic drawing shows the position of the subcortical abscess in relation to the dura.

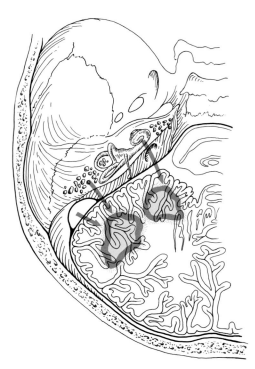

Fig. 9.**4**   Potential locations of cerebellar abscesses. The lateral abscess *(below)* is developing from the mastoid process and sinus,the medial abscess *(above)* from the labyrinth via the internal acoustic meatus.

scess may form next to Trautmann's triangle in the lateral occipital area, or it may develop from a purulent sinus thrombosis that has penetrated the inner layer of the sinus wall. If the abscess arises from suppuration in the labyrinth or the paralabyrinthine cells, it develops in the mediorostral portion of the cerebellum and thus involves an area that is difficult to reach and is dangerously close to vital brain areas (Figs. 9.**3** and 9.**4**).

Preoperative Diagnostic Procedures

General cerebral symptoms: Otogenic brain abscess should be suspected in any patient with otologic disease who develops cerebral symptoms. These symptoms may be mild initially (headache, somnolence, apathy, vomiting without nausea). With extension of the abscess, these symptoms become more prominent as the intracranial pressure rises (dullness, loss of consciousness, bradycardia).

Because the abscess develops via the meninges, CSF examination almost always shows a slight increase in cellularity and an elevated protein level. If intracranial pressure is increased, as evidenced by papilledema, lumbar of occipital puncture may induce herniation of the cerebellar tonsils. In these cases CSF should be sampled by ventricular puncture.

Focal symptoms: A *temporal lobe abscess* causes typical focal signs only if located in the dominant cerebral hemisphere (the left hemisphere in right–handed patients). Word–finding difficulty (amnestic aphasia) is present. Abscesses in the temporal lobe of the nondominant hemisphere do not produce this phenomenon. Large abscesses, moreover, can produce an array of neurologic signs (contralateral facial paralysis, ophthalmoplegias, pyramidal signs). Involvement of the superior temporal gyrus can cause impairment of word comprehension (sensory aphasia).

Cerebellar abscesses are characterized by cerebellar ataxia, dysdiadochokinesia that is more pronounced on the affected side, and a tendency to fall to the affected side. Ocular examination reveals a coarse nystagmus beating toward the side of the lesion. Rotatory and vertical nystagmus are also seen.

The definitive studies for confirming or excluding a suspected brain abscess are CT and MRI. Either modality can reliably demonstrate the location and extent of the abscess. Other neuroradiologic procedures (ventriculography, angiography, radionuclide scanning) and EEG are of lesser importance.

The principal differentiating features of *otitic hydrocephalus* (otogenic intracranial hypertension) are discussed page 271.

Surgical Treatment: Indications and Principle

Otogenic brain abscess always constitutes an urgent indication for operative treatment. In any given case, it must be decided whether therapy for the abscess should take precedence over treatment of the primary otologic focus, or vice–versa.

Treatment of the brain abscess always takes precedence if the predominant clinical symptoms are based on the mass effect of the abscess. Primary neurosurgical treatment follows precise localization of the abscess (by CT and/or MRI) and consists of aspiration and drainage of the abscess through a burr hole placed alongside the diseased temporal bone combined with intensive antibiotic treatment. Abscesses with a well–defined capsule can subsequently be excised through a craniotomy flap. Eradication of the primary otologic focus is deferred for a second sitting.

In patients who do not exhibit signs of intracranial hypertension, the temporal bone surgery may be performed first. Its goal is to prevent the further spread of septic material to the cranial cavity by primary eradication of the original bacterial focus.

The following description of abscess treatment during the course of temporal bone surgery (Körner: "attacking the abscess by the route along which it formed") is appropriate today only if a brain abscess near the dura, recognized by purulent drainage through a tract in the pathologically altered dura, is discovered incidentally during otologic surgery, and if circumstances preclude neurosurgical consultation and neuroradiologic evaluation. That is the only situation that justifies aspiration and instillation of antibiotics (closed treatment) or drainage of the abscess (open treatment) through the operated temporal bone. This approach is facilitated by the fact, noted above, that otogenic brain abscesses are situated close to the dura and therefore do not have to be approached through healthy brain tissue.

Preoperative Preparations and Anesthesia

See p. 265.

Special Instruments

The following special instruments are needed in addition to the standard instruments for otologic surgery:

- Brain needles, straight and curved, with stylet and depth markings. A Cushing needle can also be used.
- Drainage material (PVC tubing, perforated glass tubing).

Operative Technique

Closed treatment: If the otologic surgery reveals dural changes suspicious for brain abscess, especially blackish–yellow discoloration of the dura with a draining fistula located below an epidural abscess, the first step is to expose the dura with a generous margin of normal-appearing dura as described above. Following antiseptic preparation of the dural surface, the brain needle is inserted to a depth of 1–1.5 cm at the site of the fistula. If pus is not obtained when the stylet is removed, a syringe with connecting tube is attached to the needle, and *gentle* suction is applied (Fig. 9.**5**). The aspiration should be done slowly and carefully, as there is risk of ventricular rupture when a large temporal lobe abscess is present. A curved brain needle should be used to aspirate an abscess located in the medial part of the cerebellum.

If the expected abscess is found, the pus is sent for bacteriologic study and sensitivity testing. Meanwhile the needle is left in place, and antibiotic solution warmed to body temperature is instilled without pressure in a volume less than that of the aspirated pus.

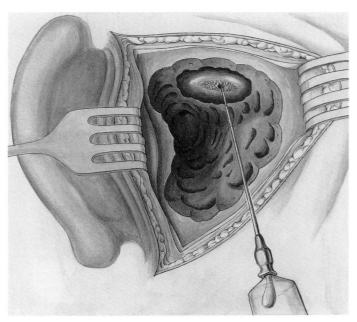

Fig. 9.**5**   Aspiration of a temporal lobe abscess that has penetrated the dura.

There are no definite rules for the further closed management of an abscess. If the patient recovers and cerebral symptoms resolve, further aspiration may be omitted. Otherwise the puncture can be repeated one or two days later. If the repeated aspiration still yields copious pus, the surgeon may proceed with open treatment, but again only if circumstances preclude neuroradiologic evaluation and consultation with a neurosurgeon.

If the initial aspiration, perhaps supplemented by one or two superficial punctures in adjacent brain, does not disclose an abscess, we caution against the old practice of puncturing in a deep, fanlike pattern due to the risk of transmitting infection to healthy brain. Instead, further diagnostic procedures should be carried out.

Open drainage: If needle aspiration does not provide sufficient evacuation, the dura is incised at the puncture site with a sickle knife, and a cruciate opening is made with a blunt–ended knife. A slender Killian speculum is carefully inserted to the depth of the previous puncture, and its blades are opened. The pus within the abscess is then suctioned from the speculum rather than from the abscess itself. Following evacuation of the pus, a fine–gauge tube armed with a suture or safety pin is inserted for further drainage (Fig. 9.**6**). A useful maneuver in the open method is to raise the patient's head to an upright position, as this will help to open the abscess and promote drainage (Herrmann, 1968).

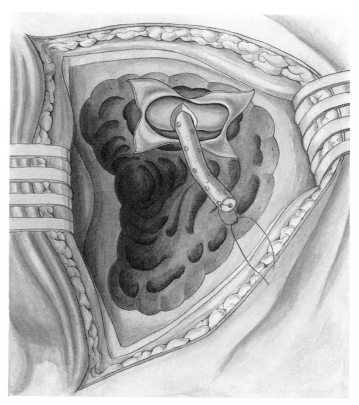

Fig. 9.**6**   Open drainage of a temporal lobe abscess.

The wound is left open postoperatively. Pressure from the ear dressing on the indwelling tube is avoided by placing a gauze–wrapped cotton ring around the ear and operative site to support the final dressing. See also p. 100.

Errors and Hazards

As noted earlier, the above measures are appropriate only if an unexpected abscess is encountered at operation, and circumstances prohibit neurosurgical consultation and a thorough evaluation by CT or MRI.

All operative procedures should be performed very gently and carefully to avoid unnecessary brain trauma. A "vigorous attack" on the abscess is to be condemned.

Large temporal lobe abscesses pose a danger of ventricular rupture. The risk of this complication is increased by the fall of pressure within the abscess caused by needle aspiration or drainage. Ventricular rupture is manifested by a deterioration in the patient's condition (increased vomiting, loss of consciousness) with an increased cellularity in the CSF. In cases managed by open treatment, soaked dressings provide evidence of CSF leakage into the abscess cavity. Occasionally, air

may be aspirated into the ventricles through the drain. This appears as a pneumocephalus on imaging.

Cerebral prolapse is a potential hazard following open treatment of brain abscess. This complication results from a persistence of brain swelling, which often is combined with additional abscesses or walled–off pockets of pus. These cases require further evaluation in conjunction with intensive osmotherapy. The prolapsed tissue should not be resected. Some time may pass before the prolapse reduces and duraplasty can be considered. As with brain abscess, neurosurgical consultation is indispensable.

Postoperative Care

If closed treatment of the abscess has been successful, it is necessary only to change the packing in the wound cavity at intervals of 2–3 days until such time as the wound is closed secondarily. The neurosurgeon should decide whether the putatively sterile abscess remnant needs to be removed.

In patients who are doing well following open treatment of the abscess, the patency of the drainage tube should be checked after 2–4 days, and the tube should be suctioned clear. When all discharge from the tube has subsided, the tube may be removed. The dural opening is left to close by granulation.

The patient should always be monitored in an intensive care setting (respiration, circulation, electrolytes, renal function). Osmotherapy is given to control brain edema, and antibiotics matched to pathogen sensitivity are administered in high dosage.

Otogenic Sinus Thrombosis

Pathogenesis and Course

If a bone–destroying infection of the temporal bone (mastoiditis, petrositis, or infected cholesteatoma) spreads to involve an adjacent dural sinus, it may damage the sinus wall and incite thrombus formation within the vessel. Sepsis can result if the thrombus becomes colonized by bacteria and periodically releases septic emboli into the circulation.

The disease may affect any sinus segments close to the ear (Fig. 9.**7**) but most commonly involves the sigmoid sinus. Less commonly the disease arises from the pyramidal petrosal sinuses, and primary thrombosis of the jugular bulb is uncommon. There may be retrograde extension of the thrombus into the transverse sinus or antegrade extension to the internal jugular vein, possibly leading to otogenic cavernous sinus thrombosis via the pyramidal sinuses. Rarely the disease is complicated by a cerebellar abscess, and a temporal lobe abscess may result from involvement of the arachnoid veins (vein of Labbé).

Preoperative Diagnostic Procedures

Signs of sepsis: As septic emboli are swept into the circulation, they produce intermittent, high fever spikes with chills. Blood studies demonstrate a left shift with an eosinophilia, and the spleen is enlarged. The causative organisms can be identified by blood culture, provided antibiotic therapy has not suppressed bacterial growth. Septic material entering the lung can lead to pulmonary abscesses, and septic metastasis via the systemic circulation can incite abscess formation in numerous organs.

Local findings: It may be assumed that the sepsis is otogenic if the history, otoscopic examination, and imaging findings are consistent with one of the bacterial temporal bone diseases noted above. An occluding thrombus can be demonstrated by magnetic resonance imaging or magnetic resonance angiography; retrograde jugular venography, an invasive procedure, is less common today. CSF examination frequently demonstrates a mild pleocytosis, and pressure on the internal jugular vein of the affected side does not increase the rate of fluid discharge from the puncture needle, as it does on the healthy side. With extensive thrombosis causing massive impairment of venous drainage, papilledema is observed.

Otitic hydrocephalus: This form of intracranial pressure elevation, termed "otitic hydrocephalus" by Symonds, results from apparently bland but extensive thrombus formation in multiple venous sinuses on one

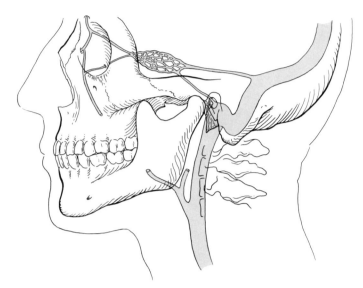

Fig. 9.**7** Relative position of the internal jugular vein and the venous sinuses in the temporal bone.

side. Though rare, its incidence is higher in patients treated with antibiotics. It is characterized by bilateral papilledema, which may increase alarmingly, and unilateral abducens nerve palsy. It is believed (and has been operatively confirmed in some cases) that many of these patients have had a previous otogenic sinus thrombosis that resolved spontaneously or in response to antibiotic treatment. Generally these cases do not require otologic surgery, although the papilledema, which (like the ophthalmoplegia) is slow to regress, may necessitate a decompressive craniotomy because of the threat posed to vision.

Indications for Surgical Treatment

Because a destructive purulent focus in the temporal bone and cholesteatoma cannot be effectively managed by medical treatment, the presumption of otogenic sepsis is an indication for surgery, which also serves to confirm the putative link between sepsis and otologic disease. Since antibiotics in suitable doses can inhibit further spread of the sepsis, it is appropriate to undertake staged procedures on the sinus itself once the infecting focus in the temporal bone has been eliminated.

Principle of the Operation

The goal of the operation following elimination of the primary focus is to remove the infected thrombus and prevent the further dissemination of septic material into the bloodstream.

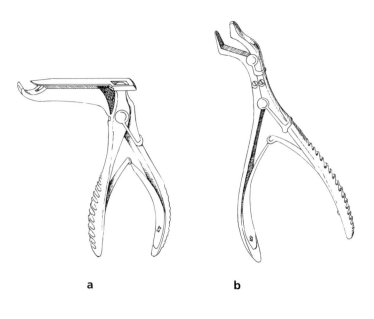

a   **b**

Fig. 9.**8**   Brünings (**a**) and Beyer (**b**) sinus punches.

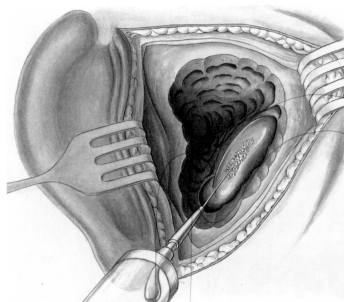

Fig. 9.**9**   Puncture of the thrombosed sigmoid sinus.

Preoperative Preparations

See p. 80

- A larger area than usual should be shaved due to the occasional need to expose the sinus far posteriorly.
- Given the potential for substantial blood loss in sinus operations, plasma expanders and/or units of whole blood should be made available.

Anesthesia

Since air may be aspirated when the sinus is opened, general endotracheal anesthesia, which allows for positive–pressure ventilation, is most suitable. If local anesthesia must be used, special steps must be taken to keep air from entering the sinus.

Special Instruments

The instruments used to treat the primary disease (see Chap. 4) should be supplemented by the following:

- A Beyer or Brünings sinus punch (Fig. 9.**8**) (advantageous but not absolutely essential),
- A high–performance suction unit with tips of assorted sizes,
- 2–cm–wide strips of gauze, rolled up at one end to form a spherical pea–size to bean–size pack.

Operative Technique

Otosurgical eradication of the primary focus should always be completed before sinus surgery is undertaken. Otherwise the sinus packing would hamper excavation of the otosurgical cavity.

Exposure of the Sinus

Almost invariably the disease has caused significant destruction of the overlying bone, and the sinus lies exposed at the base of an episinus abscess. Less commonly there is a fistulous tract leading to the affected sinus. The sinus wall is thickened and covered with granulations. Blackish necrotic foci are commonly found, and there may be a pulsatile discharge of pus. The boundaries between the sinus and adjacent dura are often difficult to discern.

The residual bony plate still covering the sinus is thinned with a burr, and the bone remnants are fractured and removed piecemeal with a bone curette or sinus punch. In this way the sinus is progressively unroofed proximally and distally until about a ¹/₂–cm margin of normal, bluish sinus wall has been exposed. In some cases the exposure must be carried far posteriorly, and it may be necessary to extend the retroauricular incision in a T–shaped fashion. Distally, the exposure may have to be carried to the second genu of the sigmoid sinus. While exposing the sinus, the surgeon must have a clear concept of its course so that, when he subsequently opens the sinus, he can preserve the adjacent, often pathologically altered dura and can accurately position the extraluminal pack between the vessel wall and overlying bone.

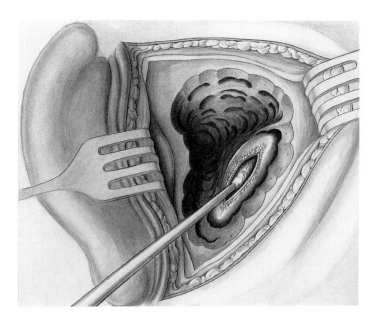

Fig. 9.**10** Aspiration of a thrombus from the sinus.

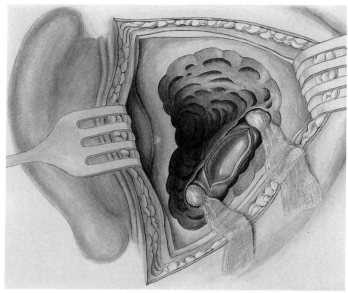

Fig. 9.**11** Extraluminal packing of the evacuated sinus.

Aspiration from the sinus lumen

The diseased sinus wall is antiseptically prepared, and a large–gauge, short–bevel needle connected to an injection syringe is inserted into the lumen. The needle is introduced at the site of the most conspicuous wall change. If findings at that point are equivocal, the needle may be reinserted at adjacent sites. While continuous aspiration is maintained, the needle is introduced at a very low angle, keeping the needle axis strictly in line with the course of the sinus (Fig. 9.**9**). If the sinus has been well exposed, inadvertent puncture of the dura is easily avoided. The needle should stop short of piercing the medial sinus wall. When estimating the depth of insertion, it is helpful to note that the diseased sinus wall may be several millimeters thick.

If copious blood can be aspirated from the sinus, it may be assumed that the interior of the sinus is healthy or that, at most, a mural thrombus is present. In this case it is appropriate to terminate the operation and take a wait–and–see approach while antibiotic therapy is maintained. Bleeding from the puncture site tends to subside after brief packing. The cavity is then loosely packed with a gauze strip, and two–thirds of the wound is closed.

If an unexpected episinus abscess is discovered incidentally during otologic surgery in a patient exhibiting no signs of sepsis, aspiration of the sinus may be withheld. If sinus aspiration is still performed, and blood cannot be aspirated, it should be assumed that an aseptic, noninfected sinus thrombosis is present, and further surgery should be withheld. These patients should be closely observed postoperatively for possible signs of septic complications.

Evacuation of the Sinus

If aspiration reveals a nonperfused sinus in a patient with marked symptoms of sepsis, the sinus should be evacuated. An incision 1–2 cm long in the altered lateral sinus wall should expose the blackish thrombus, which often displays ichorous change. At this point the surgeon introduces a large–caliber suction tip into the incision with one hand and, starting proximally and working distally, progressively aspirates the clot (Fig. 9.**10**). The other hand holds the rolled gauze pack with a forceps. Once the proximal (occipital) part of the thrombus has been aspirated, and a brisk flow of venous blood has commenced, the pack is placed at once between the exposed sinus wall and the overlying bone (Fig. 9.**11**). A sufficiently large pack placed in the correct position will arrest the bleeding. If all of the clot cannot be aspirated, the sinus must be exposed farther proximally until a profuse flow of blood is obtained.

Now the thrombus is aspirated toward the jugular bulb until a flow of blood is obtained distally. Again, a small gauze roll is packed between the bone and sinus wall. If extraluminal packing is not entirely effective over the more distal part of the sinus, packing may be carefully placed within the lumen. This presents no difficulties because the blood flow tends to be less vigorous distally.

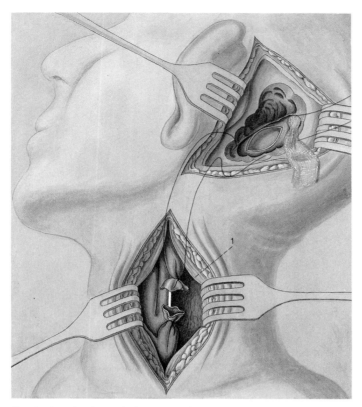

Fig. 9.**12** Ligation of the internal jugular vein during the sinus operation.
1: Vagus nerve

If a retrograde flow of blood is not obtained, it must be assumed that the clot extends farther toward the jugular bulb. The operation may still be discontinued at this point, however, if deep aspiration does not yield any purulent material, indicating that the clot is aseptic and will not generate additional septic emboli.

As a final step, the necrotic lateral wall of the sinus is removed (Fig. 9.**11**), creating an opening which is packed with a continuous gauze strip or oxidized regenerated cellulose (Surgicel). The entire bony cavity is similarly packed. The retroauricular wound is left open except for the portion covering the upper extraluminal pack. That part is closed to hold the pack securely in place.

Ligation of the Jugular Vein

Jugular vein ligation is indicated if there is reason to suspect residual infected thrombus extending to the jugular bulb, and septic symptoms persist following the operation. The sternocleidomastoid muscle is exposed by a longitudinal incision through the skin and platysma at its anterior border, and the muscle is retracted posteriorly. Attention is given to the external jugular vein coursing over the muscle. The exposed vascular sheath is isolated by blunt dissection, remov-

ing swollen lymph nodes as required. If the exposed jugular vein is bluish, soft, and perfused, it is underrun above the entrance of the facial vein, doubly ligated, and divided (Fig. 9.**12**). The vagus nerve segment accompanying the vein is carefully spared.

If the internal jugular vein is found to be thrombosed, as evidenced by a firm consistency and reddish–gray discoloration, the ligature should be placed in a lower, healthy segment of the vein.

For a venous thrombus extending down into the supraclavicular fossa, Seiffert suggests removing the clot by aspiration. A plastic tube is passed into the vein, loosely encircled with a silk ligature, and strong suction is applied. As the tube is withdrawn, the thrombus is dislodged and extracted. Positive–pressure ventilation should be initiated as the tube exits the venous opening to prevent the aspiration of air. The ligature is tightened. The experience of recent decades has shown that this maneuver, like other manipulations in the supraclavicular area, is no longer necessary when appropriate antibiotic therapy was provided.

Irrigation of the Jugular Bulb

Irrigation of the jugular bulb may be considered as an adjunct in the small percentage of patients with a non-perfused bulb who still exhibit septic signs following sinus evacuation despite jugular vein ligation and antibiotic therapy. The upper end of the ligated jugular vein is identified, and a thin tube is introduced into the lumen above the ligature and secured with a loop of thread. Irrigating antibiotic solution is then infused under gentle pressure until the fluid emerges at the end of the exposed sinus near the jugular bulb.

Surgery on the Jugular Bulb

Exposure of the jugular bulb is rarely necessary today because of the good results achieved with the above procedures combined with antibiotics. The operation, developed in the preantibiotic era (Gruner, Voss), is described here for the sake of completeness and because it may be of interest for other reasons (e. g., the treatment of glomus tumors).

The first step in exposing the jugular bulb is to join the postauricular wound with the incision used to expose and ligate the jugular vein. The tip of the mastoid process is resected, and the sternocleidomastoid muscle and the posterior belly of the digastric muscle are released. The jugular vein is now traced upward, and the occipital artery that crosses it is doubly ligated and divided. Care is taken to protect the accessory nerve, which descends across the vein in an anterosuperior to posteroinferior direction. The vagus and hypoglossal nerves run anterior to the vein (Fig. 9.**13**).

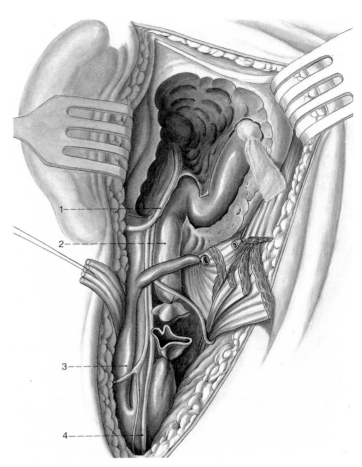

Fig. 9.**13** Exposure of the jugular bulb.
1: Facial nerve
2: Jugular vein
3: External carotid artery
4: Vagus nerve

Access to the jugular bulb by this approach (which corresponds to Grunert's operation) is still obstructed by the bony portions of the tympanic plate that remain after resection of the mastoid tip. They form the posterior wall and floor of the external auditory meatus and harbor the facial nerve. They must be partially resected. It is advisable, especially if space is limited, to visualize the facial nerve segment from approximately the origin of the chorda tympani to its emergence from the stylomastoid foramen. This is done by thinning the overlying bone with a diamond burr until the nerve is seen. (For clarity, the nerve is pictured in Fig. 9.**13** without its bony covering.)

Posteriorly, the transverse process of the first cervical vertebra can still restrict access to the jugular bulb at the skull base. Resection of the transverse process is rarely necessary, but when it is done, great care must be taken to preserve the vertebral artery.

The jugular bulb is reached by tracing the sinus distally, proceeding tangentially to the skull base, as de-

scribed by Voss. The bone covering the sinus is thinned with a diamond burr and then removed. Once the last bridge of bone has been removed to expose the bulb at the jugular foramen, the bulb and the stump of the internal jugular vein can be incised with a sickle knife. The thrombus is evacuated with a suction tip and curette. Venous tributary bleeding at this stage is controlled with packing. The wound may be closed partially or completely over a drain.

Errors and Hazards

A serious error during puncture and incision of the sigmoid sinus is to miss the sinus and damage the cerebellar dura. This underscores the importance of carefully exposing the sinus until its course and topography are clearly appreciated.

It is also a mistake to place the rolled pack *into* the proximal sinus lumen. This can injure the medial dural wall, and subsequent removal of the pack may dislodge the newly–formed, occluding thrombus. The pack should be placed extraluminally, as described, between the sinus wall and overlying bone, and it should compress the sinus to promote adhesion of its walls.

The danger of air aspiration and air embolism during sinus evacuation was noted above. This is prevented by applying positive–pressure ventilation and laying the patient flat during certain stages of the operation.

Postoperative Care

Besides appropriate antibiotic therapy, the general management of sepsis includes monitoring and observation for possible sequelae (lungs, renal and liver function, etc.).

Thrombolytic agents are discouraged because they inhibit the desired obliteration of the treated sinus.

Enough of the retroauricular wound is left open to provide access to the Meier–Whiting pack, which can be removed on day 10. Since sinus bleeding may recur at that time, the pack should be removed in the operating room so that the sinus can be repacked at once should the need arise. Suction tips, retractors, and new packs should be laid out and ready.

Closure of the wound should be deferred until all clinical findings have returned to normal.

Bibliography

Beck C. Otogene Sinusthrombose. In: Hals-Nasen-Ohren-heilkunde in Praxis und Klinik, 2nd edn, Vol. 6, Eds J. Berendes, R. Link, F. Zöllner. Stuttgart: Thieme, 1980.

Blohmke A, Link R. Die transmastoidale Zisternendrainage und ihre Bedeutung bei schwerer otogener Meningitis. Acta oto-laryng 1954; 44: 312.

Bradley P J, Manning K P, Shaw M D M. Brain abscess secondary to otitis media. J Laryng Otol 1984; 98: 1185

Brand B, Caparosa R J, Lubic L G. Otorhinolaryngological brain abscess therapy – past and present. Laryngoscope 1984; 94: 15.

Courville C B. Intracranial complications of otitis media and mas-toiditis in the antibiotic era. Laryngoscope 1955; 65: 31.

Denecke H J. Die otorhinolaryngologischen Operationen. In: All-gemeine und spezielle chirurgische Operationslehre, 2nd edn, Vol. V, Eds R. Zenker, G. Heberer, G. Hegemann. Berlin: Springer, 1953.

Fremel F. Der otogene Hirnabszeß. Mschr Ohrenheilk 1971; 105: Issues 8–12.

Ganz H. Der derzeitige Stand von Klinik und Behandlung der oto-genen und rhinogenen Hirnkomplikationen. Otologische Betrachtungen. HNO (Berlin) 1972; 20: 33.

Ganz H. Otogener Hirnabszeß. In: Hals-Nasen-Ohrenheilkunde in Praxis und Klinik, 2nd ebd, Vol. 6, Eds J. Berendes, R. Link, F. Zöllner. Stuttgart: Thieme, 1980.

Gower D, McGuirt W F. Intracranial complications of acute and chronic infections ear disease, a problem still with us. Laryngo-scope 1983; 93: 1028.

Grunert H. Die operative Ausräumung des Bulbus venae jugularis (Bulbusoperation) in Fällen otogener Pyämie. Leipzig: F. C. W. Vogel, 1904.

Harpman J A. On the management of otorhinogenic intracranial infections. J. Laryng. Otol. 1955; 69: 180.

Herrmann A. Gefahren bei Operationen an Hals, Ohr und Gesicht und die Korrektur fehlerhafter Eingriffe. Berlin: Springer, 1968.

Kellerhals B, Pfaltz C R. Entstehung und Verlauf otogener en-docranieller Komplikationen im Zeitalter der Antibiotika. HNO (Berlin) 1969; 17: 42.

Kornmesser H J. Otogene Meningitis. In: Hals-Nasen-Ohren-heilkunde, 2nd edn., Vol. 6, Eds J. Berendes, R. Link, F. Zöllner. Stuttgart: Thieme, 1980.

Körner O. Die ototischen Erkrankungen des Hirns, der Hirnhäute und der Hirnblutleiter. 3rd edn. München: Bergmann, 1902.

Mathews T J. Lateral sinus pathology. J Laryng Otol 1988; 102: 118.

Mündnich K. Ist der Otologe heute noch zur Behandlung der Hirnabszesse berechtigt? Arch Ohr- Nas- u Kehlk-Heilk 1964; 183: 205.

Pospiech J, Kalff R, Polyzoidis T, Reinhardt V, Grote W, Kocks W. Intrakranielle Komplikationen entzündlicher Ohrerkrankun-gen. HNO (Berlin) 1990; 63: 38.

Samuel J, Fernandes C M C. Lateral sinus thrombosis. A review of 45 cases. J Laryng Otol 1987; 101: 1227.

Schadel A, Böttcher H D, Haverkamp H D. Computertomo-graphische Diagnostik der epiduralen Abszesse, subduralen Empyeme Meningitiden und Hirnabszesse. Laryng Rhinol Otol 1983; 62: 164.

Seiffert A. cited by Denecke (1953).

Shambaugh G E. Surgery of the ear, 2nd edn. Philadelphia: Saunders, 1970.

Stroobandt G, Zech G, Thauvoy C, Mathurin P, de Nijs C, Gilliard C. Treatment by aspiration of brain abscess. Acta Neurochir (Wien) 1987; 85: 138.

Symonds C P. Otitic hydrocephalus. Brain 1931; 54: 55.

Voss O. Zur operativen Freilegung des Bulbus venae jugularis. Z Ohrenheilk 1904; 48: 265.

Zülch K J. Neurologische Diagnostik bei endocraniellen Kom-plikationen von oto-rhinologischen Erkrankungen. Arch Ohr-Nas- u Kehlk- Heilk 1964; 183: 1.

10 Surgery of the Labyrinth and Internal Auditory Canal for Disequilibrium

Jan Helms

Endolymphatic Sac Surgery

Preoperative Diagnostic Studies

Ménière's disease is diagnosed by exclusion, so other disorders that could account for the patient's symptoms have to be excluded before endolymphatic sac surgery is elected. A mass lesion in the cerebellopontine angle is ruled out by brainstem audiometry and, if necessary, by neuroradiologic studies and magnetic resonance imaging. Viral infections, autoimmune disorders, and other infections should also be evaluated. The history and micro–otoscopic findings should confirm or exclude a traumatic etiology or middle ear disease. Appropriate consultation is sought to evaluate for neurologic, systemic, or orthopedic disorders that may have causal significance.

Indications

The indication for endolymphatic sac surgery is based on evidence of endolymphatic hydrops, manifested by the typical triad of fluctuating hearing loss, tinnitus, and vertiginous attacks. The patient may also report a feeling of aural fullness or pressure or a "plugged" sensation in the ear.

Reports indicate that conservative trials with antivertiginous drugs, histamine analogs, hemorrheologic agents, and calcium antagonists are of little or no value in relieving complaints.

Currently available neurophysiologic tests for the detection of endolymphatic hydrops (electrocochleography, low–frequency biasing), if applicable, should demonstrate the presence of hydrops.

Principle of the Operation

The surgery involves decompressing the labyrinth at the level of the endolymphatic sac, and thus at a distance of more than 1 cm from the sensory organelles of the labyrinth. To avoid unnecessary surgical trauma such as opening the posterior fossa dura, damaging the facial nerve, or opening a semicircular canal, the surgeon must have a detailed knowledge of the topographic anatomy of the region, reinforced by practice on petrous specimens. Figures 10.1 and 10.2 illustrate the close proximity of the endolymphatic sac, sigmoid sinus, posterior semicircular canal, and facial nerve to one another in the operative field.

Preoperative Preparations

The patient is informed about the prospects for success (two–thirds to three–fourths of patients are free of vertigo attacks at three years after surgery) and the risks of the procedure (usual otosurgical risks: total hearing loss, tinnitus, vertigo, facial nerve palsy). A sleep aid is given as needed on the eve of the operation. Just before the local anesthetic is administered, a strip of skin about 2 cm wide is shaved above and behind the ear. A large adhesive dressing will be placed over this site postoperatively to keep hair from falling into the wound area.

Anesthesia

The surgery is performed under local anesthesia. General anesthesia is seldom required.

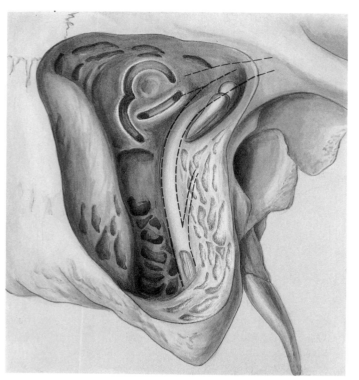

Fig. 10.**1**

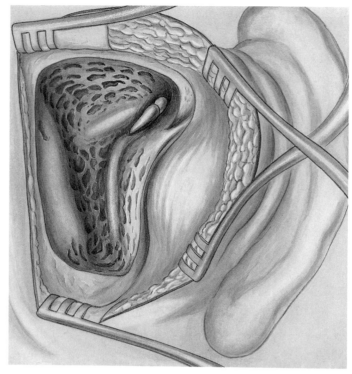

Fig. 10.**3**

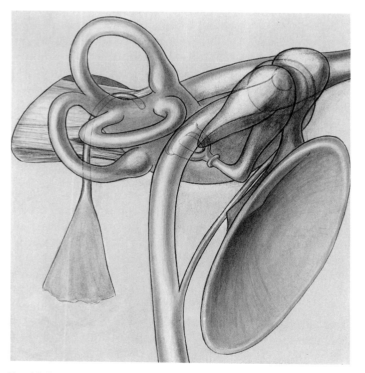

Fig. 10.**2**

Operative Technique

A postauricular transmastoid approach is used (Fig. 10.**3**). When the horizontal (lateral) semicircular canal has been positively identified, the aditus and antrum is plugged with a small piece of antibiotic–impregnated gelatin sponge to keep bone dust out of the middle ear. The horizontal semicircular canal is followed posteriorly with the burr, without exposing its blue line. The center of the posterior semicircular canal is located at a point about twice the thickness of the canal bone posterior to the greatest lateral projection of the horizontal semicircular canal. The posterior semicircular canal is usually located about 2 mm farther medially than the lateral border of the horizontal canal.

If the sigmoid sinus is far enough anterior to obstruct access to Trautmann's triangle, the bony covering of the sinus is burred down laterally and medially with a large diamond burr until there is room to insert a small blade and retract the sinus posteriorly during dissection of the endolymphatic sac.

As the bony posterior semicircular canal is followed inferiorly, the burr closely approaches the facial nerve. This proximity of the semicircular canal to the upper part of the mastoid segment of the facial nerve should be kept in mind to avoid facial nerve injury.

The dissection is performed medial to the sigmoid sinus. Sinus exposure is necessary only if it is covered by

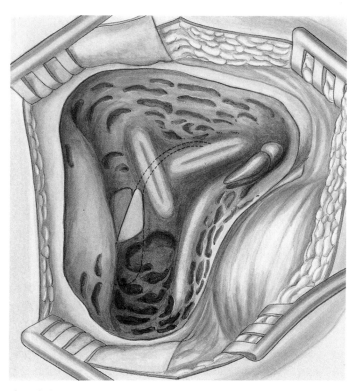

Fig. 10.**4**

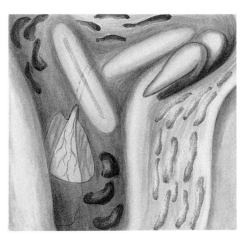

Fig. 10.**5 a**
1 Endolymphatic duct
2 Endolymphatic sac
3 Surgical approach

a bony overhang that restricts access to the endolymphatic sac region. If the course of the facial nerve below the horizontal semicircular canal is uncertain, we favor exposing the nerve so that it can be protected from injury.

The bony posterior semicircular canal is gently thinned with the diamond burr until its blue line is exposed (Fig. 10.**4**). The blue line is traced inferiorly to its lowest point. It is not strictly necessary to obtain a blue line on the horizontal semicircular canal. Meanwhile, the bone at the posterior surface of the pyramid is thinned until the dura is just visible through the bone. If the petrous bone is well pneumatized, a whitish area with well–defined upper margins, visible under the bluish dura, can be seen in the lower part of the field behind the inferior half of the posterior semicircular canal. This feature represents the upper border of the endolymphatic sac.

Using progressively smaller diamond burrs, the surgeon removes the bone behind the blue line of the posterior semicircular canal and its inferior half and traces the pale upper border and lateral surface of the endolymphatic sac as far as possible behind the posterior semicircular canal. The schematic drawing in Figure 10.**5 a** shows the endolymphatic duct (1) and endolymphatic sac (2) in transverse section. The arrow (3) indicates the route of the surgical approach.

Fig. 10.**5 b**

In slightly more than half of cases, an intratemporal component of the endolymphatic sac can be identified (Fig. 10.**5 b**). It corresponds to the pars rugosa. In the remaining cases a thickening of the dura is encountered below the posterior half of the posterior semicircular canal.

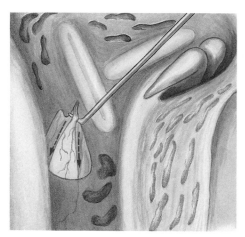

Fig. 10.**6**

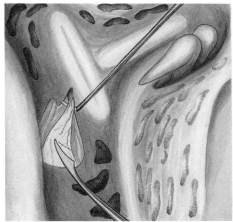

Fig. 10.**7**

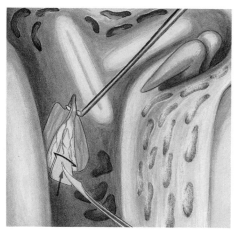

Fig. 10.**8**

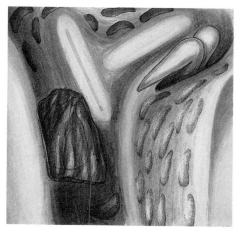

Fig. 10.**9**

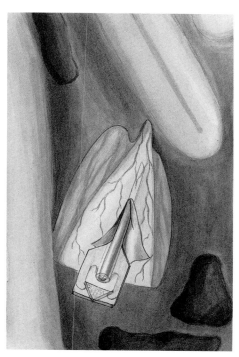

Fig. 10.**10**

The lateral wall of the endolymphatic sac is of variable thickness and shows variable adherence to the opposing petrous bony surfaces. Burring at the junction of the petrous bone and endolymphatic sac must be done very slowly to ensure that the lumen of the sac is not entered prematurely. The sac lumen is more difficult to identify when it has been traumatized with a burr.

If the surgeon has been able to demonstrate the intratemporal portions of the endolymphatic sac without destroying its lateral wall, the sac can be followed laterally and partially separated from the dura, to which it is firmly adherent (Fig. 10.**6**). Biopsies can be taken, and the "true lumen" of the endolymphatic sac (Arenberg) can be entered by incision of the lateral sac wall (Fig. 10.**7**). This avoids the error of incising the posterior fossa dura without opening the endolymphatic sac ("false sac lumen" after Arenberg).

After incision of the sac, a piece of silicone film cut to a sharp angle is inserted into the lumen (Fig. 10.**8**). The film and sac can be covered with a piece of lint–free connective tissue taken from behind the auricle. This graft is placed loosely at the base of the operative field (Fig. 10.**9**).

The site is inspected with the operating microscope to verify that the surfaces of the silicone film and connective–tissue graft are free of lint, metallic particles, and other contaminants that could incite foreign body granuloma formation with damage to the labyrinth.

The pieces of gelatin sponge packed into the antrum at the start of the operation are completely suctioned out. The ear is closed with subcutaneous and cutaneous sutures. It is unnecessary to pack the auditory canal.

Modifications

Instead of plain silicone film, a special silicone–coated valve implant can be inserted into the lumen of the endolymphatic sac (Arenberg). The heparin–filled valve is designed to provide continuous decompression of the hydrops with better efficiency than silicone film alone (Fig. 10.**10**). Other alternatives to silicone film are thin catheters or films made of other material. All plastic materials must be bioinert and free of monomers.

Landmarks and Pitfalls

The principal landmark in the opening phase of endolymphatic sac decompression is the horizontal semicircular canal, located at the base of the antrum. After identifying this canal and defining its course, the surgeon can estimate the position of the endolymphatic sac posterior to the lower half of the posterior semicircular canal and behind the mastoid segment of the facial nerve.

Difficulties arise only if the sigmoid sinus is in a far anterior position that restricts access to the deep portion of the mastoid. There is the risk in this situation that the surgeon may inadvertently open the sinus or damage the facial nerve by carrying the dissection too far anteriorly. The inner ear, already damaged by the endolymphatic hydrops, is particularly susceptible to additional trauma. It is important, therefore, to avoid opening the semicircular canals.

The surgeon should be familiar with potential variations in the course of the facial nerve so that, when such a variation is present, he can avoid traumatizing the nerve while dissecting about the inferior portion of the posterior semicircular canal.

Rules, Hints, and Common Errors

Reoperations after unsuccessful endolymphatic sac decompression have generally shown that the sac was neither opened nor drained in the original operation. Identification of the "true sac" is facilitated by routinely obtaining a blue line on the posterior semicircular canal and following the canal to its maximum inferior extent. The labyrinthine bone behind this blue line is removed without opening the perilymphatic space, and bone removal is continued posteriorly until the dura is exposed. In this way the intratemporal portion of the endolymphatic sac can consistently be identified in normally pneumatized ears. This may not succeed in ears with less pneumatization, where the only clues may be the localized, whitish thickening of the dura and the presence of blood vessels in the lateral sac wall coursing toward the pars rugosa and the intratemporal portion of the sac.

The last bony layer covering the lateral sac wall is removed very slowly using high magnification and small diamond burrs to preserve the lateral connective–tissue investment of the sac that will facilitate identification of the sac lumen.

Of course, a slitlike lumen can be developed anywhere in the dura, not just in the endolymphatic sac, so the dissection of an apparent "lumen" does not prove that the true sac has been entered.

Postoperative Care

No special postoperative care is necessary besides the single perioperative administration of an antibiotic. Hearing is tested daily with C2 and C3 tuning forks, or a bone conduction audiogram may be obtained. Frenzel glasses are used to check for nystagmus.

Postoperative Complications

Inadvertent incision of the dura may result in a CSF fistula. If the opening is small, it can be repaired intraoperatively by inserting a small piece of connective tissue into the subarachnoid space and pulling it back toward the mastoid. Larger defects are repaired, after CSF decompression, by gluing on a piece of banked dura and obliterating the mastoid with autogenous tissue (e. g., a postauricular soft–tissue flap or free abdominal fat).

If rapidly progressive hearing loss, nystagmus, or both are noted from two to five days postoperatively, the ear should be reopened and explored for a foreign body granuloma. If uncertainty exists, infusion therapy should be initiated with anti–inflammatory and hemorrheologic agents.

Functional Sequelae

Endolymphatic sac surgery relieves vertiginous attacks in about three–fourths of patients. Its effects on hearing and tinnitus as not so positive. Dramatic hearing gains are occasionally reported. There is about a 5% incidence of total hearing loss following endolymphatic sac surgery, mostly in patients with significant pre–existing sensorineural hearing loss.

Some patients who are essentially free of vertigo after surgery may occasionally experience subjective unsteadiness or a renewed attack of vertigo, but a true whirling sensation should not recur. These patients should receive several months' adjunctive medical treatment with a calcium antagonist, antihistamine, or other effective medication.

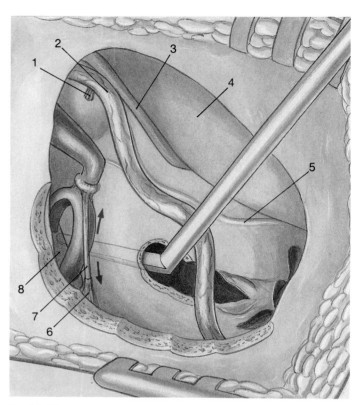

Fig. 10.**11**
1   Tensor tympani tendon
2   Chorda tympani
3   Malleus handle
4   Tympanic membrane
5   Jacobsons nerve
6   Pyramidal process
7   Stapedial tendon
8   Footplate

Alternative Methods

Numerous treatments have been devised as alternatives to endolymphatic sac surgery. Partial destruction of the vestibular labyrinth by the instillation of gentamycin into the middle ear is certainly an option. The technique of Lange (1977) involves the repeated transtympanic administration of a defined dose of gentamycin into the middle ear cleft through a myringotomy tube (see Chapter 4). This vestibulotoxic drug mainly diffuses through the round window and damages the vestibular sensory organelles while causing relatively little harm to the cochlea. Lange (1977) published detailed directions that, if followed precisely, will minimize the risks of the procedure.

Ultrasonic and cryosurgical procedures have not been consistently successful in effecting partial destruction of the vestibular sensory organelles. Nor has drainage of the saccule through the stapes footplate, as described by Fick and modified by Cody, or Arslan's technique of applying sodium chloride crystals to the round window. It is interesting to note the observation of Montandon and Arnold in patients frequently subjected to altitude extremes and suffering from Ménière's disease; these authors found that the insertion of a myringotomy tube (see Chapter 4) could improve symptoms without further medication.

Schuknecht decompresses the endolymphatic space by creating an endocochlear shunt between the endolymphatic and perilymphatic systems (Fig. 10.**11**). In this technique the round window niche is exposed through a transtympanic approach like that used for stapedectomy (see Chapter 8). The bony overhang in front of the round window membrane is removed with a fine diamond burr, and a 3–mm–long hook is passed through the round window membrane and bony spiral plate to create a permanent communication between the endolymphatic duct and perilymphatic duct. The hydropic saccule in the vestibule is also punctured by advancing the tip of the hook to a point below the center of the footplate. This procedure is associated with a markedly higher incidence of total hearing loss than endolymphatic sac surgery.

Labyrinthectomy

Preoperative Diagnostic Studies

The diagnostic studies prior to labyrinthectomy are the same as those preceding endolymphatic sac surgery.

Indications

The indications for labyrinthectomy in patients with vertigo and no apparent middle ear pathology include high–grade labyrinthine failure, repeated or persistent incapacitating vertigo, and a presumed inability to tolerate the general anesthesia that would be required for a neurectomy.

Surgical labyrinthectomy, which may be combined with ototoxic medications, does not ablate labyrinthine function as effectively as neurectomy.

Principle of the Operation

The object of the surgery is to remove and destroy as many labyrinthine organelles as possible, including both the vestibular and cochlear sensory cells. Because surgery is only partially effective in destroying these structures, an ototoxic antibiotic such as gentamycin is instilled into the surgically ablated labyrinth. The use of alcohol or other destructive agents is not recommended, as they may cause collateral damage to the facial nerve.

Preoperative Preparations

The preparations are the same as those for endolymphatic sac surgery (see page 277).

Anesthesia

The surgery is usually performed under general anesthesia, although local anesthesia may be used.

Operative Technique

The ear is opened through an endaural, transcanal approach like that for a stapedectomy. The oval and round window niches are identified (see Chapter 8). After removal of the stapes, the bony bridge between the lower part of the oval window and the round window niche is completely removed, establishing a broad connection between both windows (Fig. 10.**12**). All accessible soft–tissue elements are then removed from the labyrinth using very fine hooks and grasping forceps. The ex-

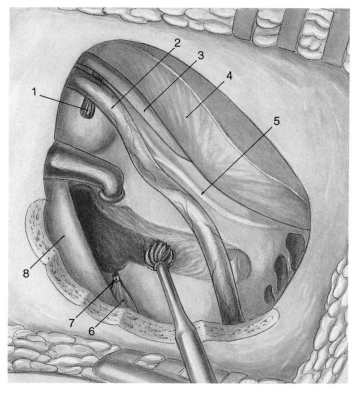

Fig. 10.**12**
1 Tensor tympani tendon
2 Chorda tympani
3 Malleus handle
4 Tympanic membrane
5 Jacobsons nerve
6 Pyramidal process
7 Stapedial tendon
8 Facial nerve

enterated cavity is suctioned clear and filled with an ototoxic antibiotic powder.

The labyrinthine defect is closed with fascia or perichondrium, and the tympanic membrane is returned to its anatomic position along with the attached meatal flap. The rest of the closure is like that following stapedectomy (see Chapter 8).

Modifications

One modification is to destroy the semicircular canals and vestibule through a postauricular transmastoid approach. This is more technically demanding, however, and the advantage of leaving the tympanic membrane in place is relatively minor considering the good healing that is achieved after stapedectomy and other transcanal procedures.

Other modifications involve the use of toxic substances to destroy labyrinthine structures not accessible to mechanical ablation. Care is taken to avoid using substances that might diffuse into the facial canal and damage the nerve.

Landmarks and Pitfalls

The critical landmarks and pitfalls are the same as in the opening phase of stapedectomy (see Chapter 8).

Additionally, the surgeon should be aware that the medial wall of the labyrinth is formed by the fundus of the internal auditory canal (IAC). It may be so thin that the bluish color of the underlying CSF is visible through the bone. Damage to this bony plate would lead to copious CSF leakage, so drilling of the bony bridge between the oval and round windows should be done in a way that does not damage the medial labyrinthine wall.

Rules, Hints, and Common Errors

Authors have reported a 15 to 40% recurrence rate of vertiginous symptoms after surgical labyrinthectomy. Hence, surgical labyrinthectomy alone is not recommended for the control of Ménière's disease or other intractable vertigo and should always be combined with ototoxic ablation of the labyrinthine organelles. Inadvertent opening of the fundus of the IAC is a common error.

Postoperative Care

Postoperative care is the same as that following stapedectomy (see Chapter 8).

Postoperative Complications

Facial nerve palsy can developif dehiscences between the labyrinth and facial canal allow the transmission of destructive surgical forces and/or chemical toxicity to the facial nerve from the labyrinth. This would necessitate a second operation to aspirate the toxic material from the labyrinth.

Functional Sequelae

Vertiginous symptoms may recur following a technically flawless labyrinthectomy, usually with a latency of months or years, resulting from some residual function of vestibular organelles left in the exenterated labyrinth or perhaps from irritation of Scarpa's ganglion. A neurectomy is indicated in these cases.

Alternative Methods

One alternative to surgical and ototoxic labyrinthectomy is neurectomy. If the patient cannot tolerate the general anesthesia required for this procedure, other options are cryosurgical or ultrasound ablation performed under local anesthesia. The risks to the facial nerve must be considered when cryosurgery or ultrasound is used.

Transtemporal Neurectomy

Preoperative Diagnostic Studies

The diagnostic procedures are the same as those preceding endolymphatic sac surgery (see page 277).

Indications

Because neurectomy is a permanent, destructive procedure, it is appropriate only if other, function–conserving nonoperative or operative treatment options are not available in the given situation. Transtemporal neurectomy is performed if hearing is to be preserved. The risk of total hearing loss with this procedure is in the order of less than 5% — the same as with endolymphatic sac surgery.

Candidates for neurectomy are patients with Ménière's disease and patients with serviceable hearing who have vertigo of labyrinthine origin.

Principle of the Operation

Through an essentially transpetrous approach, the IAC is opened medial to the superior semicircular canal, and Scarpa's ganglion is resected. This approach requires slight extradural elevation of the temporal lobe. Also, it provides the surgeon with a somewhat unaccustomed view of anatomic structures in the petrous bone, so special training is required.

Relevant landmarks and topographic details are illustrated in Figures 10.**13** and 10.**14**. In Fig. 10.**13** the red line indicates the translabyrinthine approach.

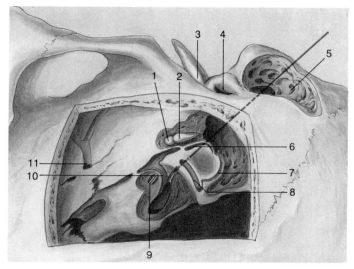

Fig. 10.**13**

1	Head of malleus	6	Horizontal sem. canal
2	Body of incus	7	Posterior sem. canal
3	Styloid process	8	Superior sem. canal
4	Outer ear canal	9	Cochlea
5	Mastoid	10	Facial nerve canal, labyrinth. part
		11	Foramen spinosum

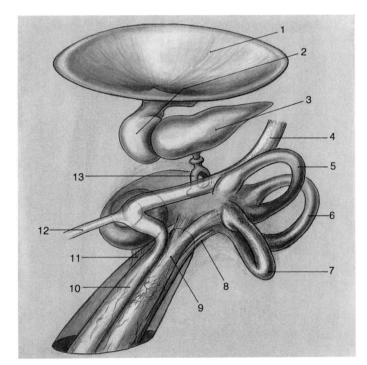

Fig. 10.**14**

1	Ear drum	7	Superior sem. canal
2	Head of malleus	8	Singular nerve
3	Body of incus	9	Sup. vestibular nerve
4	Facial nerve	10	Facial nerve
5	Horizont. sem. canal	11	Cochlear nerve
6	Posterior sem. canal	12	Greater petrosal nerve
		13	Stapes

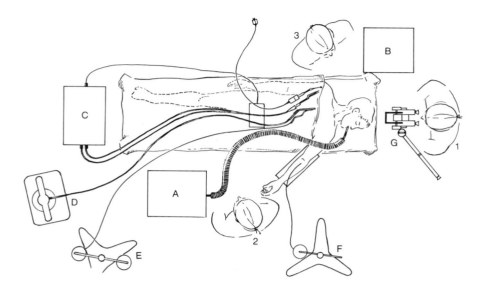

Fig. 10.**15**
1   Surgeon
2   Anesthesiologist
3   Scrub nurse
A   Anesthesia unit
B   Instrument stand
C   Coagulation
D   Suction
E   Irrigating solution
F   Infusion stand
G   Microscope

Preoperative Preparations

An area 10 cm × 10 cm above the ear is shaved prior to induction of general anesthesia (preferably neuroleptanalgesia). The area of the incision is also infiltrated with a standard local anesthetic solution containing epinephrine.

The patient is positioned supine with the head turned to the side. The head should not be turned to a degree that would cause circulatory impairment. If necessary, the operating table is rotated on its long axis to achieve the desired head position (corresponding chest and pelvic supports are preplaced on the side of the table that will be lowermost).

Our preferred arrangement of equipment and operating room personnel is shown in Figure 10.**15**.

Anesthesia

The surgery is performed under general anesthesia, preferably in the form of neuroleptanalgesia to minimize diffuse bleeding. The patient is hyperventilated to lower the intracranial pressure and facilitate elevation of the temporal lobe and dura. Pharmacologic reduction of intracranial pressure is not required. Details may be found in the chapter on Anesthesia (see p. 1 ff).

Operative Technique

The approach is made through a slightly curved skin incision about 8–10 cm long that passes in front of the ear and over the root of the zygomatic arch toward the vertex (Fig. 10.**16**). The temporalis fascia is incised, and the temporal artery is ligated as required. Simple coagula-

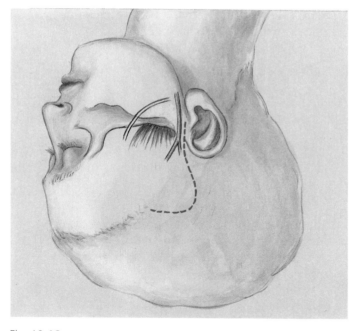

Fig. 10.**16**

tion cannot reliably prevent the formation of a large postoperative hematoma. The temporalis muscle is incised vertically upward from the root of the zygomatic arch. An inferiorly based muscle flap about 2 cm wide at the base is outlined for subsequent use in covering the craniotomy, and a free temporalis muscle graft is harvested for later use in establishing closure of the IAC (Fig. 10.**17**).

The periosteum is stripped from the petrous squama to the squamous suture, and hemostasis is secured throughout the wound area with bipolar cautery. A broad retractor is then inserted so that the surgeon can work on the craniotomy site without soft–tissue interference. A 2.5 × 3.5-cm craniotomy is outlined with a

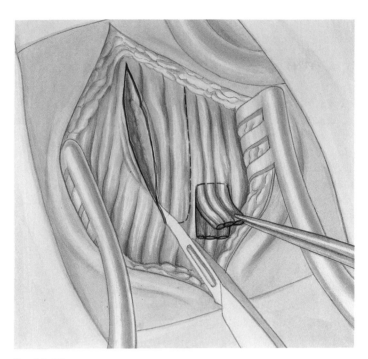

Fig. 10.**17**

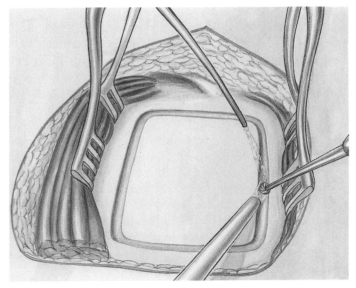

Fig. 10.**18**

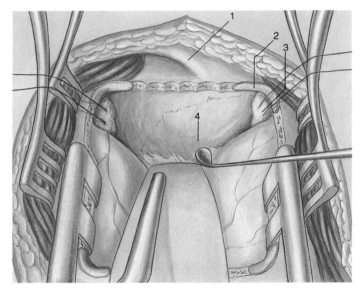

Fig. 10.**19**
1   Zygomatic arch
2   Bone wax
3   Neurosurgical cotton
4   Floor of middle cranial fossa

small cutting burr, or it may be performed using burr holes and a craniotome (Fig. 10.**18**). The bone flap is elevated and placed with the free muscle graft in a dry dish covered with a moist cloth. Physiologic saline solution is a less satisfactory storage medium, as it can cause elution of the tissues.

The craniotomy should be centered over the root of the zygomatic arch (1 in Fig. 10.**19**).

After bipolar coagulation of fine branches of the middle meningeal artery or, if necessary, coagulation of the artery itself, sharp bone spurs are removed from the margins of the craniotomy with suitable forceps or punch ronguers, and the opening is extended inferiorly to the level of the floor of the middle cranial fossa by craniectomy. At this inferior level considerable bone can be nibbled from the anterior and posterior margins of the opening, establishing broad access to the floor of the middle fossa. Bleeding from the cancellous bone is controlled with a diamond burr or bone wax (2 in Fig. 10.**19**).

The dura is gently and progressively elevated from the floor of the middle fossa using a moderately small elevator whose edge is kept in constant contact with the bone. Firm connective–tissue strands are coagulated before they are divided. The dissection is carried posteriorly until the posterior margin or sulcus of the superior petrosal sinus is palpable at the posterior border of the pyramid. Venous bleeding is usually scant and is controlled with Tabotamp and cottonoids (3 in Fig. 10.**19**). Dural elevation is carried anteriorly to near the foramen spinosum and medially to a point above the greater and lesser petrosal nerves. If the hiatus of the corresponding bony canal is close to the geniculate ganglion, the very firm connective–tissue attachments between the epineurium of the greater petrosal nerve and the dura should be progressively freed, working forward, to create sufficient room at the petrous apex and to permit dural elevation from the meatal plane, i. e., the floor of the middle fossa covering the IAC (Fig. 10.**19**). As the dissection is carried posteriorly, the dura is separated from the arcuate eminence (4 in Fig. 10.**19**) and, behind the eminence, is progressively elevated as far as the posterior border of the pyramid. Cottonoids are placed between the dura and calvarium at the sides of the field after elevation of the temporal lobe dura to help restrict mass movements of the temporal lobe itself.

When the arcuate eminence has been well exposed and sufficient access has been established to the meatal plane farther medially, a self–retaining retractor is placed into the craniotomy defect and tightened. A dural retractor is placed on the floor of the middle fossa medial to the porus acousticus and locked in place. Any troublesome bleeding, usually venous, below the calvarium at the sides of the field is controlled with Tabotamp and cottonoid pressure.

After the floor of the middle fossa has been exposed, the next landmark to be identified is the blue line of the superior semicircular canal (Fisch) (Fig. 10.**20**). It is exposed by gently taking down the arcuate eminence with a medium–size diamond burr. The labyrinthine bone (the bony superior semicircular canal) has a somewhat more yellow cast than the rest of the pyramidal bone, which is pale pink, and it is consistently identifiable by this color difference. If gray streaks are encountered in the bone as the arcuate eminence is burred down, the surgeon must decide whether they represent the blue line of the superior semicircular canal or pneumatized cell tracts. A Stenvers radiograph is helpful in making this differentiation. If the film shows extensive pneumatization, it is likely that the superior semicircular canal is obscured by pneumatized petrous bone.

If the petrous apex is moderately or poorly pneumatized, the superior semicircular canal may lie directly in the floor of the middle fossa. In rare cases the blue line of the superior semicircular canal will be visible as soon as the dura is elevated. An even less common situation is to find the superior semicircular canal only partially covered by bone, so there is a danger of entering the perilymphatic space during dural elevation. The blue line is consistently oriented at about a 90° angle to the posterior border of the pyramid, and its oblong shape helps to distinguish it from the irregularly shaped pneumatic cells.

The position of the arcuate eminence does not strictly coincide with that of the superior semicircular canal. The summit of the arcuate eminence may deviate up to 5 mm from the blue line of the superior canal in the mediolateral direction (Fig. 10.**21**). To allow for this deviation when attempting to locate the superior semicircular canal, the surgeon should drill over a broad area of the arcuate eminence using a moderately large diamond burr. By palpating the posterior border of the pyramid below the inferior petrosal sinus, one can keep from drilling too far anteriorly in the petrous floor, jeopardizing such structures as the temporomandibular joint, geniculate ganglion, or superior petrosal nerve. The bone of the superior semicircular canal is located about 10–15 mm in front of the posterior border of the pyramid.

Once the initial portion of the blue line has been exposed, it can be traced anteriorly and posteriorly to confirm the identify of the superior semicircular canal. It is not sufficient to obtain the "blue line" at a single point.

Medial to the superior semicircular canal is the meatal plane. An area of the meatal plane measuring about 1.5×1 cm is burred open just medial to the blue line. The deepest penetration into the bone should be directed at about a 60° angle (Fisch) over the superior vestibular nerve. The apex of the angle is defined by the segment of the superior semicircular canal that runs forward and downward over the superior ampulla. Bone removal farther anteriorly could jeopardize the facial nerve and even the basal turn of the cochlea.

When the dura of the IAC is identified, bone removal is first continued posteriorly toward the posterior fossa and then medially toward the porus acousticus to determine the exact course of the IAC and its greatest posterior extent. The cutting burr should be oriented so that its direction of rotation will not allow it to skip abruptly over a bony ridge and enter the IAC.

Next, the bone removal is continued anteriorly and laterally over the facial nerve to near the fundus, where the posterior wall of the entrance to the facial canal is identified as a vertical crest of bone (Bill's bar). The facial nerve enters the fallopian canal anterior to this bony vertical crest in the superior part of the fundus of the IAC. Posterior to the facial nerve is the superior vestibular nerve.

For the neurectomy itself, the dura of the IAC is exposed near the porus acousticus, avoiding bony overhangs (Fig. 10.**22**). If an acoustic neuroma, for example (see page 313), is to be removed by the transtemporal route, the dissection extends to the fundus, and the posterior fossa dura above and behind the porus acousticus is broadly dissected (Wigand's extended approach to the IAC).

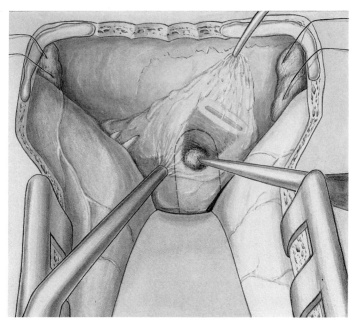

Fig. 10.**20**

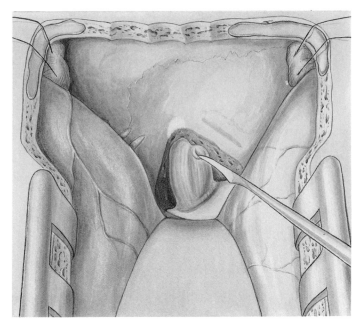

Fig. 10.**22**

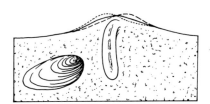

Fig. 10.**21**

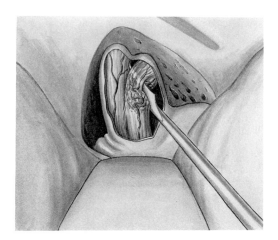

Fig. 10.**23**

After identification of Bill's bar and adequate dural exploration toward the porus acousticus, the dura is incised from laterally to medially over the vestibular nerve, i. e., in the posterior half of the IAC (Fig. 10.**22**). All bleeding points are coagulated with low–intensity bipolar current to maintain full visibility. The initially brisk CSF discharge from the dural incision will subside within minutes, allowing further dissection of the nerves in the IAC. If the dura has been inadvertently incised over the anterior part of the IAC, and if CSF pressure sweeps the facial nerve into the incision, the surgeon should quickly extend the incision to protect the nerve from damage.

After broad incision and partial resection of the dura, the superior vestibular nerve is mobilized posterior to Bill's bar and above the transverse crest (Fig. 10.**23**) and retracted medially upward with a fine suction tip. This places tension on the vestibulofacial anastomotic branches as well as the two inferior vestibu-

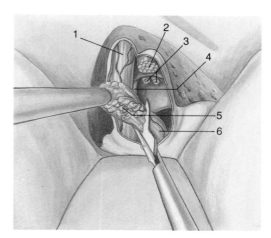

Fig. 10.**24**
1   Facial nerve
2   Superior vestibular nerve
3   Inferior vestibular nerves
4   Cochlear nerve
5   Scarpa's ganglion
6   Vestibular nerve

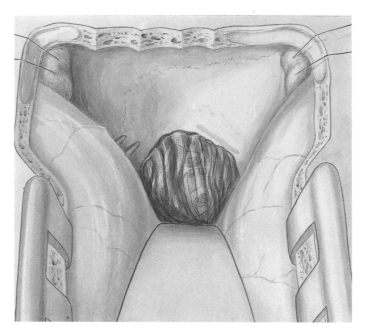

Fig. 10.**25**

lar nerves below the transverse crest in the posterior part of the fundus. In a patient with typical Ménière's disease of long standing, Scarpa's ganglion is conspicuous by its yellowish discoloration and tortuous vasculature just medial to the site where the superior vestibular nerve is divided. The inferior vestibular nerves, which transmit information from the saccule and the posterior semicircular canal ampulla, are also peripherally mobilized and retracted upward with the previously mobilized portion of the vestibular nerve, and the vestibular nerve is progressively sectioned medial to Scarpa's ganglion (Fig. 10.**24**).

Following resection of Scarpa's ganglion, the facial nerve is visible anterosuperiorly and the cochlear nerve anteroinferiorly, along with accompanying vessels that course directly on the nerve. Usually it is possible at this stage to look through the porus acousticus into the posterior fossa, where a loop of the anterior inferior cerebellar artery can often be identified. If part of the artery bulges into the IAC, it can be gently freed from surrounding arachnoid tissue and transposed through the porus into the posterior fossa to minimize compression effects in the IAC.

The defect in the IAC is covered with the free graft of temporalis muscle taken at the start of the operation. The graft is trimmed to the proper size, coated with fibrin glue, and pressed gently over the defect in the floor of the middle fossa (Fig. 10.**25**). The repair is reinforced by gluing a larger piece of banked dura over the floor of the middle fossa (Fig. 10.**26**). This ensures that any small CSF leaks produced in the delicate temporal lobe dura by the retractor, burr, or other instruments will not lead to CSF otorrhea.

All neurosurgical cottonoids are removed, leaving the hemostatic Tabotamp in place. A suction drain is placed to preclude any possibility of extradural hematoma (Fig. 10.**26**). It is left in place for two or three days while a constant, low-level suction is maintained.

The temporal bone flap is replaced, and the anteroinferiorly based temporalis muscle flap outlined at the start of the operation is swung into the lower part of the craniotomy to cover the craniectomized area and also promote vascularization of any scar tissue resulting from hematoma formation. The muscle and fascia are closed with continuous sutures (Fig. 10.**27**). Reapproximation of the fascia is often imperfect due to intraoperative shrinkage, but it is adequate. The wound is closed with continuous subcutaneous and cutaneous sutures.

Modifications

Various skin incisions have been described for the transtemporal approach to the IAC (see red lines in Fig. 10.**28**). Other modifications relate to the landmarks used to locate the IAC at the petrous apex. Some authors use the course and position of the greater superficial petrosal nerve, the direction of the superior petrosal sinus, and distance measurements from the surface of the calvarium.

Landmarks and Pitfalls

The principal landmark for the temporal craniotomy is the root of the zygomatic arch. The blue line of the superior semicircular canal (or greater petrosal nerve) is the essential landmark for locating the IAC, also the poste-

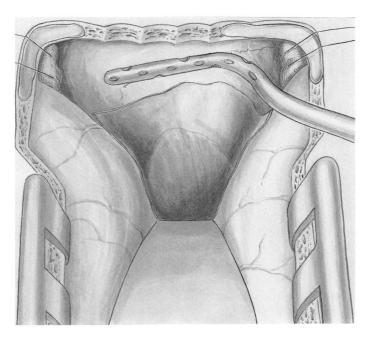

Fig. 10.**26**

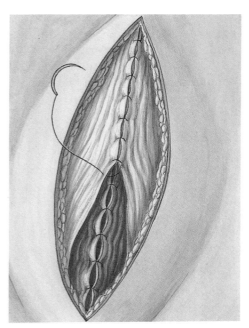

Fig. 10.**27**

rior border of the pyramid below the superior petrosal sinus. Hazards include undesired opening of the superior semicircular canal or cochlea or inadvertent injury to the facial nerve. Bleeding from the superior petrosal sinus is controlled with Tabotamp and cottonoids.

In about 10 to 20% of patients the geniculate ganglion lacks a bony covering or is covered only by a very thin shell of bone. Thus, when elevating the dura from the floor of the middle fossa, the surgeon should be careful to exert minimal pressure on the underlying bone in this area and keep in mind the potential vulnerability of the ganglion. Rarely, arachnoidal granulations in the same area can make the dissection more difficult. These very vascular dural appendages are always firmly adherent to the dura. By contrast, the dura is relatively easy to elevate from the geniculate ganglion.

The best way to avoid opening the superior semicircular canal, the cochlea, or even the labyrinthine segment of the fallopian canal is to use a precise dissection technique in which minimal pressure is applied to underlying structures and bone removal is performed gently and carefully over a relatively broad area.

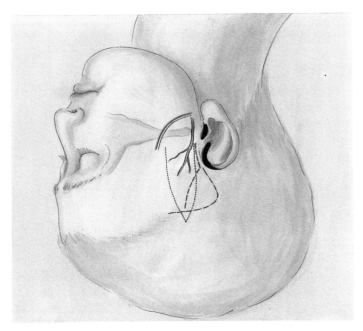

Fig. 10.**28**

It should be emphasized that the basal turn of the cochlea is very close to the floor of the middle fossa medial to the geniculate ganglion and anterior to the labyrinthine segment of the fallopian canal, and that the labyrinthine portion of the facial nerve may come within 1–3 mm of the floor of the middle fossa. Both the facial nerve and the basal turn of the cochlea can be promptly identified if bone is removed over a broad area using adequate irrigation and a reasonably large burr that is applied with minimal pressure.

The superior petrosal sinus may be opened during dissection at the posterior border of the pyramid. Since the pressure in this sinus is relatively low, firm Tabotamp packing is adequate for permanent and effective hemostasis. Coagulation alone is insufficient due to the tension exerted on this area by the retractor.

Rules, Hints, and Common Errors

If continuous irrigation is not maintained during bone removal, the burr can easily generate temperatures high enough to coagulate the bone at the drilling site. Constant irrigation is especially important near the labyrinth and the nerves in the IAC. An added benefit of irrigation is that it keeps the burr functioning effectively by clearing the flutes of bone debris.

When bipolar coagulation is used close to nerves, a relatively low current intensity should be applied while constant, gentle irrigation is maintained. The vessel should not be compressed between the tips of the coagulation forceps, as this might cause a forceps blade to stick to the vessel and tear it at an indeterminate site when the forceps is withdrawn. Hemostasis in these cases can be complicated, time–consuming, and hazardous.

Common errors include imperfect positioning of the craniotomy opening, imprecise dural elevation from the bone with tearing, and poor hemostasis in the area surrounding the actual operative field, so that dissection of the dura and nerves is obscured by bloody CSF.

Postoperative Care

Whenever the cranial cavity has been opened, especially under neuroleptanalgesia, the patient should be closely monitored for about the first 6 h postoperatively. Pulse and blood pressure are recorded at 30–min intervals for the first 12 h, then at 1–h intervals for the next 12 h. A bladder catheter is inserted for at least 12 h, and respiratory monitoring is advised. These measures are helpful for the early detection of intracranial hematoma.

Since the surgery involves slight elevation of the temporal lobe, a corticosteroid is given prophylactically on the day of the operation (e. g., 3×4 mg dexamethasone or 3×25 mg hydrocortisone). Also, sulpiride (e. g., 4×100 Dogmatil) may have to be administered for 2 to 5 days for relief of postneurectomy vertigo, depending on the severity of the complaints.

Postoperative Complications

Potential complications include CSF leak, extracranial or intracranial hematoma, and secondary infection.

A CSF leak following the transtemporal neurectomy will generally resolve spontaneously, and the surgeon should wait at least 2 weeks before considering reoperation. Lasix can be given in an attempt to reduce CSF production, and several days of lumbar CSF drainage may be appropriate.

Extracranial hematoma is usually due to bleeding from the temporal artery or one if its branches. If continued swelling is noted after a pressure dressing has been applied for 24 h, the wound should be reopened and explored under general anesthesia. If the bleeding persists, the hematoma will spread into the intracranial space and produce the clinical symptoms and risks of an extradural hematoma. Postoperative intracranial hemorrhage requires appropriate neuroradiologic or MRI assessment in consultation with a neurosurgical colleague before reoperation is considered.

Functional Sequelae

The neurectomy abolishes all vestibular impulses from the operated side, assuming that the surgery has removed all portions of the vestibular nerve and associated ganglion cells. If this has been accomplished, the patient will experience severe vertiginous symptoms for several days postoperatively. Most of this will subside within a few weeks or perhaps longer (several months) in older patients. If the surgery has been correctly performed, hearing is preserved in 95% of cases. The surgery improves hearing in some patients, and it may improve tinnitus as well as aural pressure and fullness. This is difficult to predict in advance, however.

Alternative Methods

Alternatives to transtemporal neurectomy are translabyrinthine neurectomy and retrolabyrinthine or retrosigmoid–suboccipital neurectomy in the posterior fossa. Another option is labyrinthectomy (see page 283).

Translabyrinthine Neurectomy

Preoperative Diagnostic Studies

The preoperative studies are the same as those preceding transtemporal neurectomy (see page 285).

Indications

The indications for translabyrinthine neurectomy are basically the same as for transtemporal neurectomy (page 285), but the translabyrinthine procedure is used in patients who lack serviceable preoperative hearing.

Principle of the Operation

Scarpa's ganglion and the acoustic nerve are exposed through a transmastoid–translabyrinthine approach and are either sectioned or removed.

Preoperative Preparations

The preparations are like those for transtemporal neurectomy (page 285). Also, the patient is told explicitly that the surgery will produce total, irreversible hearing loss on the operated side.

Initial preparation of the operative field is similar to that for mastoidectomy (see Chapter 4). The shaved postauricular area is about 1 cm wider. The positions of the patient, surgeon, scrub nurse, anesthesiologist, instrument stands, and auxiliary equipment are the same as for mastoidectomy (see Chapter 4).

Anesthesia

The surgery is performed under general endotracheal anesthesia. Since this procedure, unlike transtemporal neurectomy, does not require reduced intracranial pressure, hyperventilation is not essential. General anesthesia is supplemented by local infiltration of the operative field, as in mastoidectomy.

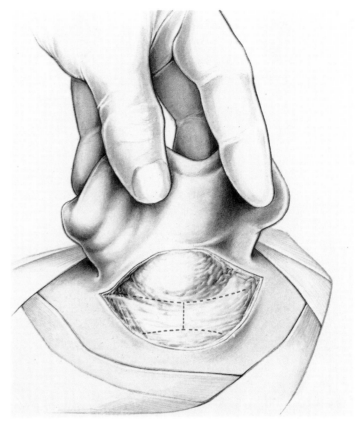

Fig. 10.**29**

Operative Technique

Since a very broad mastoidectomy is required, the post-auricular incision is extended somewhat to allow a tension–free retraction of the soft tissues (Fig. 10.**29**). The skin and subcutaneous tissues are left based on the auricle, while the periosteum, connective tissue, and muscles over the mastoid cortex are opened with an H–shaped incision and retracted upward, downward, and backward.

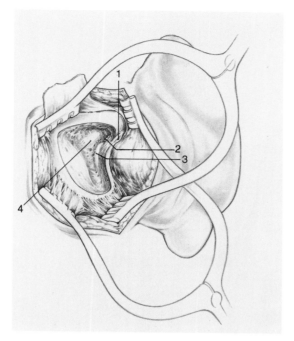

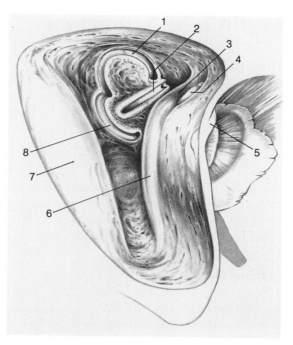

Fig. 10.**30a**
1 Suprameatal spine
2 Incus
3 Facial canal
4 Horizontal semicircular canal

Fig. 10.**30b**
1 Superior semicircular canal
2 Horizontal semicircular
   canal
3 Facial canal
4 Incus

5 Suprameatal spine
6 Mastoid portion of facial
   canal
7 Sigmoid sinus
8 Posterior semicircular canal

Further dissection of the mastoid is the same as for endolymphatic sac surgery (page 277). The horizontal, posterior, and then the superior semicircular canals are opened so that their course can be identified. They will serve as topographic landmarks (Fig. 10.**30a, b**).

The fundus of the IAC is projected between the opened superior and posterior ampullae. The endolymphatic duct can be seen in the bone on the posterior wall of the pyramid. It is visible through the medial wall of the common crus of the semicircular canals, and it can be seen entering the vestibule at the root of the common crus (Figs. 10.**31**, 10.**32**).

As bone is removed from the semicircular canals and mastoid bone, the facial nerve can be identified from about the cochleariform process to just before the stylomastoid foramen. A thin shell of bone is left over the nerve to protect it from inadvertent contact with a burr or other instrument. Except for an eggshell thickness of bone, the nerve must be skeletonized in order to approach and expose the fundus of the IAC, i. e., the medial wall of the vestibule. The same purpose is served by widely excavating the sinodural angle superiorly and posteriorly. These measures provide a clear view into the fundus of the IAC.

The bone between the inferior part of the mastoid portion of the facial nerve above the stylomastoid foramen and the anterior border of the sigmoid sinus is re-

moved to establish broad access to the posterior semicircular canal ampulla. Diamond burrs should be used close to the facial canal and on the sigmoid sinus to respect the occasional proximity of these structures. Medial to the sinus, the bony posterior wall of the pyramid is thinned down until the dura is faintly visible through the bone. In this way a broad access cavity can be created toward the petrous apex to facilitate later dissection at the IAC.

While the fundus of the IAC borders directly on the medial wall of the vestibule, the porus acusticus is located far medially, making it necessary to remove an additional 1 cm or more of hard labyrinthine bone in the posterior portion of the pyramid.

As bone is sparingly removed from the medial wall of the vestibule and superior semicircular canal ampulla near the fundus of the IAC, the bone assumes a more whitish color. This marks the site where the superior vestibular nerve enters the IAC at "Mike's dot" (Fig. 10.**32**).

Bone removal medial to the posterior semicircular canal ampulla exposes the delicate singular nerve, which enters the IAC fundus in a thin bony canal (the singular canal) (Fig. 10.**33a, b**). This nerve is the portion of the vestibular nerve that originates from the posterior semicircular canal ampulla. Between the posterior and superior ampullae, near the fundus, is the poste-

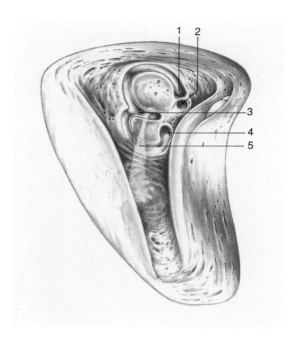

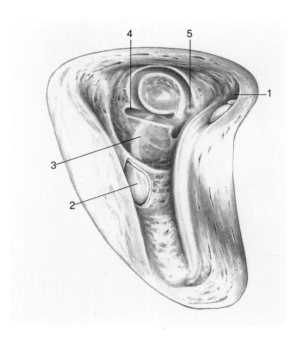

Fig. 10.**31**
1 Superior ampulla
2 Horizontal ampulla
3 Common crus
4 Posterior ampulla
5 Endolymphatic duct

Fig. 10.**32**
1 Geniculate ganglion
2 Endolymphatic sac
3 Endolymphatic duct
4 Projected IAC (broken line)
5 Mike's dot

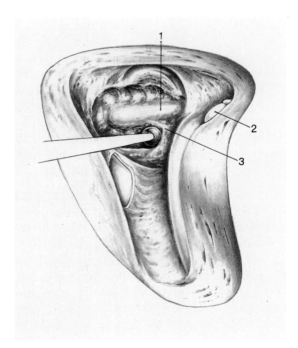

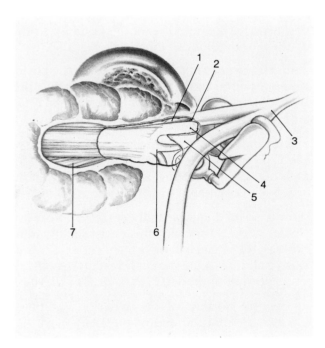

Fig. 10.**33 a**
1 Lateral wall of the IAC
2 Incus
3 Singular canal

Fig. 10.**33 b**
1 Facial nerve
2 Vertical crest (Bill's bar)
3 Geniculate ganglion
4 Superior vestibular nerve
5 Transverse crest
6 Inferior vestibular nerves
7 Cochlear nerve

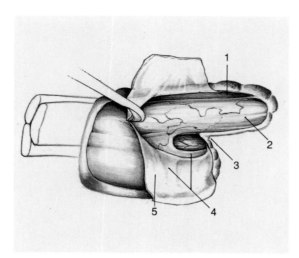

Fig. 10.**34 a**
1 Facial nerve
2 Superior vestibular nerve
3 Transverse crest
4 Inferior vestibular nerves
5 Dura

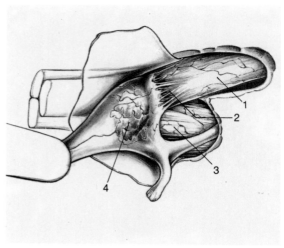

Fig. 10.**34 b**
1 Facial nerve
2 Anastomotic branches
3 Cochlear nerve
4 Scarpa's ganglion

rior wall of the IAC. It is exposed and followed to the posterior fossa. The dissection is carried to near the porus acousticus, as the dura on the posterior wall of the IAC is broadly separated from the bone up to the roof and down to the floor of the canal (Fig. 10.**33 a**).

The neurectomy does not require exposing the posterior fossa dura lateral to the porus acousticus, but this would be necessary for the excision of a neuroma, for example (Fig. 10.**33 b**).

After sufficiently broad access has been established to the IAC, and the dura has been adequately exposed, the dura is incised, producing a gush of CSF. Dural blood vessels are coagulated with low–intensity current.

The dura is opened and partially resected to expose the vestibular nerve. Displacing this nerve slightly inferiorly exposes the facial nerve, which enters the fallopian canal anterior to the vertical crest (Bill's bar) in the superior portion of the IAC (Figs. 10.**33 b**, 10.**34 a**).

The peripheral portion of the superior vestibular nerve is removed from the end of the IAC above the transverse crest and grasped with a fine suction tip (Fig. 10.**34 b**). The inferior vestibular nerve branches are similarly mobilized below the transverse crest (Fig. 10.**35**). This places tension on the vestibulofacial anastomoses (Fig. 10.**34 b**), which are coagulated and divided. A loop–like network of delicate blood vessels is often found between Scarpa's ganglion and the facial and cochlear nerves; bleeding from these vessels is controlled with bipolar cautery.

Scarpa's ganglion, recognized by its yellowish tinge and the tortuous blood vessels on its surface, is resected (Fig. 10.**36**). The vestibular nerve is sectioned medial to the ganglion, preferably using a fine neurectomy scissors.

Vessels traversing the center of the vestibular nerve are coagulated to clarify the CSF and afford a clear view of the IAC. The facial nerve courses above the transverse crest and the cochlear nerve below it. With a fine hook or sickle knife, the cochlear nerve is either avulsed from its bony canal near the fundus or divided (Fig. 10.**37**).

This alone is sufficient to disrupt the cochlear pathways, since the spiral ganglion is located in the modiolus. A small piece of the cochlear nerve can be taken if desired for histologic examination (Fig. 10.**38**). The skeletonized facial nerve, covered by a few delicate blood vessels, remains in its natural position within the fallopian canal. The central stumps of the vestibular nerve and cochlear nerve are visible in the inferior portion of the IAC. All bleeding, even from very fine vessels, is controlled with bipolar cautery.

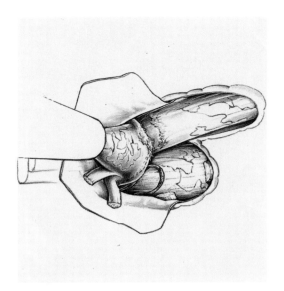

Fig. 10.**35**

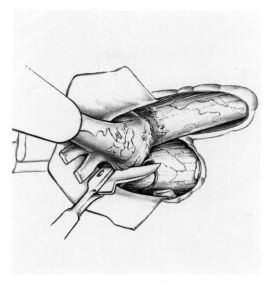

Fig. 10.**36**

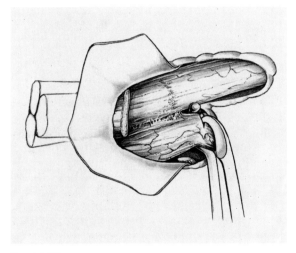

Fig. 10.**37**

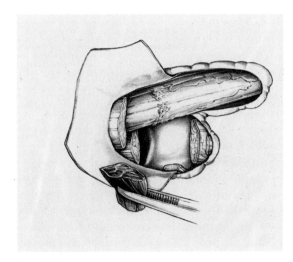

Fig. 10.**38**

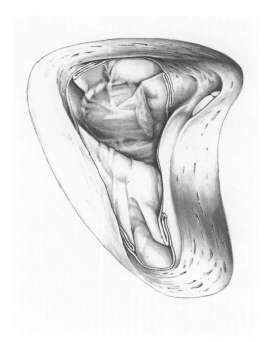

Fig. 10.**39**

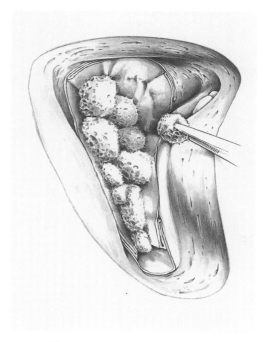

Fig. 10.**40**

The IAC is closed with a small, postauricular free muscle graft secured with fibrin glue (Fig. 10.**39**).

The funnel–shaped cavity in the petrous bone from the sigmoid sinus to the antrum is lined with folded banked dura, which is glued to the bony walls that are still intact (Fig. 10.**39**). The cavity is packed with dried, antibiotic–impregnated gelatin sponge, leaving the antrum open to maintain a communication with the middle ear (Fig. 10.**40**). We recommend overlapping cover of the attached dura with bone cement that leaves the antrum clear and provides a CSF–tight closure of the petrous apex.

If large portions of the dura on the posterior aspect of the pyramid (near the porus acousticus) have been removed to permit the removal of an acoustic neuroma, for example, then autologous abdominal fat can also be used to obliterate the transmastoid cavity.

The periosteal–connective tissue flaps elevated in the opening phase of the operation are repositioned and secured with absorbable sutures (Fig. 10.**41a**). Then subcutaneous and cutaneous sutures are placed (Fig. 10.**41b**), and a light, circumferential pressure dressing is applied.

Modifications

The only modifications relate to minor technical details and do not require any further description.

Landmarks and Pitfalls

The landmarks and pitfalls in the opening phase of the translabyrinthine neurectomy are the same as in endolymphatic sac surgery (page 277). The risks are minimized by following the facial nerve centrally below the semicircular canal, leaving a thin shell of bone over the nerve, and maintaining a constant irrigating stream to prevent thermal injury.

If the sigmoid sinus is so far anterior that it restricts access to the petrous apex, bone is removed from the sinus so that it can be retracted with a special blade.

Undesired opening of the dura can be avoided by using large diamond burrs when removing bone in proximity to the dura.

Rules, Hints, and Common Errors

These are the same as described for transtemporal neurectomy (page 285).

Postoperative Care

Since the subdural space has been entered, posing a slight but definite risk of intracranial hemorrhage, the patient requires an adequate period of postoperative surveillance with pulse and blood pressure monitoring, bladder catheterization, and treatment with antivertiginous medications. Cerebral tissues were not significantly displaced during the operation, so there is no

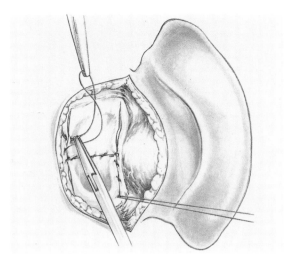

Fig. 10.**41 a**

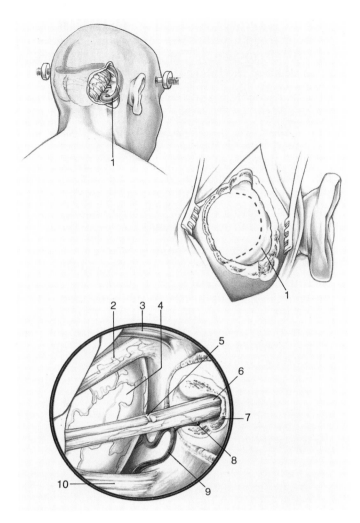

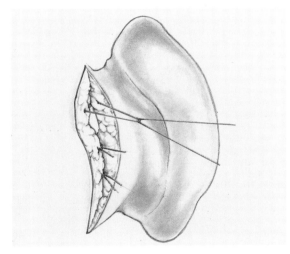

Fig. 10.**41 b**

Fig. 10.**42**

1	Sigmoid sinus	7	IAC opened
2	Trigeminal nerve	8	Labyrinthine arteries
3	Petrocel vein	9	Anterior inferior cerebellar artery
4	Pons	10	Glossopharyngeal nerve,
5	Facial nerve		vagus nerve, accessory nerve
6	Vestibular nerve		

need to give corticosteroids for prevention of brain edema.

Postoperative Complications

A CSF leak or facial nerve palsy may develop postoperatively. For CSF leakage, we recommend at least a 10–day period of observation and medical therapy (e. g., Lasix); a lumbar drain may be inserted if required. Many of these leaks will resolve spontaneously. If the leak persists, the site should be surgically reexposed and definitively sealed.

Facial nerve palsy developing within days after the operation has a favorable prognosis. It is unclear whether conservative treatment will improve the prognosis, but patients may be treated as needed with anti–inflammatory and hemorrheologic infusions of cortisone and pentoxifylline (after Stennert).

Functional Sequelae

The surgery produces a total loss of labyrinthine function on the operated side. Most patients with Ménière's disease experience vertiginous symptoms for only a few days after surgery. However, older patients and especially patients with non–Ménière–related vertigo may have mild complaints that persist for months or even years.

Alternative Methods

A complete cochleovestibular neurectomy can also be performed through a posterior fossa approach (Fig. 10.**42**), which may involve a transmastoid retrolabyrinthine approach or a suboccipital, retrosigmoid neurosurgical approach. The individual nerves are more difficult to identify in this type of approach, however, than in the internal auditory canal.

In the transcochlear approach (of Alvarez de Cozar), the fundus of the IAC is exposed through a transmeatal approach involving resection of the promontory inferior to the tympanic segment of the facial nerve and anterior to the highest portion of its mastoid segment. This provides a straight–on view of the fundus of the IAC, making it more difficult to identify the individual nerves and to identify and resect Scarpa's ganglion than in the translabrinthine approach described above.

The seventh and eighth cranial nerves can also be exposed through a suboccipital retrosigmoid approach like that used by neurosurgeons to access the cerebellopontine angle. Again, however, the individual nerves are more difficult to identify than in the IAC, because they form a densely packed bundle and are not conveniently separated from one another by bony ridges as they are in the internal meatus.

Bibliography

Arenberg I K, Stahle J. Unidirectional inner ear valve implants: a nondestructive alternative to labyrinthectomy in Ménière's disease, Am J Otol 1981; 3: 9–10.

Fisch U. Chirurgie im inneren Gehörgang und an benachbarten Strukturen. In: Naumann H H (ed) Kopf- und Hals-Chirurgie, Vol 3. Stuttgart: Thieme, 1976, pp. 457–543.

Helms J. Die chirurgische Therapie des Morbus Ménière. Arch Oto-Rhino-Laryng 1985; 68–118.

House W F, Owens F D. Long-term results of endolymphatic-subarachnoid shunt surgery in Ménière's disease, J Laryngol Otol 1973; 87: 521–7.

Lange G. Die intratympanale Behandlung des Morbus Ménière mit ototoxischen Antibiotika. Laryngol Rhinol Otol 1977; 56: 409–14.

Nadol J B. (Ed): Ménières Disease, Kugler and Ghedini, 1989, Proceedings of the second Ménière's Symposium.

Plester D, Hildmann H, Steinbach E. Atlas der Ohrchirurgie. Stuttgart: Kohlhammer, 1989.

Portmann G. The old and new in Ménière's disease – over 60 years in retrospect and a look to the future. Otolaryngol Clin North Am 1980; 13: 567.

11 Removal of Acoustic Neuroma through the Retrosigmoid (Lateral Suboccipital) Approach

Madjid Samii

Acoustic Neuroma

"Acoustic neuroma" actually arises from the Schwann cells investing the vestibular nerve (vestibular schwannoma). It is typically manifested by symptoms of vestibulocochlear dysfunction. Growth of the lesion leads to concomitant involvement of the trigeminal, facial, and lower cranial nerves. Visual disturbance and impaired consciousness can develop in the late stage as a result of cerebellar compression, brain–stem compression, and obstructive hydrocephalus.

Preoperative Diagnostic Measures

A detailed history is taken with regard to the onset, course, duration, and severity of symptoms, especially with respect to hearing loss, tinnitus, and vertigo, and a neurologic evaluation is performed. This is supplemented by function tests such as pure tone audiometry, speech discrimination, vestibular testing, and, if necessary, facial nerve testing by EMG or MEP (motor evoked potentials). The radiologic workup includes CT or MRI with contrast enhancement to define the extent of the tumor in the internal auditory canal (IAC), define its relation to the brain stem, detect possible compression or edema, and determine the primary direction of tumor growth. Additionally, the bony walls of the posterior cranial fossa should be imaged by high–resolution bone window CT to evaluate the generally widened IAC, assess the position of the labyrinthine system, and check for a high position of the jugular bulb.

Indications

As a general rule, the detection of an acoustic neuroma constitutes an indication for surgical removal. The earlier this can be done, the lower the morbidity (es-

pecially with regard to cranial nerve function) and mortality.

With the advent of microsurgery and numerous technical refinements in recent years, the *lateral suboccipital approach* now offers the most comprehensive means of removing even large acoustic neuromas while ensuring a reasonable chance of functional preservation.

Principle of the Operation

By the 1960's, three basic objectives had emerged in the surgical treatment of acoustic neuroma:
(1) complete removal of the tumor,
(2) the reduction of mortality, and
(3) preservation of the facial nerve.

A fourth basic goal has emerged since the early 1980's: preservation of the cochlear nerve. All of these goals can be achieved by removing the tumor through the lateral suboccipital approach, which provides an excellent view of the tumor–distorted anatomy and permits a complete tumor removal with maximum chance of preservation of neurovascular structures and functions.

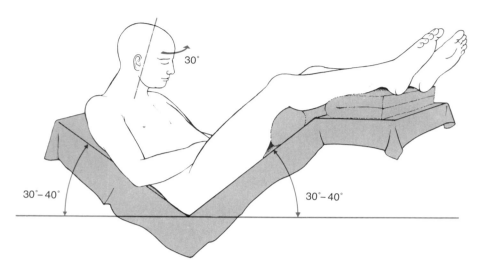

Fig. 11.**1**

Preoperative Preparations

Patient Positioning

The anesthetized and intubated patient is placed in a semisitting position in which the upper body and the lower extremities, wrapped with elastic tape, are angled 30–40° relative to the horizontal plane (Fig. 11.**1**). The knees are slightly flexed, and the table is tilted head–down until the proposed operative field is below the level of the patient's feet. All joint areas should be well padded before the start of the operation to prevent local neurovascular compression.

The patient's head, immobilized in a three–point Mayfield clamp, is anteroflexed 30° and rotated 30° toward the affected side to gain optimum posterior access to the suboccipital region on the side of the tumor (Fig. 11.**2**). There should be at least 2 cm clearance between the chin and sternum to avoid pressure on the trachea and jugular vein.

Alternatively, the patient may be positioned supine with the head turned to the opposite side or in a lateral position with little or no head rotation. Although these horizontal positions are widely used, the semisitting position offers one key advantage to the neurosurgeon. While the lateral position keeps one of the surgeon's hands busy suctioning blood and irrigating fluid from the operative field, leaving only one hand free for active tumor dissection and removal, the semisitting position allows fluids to drain from the operative field spontaneously, freeing both of the surgeon's hands for tumor and nerve dissection while an assistant (the "third hand") irrigates the operative site. Beyond this practical aspect, the reduced need for suction and for

bipolar cautery to control small bleeding tumor vessels results in less intraoperative trauma to nervous tissues.

Anesthesia

Neuroanesthesiologic Monitoring for the Detection, Treatment, and Prevention of Venous Air Embolism in the Semisitting Position

While advantageous for the surgeon, the semisitting position has certain inherent risks that can be minimized through appropriate primary measures. The principal hazard is intraoperative venous air embolism, which becomes a risk as soon as the skin incision has been made and veins have been transected (Hey et al., 1983). The following precautionary measures are applied routinely when neurosurgery is performed in the semisitting position.

- The central venous pressure is increased by the positioning measures noted above and by the administration of plasma volume expanders. This serves to reduce the pressure gradient between the operative area and the heart (Colohan et al., 1985).
- Positive end expiratory pressure (PEEP) ventilation is applied to reduce the pressure difference between the operative area and the right atrium (Pearl, 1986; Perkins, 1984).
- Continuous precordial Doppler ultrasound monitoring is used for the early detection of turbulence caused by air embolism (Furuya et al., 1983).
- The end expiratory carbon dioxide concentration is continuously monitored to permit rapid detection of air embolism.

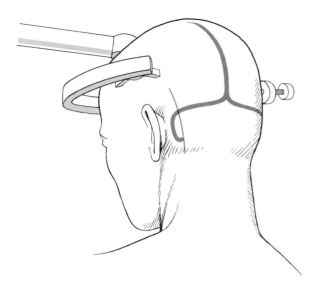

Fig. 11.**2**

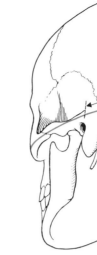

Fig. 11.**3**

- A central venous catheter is positioned in the right atrium for local pressure monitoring and, if necessary, for recovery of air from the atrium (Bedford et al., 1981).
- A continuous ECG (electrocardiogram) trace is obtained, and the radial artery pressure is continuously measured to monitor the patient's vital signs.

As soon as intraoperative monitoring signals *the presence of venous air embolism,* two parallel measures are instituted: The head–down table tilt is increased to raise the venous pressure, especially in the operative area, and the anesthesiologist manually compresses the jugular vein so that the presumed venous leak can be identified and controlled.

Recovery of air from the atrial catheter is attempted to reduce the damaging effects of the embolus. Also, as soon as a decrease in the end expiratory CO_2 concentration signals the presence of significant intravenous air, pure oxygen ventilation is initiated. The operation is discontinued until the venous leak can be identified and controlled.

Operative Technique

Skin Incision

The skin is opened with a vertical incision 6–10 cm long placed 2 cm behind the mastoid and auricle. The position of the transverse sinus, which runs between the external occipital protuberance and external auditory canal, is a factor to be considered in planning the skin incision. The skin incision may be shifted laterally or medially by 0.5 to 1 cm, depending on the location and pri-

mary growth direction of the tumor. The insertions of the short posterior neck muscles are released from the area of the craniotomy.

Craniotomy

The initial burr hole for the small craniotomy is placed at a site that respects the transverse and sigmoid sinuses (Lang and Samii): the "Frankfurt horizontal" (FH) is drawn from the suprameatal spine to the external occipital protuberance, and the center of the initial 12–mm burr hole is positioned 11.5 mm below the FH and 45–50 mm behind the suprameatal spine (45–50 mm in women, 50 mm in men). This places the bony opening safely within the angle formed by the junction of the transverse and sigmoid sinuses (Fig. 11.**3**). From there the burr hole is enlarged to a craniotomy 3 cm in diameter, with progressive exposure of the margin of the sigmoid sinus and the lower border of the transverse sinus. If the craniotomy is performed in the manner described, its size does not need to be varied as a function of tumor size.

During exposure of the craniotomy site and during the craniotomy itself, the anesthesiologist and neurosurgeon should respect the potential for air embolism by immediately closing emissary veins as they are opened. The opened mastoid cells are sealed with muscle and fibrin glue at the end of the operation to prevent leakage of CSF through the mastoid cells.

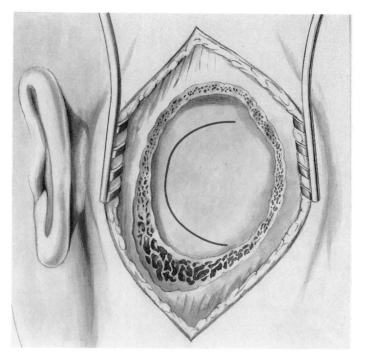

Fig. 11.**4**

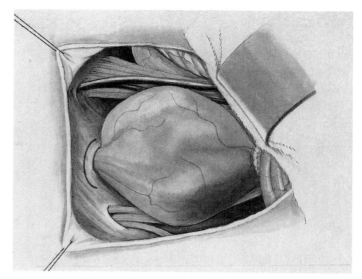

Fig. 11.**5**

Incision of the Dura

Before the intradural phase of the operation is begun, the anesthesiologist should compress the jugular vein to check the operative field for previously undetected opened veins. Once bleeding veins have been secured, the surgeon opens the dura 2 mm from the sigmoid and transverse sinuses with a laterally convex C-shaped incision, aided by the operating microscope (Fig. 11.**4**). The lateral dural margins at the sigmoid sinus are retracted laterally with two stay sutures to increase the exposure of the field (Fig. 11.**5**). The lateral cerebellomedullary cistern is opened, producing a gush of CSF that serves to enlarge the accessible field. Next the cerebellum is covered with protective cotton patties and retracted medially upward with a brain retractor with a 2–cm–wide blade.

Opening the Internal Auditory Canal

Before any intradural dissection is performed, the IAC must be opened so that the lateral, intrameatal extent of the tumor can be assessed. First the dura over the petrous bone is coagulated posterior and lateral to the IAC and resected with a semicircular incision. Occasionally a loop of the anterior inferior cerebellar artery (AICA) is adherent to the dura over the porus; this arterial loop must be protected and, if necessary, separated from the bone and displaced medially along with the dura. Starting from the porus and proceeding toward the fundus, the posterior lip of the IAC is progressively taken down with a diamond burr. We start with a 4– to 5–mm burr and exchange it for progressively smaller burrs as opening of the IAC proceeds. Continuous saline irrigations is maintained to prevent overheating and remove the debris.

Tumor Resection

The size and location of the tumor will determine the displacement of nerves and vessels in the cerebellopontine angle. With an extensive acoustic neuroma, cranial nerves V through XII may be significantly displaced and covered by tumor tissue. After the IAC has been adequately opened, the dura surrounding the tumor is opened and widely resected. The identification, protection, and preservation of the AICA are among the most important primary goals in the removal of acoustic neuroma. If this artery courses on the posterior surface of the tumor, it must be mobilized while small vessels en-

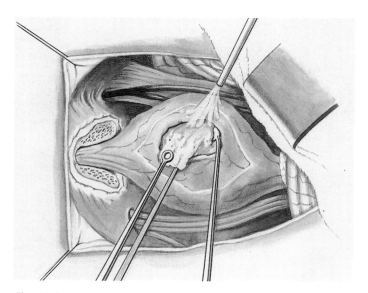

Fig. 11.**6**

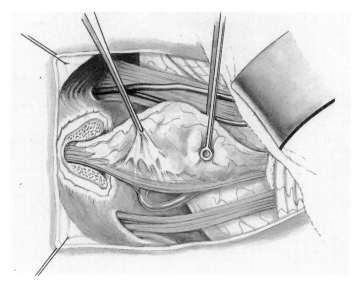

Fig. 11.**7**

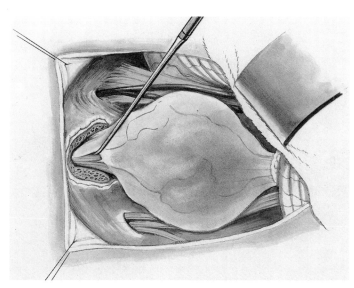

Fig. 11.**8**

tering the tumor are coagulated and divided. After the vessel has been freed from the posterior tumor aspect, that area can be coagulated with bipolar current, and tumor removal can be started at the coagulated site. We start by debulking the tumor to relieve pressure on surrounding structures. Once this has been accomplished and the surrounding structures are less tense, it is much easier to dissect the tumor capsule from the brain stem and surrounding cranial nerves. The core of the tumor can be debulked with sharp microdissectors or with an ultrasonic aspirator (CUSA; Fig. 11.**6**). The adequacy of the enucleation is assessed by noting the relative ease or difficulty of mobilizing the tumor capsule. The tumor core should be debulked evenly in all directions to avoid uncontrolled perforation of the capsule from the inside. During the subsequent dissection of the tumor capsule, special attention should be given to the arachnoid layer between the tumor and adjacent structures. Maintaining a plane of dissection along the arachnoid layer significantly reduces the likelihood of nerve injury or damage to the adjacent brain stem. The surgeon does this by grasping the capsule with a tumor forceps and applying gentle traction while carefully separating the arachnoid from the tumor capsule with a dissecting forceps (Fig. 11.**7**). Meanwhile the assistant continuously irrigates the site with warm saline solution to maintain visibility of the tumor–nerve boundary and avoid the need for constant, time–consuming coagulation of small bleeders.

When the inferior portion of the tumor has been adequately resected, cranial nerves IX through XII are freed from the tumor capsule. Dissection of the capsule then moves to the brain stem, where the origins of the vestibulocochlear and facial nerves are identified. As the tumor is progressively dissected from the brain stem, the resection is continued rostrally along the nerves. When the brain stem has been completely freed of tumor tissue, dissection of the facial nerve should not be continued on laterally towards the porus internus; experience shows that the tumor tends to adhere very firmly to the facial nerve at the entrance to the porus, so dissection in that area should be saved for last. It is better to stop short of the porus and move to the IAC, where tumor is first removed from the lateral portion of the fundus (Fig. 11.**8**).

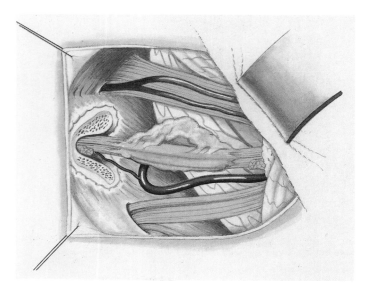

Fig. 11.**9**

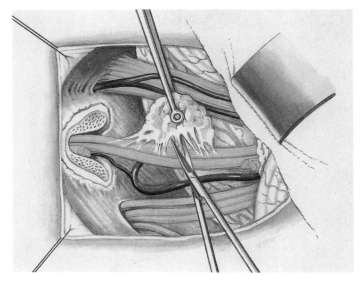

Fig. 11.**10**

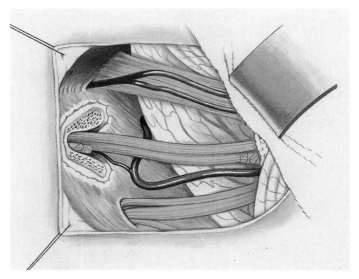

Fig. 11.**11**

Most acoustic neuromas arise from the vestibular nerve (vestibular schwannoma), which may be divided if it is found to be infiltrated by tumor in the fundus region. After the facial nerve has been identified in the anterosuperior portion of the IAC and the cochlear nerve anteroinferiorly, tumor removal is continued in the direction of the cerebellopontine angle. On encountering a very firm adhesion between the tumor capsule and facial nerve at the porus (Fig. 11.**9**), the surgeon should first debulk the tumor to improve vision and gain additional working space for this most difficult part of the facial nerve dissection (Fig. 11.**10**).

After all tumor has been removed (Fig. 11.**11**), the facial nerve is electrically stimulated just distal to its origin from the brain stem, and the motor response is

checked intraoperatively by watching for facial contraction or by electromyographic monitoring. The C–shaped dural incision is closed with two interrupted sutures and one running suture (Figs. 11.**12** and 11.**13**). Then the wound is closed in anatomic layers: muscle, fascia, subcutaneous tissue, and skin.

Modifications

Local Intraoperative Findings

Although acoustic neuromas are a well–defined neuroradiologic and pathohistologic entity, some tumor parameters can only be assessed intraoperatively after incision of the dura. These parameters, listed below, critically influence the conduct and difficulty of the operative procedure.

- Tumor size,
- The degree of tumor adherence to the cranial nerves, vessels, and brain stem,
- Tumor vascularization,
- Tumor consistency, including possible cystic changes,
- Reactive perifocal edema in the region of the cerebellum or brain stem,
- Displacement of the brain stem with obstructive hydrocephalus,
- The relation and adherence of the AICA to the tumor, cranial nerves VII and VIII, the IAC, and the petrous dura,
- The relation and adherence of the tumor to the trigeminal nerve and lower cranial nerves,
- The height of the jugular bulb.

Despite these parameters, it is generally sound practice to follow the sequence of intradural operative steps as they are outlined above (page 304). Several modifications will be noted below.

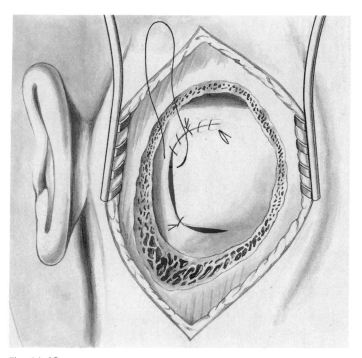

Fig. 11.**12**

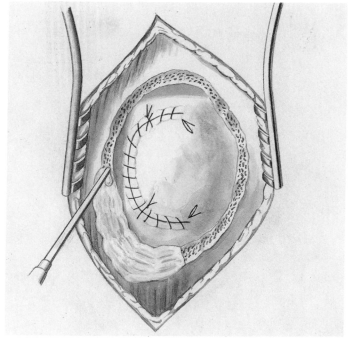

Fig. 11.**13**

High Jugular Bulb

With a high position of the jugular bulb, the IAC cannot be adequately opened without exposure of the bulb. This is done by burring down the posterior bony encasement of the bulb with a diamond burr and transposing the bulb downward, covering it if necessary with a small piece of muscle. A high jugular bulb can extend to various levels and in extreme cases may even project to the roof of the IAC (Shao et al., 1993).

Facial Nerve Discontinuity with Immediate Reconstruction

In approximately 10% of cases the tumor is so densely adherent to the facial nerve that it cannot be totally removed without resecting the involved facial nerve segment. Preserving facial nerve continuity in such a case would necessitate leaving residual tumor on the nerve, creating an unacceptable risk of recurrence. Thus, to achieve total removal, the affected facial nerve segment is generally resected (Fig. 11.**14**), and the nerve is repaired or reconstructed in the same sitting. If the missing segment is small, a tension–free end–to–end nerve repair can be performed. Especially with larger tumors, the facial nerve is often in a stretched and elongated condition that permits about a 1 cm defect to be bridged without tension by a direct end–to–end anastomosis. Larger defects are reconstructed by nerve grafting. The donor nerve generally consists of the distal portion of the sural nerve just behind the lateral malleolus. If both a central and peripheral facial nerve stump are available in the cerebellopontine angle, a sural nerve

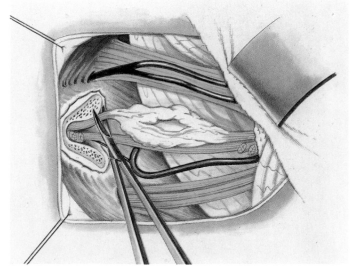

Fig. 11.**14**

graft 1–3 cm long can be interposed at that level (Fig. 11.**15**). With larger defects in which the distal facial nerve stump cannot be found in the cerebellopontine angle or the opened IAC, the mastoid must be opened to expose the mastoid segment of the facial nerve below the geniculate ganglion so that an intracranial–intratemporal graft can be performed. After the intracranial end of the graft has been anastomosed to the proximal facial nerve stump, the graft is brought out to the mastoid through a dural incision just anterior to the sigmoid sinus (Fig. 11.**16**). If the patient has a sig-

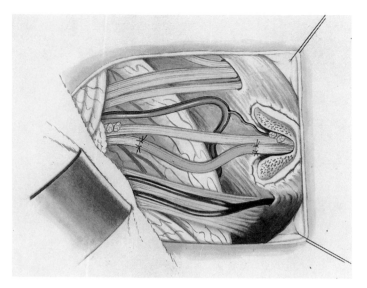

Fig. 11.**15**

Fig. 11.**16**

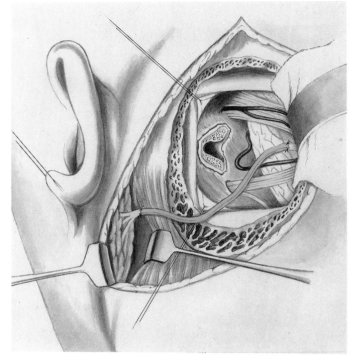

Fig. 11.**17**

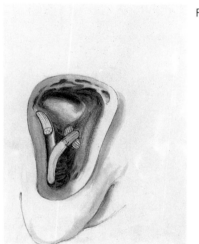

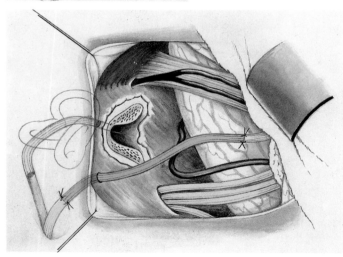

nificant prior history of mastoid disease (e. g., frequent middle ear inflammations, cholesteatoma, etc.), the distal anastomosis should not be performed in the mastoid segment. It is better to perform an intracranial–extracranial nerve graft (Dott, 1958) in which a graft 12–15 cm long is brought out through the dura, passed through a subcutaneous tunnel to the stylomastoid foramen, and anastomosed to the extracranial stump of the facial nerve (Fig. 11.**17**). The anastomoses are performed with 10/0 suture material or an externally applied drop of fibrin glue.

Landmarks and Pitfalls

Opening of the IAC should be carried to the full lateral extent of the tumor, if necessary to the fundus. Trauma to the posterior semicircular canal or vestibule should be avoided, since opening the vestibular system could lead to hearing impairment or total hearing loss despite preservation of the cochlear nerve. This approach lacks a well-defined anatomic landmark by which the surgeon can accurately assess the depth of these structures. The blue lines that guide the surgeon in the transtemporal approach to the IAC are far more difficult to see in the retrosigmoid approach due to the more tangential line of vision. The best orientation is provided by accurate CT views of the bony anatomy, which will demonstrate the relations of the semicircular canals, vestibule, IAC, and fundus. An imaginary line can be drawn from the medial border of the sigmoid sinus (the margin of the craniotomy) to the fundus of the IAC (the most lateral extent of the tumor) to see whether the line crosses the vestibule or posterior semicircular canal and determine how much of a protective bony bridge can be left between the fundus and the vestibule. If the vestibular structures are lateral to the imaginary line, they will not be harmed by the bony exposure of the fundus. If the vestibular structures are located more medially, the line should be placed farther medially so that it will bypass the vestibular structures and leave several millimeters of the posterior canal wall intact. As opening of the IAC progresses, we use angled microdissectors with round blade sizes of 1–5 mm to measure the remaining thickness of posterior canal wall (Fig. 11.**18**). Repeated measurements during the burring allow the IAC to be safely opened with no danger to vestibular structures.

If considerable lateral tumor extension into the fundus region is encountered, one option is to open the bony bridge remaining between the fundus and vestibule with a 1–mm diamond burr, working from the IAC toward the vestibule. Additionally, a micromirror or microendoscope can be used to facilitate the lateral dissection. It is also helpful at the outset to extend the craniotomy 1 cm medially to obtain a more favorable viewing angle from the medial side.

Rules, Hints, and Common Errors

Preservation of the cochlear nerve has become a basic goal in the neurosurgical treatment of acoustic neuroma (Cohen, 1981; Lehnhardt, 1982; Matthies, 1994; Samii, 1985; Smith, 1977; Glasscock, 1993; Harner, 1990; Nadol, 1992; Post, 1995; Samii and Matthies, 1995; Silverstein, 1993). Through microsurgical technique, anatomic preservation of the cochlear nerve has become feasible in the great majority of patients. This is not synonymous with functional integrity, however, and the postoperative functional status of the vestibulo-cochlear nerve depends on various factors such as pre–existing impairment caused by the tumor, objective preoperative hearing, and demonstrable changes in pre- and perioperative auditory evoked potentials. An analysis of the last 700 acoustic neuroma cases operated by the author indicates that cochlear nerve function can be preserved in up to 64% of cases if preoperative hearing loss does not exceed the 30 dB limit and the tumor diameter, including the intrameatal portion, is smaller than 30 mm. The rate of hearing preservation is inversely proportional to tumor size and the degree of preoperative hearing impairment. Since the chance of preserving auditory function is significantly higher in patients with small tumors and good preoperative hearing, a conservative, expectant approach is a less viable

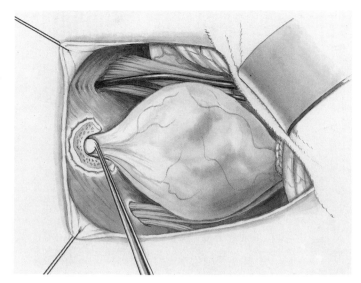

Fig. 11.**18**

option than early operative intervention, especially in patients with bilateral acoustic neuromas.

Brain Stem Auditory Evoked Potentials

Brain stem audiometry, or the continuous recording of brain stem auditory evoked potentials (BAEP, also called auditory brain stem response), is routinely performed prior to surgical procedures in the cerebellopontine angle. Changes such as a conduction delay or loss of specific waves signifying impairment of the cochlea, vestibulocochlear nerve, or auditory nuclei and pathways of the brain stem and midbrain are reported to the neurosurgeon, who modifies the microsurgical procedure accordingly.

Wound Closure

After complete tumor removal and the electrophysiologic testing of facial nerve function, it is prudent to make some final checks before proceeding with wound closure. The initial drainage of CSF leads to a slight descent of the cerebellum, producing a traction effect that may cause tearing of the bridging veins in the region of the tentorium. Unrecognized, these tears can lead to postoperative subdural hemorrhage and are probably its most frequent cause. As a precaution, therefore, jugular vein compression should be applied at the end of the operation to test the integrity of the bridging veins and other veins in the operative region. Small tears or bleeding points are coagulated with bipolar current.

Air cells are frequently opened during exposure of the IAC. The opened cells should be securely sealed with fascia and fibrin glue to prevent CSF leakage. A small piece of fascia is harvested, cut to size, and se-

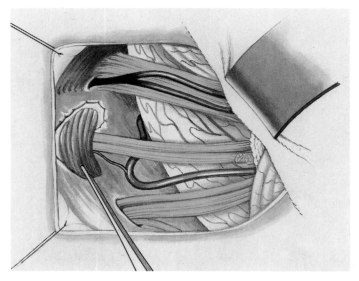

Fig. 11.**19**

cured with fibrin glue over the opened bony and dural defect to establish a watertight seal (Fig. 11.**19**).

A few small, thin pieces of fascia are glued over mastoid cells that were opened during the craniotomy. If leakage is noted at needle tracks in the reapproximated dura, the site should be covered with thin muscle strips secured with fibrin glue. A watertight dural closure serves to prevent epidural pooling of CSF and avoid paradoxical CSF rhinorrhea through the mastoid cells. When the retractors are removed, the anesthesiologist should have jugular vein compression reapplied to ensure that complete hemostasis is achieved.

Postoperative Bleeding

The immediate postsurgical patient should remain in the intensive care unit for one night to allow monitoring by neurosurgically trained personnel. Recovery from anesthesia may proceed swiftly, and generally the patient is extubated right away or within two hours. This permits an accurate clinical assessment to be made in the early postoperative period and allows the patient to be ambulated from bed on the day after surgery. Early follow–up examinations for 8–10 days after the operation should include neurologic function tests, audiometric tests, and cranial CT. Generally, the patient is ready for discharge by 8–14 days and can return to work at 2–3 months. Long–term clinical and radiologic follow–up should be scheduled at one, two, and five years.

Postoperative Complications

Early postoperative bleeding occurring within the first 12 hours after surgery may be subdural, epidural, or may occur within the cerebellopontine angle. The incidence is approximately 2%. Cranial nerve function and state of consciousness should be closely monitored in the intensive care unit so that problems can be detected quickly and CT scans can be obtained for a definitive assessment. The need for surgical exploration depends essentially on the clinical condition of the patient. If the patient shows increasing impairment of consciousness as a result of mass hemorrhage or becomes secondarily obtunded following good initial recovery, the hematoma should be evacuated at once and the source of the bleeding secured.

Paradoxical CSF rhinorrhea has an incidence of 8–10% in the first two postoperative weeks. It results from the epidural pooling of CSF, which drains through the mastoid, middle ear, and finally the eustachian tube to present as CSF rhinorrhea. Half of these cases are adequately managed by applying a local compression dressing for five days to inhibit CSF pooling. The remaining half additionally requires lumbar drainage for 7–10 days to reduce the local CSF pressure during the healing period.

Purulent meningitis is extremely rare and occurs chiefly in predisposed patients (e. g., diabetes mellitus).

Functional Sequelae

Preserving the function of the cranial nerves in the cerebellopontine angle is the ideal goal of this operation. While it is achieved in increasing numbers of cases, functional deficits are very likely to occur in patients with pre–existing dysfunction and in patients with tumors larger than 3 cm. Some auditory function can be preserved in an average of 40% of patients; the quality of hearing in these cases is highly variable and depends on the severity of the pre–existing deficit. Sixty percent of patients have normal facial function immediately after surgery, and a total of 80% have normal facial function by several months postoperatively. In approximately 10% of cases where the facial nerve has been anatomically preserved at operation, a severe or complete facial paralysis develops in the immediate postoperative period. Generally this resolves over a period of 1–2 years, leaving the patient with varying degrees of residual dysfunction. Minor corrective plastic surgical measures are occasionally indicated. Only 2% of patients will require a secondary facial reanimation procedure, preferably in the form of a hypoglossal–facial anastomosis. Generally a very acceptable functional and cosmetic result is achieved within 6–12 months. Patients who undergo facial nerve grafting at the time of operation show initial signs of facial reinnervation at 6–12 months and in the long term achieve good rest symmetry and acceptable symmetry of facial movements. About 6% of patients in whom the proximal facial nerve stump could not be preserved are selected for hypoglossal–facial anastomosis several weeks after the operation. A very satisfactory functional result is achieved in these cases.

Alternative Methods and Techniques

Two other surgical approaches are available: the *middle fossa approach* and the *translabyrinthine approach.* Tumors 2–3 cm in size can be approached through the middle cranial fossa, and the cochlear nerve and facial nerve can be preserved by this route. One disadvantage is the need for temporal lobe retraction.

Tumors of any size can be removed by the translabyrinthine route, but destruction of the labyrinth invariably results in total hearing loss.

An *alternative* to complete microsurgical resection is radiotherapy (with a linear accelerator or gamma knife), which can influence the growth of tumors up to 3 cm in size. Radiotherapy provides arrest of tumor growth ("tumor control") in about 60% of patients with acoustic neuroma. Twenty percent of tumors show a reduction in size, and another 20% show no apparent change in growth rate. Delayed side effects occurring at 6–12 months may include facial paralysis, trigeminal dysfunction, and hearing impairment or total hearing loss, presumably due to scarring and microvascular pathology.

For *curative* treatment, then the ideal concept is still early, complete surgical tumor removal with preservation of nerve functions.

Bibliography

Bedford R F, Marshall W K, Butler A, Welsh J E. Cardiac catheters for diagnosis and treatment of venous air embolism, J Neurosurg 1981; 55: 610–4.

Cohen N L. Preservation of hearing in acoustic neurinoma surgery, The Cranial Nerves. Samii, M. (ed), pp. 561–8, Berlin, Heidelberg, New York: Springer Verlag 1981.

Colohan A R T, Perkins N A K, Bedfor R F, Jane J A. Intravenous fluid loading as a prophylaxis for paradoxical air embolism, J Neurosurg 1985; 62: 839–42.

Cushing H. Tumors of nervous acusticus and syndrome of cerebellopontine angle. Philadelphia: Saunders, 1917.

Dandy W E. An operation for the total removal of cerebellopontine (acoustic) tumors. Surg Gynecol Obstet 1925; 41: 129–48.

Di Tullio M V. et al. A critical comparison of neurosurgical and otolaryngological approaches to acoustic neuromas. J Neurosurg 1978; 48: 1–12.

Dott N M. Facial paralysis. Restitution by extrapetrous nerve graft. Proc R Soc Med 1958; 51: 900–2.

El Azm M, Samii M, Bini W, Stanley L. Computed Tomographic Studies in Acoustic Neurinomas in Relation to the Vestibular Organ and Hearing Function, Neurinomes de l'Acoustique, aquisitions et controverses, Fraysse B,, Lazorthes Y. (eds), Editions Médicales Pierre Fabre, 1: 81–89, 1988.

Furuya H, Suzuki T, Okumura F, Kishi Y. Yefuji T. Detection of air embolism by transesophageal echocardiography. Anesthesiology 1983; 58: 124–31.

Glasscock III M E, Hays J W, Minor L B, Haynes D S, Carrasco V N. Preservation of hearing in surgery for acoustic neuromas. J Neurosurg 1993; 78: 864–70.

Harner S G, Beatty C W, Ebersold M J. Retrosigmoid removal of acoustic neuroma: Experience 1978–1988. Otolaryngol Head Neck Surg 1990; 103: 40–5.

Hey O, Fischer F, Reinery G, Steingass, U, Knorre D. Erkennung und Verhütung von Luftembolien während neurochirurgischer Eingriffe in sitzender Position. In: Ahnefeld, F. W., Dick, W., Kilian, J. (eds), Anästhesie in der Neurochirurgie, Berlin, Heidelberg, New York: Springer, 1983.

House W F, Hitselberger W W. Preservation of the facial nerve in acoustic tumor surgery. Arch Otolaryngol 1968; 88: 655–8.

Krause F. Zur Freilegung der hinteren Felsenbeinfläche und des Kleinhirns, Beitr Klin Chir 1903; 37: 728–64.

Lang J jr., Samii A. Retrosigmoidal approach to the posterior cranial fossa. An anatomical study. Acta Neurochirurgia (Wien) 1991; 111: 147-53.

Lehnhardt E, Samii M. Neurotologische Diagnostik bei Tumoren der hinteren Schädelgrube – verzögerte akustisch evozierte Potentiale auch auf der Gegenseite, Laryng Rhinol Otol 1982; 61: 501–4.

MacCarty C S. Acoustic neuroma and the suboccipital approach (1967–1972). Mayo Clin Proc 1975; 50: 15–6.

Matthies C, Samii M. Intraoperative Monitoring in Acoustic Neurinoma Surgery in the Semi-Sitting Position. Electroencephalography and Clinical Neurophysiology 1993; 2: 105.

Matthies C, Samii M. Surgical Action and BAEP Monitoring in Acoustic Neurinoma Removal. Proceeding of the First International Skull Base Congress, 1992, Karger, 1994.

Nadol J B Jr, Chiong C M, Ojemann R G, McKenna M J, Martuza R L, Montgomery W W, Levine R A, Ronner S F, Glynn R J. Preservation of hearing and facial nerve function in resection of acoustic neuroma. Laryngoscope 1992; 102(10): 1153–8.

Olivecrona H. Acoustic tumors. J Neurol Neurosurg Psychiatry 1940; 3: 141–6.

Pearl R G, Larson P. Hemodynamic effects of positive end-expiratory pressure during continuous venous air embolism in the dog. Anesthesiology 1986; 64: 724–9.

Perkins N A K, Bedford R F. Hemodynamic consequences of PEEP in seated neurological patients: Implications for paradoxical air embolism. Anesthesiol Analg. 1984; 63: 429–32.

Post K D, Eisenberg M B, Catalano P J. Hearing preservation in vestibular schwannoma surgery: what factors influence outcome? J Neurosurg 1995; 83(2): 191–6

Rand R W, Kurze T L. Facial nerve preservation by posterior fossa transmeatal microdissection in total removal of acoustic tumors. J Neurol Neurosurg Pyschiatry 1965; 28: 311–6.

Rand R, Kurze T. Preservation of vestibular, cochlear and facial nerves during microsurgical removal of acoustic tumors: Report of 2 cases. J Neurosurg 1968; 28: 158–61.

Rand R W. Microneurosurgery for acoustic tumors. Microneurosurgery, pp. 126–155, St. Louis: Mosby 1969.

Rhoton A L. Microsurgery of the internal acoustic meatus. Surg Neurol 1974; 2: 311–8.

Rhoton A L. Microsurgical removal of acoustic neuromas. Surg Neurol 1976; 6: 211–9.

Samii A. Retrosigmoidal approach to the posterior cranial fossa. An anatomical study. Acta Neurochir (Wien). 147–53, 1991; 111 (3–4).

Samii M. Neurochirurgische Gesichtspunkte bei der Behandlung der Akustikusneurinome mit besonderer Berücksichtigung des N. facialis. Laryng Rhinol 1979; 58: 97–106.

Samii M. Facial Nerve Grafting in Acoustic Neurinoma, Clinics in Plastic Surgery, Vol. 11, 1: 221–225, 1984.

Samii M. Microsurgery of acoustic neurinomas with special emphasis on preservation of seventh and eighth cranial nerves and the scope of facial nerve grafting. Rand R W. (ed), Microneurosurgery, 4rd edn, 366–388, Mosby, 1985.

Samii M, Matthies C. Hearing preservation in acoustic tumour surgery. In: Symon L. (ed.), Advances and Technical Standards in Neurosurgery, Vol. 22. Springer, Berlin, Heidelberg, New York: 343–373, 1995.

Samii M, Turel K E, Penkert G. Management of Seventh and Eighth Nerve Involvement by Cerebellopontine Angle Tumors. Clinical Neurosurgery Vol. 32, 13: 242–271, 1985.

Samii M, Matthies C, Tatagiba M. Intracanalicular Acoustic Neurinomas. Neurosurgery, Vol. 29, 2: 189–199, 1991.

Samii M, Penkert G. Ergebnisse von 110 mikrochirurgischen Akustikusneurinom-Operationen. Eur Arch Psychiatr Sci, 1984; 234 42–7.

Shao K-N, Tatagiba M. Samii, M. Surgical Management of High Jugular Bulb in Acoustic Neurinoma Via Retrosigmoid Approach. Neurosurgery 1993; 32(1): 32–7.

Silverstein H, Rosenberg S I, Flanzer J M, Wanamaker H H, Seidman M D. An algorithm for the management of acoustic neuromas regarding age, hearing, tumor size, and symptoms. Otolaryngol Head Neck Surg 1993; 108(1): 1–10.

Smith M F W, Clancy T P, Lang J S. Conservation of hearing in acoustic neurilemmoma excision. Trans Am Acad Ophthal & Otolaryng 1977, 84: 704.

Sterkers J M. Facial nerve preservation in acoustic neuroma surgery. In: Samii M, Jannetta P J (eds), The cranial nerves. Berlin, Heidelberg, New York: Springer, 451–455, 1981.

Tatagiba M, Samii M, Matthies C, Ell Azm M, Schönmayr R. The Significance for postoperative hearing of Preserving the Labyrinth in Acoustic Neurinoma Surgery. J Neurosurg 1992; 77: 677–94.

von Gösseln H, Bini W, Suhr D, Samii M. The lounging position: advantages outweight risks? Tos M, Thomsen J (eds), Acoustic Neuroma, Proceeding of the First International Conference on Acoustic Neuroma, Copenhagen, Denmark, August 25–29, 1991. Amsterdam, New York: Kugler Publications; 1992.

Yasargil M G, Fox J L. The microsurgical approach to acoustic neuromas. Surg Neurol. 1974; 2: 393–8.

12 Acoustic Tumor Removal: Middle Fossa and Translabyrinthine Approaches

Derald E. Brackmann

Physicians of the House Ear Clinic (formerly Otologic Medical Group) have surgically removed over 3,200 acoustic neuromas as of September 1994.

The translabyrinthine approach has been used for the majority of these cases with the middle fossa and retrosigmoid approaches used for the remainder. In this chapter, the middle fossa and translabyrinthine approaches are detailed.

Middle Fossa Approach

The middle fossa approach for the removal of the acoustic tumors was developed by William F. House in the early 1960s. It has been shown to be a safe approach with a minimum of mortality and morbidity.

Diagnosis and Preoperative Evaluation

Progressive unilateral sensorineural hearing impairment, unilateral tinnitus, or dizziness are indications for a neurotologic evaluation. Pure–tone and speech audiometry and auditory brainstem response audiometry (ABR) have now replaced other site–of–lesions tests. The definitive test for an acoustic neuroma is gadolinium–enhanced magnetic resonance imaging. This test will detect even the smallest acoustic neuroma. After acoustic tumor detection, preoperative evaluation includes a complete general physical examination, routine chest X–ray, ECG, and blood chemistries. A bleeding and clotting time is also obtained.

Indications

The indication for the middle fossa approach is a small acoustic tumor that extends no further than 1 cm into the cerebellopontine angle. If the tumor is medially placed and does not extend to the fundus of the internal auditory canal, the retrosigmoid approach is preferred.

Tumors that involve the distal end of the internal auditory canal are better approached via the middle fossa.

The middle fossa approach offers several advantages for the removal of small, laterally placed acoustic tumors. First, the majority of the dissection is extradural thereby lowering morbidity. Secondly, the lateral end of the internal auditory canal is exposed which assures removal of all tumor. With the retrosigmoid approach, the most lateral end of the internal auditory canal cannot be exposed safely without entering the labyrinth. Thirdly, positive identification of the facial nerve is possible at the lateral end of the internal auditory canal. This facilitates tumor dissection from the facial nerve in this area (Brackmann et al., 1985).

Candidates for hearing preservation surgery are those that have serviceable hearing, usually no greater than a 50 dB puretone loss with speech discrimination of at least 50%. Preservation of waveforms with only a slight increase of latencies on ABR is a favorable prognostic sign. Loss of function of the superior vestibular nerve as indicated by a reduced vestibular response on electronystagmography is also a favorable sign indicating a tumor in the superior compartment of the internal auditory canal. Tumors in the superior compartment are less likely to intimately involve the cochlear nerve and are also more likely to displace the facial nerve anteriorly rather than be located beneath the facial nerve.

Goal of the Operation

The goal of middle fossa acoustic tumor removal is complete tumor removal without increasing the neurologic deficit. One hopes to preserve residual hearing and not produce facial paralysis or other neurologic deficits.

Preparation for Surgery

Positioning

The patient is placed supine on the operating table with the head turned so that the operated ear is upmost. No external fixation is utilized. The surgeon is seated at the head of the table. The remainder of the operating room setup is shown in Figure 12.**1**.

A large area of hair removal is required because the incision extends far superiorly. The area of preparation extends nearly to the top of the head and far anteriorly and posteriorly. The skin is prepared with a povidone–iodine (Betadine) scrub and self–adhering plastic drapes are applied.

Special Instruments

The instruments utilized for neurotologic procedures are shown in Figure 12.**2 a-c**. The only special instrument required for the middle fossa approach is the House/Urban Middle Fossa Retractor (Fig. 12.**3**).

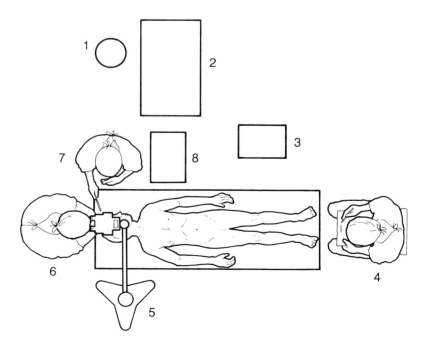

Fig. 12.**1** Operating room arrangement. The surgeon is seated at the head of the table.
1 = bucket
2 = back table
3 = bovie
4 = anesthetist
5 = microscope
6 = surgeon
7 = instrument nurse
8 = Mayo stand

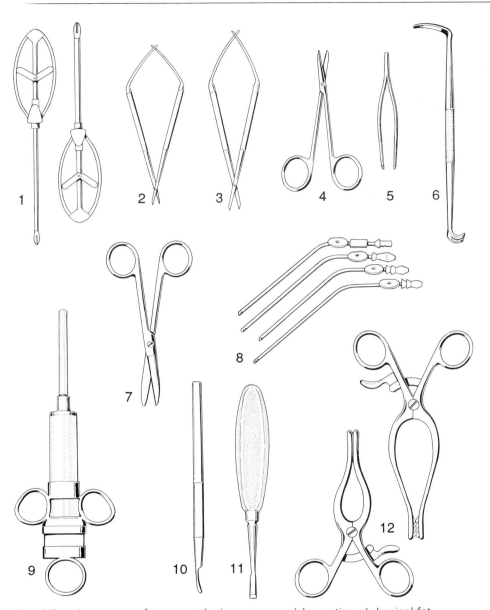

Fig. 12.**2 a** Instruments for neurotologic surgery and harvesting abdominal fat.

1	=	Weck micro clip applier	7	=	Suture scissors
2	=	Jacobson scissors	8	=	Brackmann suctions # 5 and # 7 (2 of each)
3	=	Malis titanium scissors	9	=	10cc Luer lock syringe
4	=	Lahey scissors	10	=	House endaural elevator
5	=	Adson forceps with teeth	11	=	Lempert elevator
6	=	Senn retractor	12	=	Weitlaner self retaining retractor large and small

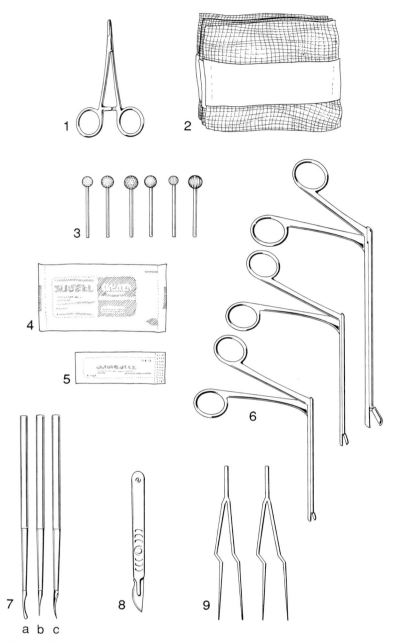

Fig. 12.**2b** Instruments for neurotologic surgery and harvesting abdominal fat.

1 = Halsted mosquito forceps
2 = Raytex sponges
3 = Drill bits, various sizes diamond and carbide cutting
4 = Surgicel
5 = Bone wax
6 = Cup forceps 2 mm, 3 mm, 5 mm
7 = Various micro instruments
       a. anulus elevator (gimmick)
       b. rosen needle
       c. sickle knife (# 1 knife)
8 = # 3 Knife handle with # 15 Bard-Parker blade
9 = Bayonet forceps

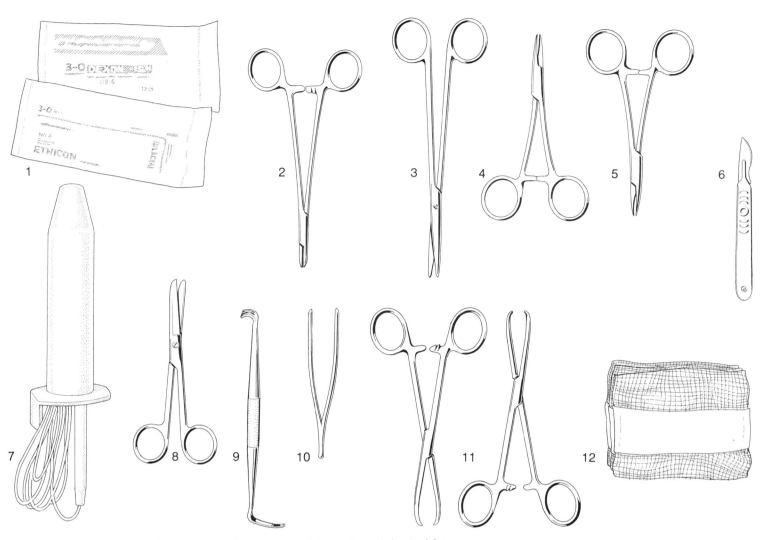

Fig. 12.**2c**   Instruments for neurotologic surgery and harvesting abdominal fat.

1 = Suture, 2–0 dexon, 3–0 dexon
2 = Crile wood needle holder
3 = Metzenbaum scissors
4 = Halsted mosquito forceps
5 = Kelly forceps
6 = # 3 Knife handle with # 15 Bard-Parker blade

7 = Bovie cautery
8 = Suture scissors
9 = Senn retractor
10 = Adson forceps with teeth
11 = Allis forceps
12 = Raytex sponges

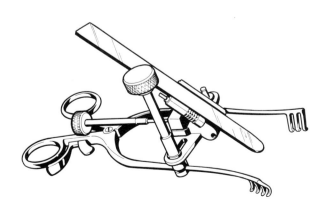

Fig. 12.**3**   The House/Urban middle fossa retractor. Three adjustments allow accurate placement of retractor blade.

Anesthesia

This operation is performed under general endotracheal anesthesia using inhalation agents. Facial nerve monitoring is routinely utilized so that relaxation is not used except for the initial induction of anesthesia. Diuretics and mannitol are usually used to promote diuresis. Arterial monitoring is not routinely utilized but may be employed for patients who are at greater than usual risk.

Far field auditory brainstem responses and direct eighth nerve potentials are monitored.

Operative Techniques

Incision

The middle fossa incision begins in the natural hairline just anterior to the base of the helix and extends superiorly approximately 10 to 12 cm, curving first posteriorly and then anteriorly (Fig. 12.**4**). Curving the incision allows the surgeon to spread soft tissue widely to gain more access anteriorly. Bleeding vessels are controlled with cautery. The surgeon often encounters a branch of the superficial temporal artery which is ligated with nonabsorbable suture to avoid late postoperative bleeding and hematoma (Fig. 12.**5**).

The initial incision extends to the level of the temporalis fascia. Finger dissection develops the plane of the temporalis fascia along the temporal line. An incision is then made posteriorly/superiorly along the insertion of the temporalis muscle onto the squamous portion of the temporal bone (Fig. 12.**6**). The temporalis muscle is freed from the temporal bone and retracted anteriorly/inferiorly (Fig. 12.**7**). Elevation of the temporalis muscle in this fashion preserves its nerve and blood supply so that it could be later utilized for a temporalis muscle transfer to the lower face in case of persistent facial paralysis. The temporalis muscle is elevated to the temporal line and held in place with self-retaining retractors and a stay suture.

Elevation of the Bone Flap

A craniotomy opening is made in the squamous portion of the temporal bone (Fig. 12.**8**). The opening is approximately 5 cm square and is located two-thirds anterior and one-third posterior to the external auditory canal. It is important to place the craniotomy opening as near as possible to the floor of the middle fossa. This usually requires hand retraction of soft tissue by an assistant.

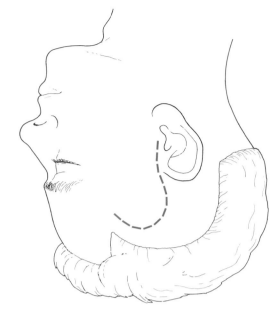

Fig. 12.**4**

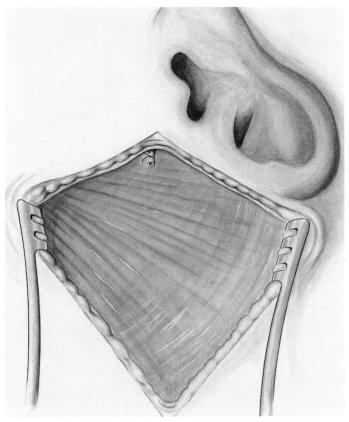

Fig. 12.**5**

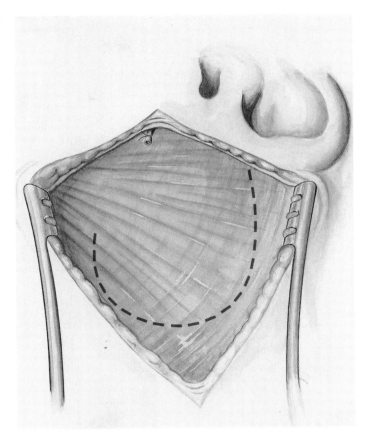

Fig. 12.**6**

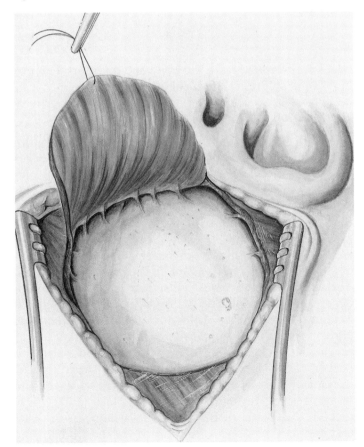

Fig. 12.**7**

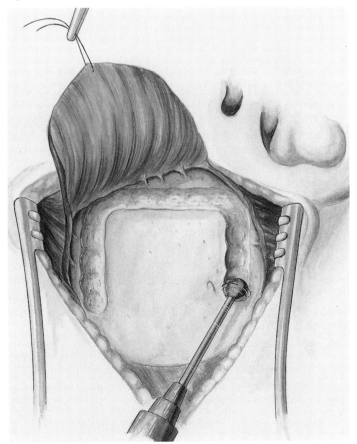

Fig. 12.**8**

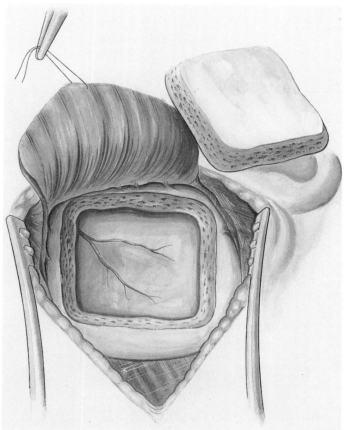

Fig. 12.**9**

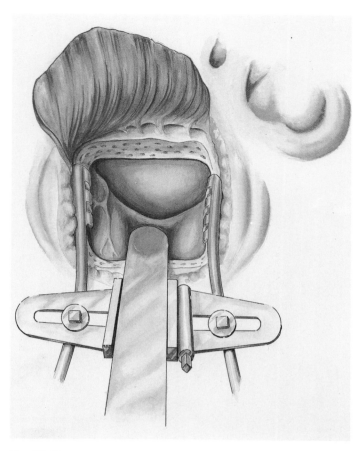

Fig. 12.**10**

A medium cutting burr and continuous suction–irrigation are used. The bone flap is thicker superiorly as the squamo–parietal suture is approached. It is important not to lacerate the dura during the bone removal for this could allow herniation of the temporal lobe. Herniation can best be avoided by leaving a thin plate of bone over the dura. The bone can then easily be fractured and removed. The bone flap can also be made using a high–speed drill with a footplate attachment. We prefer to make a bone flap rather than a burr hole and rongeur enlargement so that the temporal bone flap can be replaced at the end of the procedure. This results in less retraction in the area of the incision thus improving the cosmetic appearance. Replacement of the bone flap also reduces the possibility of transmission of brain pulsations to the skin which is cosmetically undesirable.

Bone bleeders are commonly encountered and are controlled with bone wax. It is important to keep the edges of the bone flap parallel. This facilitates placement of the middle fossa retractor.

Once the surgeon has drilled nearly through the temporal bone flap, a joker elevator is used to separate the underlying dura and the bone flap is removed. Sharp edges are trimmed from the bone and it is placed in normal saline solution during the operation.

Elevation of the Dura

The dura is separated from the margin of the craniotomy defect with the joker elevator. Any sharp edges are removed with the rongeur. Occasionally, the inferior bone cut is above the floor of the middle fossa. This excess bone is removed with the rongeur. At times, there will be bleeding from the branches of the middle meningeal artery on the surface of the dura (Fig. 12.**9**). This is best controlled with bipolar cautery with care being taken not to burn a hole in the middle fossa dura. The level of cautery must be reduced to the minimum necessary to coagulate the vessel. It is important to maintain the integrity of the dura since any defect may allow herniation of the temporal lobe. If a small tear is produced, it should be closed with dural silk suture to prevent extension and herniation. After separation of the dura from the edges of the craniotomy defect, the House/Urban retractor is put in place and firmly locked. The blade of the retractor is then set in place and gentle elevation of the dura from the floor of the middle cranial fossa is begun (Fig. 12.**10**).

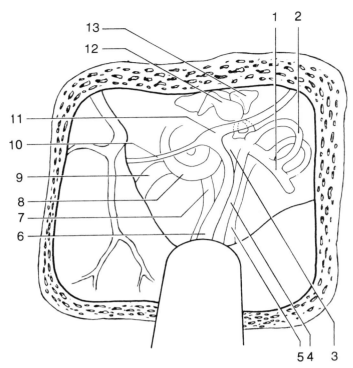

Fig. 12.**11** Relationship of structures within the temporal bone as viewed from the middle fossa.
 1 = superior semicircular canal
 2 = lateral semicircular canal
 3 = Bill's bar
 4 = superior vestibular nerve
 5 = inferior vestibular nerve
 6 = facial nerve
 7 = cochlear nerve
 8 = cochlea
 9 = carotid artery
10 = greater superficial petrosal nerve
11 = geniculate ganglion
12 = malleus
13 = incus

The House/Urban retractor contains three adjustments, allowing for the desired placement of the retractor. The first adjustment affords movement of the entire blade mechanism in an inferior/superior direction. Once the blade is properly centered at the depth of the middle fossa dissection, this adjustment is secured at a position that gives maximum exposure but does not impinge on the superior edge of the craniotomy opening.

Dural elevation is carefully begun from posterior to anterior. As the dura is elevated, the tip of the blade is advanced. The two other adjustments are arranged appropriately. One adjustment allows for anterior to posterior movement of the tip of the retractor blade. The other adjusts the placement of the tip of the blade in a superior/inferior direction (Fig. 12.**3**).

The structures within the temporal bone as viewed from above are shown diagrammatically in Figure 12.**11**. The first landmark to be identified is the cranial entrance of the middle meningital artery at the foramen spinosum. This marks the anterior limit of the dural elevation. Frequently venous bleeding is encountered in this area. It may be necessary to control this bleeding by placing a firm pack of Surgicel into the foramen spinosum.

The surgeon's attention is then directed posteriorly and the medial elevation of the dura is accomplished from posterior to anterior. First the petrous ridge is identified posteriorly. Care is taken in this area because the petrous ridge is grooved by the superior petrosal sinus which the surgeon must avoid entering. If the sinus is inadvertently entered, bleeding can usually be controlled by extraluminal packing with Surgicel. It is best to use large pieces of Surgicel as small pieces could enter the sinus lumen and produce a pulmonary embolus.

The dura is then elevated from the floor of the middle fossa medially from posterior to anterior. In approximately 5% of cases, the geniculate ganglion of the facial nerve will not be covered by bone. Blind or rough elevation of the dura in such cases can result in damage to the facial nerve. It is best to gently elevate the dura from the temporal bone rather than to scrape the elevator along the bone of the middle fossa.

The posterior to anterior elevation avoids raising the greater superficial petrosal nerve. If this nerve were elevated and the dissection carried posteriorly, the geniculate ganglion and facial nerve would again be subject to injury. In the literature on the middle fossa approach to the gasserian ganglion an up to 5% incidence of facial paralysis has been reported. With careful dural elevation performed with the aid of the surgical microscope, this complication can be avoided in all cases.

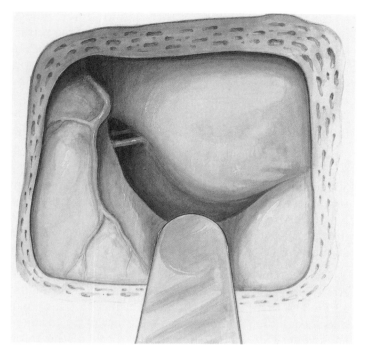

Fig. 12.**12**

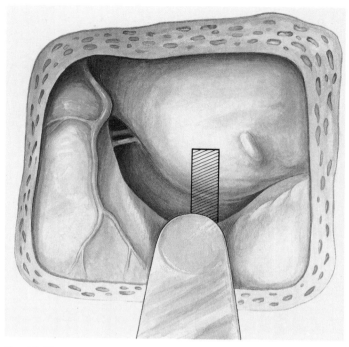

Fig. 12.**13**

As dural elevation proceeds, the arcuate eminence is encountered. At times, this is an obvious landmark but sometimes it is indistinct. The positive landmark is the greater superficial petrosal nerve which passes parallel to the petrous ridge from the geniculate ganglion anteriorly. This nerve lies medial to the middle meningeal artery. Once the greater superficial petrosal nerve has been identified, it is carefully followed to the hiatus of the facial nerve and the blade of the middle fossa retractor is readjusted (Fig. 12.**12**).

A word of caution is necessary regarding pressure on the bone of the floor of the middle fossa. Both in the area of the tegmen and over the internal carotid artery the bone may be very thin and, rarely, even dehiscent. Although injury to the internal carotid artery has not occurred in our cases, care must be taken to avoid this complication. At this point the major landmarks of the middle fossa approach have been identified. These are the middle meningeal artery, arcuate eminence, and the greater superficial petrosal nerve and facial hiatus.

Therefore, the surgeon is ready to begin bone removal over the internal auditory canal. There is often considerable bleeding from small vessels on the surface of the dura and the floor of the middle fossa. This bleeding is particularly troublesome since it pools into the most dependent portion of the wound where the bone removal is to begin. Considerable bleeding from any one vessel must be controlled. It is usual however for oozing to occur from multiple sites. We have found that

such bleeding will stop spontaneously and it is best to proceed with the operation at this point.

Exposure of the Internal Auditory Canal

Dr. William House originally described identification of the internal auditory canal by following the greater superficial petrosal nerve to the geniculate ganglion and then the geniculate ganglion through the labyrinthine segment of the facial nerve to the internal auditory canal. This method is still used for middle fossa procedures involving the facial nerve.

For acoustic tumor removal, however, a different technique is now used. The area of the porus acousticus is estimated by bisecting an angle formed by the greater superficial petrosal nerve and the arcuate eminence (Fig. 12.**13**). Drilling commences at the medial aspect of this line with a large diamond burr and proceeds deeper until the dura of the internal auditory canal is detected (Fig. 12.**14**). The bone around the porus acousticus is removed widely in an arc of approximately 270° using diamond burrs with continuous suction irrigation. A great deal of exposure can be obtained by drilling anteriorly and posteriorly at the medial aspect of the internal auditory canal without risking violation of the superior semicircular canal posteriorly or the cochlea anteriorly (Fig. 12.**15**).

The internal auditory canal is then followed laterally to the fundus using progressively smaller diamond

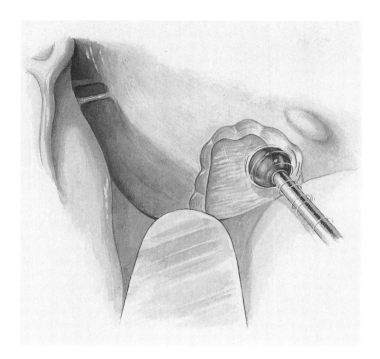

Fig. 12.**14**

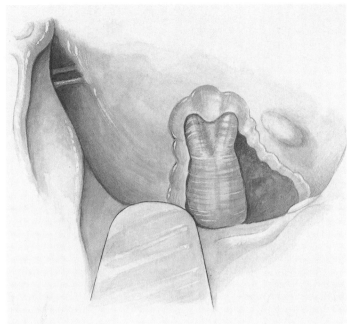

Fig. 12.**15**

burrs with a tapering effect such that only the superior 90° of the internal auditory canal is exposed at the fundus to avoid entry into the cochlea or the ampulla of the superior semicircular canal. The proximal labyrinthine portion of the facial nerve is decompressed approximately 3 mm to allow for swelling that may occur as a result of the dissection of the tumor from the facial nerve. The labyrinthine segment of the facial nerve courses in a direction parallel to the plane of the superior semicircular canal. A smaller diamond burr is necessary for this bone removal since the ampullated end of the superior semicircular canal and vestibule lie only a few millimeters posterior to the facial nerve at this point and the cochlea lies only few millimeters anteriorly. Continuous facial nerve monitoring alerts the surgeon when the facial nerve is exposed.

The dissection then is carried posteriorly and the bar of bone separating the facial nerve from the superior vestibular nerve (Bill's bar) is identified. This marks the lateral limit of bone removal. The vestibule lies immediately lateral to Bill's bar. Great care must be taken to remove the bone without entering the dura because the facial nerve lies directly against the dura. It is best to leave an eggshell thickness of bone over the entire surface of the internal auditory canal until all bone removal has been completed.

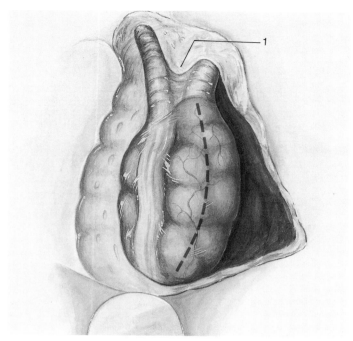

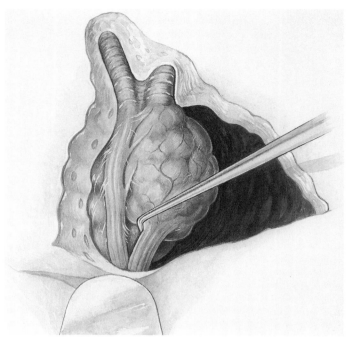

Fig. 12.**16** The fundus of the internal auditory canal and Bill's bar has been exposed. The labyrinthine segment of the facial nerve has been decompressed. The dura is opened posteriorly.
1 = Bill's bar

Fig. 12.**17**

Bone removal must be extensive for middle fossa acoustic tumors. The superior petrosal sinus will be lying free in the dura following removal of the petrous ridge. Care must be taken to avoid bleeding but should it occur it may be controlled with extraluminal packing of Surgicel or with clips.

This completes the bone removal. The fine eggshell of bone is then removed and the dura is opened along the posterior aspect of the internal auditory canal (Fig. 12.**16**). The facial nerve lies anteriorly and the first exposure of internal auditory canal should be away from the facial nerve. The dural flap is carefully elevated from the underlying tumor and the facial nerve is identified at the lateral end of the internal auditory canal where the vertical crest of bone (Bill's bar) allows positive identification.

Tumor Removal

The first objective in tumor dissection following wide exposure is to preserve the facial nerve while removing the entire tumor. Under 25 or 40 power magnification the fibers of the facial nerve are dissected free from the adhered portions of the tumor. The high magnification allows more precise dissection using fine hooks and scissors. In larger tumors the bulk of tumor mass is removed at this point leaving the tumor capsule in place. In smaller tumors the debulking step is omitted. The

tumor is freed from the contents of the internal auditory canal preserving all vascular and neural elements possible. The dissection of the tumor within the internal auditory canal is always in a medial to lateral direction. This avoids tension on the facial nerve in the area where it is fixed at the entry into its labyrinthine segment (Fig. 12.**17**).

After the facial nerve is freed from the tumor, the next step is to separate it from the cochlear nerve. It is also important to conduct this dissection in a medial to lateral direction to avoid traction on the cochlear nerve as it enters the modiolus. The nerve divides into many fibers in this area and is very fragile. It is also likely that medial traction could interrupt the vascular supply to the cochlea. Care to avoid medially directed dissection is considered critical in preserving hearing.

Previously both the superior and inferior vestibular nerves were cut. Now all non–involved structures are preserved to aid in maintaining the cochlear blood supply. Leaving vestibular nerve fibers intact does increase the risk for postoperative unsteadiness. This has not been a problem in recent cases although one patient in an earlier series required a vestibular nerve section because of disabling unsteadiness following acoustic tumor removal where some vestibular fibers were left. Even though there is an increased risk of postoperative unsteadiness, the risk is small and worth taking for

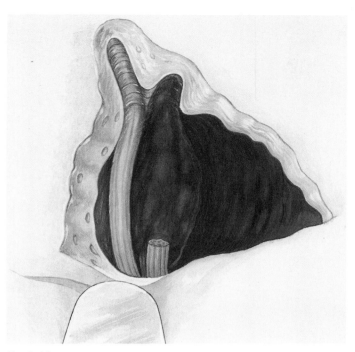

Fig. 2.**18**

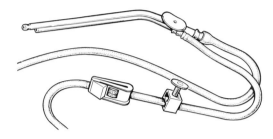

Fig. 12.**19**   Fenestrated neurotologic suction: multiple openings reduce suction to protect neural tissue.

the improved possibility of hearing preservation (Fig. 12.**18**).

During tumor dissection the anterior/inferior cerebellar artery is identified and carefully preserved. The artery may loop into the internal auditory canal inferior to the cochlear nerve or the tumor may displace it into the cerebellopontine angle. Great care must be taken to identify and not injure this most important artery.

During the course of the dissection the surgeon must be careful not to injure the facial nerve with the suction. This possibility is reduced by the use of the fenestrated neurotologic suction (Fig. 12.**19**) (Brackmann, 1977).

After total removal of the tumor is accomplished, a Gelfoam pledget soaked with papavarine is placed on the cochlear nerve in the internal auditory canal and at the modiolus. We sometimes use the same medication during tumor dissection if the direct VIII nerve action potentials, which are continuously recorded, begin to deteriorate. Papavarine is a non–specific smooth muscle relaxant. The vasodilator effects of papavarine help increase cochlear blood flow as well as flow to the cochlear nerve itself and we believe this is beneficial in preserving hearing.

Bleeding from small vessels usually subsides during irrigation of the wound bed. At times larger vessels will require bipolar cautery for control of bleeding.

Inadvertent injury to the anterior/inferior cerebellar artery is always a possibility during removal of the medial aspect of the tumor. Control of bleeding would be extremely difficult in this situation because of limited access. Fortunately this has not occurred in our experience: but if it should, it might be necessary to remove more bone in the area of the superior semicircular canal to expose more of the posterior fossa dura in order to gain access for the application of a clip. If bleeding should still not be controlled, it might be necessary to perform a postauricular approach and translabyrinthine exposure of the cerebellopontine angle to achieve this control.

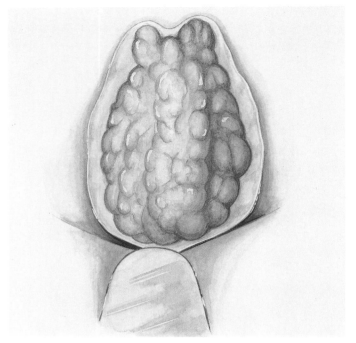

Fig. 12.**20**

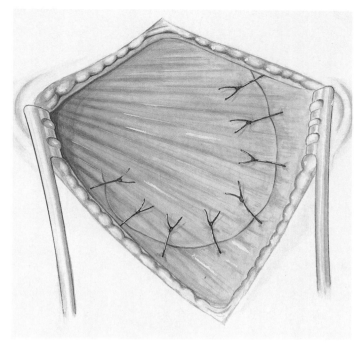

Fig 12.**21**

Wound Closure

Closure of the defect in the internal auditory canal is accomplished with a free graft of abdominal fat (Fig. 12.**20**). The temporal bone flap is then replaced and the temporalis muscle resutured to its insertion (Fig. 12.**21**). The subcutaneous tissue and skin are closed in layers and a sterile dressing is applied. If there is excessive oozing, a Penrose drain is utilized.

Surgical Landmarks and Danger Points

Positive identification of the greater superficial petrosal nerve and arcuate eminence are necessary for orientation to the internal auditory canal.

The geniculate ganglion may be congenitally dehiscent of bone and may be subject to injury during dural elevation.

The bone flap must be placed anteriorly to allow access to the internal auditory canal.

At the fundus of the internal auditory canal, the ampullated end of the superior canal and the cochlea lie in very close proximity to the internal auditory canal. Dissection must be limited to the roof of the internal auditory canal to avoid injury to these structures.

Rules, Tips, and Pitfalls

1) Place the temporal craniotomy far enough anteriorly to allow access to the porus acousticus.
2) Avoid the frontal branch of the facial nerve with the initial incision by staying posteriorly.
3) Avoid dural laceration during elevation from the floor of the middle fossa.
4) Avoid injury to the geniculate ganglion during dural elevation by progressing from a posterior to anterior direction.
5) Avoid a postoperative epidural hematoma by controlling epidural arterial bleeding.
6) Avoid excessive brain retraction by proper placement of the middle fossa retractor.
7) Do not lacerate the superior petrosal sinus on elevating the dura from the petrous ridge.
8) Use sharp dissection to remove the tumor from the facial nerve during tumor removal.
9) Carefully identify the anterior/inferior cerebellar artery and separate it from the medial aspect of the tumor to avoid serious posterior fossa hemorrhage.
10) Dissect only the roof of the internal auditory canal at the fundus to avoid entering the superior semicircular canal or cochlea.

Postoperative Management

The patient is observed in the intensive care unit for 24 hours postoperatively with the usual monitoring techniques. Postoperative antibiotics are not routinely employed. The Foley catheter and nasogastric tube are removed on the first postoperative day as is the abdominal drain. The middle fossa wound drain is also removed if one has been used. Early ambulation is encouraged depending upon the amount of unsteadiness.

Postoperative Complications

An epidural hematoma is an uncommon early postoperative complication. The incidence of this may be reduced by the use of a Penrose drain where there is excessive oozing. Meticulous attention to hemostasis is a necessity. Patients with this complication will exhibit signs of increasing intracranial pressure. Treatment is immediate evacuation of the hematoma in the intensive care unit. The patient is then taken to surgery where more definitive control of the bleeding is accomplished.

Other complications are those which are common to any intracranial procedure, such as meningitis. Temporal lobe injury from retraction on the temporal lobe was an early concern but has not been a problem in our series. We have had no patients who have had signs of a cortical injury such as hemiparasis or aphasia. Hearing loss and facial paralysis are expected complications in some of these patients as with any acoustic tumor removal.

Results of Surgery

The middle fossa approach was used to remove 106 acoustic neuromas as of December 1986 and this series was reported by Shelton et al. (1989). The size of these tumors has varied from 0.4 to 2 cm. Hearing was preserved in 63 patients (59%). In 37 patients (35%), hearing was the same as before surgery. There was a partial loss of hearing in 26 patients (25%). In the remainder a total sensorineural hearing loss occurred despite preservation of the cochlear nerve in 89% of patients. Hearing preservation roughly correlated with tumor size: hearing preservation is better for smaller tumors.

Eighty percent of patients had normal facial nerve function one year after middle fossa surgery for removal of acoustic tumors. Another 9% had grade II function and the remainder a greater degree of weakness. No patient had a total facial nerve paralysis.

Other than hearing loss and facial weakness, there were no other serious complications or deaths in this series.

A more recent series was recently reported (Brackmann et al., 1994). Twenty-four consecutive patients operated for acoustic tumor via the middle fossa approach between January and December 1992 were reviewed. Hearing was preserved at or within 10 dB of the preoperative levels in 71% of patients. An additional three patients, 12%, had some hearing preserved whereas 16% lost all hearing.

Facial nerve function was grade I in 79% of patients, grade II in 17% and grade III in one. No patient had poorer than grade III recovery.

There was one patient with an epidural hematoma which required early evacuation. There were no sequelae to this complication and there were no other serious complications or deaths in either of the middle fossa series reviewed.

Alternative Techniques

The alternative technique for acoustic tumor removal with attempt at hearing preservation is the retrosigmoid approach. This is discussed in detail in another chapter in this volume. The advantages of the middle fossa approach are:
1) Primarily extradural dissection, thereby lowering morbidity.
2) Exposure of the most distal end of the internal auditory canal assuring complete tumor removal.
3) Positive identification of the facial nerve in the lateral end of the internal auditory canal facilitating tumor dissection in this area.

When hearing preservation is not a goal, the translabyrinthine approach is the preferred method for acoustic tumor removal.

Conclusion

The middle fossa approach is the preferred method for removal of small, laterally placed acoustic neuromas.

Translabyrinthine Approach

The translabyrinthine approach is the most direct route to the cerebellopontine angle. We believe that this approach offers many advantages for acoustic tumor removal. It requires a minimum of cerebellar retraction. Exposure and dissection of the lateral end of the internal auditory canal insure complete tumor removal from that area and also allow positive identification of the facial nerve in a consistent anatomic location (Brackmann et al., 1985).

If the facial nerve is lost during acoustic tumor removal, the translabyrinthine approach offers the best opportunity for immediate repair by end to end anastomosis or interposition of a nerve graft (Brackmann et al., 1978).

Finally, and most importantly, this approach carries the lowest morbidity and mortality rates. The mortality rate for this approach is 0.4 of 1% for the last 2,300 cases.

The obvious disadvantage of the translabyrinthine approach is the sacrifice of any residual hearing in the operated ear. It is therefore reserved for patients whose hearing is poor or for large tumors when the possibility of hearing preservation is slight.

Diagnosis and Preoperative Evaluation

See Section under Middle Fossa Approach.

Indications and Patient Selection

Small tumors which extend no further than 1 cm into the cerebellopontine angle in patients with good hearing are usually approached via the middle fossa. Larger tumors where good hearing remains are approached via the retrosigmoid route. This route is ideal when the tumor arises more medially and is not impacted into the fundus of the internal auditory canal and does not expand the internal auditory canal.

In general, the outlook for hearing preservation for tumors with greater than 2 cm extension into the cerebellopontine angle is very poor. These tumors and all tumors with poor hearing are removed via the translabyrinthine approach.

There is no tumor too large to be approached via the translabyrinthine route. For large tumors more bone removal is accomplished posterior to the sigmoid sinus to gain access.

Goal of Surgery

The goal of translabyrinthine acoustic tumor removal is total tumor removal with no increase in the neurologic deficit with the exception of total loss of hearing.

Preparation for Surgery

The patient is placed supine on the operating table with the head at the foot of the table. This allows the anesthesiologist, who is seated at the patient's feet, easy access to the controls for moving the table. The patient's head is turned toward the opposite side and maintained in a natural position without fixation. The surgeon is then seated at the patient's side. This position minimizes fatigue and allows stabilization of the arms and hands during the exacting microsurgical procedures (Fig. 12.**22**).

Instruments

Standard neurotologic instruments are utilized (see pp. 316–318). One special instrument is used and will be discussed later.

Anesthesia

General endotracheal anesthesia with inhalation agents is utilized. Muscle relaxants are only used for induction of anesthesia since intraoperative monitoring of facial nerve activity is routinely utilized. Prophylactic antibiotics or steroids are not routinely used. Occasionally with very large tumors these measures are employed.

Operative Technique

The ear is prepared with Povidone–Iodine (Betadine Solution) and plastic drapes are applied. A postauricular incision is made approximately 2 cm behind the postauricular crease (Fig. 12.**23**). The incision is curved anteriorly to allow anterior retraction of the pinna. The posterior curve of the incision allows access to the area behind the sigmoid sinus. Because most of the surgical view of the cerebellopontine angle is along the plane of the posterior fossa dura, posterior access is important.

The incision first extends to the fascia temporalis, and the dissection is carried to the linea temporalis, lateral to the fascia temporalis. Incision is then made through the fascia and periosteum along the linea tem-

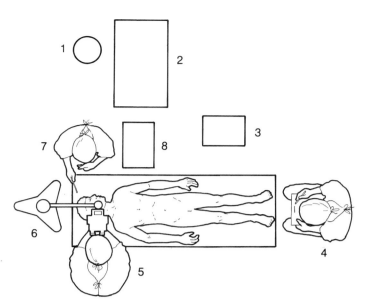

Fig. 12.**22** Room arrangement for translabyrinthine approach. Note positions of surgeon, anesthesiologist, and nurse.

1 = bucket
2 = back table
3 = bovie
4 = anesthetist
5 = surgeon
6 = microscope
7 = instrument nurse
8 = Mayo stand

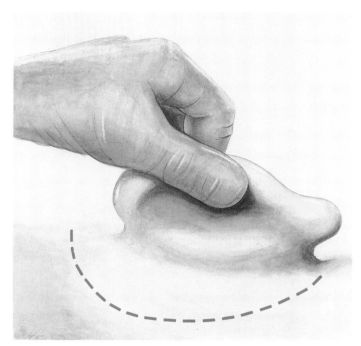

Fig. 12.**23**

poralis posteriorly to the sinodural angle and then inferiorly on the mastoid bone to the mastoid tip (Fig. 12.**24**). The Lempert periosteal elevator is used to free the postauricular tissues from the underlying cortex, posterior to the sinodural angle and forward until the spine of Henle and the external auditory canal are identified. Care must be taken not to tear into the external auditory canal, since this would introduce a possible route for infection.

Self-retaining retractors are placed to maintain the ear forward and also to elevate the temporalis muscle superiorly. Suction on the posterior blade of the retractor removes excess irrigation fluid and blood from the wound.

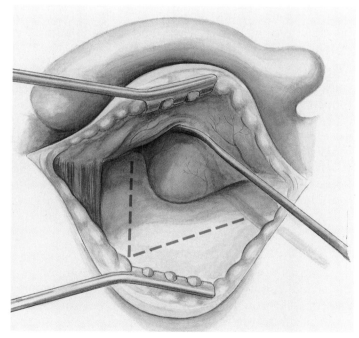

Fig. 12.**24**

Cortical Mastoidectomy

After adequate exposure of the cortex has been obtained, bone removal is carried out with continuous suction–irrigation and a large cutting burr. Bone removal is started along the external auditory canal, and then a horizontal incision is made along the temporal line (Fig. 12.**25**). The junction of these incisions will lie over the mastoid antrum. Identification of the mastoid antrum and the lateral semicircular canal therein is the key to the beginning dissection of the temporal bone.

Bone removal continues with care taken not to undercut the mastoid cortex. The external opening must be as large as possible. The middle fossa plate is identified superiorly and the sigmoid sinus posteriorly. Removal of bone is then continued over the sigmoid sinus to the area of the posterior fossa dura.

In large tumors bone removal is carried out far behind the sigmoid sinus. In some cases the bone is removed with a rongeur or drill as far as 2 or 3 cm posterior to the sigmoid sinus and inferiorly beneath the cerebellar hemisphere. This gives more decompression of the posterior fossa and allows room for retraction of the dura posteriorly. Care must be taken, however, not to injure the dura. Dural tears allow the cerebellum to herniate into the defect, which may result in infarction of that portion of the cerebellum.

Removal of bone over the sigmoid must be done carefully. If the cutting burr tears the sigmoid sinus, profuse bleeding will ensue and will require packing with oxidized regenerated cellulose (Surgicel). Large emissary veins often arise from the posterior aspect of the sigmoid sinus. They can be identified through the bone as it is removed, since the suction–irrigation keeps the bone clean. If the emissary vein is injured, bleeding must be controlled with bone wax, cautery, Surgicel packing, or in some cases suture of the emissary.

Complete, Simple Mastoidectomy

As soon as the mastoid cortex has been removed and the sigmoid sinus has been outlined, the operating microscope is brought into place. Magnification allows more accurate bone removal and exposure of all the structures of the temporal bone. A thin layer of bone is left over the sigmoid sinus and around the emissary veins, and a complete, simple mastoidectomy is performed down to the level of the horizontal semicircular canal (Fig. 12.**26**). It is important that the antrum be opened and the horizontal semicircular canal be identified. This canal is the basic landmark in temporal bone surgery. Once the position of this canal is known, the depth and three–dimensional relationship of the facial nerve and posterior and superior semicircular canals can be viewed. Expertise in temporal bone surgery depends upon a thorough knowledge of the anatomy of the temporal bone and the ability to identify the structures as they are encountered. This appreciation of the anatomy comes only after many hours of diligent temporal bone dissection.

Labyrinthectomy

After the mastoid air cells have been removed to the level of the horizontal semicircular canal, labyrinthectomy is begun. Bone is removed in the sinodural angle along the superior petrosal sinus (Fig. 12.**27**). This area, which is farthest from the facial nerve, is the key to this step in the dissection. The opening along the superior petrosal sinus is gradually deepened and widened until the labyrinthine bone is encountered. The lateral and posterior semicircular canals are then progressively removed, and the facial nerve, which lies anteriorly (Fig. 12.**28**), is carefully approached. The lateral semicircular canal is opened, and the common crus of the superior and posterior semicircular canals is identified deep in the dissection. The superior semicircular canal is followed to its ampulla. The vestibule is then opened, and the facial nerve is skeletonized from the genu inferiorly to near the stylomastoid foramen. It is not necessary to remove bone lateral to the facial nerve; rather, the facial nerve is skeletonized from a posterior direction, where access is needed to approach the cerebellopontine angle.

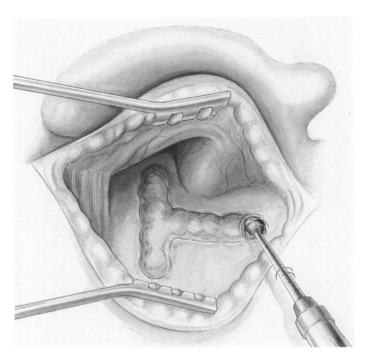

Fig. 12.**25**

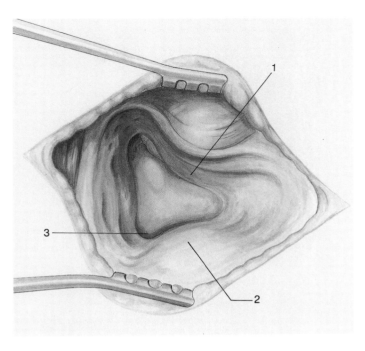

Fig. 12.**26**   Mastoidectomy is completed. Facial nerve is localized and sigmoid sinus is skeletonized.
1 = localized facial nerve
2 = sigmoid sinus
3 = sinodural angle

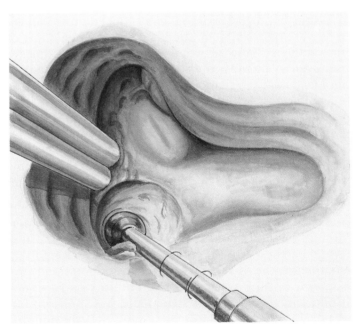

Fig. 12.**27**

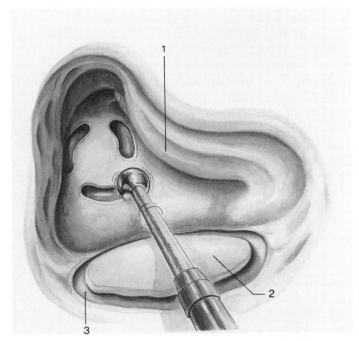

Fig. 12.**28**   Semicircular canals are opened. An island of bone over the sigmoid sinus is created.
1 = localized facial nerve
2 = Bill's island
3 = sigmoid sinus

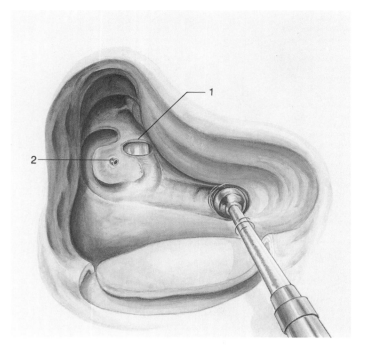

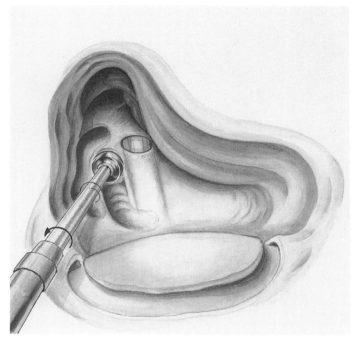

Fig. 12.**29** Lateral and posterior semicircular canals are removed, vestibule is opened, and facial nerve is skeletonized in its tympanic segment.
1 = vestibule opened
2 = subarcuate artery

Fig. 12.**30** Internal auditory canal is skeletonized. Note direction of rotation of burr.

The final removal of bone along the facial nerve is accomplished with a diamond burr. Having removed the labyrinthine bone from posterior to the nerve, the surgeon may then use the side of the diamond burr rather than the end and at all times view the plane between the side of the burr and the facial nerve. This reduces the hazard of injury to the facial nerve, which is very slight with this technique. As the facial nerve is skeletonized, the cribriform area of the superior vestibular nerve entering the vestibule will be seen. It is important to skeletonize the facial nerve adequately so that the vestibule can be seen in this area (Fig. 12.**29**).

Internal Auditory Canal Dissection

After the labyrinthine bone has been removed to the level of the vestibule, dissection of the bone surrounding the internal auditory canal is started (Fig. 12.**30**). This dissection is started along the superior petrosal sinus and then is gradually enlarged in all directions toward the internal auditory canal. The dura of the internal auditory canal is identified posteriorly, as is the dura of the posterior fossa. This bone is gently removed, with care taken to leave an eggshell thickness of bone over the dura of the internal auditory canal and the posterior fossa to prevent injury to the soft tissue. Dissection is carried inferior to the labyrinth, with removal of the retrofacial air cells, until the blueness of the dome of the jugular bulb is seen through the overlying bone.

As the bone posterior to the internal auditory canal is removed, the vestibular aqueduct and the beginning of the endolymphatic sac will be removed. Bone is further removed along the posterior fossa dura beneath the sigmoid sinus. If the sigmoid sinus is overhanging into the mastoid cavity, which makes the dissection difficult, the eggshell covering of bone over the sinus may be removed so that the sinus can be retraced posteriorly. It is good to leave an island of bone (Bill's island) over the dome of the sigmoid sinus to protect it from the rotating burr and retraction of the suction–irrigation at this point.

We complete the dissection around the inferior portion of the internal auditory canal first. This is the area that is farthest from the facial nerve, and we find that completing the dissection here makes orientation to the superior portion of the internal auditory canal easier. Bone removal is continued medially and anteriorly between the dome of the jugular bulb and the internal auditory canal until the cochlear aqueduct is identified.

The cochlear aqueduct is not always readily identifiable. In large tumors it will be occluded at its medial orifice, and spinal fluid is not likely to escape. The cochlear aqueduct enters the posterior fossa directly inferior to the midportion of the internal auditory canal above the jugular bulb. It is an important landmark because it identifies the location of the ninth, tenth, and eleventh

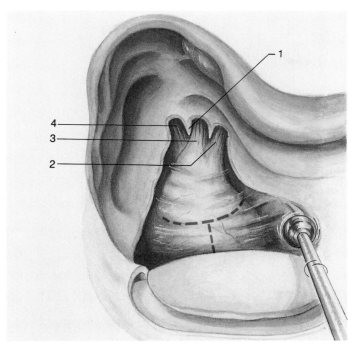

Fig. 12.**31** Superior and inferior vestibular nerves are identified in the internal auditory canal. Note transverse crest between the nerves.

1 = Bill's bar   3 = superior vestibular nerve
2 = inferior vestibular nerve   4 = facial nerve

cranial nerves in the neural compartment of the jugular foramen anterior to the jugular bulb. If the dissection is confined to the area superior to the cochlear aqueduct, these nerves will not be injured.

After the cochlear aqueduct has been identified, bone removal is continued around the internal auditory canal to the porus acousticus until the entire inferior lip of the internal auditory canal is removed. The diamond burr is used for these later parts of the dissection. The bone of the posterior fossa dura is then removed inferiorly until the sigmoid sinus is skeletonized. This completes the dissection inferiorly.

Dissection is then carried superiorly and anteriorly around the internal auditory canal. This bone removal is tedious because the facial nerve often underlies the dura along the anterosuperior aspect of the internal auditory canal. The surgeon must be very careful not to allow the burr to slip into the internal auditory canal. We prefer to remove the entire porus and the medial portion of the internal auditory canal first, leaving the dissection of the lateral end of the internal auditory canal until last. In this way the facial nerve is not exposed until most of the bone removal is completed.

Removal of the superior lip of the porus acousticus is tedious, but it is one of the most important parts of the dissection. If this is not entirely removed, the facial nerve will underlie the ridge of bone at the porus and

will make identification and removal of the tumor from the nerve in this area very difficult. Diamond burrs are used to continue the dissection until two thirds of the porus acousticus is removed. Bone removal is then carried laterally, and the end of the internal auditory canal is exposed.

Dissection of the lateral end of the internal auditory canal begins inferiorly. The singular nerve is first identified, and bone removal done inferiorly then exposes the inferior vestibular nerve. As dissection proceeds superiorly, the transverse crest is identified. The superior aspect of the internal auditory canal is then dissected, and the facial nerve is identified as it exits the internal auditory canal and begins its labyrinthine segment. Finally, the bar of bone (Bill's bar) separating the superior vestibular nerve from the facial nerve is identified. This completes the dissection around the internal auditory canal.

During the dissection of the internal auditory canal, an eggshell thickness of bone was left on the sigmoid sinus and the posterior and middle fossa dura. At this stage this is removed completely, and the surgeon is ready to open the posterior fossa dura to expose the cerebellopontine angle (Fig. 12.**31**). It is noteworthy that until this point all of the dissection has been extradural and the morbidity of the approach has been minimal.

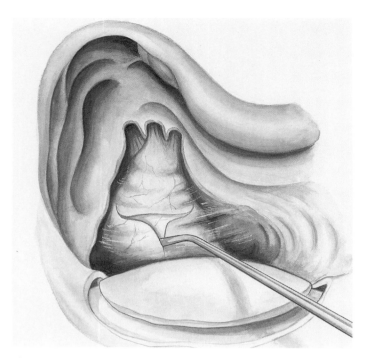

Fig. 12.**32**

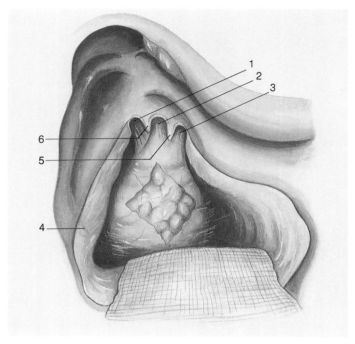

Fig. 12.**33** Facial nerve is identified by localizing Bill's bar. Tumor capsule is incised.

1	=	facial nerve	4	=	dura
2	=	superior vestibular nerve	5	=	transverse crest
3	=	inferior vestibular nerve	6	=	Bill's bar

Dural Incision

The dura of the posterior fossa is then incised over the mid–portion of the internal auditory canal (Fig. 12.**32**). The incision then extends around the porus acousticus superiorly and inferiorly. Care is taken to avoid vessels on the surface of the tumor and anteriorly/superiorly care is exercised to avoid injury to the facial nerve which lies directly beneath the dura in this area. Posteriorly the petrosal vein lies just beneath the dura and insertion of a Rosen elevator will separate underlying blood vessels from the dura prior to incision. Keeping the deep blade of the scissors just beneath the dura prevents injury to underlying blood vessels as the incision progresses. The dural flaps are then retracted superiorly and inferiorly and cottonoids are placed between the tumor and the cerebellum posteriorly.

An arachnoid cyst is often encountered around the posterior aspect of the tumor. The cyst is opened and the plane of the tumor and cerebellum is further developed around the posterior aspects of the tumor. Cottonoids are advanced into this plane. It is extremely important to accurately develop this plane, since doing so will separate the major vessels of the cerebellopontine angle from the tumor. The operating microscope makes it possible to follow this proper plane and to a large extent has eliminated the major bleeding often associated with cerebellopontine angle tumor removal.

Bleeding from the proximal portion of the petrosal vein can be controlled by a clip. However, bleeding from the superior petrosal sinus is often much more difficult to manage. One means of controlling this bleeding is to fill the superior petrosal sinus with Surgicel. Another technique is to pack Surgicel extradurally over the petrous ridge at the anterior limit of the dissection. This produces extradural compression of the superior petrosal sinus and thus controls proximal bleeding. Distal back–bleeding from the sinus is controlled by placing a clip on the sinus between the sinodural angle, where it enters the sigmoid sinus, and the petrosal vein.

Partial Tumor Removal

In the case of a small tumor the surgeon can begin development of the inferior and superior planes of the tumor. With a medium or large tumor it is better to begin intracapsular removal of the tumor to reduce its size before developing the other planes.

The posterior surface of the tumor is first carefully inspected for nerve bundles. On rare occasions the facial nerve may lie on the posterior surface of a tumor. After it has been determined that no nerve bundles are present on the posterior surface of the tumor, the capsule of the tumor is incised (Fig. 12.**33**), and intracapsular removal of the tumor is begun with the House/Urban dissector (Fig. 12.**34**). During intracapsular removal of the

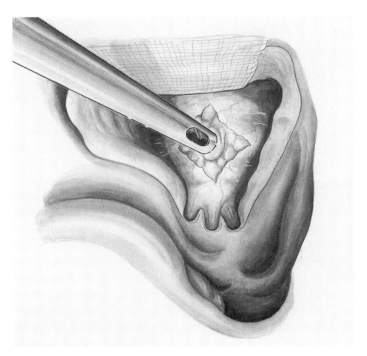

Fig. 12.**35** House/Urban rotating vacuum dissector starts gutting the tumor within its capsule.

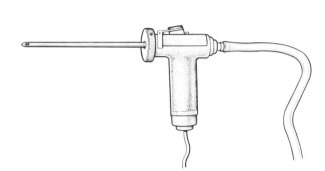

Fig. 12.**34** House/Urban dissector. The rotating blade cuts small pieces of tissue pulled into it by suction.

tumor it is important to avoid excessive movement and pressure on the tumor because this may stretch and injure the facial nerve (Fig. 12.**35**).

Isolating the Tumor

Once the interior of the tumor has been extensively gutted, the development of the tumor plane is carried out further inferiorly and superiorly. Small cottonoids are used to develop the plane of the tumor and to separate surrounding structures. Avoidance of injury to surrounding structures is greatly facilitated by use of the fenestrated neurotologic suction tip. Since the tumor has been extensively gutted, the capsule is displaced into the interior of the tumor. The surface of the capsule is then followed to the brainstem. We attempt to develop the posterior aspect of the tumor to the point where it can be seen at the brainstem, and cottonoids are placed into this plane.

Inferiorly, an attempt is made to localize the ninth cranial nerve, which can be best identified near its exit medial to the jugular bulb. In larger tumors the ninth cranial nerve may be stretched over the surface of the tumor. This plane is carefully developed, and the ninth cranial nerve is isolated from the field with cottonoids. During manipulation of the ninth and tenth cranial nerves there are often changes in the pulse rate. If these occur, we stop manipulation of the nerves and allow the vital signs to stabilize.

Often large vessels are located around the inferior aspect of the tumor, and these must be carefully separated from the tumor capsule and preserved. After the inferior aspect of the tumor has been developed down to the brainstem, additional debulking of the tumor and removal of a portion of the capsule can be completed.

The superior aspect of the tumor capsule is next developed. The petrosal vein will be encountered in this location and must be carefully separated from the tumor. The facial nerve usually lies more anteriorly, but it is not unusual for it to come over the top of the tumor. The fifth cranial nerve is identified at the medial superior aspect of the tumor, and all these structures are carefully separated from the capsule and packed away from the field with cottonoids (Fig. 12.**36**).

Identification of the Facial Nerve

The lateral end of the internal auditory canal is dissected, and the plane of the facial nerve is established. During bone removal the vertical crest of bone (Bill's bar) separating the facial nerve from the superior vestibular nerve has been clearly identified. A long fine hook is then inserted lateral to Bill's bar to identify the superior vestibular nerve. The hook is gently passed medially and slightly anteriorly until it falls over Bill's bar into the facial nerve canal, which positively identifies the facial nerve. The hook is then withdrawn and placed beneath the superior vestibular nerve, turned inferiorly, and the superior vestibular nerve is pulled out from its canal (Fig. 12.**37**). At this point the underlying facial nerve is seen, and the plane of the facial nerve from the tumor is definitely identified. Positive identification of the facial nerve at the lateral end of the internal auditory canal is one of the principal advantages of the translabyrinthine approach. Continuous intraoperative facial nerve monitoring is routinely used.

Next the hook is used to remove the inferior vestibular nerve, and the dura of the internal auditory canal is opened along the inferior aspect of the tumor. The dura is also opened superiorly, with great care taken to avoid the facial nerve. Incision of the dura of the internal auditory canal frees the tumor so that it can be gently retracted posteriorly away from the facial nerve. The Rosen separator and hooks are used to carefully develop the plane between the facial nerve and the tumor. The tumor is gently retracted posteriorly to bring this plane into relief. After the lateral end of the facial nerve has been definitely identified and separated from the tumor, all tumor remnants are removed from the lateral end of the internal auditory canal. The cochlear nerve is usually removed along with the tumor and the vestibular nerve.

Facial Nerve Dissection

Usually it is relatively easy to develop the plane along the facial nerve within the internal auditory canal, but considerable difficulty often arises when the porus acousticus is reached. Dural adhesions to the surface of the tumor at the porus acousticus invariably make dissection of the facial nerve from the tumor very difficult

in this area. The facial nerve usually can be followed past the area of adhesions without undue difficulty. At times, however, this plane becomes very difficult, and we rotate the tumor posteriorly to identify the facial nerve on the tumor medially nearer the brainstem. The facial nerve is then followed medially to laterally until the plane becomes apparent, and tumor removal can be completed at the porus acousticus (Fig. 12.**38**). During this entire dissection the surgeon must be careful not to push the tumor forward or medially which would stretch the facial nerve. It is better to gently retract the tumor posteriorly and laterally removing the stretch from the facial nerve.

Completion of Tumor Removal

Once the facial nerve has been separated from the tumor to the brainstem, the bulk of the tumor is removed with the House/Urban dissector, leaving only a small portion of tumor attached to the brainstem (Fig. 12.**39**). Removing the bulk of the tumor allows greater visibility of the tumor–brainstem plane. The last bit of tumor is then removed from the brainstem under direct vision. The adhesions between the tumor and the brainstem are usually not dense and can be easily separated. Bleeding in this area is controlled with bipolar cautery. Only those vessels that actually enter the tumor capsule are coagulated; the others are carefully freed from the tumor capsule. Often a small artery accompanies the eighth cranial nerve into the tumor. Bleeding from this artery is controlled by placing a clip on the eighth nerve and contained artery or by bipolar coagulation.

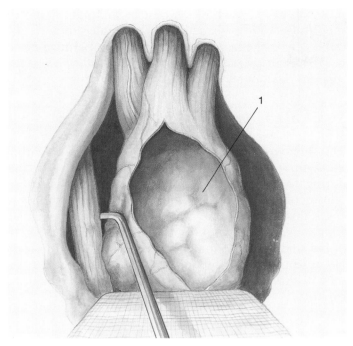

Fig. 12.**36**   Tumor is gutted and only the capsule remains. Note the size of the tumor as compared to Fig. 12.**32**.
1   =   gutted tumor, only capsule remains

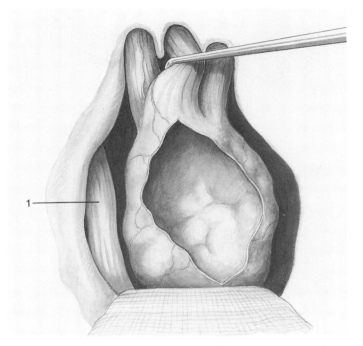

Fig. 12.**37**   Superior and inferior vestibular nerves are cut above the level of the transverse crest. Note the ninth nerve and the fifth nerve in the posterior fossa.
1   =   V nerve

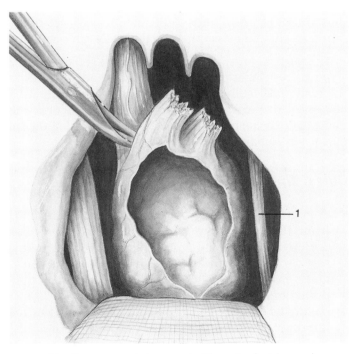

Fig. 12.**38**   Tumor capsule is separated from the facial nerve by careful cutting of the arachnoid sheath.
1   =   IX nerve

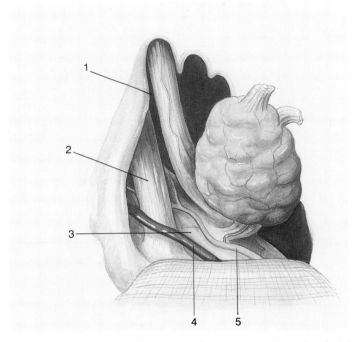

Fig. 12.**39**   Tumor capsule is carefully separated from the facial nerve.
1   =   remnants of arachnoid
2   =   V nerve
3   =   brainstem
4   =   petrosal vein
5   =   anterior inferior cerebellar artery

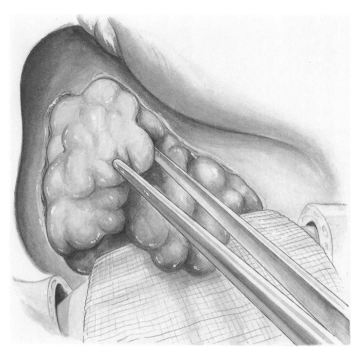

Fig. 12.**40**

Hemostasis and Closure

After total tumor removal the wound is profusely irrigated with Ringer's solution to remove any blood clots. The cottonoids are then removed, and all bleeding points are controlled with either clips or bipolar cautery. Absolute hemostasis must be obtained, and this may require considerable time and effort. It is best to control bleeding with clipping or cautery rather than Surgicel packing. Using large amounts of Surgicel must be avoided because this substance expands considerably with fluid absorption and can consequently cause pressure on surrounding vessels or the brainstem.

After hemostasis is complete, the dura is sutured and the area of the mastoidectomy obliterated with strips of fat taken from the abdomen. A small piece of muscle is used to obliterate the additus. The mastoid cavity is then filled to the surface of the cortex with strips of abdominal fat (Fig. 12.**40**), and the postauricular incision is closed in layers. The skin is closed with interrupted subcuticular sutures. The patient is kept on the operating table until responding well and then is transferred directly to the intensive are unit.

Modifications

There have been few modifications to the approach as originally described by Dr. William House. Some surgeons use the ultrasonic aspirator to debulk the tumor while others employ the CO_2 laser for the same pur-

pose. We have tried both of these techniques but prefer the House/Urban dissector, or in smaller tumors, debulking with the large cup forceps. Intraoperative facial nerve monitoring has been a significant addition to the surgical procedure.

Surgical Landmarks and Danger Points

The sigmoid sinus may be in a variable location within the temporal bone. An unusual problem that can occur during the translabyrinthine approach is inadvertent tearing of the sigmoid sinus or the jugular bulb. In most cases, this can be readily controlled by Surgicel packing. Care must be taken not to pack Surgicel into the lumen of the sinus or a portion of it may embolize to the lung. Because of the recumbent position of the patient, air embolism is not a problem. Blood loss, however, can be rapid.

If bleeding continues despite careful placement of Surgicel packs (this usually occurs only if a tear in the sinus is large), it may need to be controlled by occluding the sinus with extraluminal packing at the sinodural angle and by tying the jugular vein in the neck. Tying this vein prevents embolization of the Surgicel. Bleeding may still occur from the inferior petrosal sinus, however, and care must be taken not to pack the area of the inferior petrosal sinus too firmly or paralysis of the ninth, tenth, and eleventh cranial nerves can result.

The vertical crest of bone (Bill's bar) separating the superior vestibular nerve from the facial nerve is a critical landmark in the translabyrinthine approach. It is necessary to positively identify Bill's bar in order to identify the facial nerve and begin the removal of the superior vestibular nerve and tumor from it.

Rules, Tips, and Pitfalls

- A common pitfall is not to remove adequate bone from the middle fossa plate and posterior fossa thereby reducing the overall exposure. It is necessary to do a wide mastoidectomy in order to gain adequate exposure to the deeper portions of the temporal bone.
- Failure to identify Bill's bar at the lateral end of the internal auditory canal can result in confusion of the location of the facial nerve with inadvertent injury. It is best to identify the facial nerve in its normal location distal to the internal auditory canal to positively identify it.
- Inadequate removal of the superior lip of the internal auditory canal will hide the facial nerve in the area of the porus acousticus. It is necessary to remove $2/3$ of the circumference of the lip of the internal auditory canal to adequate expose the facial nerve at the porus.

- Meticulous sharp dissection of the tumor from the facial nerve is necessary to avoid injury to the nerve. It is particularly important not to place lateral to medial traction on the facial nerve as it is very sensitive to traction injury at the fundus of the internal auditory canal. The nerve is always very adherent to the tumor in the area of the porus acousticus. At times, it is better to identify the facial nerve medially and then dissect from medial to laterally to remove the tumor from the nerve in the area of the porus.
- Meticulous hemostasis must be secured before closure to avoid postoperative hematoma.

Postoperative Management

The patient is observed in the intensive care unit for a period of 36 hours. Steroids or antibiotics are not routinely utilized. In some patients with very large tumors that exhibit signs of cerebellar swelling we do use steroids. The mastoid dressing remains in place for four days and the patient is instructed not to lift or strain during the early postoperative period.

Complications and Management

Although rare, the most common early postoperative complication is a hematoma in the cerebellopontine angle. This is manifested by signs of cerebellopontine angle pressure and is managed by immediate opening of the wound and removal of the fat in the intensive care unit. This is a further advantage of the translabyrinthine approach in that the angle may be rapidly decompressed for this uncommon complication. The patient is then taken to surgery where complete hemostasis is obtained and the wound again closed with abdominal fat.

Meningitis is an uncommon complication and is managed in the usual manner with appropriate antibiotics following culture and identification of the offending organism.

If facial weakness occurs, eye care is provided by a consulting ophthalmologist. Conservative measures are first utilized including artificial tears, moisture chambers and soft contact lens. If these measures fail to provide adequate corneal protection a palpebral spring is inserted. The latter procedure is more commonly necessary when there is a concomitant fifth nerve deficit with corneal anesthesia. The average hospitalization is 6–7 days. The patient is advised to avoid heavy lifting or strenuous activity for approximately 3 weeks.

Results of Surgery

The House Ear Clinic series numbers over 3,200 acoustic tumors as of September 1994. The results in the first 700 patients have been previously published (House and Leutje, 1979). With experience and refinements in technique the results have improved throughout the years.

Most recently we have studied the results in 216 patients who underwent surgery for acoustic tumor in 1980 and 1981. The average age of these patients was 47.3 years, and the group was equally divided as male and female.

Tumor size, measured on cranial CT, has been reported as extension into the cerebellopontine angle. Small tumors are those that extend less than 0.5 cm into the cerebellopontine angle; 20 of the 216 (9%) fit this category. Medium tumors, which are considered as those that extend from 0.5 to 2.0 cm into the cerebellopontine angle, numbered 110 (51%). Large tumors are those extending from 2 to 4 cm into the cerebellopontine angle; this group included 67 (31%) of the tumors. Tumors that extend more than 4 cm into the cerebellopontine angle are considered to be giant tumors; 19 patients (9%) had tumors of this size.

The average length of surgery was 3 hours and 12 minutes. There was one death in this series (0.4%). The patient had a postoperative hemorrhage and, despite early evacuation of the clot, sustained brainstem infarction and died.

Facial nerve function was studied one year after surgery. At that time 180 patients (83%) had normal facial function. There was a partial paralysis in 34 patients (16%). In four of these patients the facial nerve had been divided during tumor removal; they underwent immediate facial nerve anastomosis in the cerebellopontine angle and had satisfactory recovery of facial function. Two patients had total facial paralysis one year after surgery; they then underwent hypoglossal facial anastomosis and had satisfactory recovery of facial function.

There was a direct correlation between preservation of normal facial nerve function and size of tumor. All 20 patients with small tumors had normal facial function at one year. Of the patients with medium–sized tumors, 85% had normal facial function. In the group with large tumors, 81% of the patients had normal facial function. Of those patients with giant tumors, 63% had normal facial function one year after surgery. Despite this correlation, it must be noted that some patients with relatively small tumors may have invasion of the facial nerve and thus incomplete recovery. Therefore the surgeon must be careful not to be overly optimistic in patient discussion even when the tumor is a small one.

Alternative Techniques

As previously discussed, the middle fossa and retrosigmoid approaches are alternatives to translabyrinthine acoustic tumor removal.

Conclusion

The translabyrinthine approach is the preferred method for removal of all sizes of acoustic tumors when there is non–serviceable hearing.

References

Brackmann D E. Fenestrated suction for neuro-otologic surgery, Trans Am Acad Ophthalmol Otolaryngol 1977; 84:975.

Brackmann D E, et al. Acoustic neuromas: middle fossa and translabyrinthine removal. In Rand RW (ed): Microneurosurgery, St. Louis: C V Mosby Company, 311–334, 1985.

Brackmann D E, Hitselberger W E, Robinson J V. Facial nerve repair in cerebellopontine angle surgery. Ann Otol Rhinol Laryngol 1978; 87:722–7.

Brackmann D E, House J R III, Hitselberger W E. Technical modifications to the middle fossa craniotomy approach in removal of acoustic neuromas. Am J Otol 1994; 15:614–9.

House W F, Leutje C M (eds): Acoustic Tumors, Vol. II: Management. Baltimore: University Park Press, 1979.

Shelton C, Brackmann D E, House W F, Hitselberger W E. Middle fossa acoustic tumor surgery: Results in 106 cases. Laryngoscope 1989; 99:405–8.

13 Basic Aspects of Neurosurgical Procedures in the Head Region

Frank Marguth † and Vladimir Olteanu-Nerbe

This chapter deals with the close relationships that exist between the "neighboring" specialities of otolaryngology and neurosurgery. It is intended to guide the head and neck surgeon who enters the neurosurgical domain and to furnish information on procedures in the borderline area between the specialities. With this in view, we outline basic surgical approaches to the cranial interior and briefly describe some specific procedures that are of special interest to the head and neck surgeon.

Principles of Surgery

Instrumentation

The hallmark of modern neurosurgery is the operating microscope. Its advantages include the capacity for high magnification of minute structures, stereoscopic vision, and good illumination deep in the surgical cavity. Among the many microscopes that are commercially available, the Contraves-type microscopes are particularly useful for neurosurgical applications. Their maneuverability is enhanced by electromagnetic locks built into the various articulations of the stand, and the field–of–view position can be finely adjusted by activating a mouth switch—a feature that is especially useful in prolonged operations.

The patient's head is positioned and fixed with a Mayfield clamp. With its three–point fixation system and articulated design, this device can immobilize the head in almost any desired position with few risks of pressure injury to soft tissues.

Microsurgical instruments permit the surgeon to carry out deep dissections in very small spaces: forceps, scissors, and hooks of varying lengths and shapes include self–retaining retractors that replace the human hand. Hemostasis is accomplished with bipolar coagulation. Different bipolar forceps have essentially the same design as microforceps and, to save time, can be used for dissecting very fine structures.

Increasingly, cranial burrs are supplemented by microdrills for gaining access to the skull base. These allow for an extremely precise, place–sparing approach.

Some tumors can be removed less traumatically by supplementing the standard instrument sets with accessories such as ultrasonic aspirator and laser beams. These devices are no substitute for precise microsurgical technique, however.

Preoperative Preparations

Patients with intracranial mass lesions are premedicated with steroids to prevent cerebral edema. The scalp in the operative area is shaved and washed. The eyebrows should not be shaved because of the poor cosmetic result.

Two intravenous lines, one central and one peripheral, are established so that fluid can be administered in the event of heavy blood loss. After general anesthesia has been induced, the eyes are protected with a bland ophthalmic ointment, and a compress is placed over the closed eyelids.

The head is immobilized with the Mayfield clamp. If the patient is placed in the lateral position, pillows are placed between the patient's legs, and the site where the common peroneal nerve crosses the neck of the fibula is protected with padding. If a prone position is used, the shoulders and pelvis are supported and elevated laterally to create room for respiratory excursions. Any pressure on the jugular vein should be avoided, as this would raise the intracranial pressure.

The sitting position is advantageous for operations on the posterior cranial fossa, as it provides better visibility and lowers the cranial venous pressure, with reduction of operative blood loss. The disadvantages of this position include risk of venous air embolism and possible subdural hematoma formation in the supratentorial space due to rapid intracranial decompression.

The line incision for the proposed skin flap is marked with dye. The flap should be based on a broad vascular pedicle to preserve the flap circulation. Then a local anesthetic agent or physiologic saline solution is injected beneath the scalp. This produces a compressive effect that aids in hemostasis—an effect that is enhanced by the addition of octapressin.

Operative Technique

Craniotomy and Craniectomy

Supratentorial Craniotomy

A unifrontal or bifrontal flap should be placed behind the hairline for cosmetic reasons (Figs. 13.**1** and 13.**2**). Special care is taken to protect the frontal branch of the facial nerve during dissection and elevation of the flap. If the frontal sinus is entered during the sawing of a frontal bone flap, the mucosal lining should be removed and the sinus occluded with muscle, periosteum, or fascia so that it does not communicate with the cranial interior. It is customary to use a hinged bone flap for a temporal or parietal craniotomy (Fig. 13.**3** and 13.**4**) and a free, completely detached bone flap for an occipital craniotomy (Fig. 13.**5**).

Figure 13.**6** shows the incision for a frontotemporal flap. As the scalp is incised, digital pressure is maintained to control bleeding until hemostatic clips can be applied (Fig. 13.**7**). We use hemostats on the galea and scalp clips on the skin. In frontal and temporal operations, the superficial temporal artery is ligated. In frontal and occipital craniotomies, the skin and galea are dissected from the periosteum (Fig. 13.**8**), and burr holes are placed at equally spaced intervals to define the boundaries of the craniotomy (Fig. 13.**9**). Figure 13.**10** illustrates how the Gigli saw (alternative: side-cutting drill) is used so saw out the bone flap. The areas over the middle meningeal artery and near the dural sinus are sawed last so that, if hemorrhage occurs, the bone flap can be quickly raised and hemostasis secured. A bone flap that is to be hinged frontally or temporally is

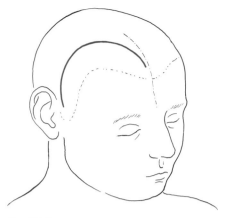

Fig. 13.**1**

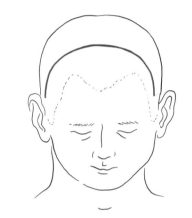

Fig. 13.**2**

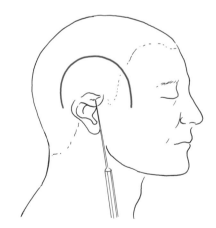

Fig. 13.**3**

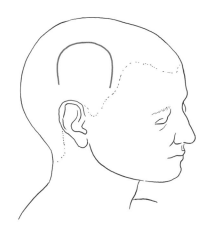

Fig. 13.**4**

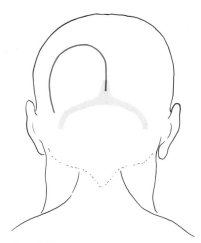

Fig. 13.**5**

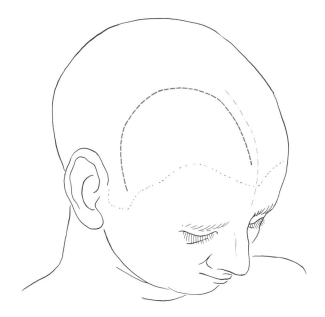

Fig. 13.**6**

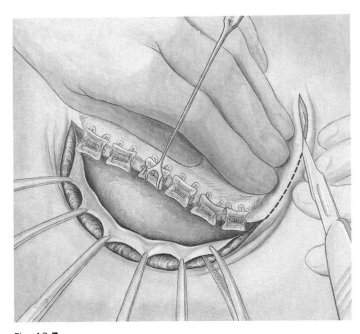

Fig. 13.**7**

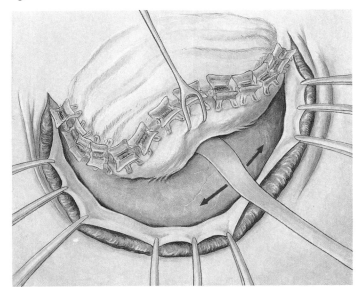

Fig. 13.**8**

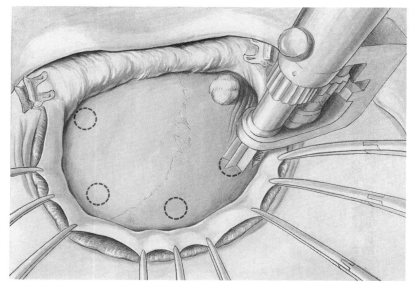

Fig. 13.**9**

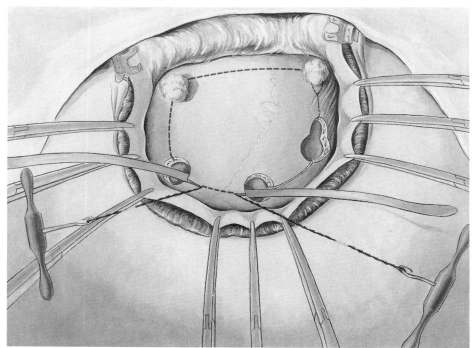

Fig. 13.**10**

ronguered and then broken across the basal side (Fig. 13.**11**). It is left attached to the temporalis muscle when raised (Fig. 13.**12**). The muscle is separated from the underlying bone before the basal part of the craniotomy is extended with a ronguer. Bleeding from the cut edge of the bone is controlled with sterile bone wax (Fig. 13.**13**).

The bone flap is wrapped in moist gauze for the remainder of the operation. The craniotomy can be extended temporally with ronguers to relieve intracranial tension. Before the dura is opened, it is carefully tacked up to the galea and periosteum with interrupted sutures

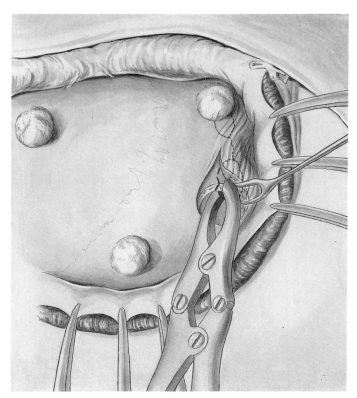

Fig. 13.**11**

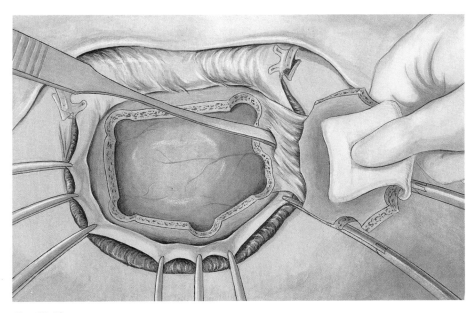

Fig. 13.**12**

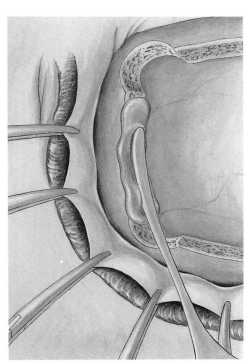

Fig. 13.**13**

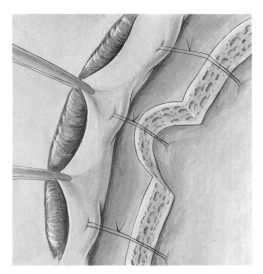

Fig. 13.**14**

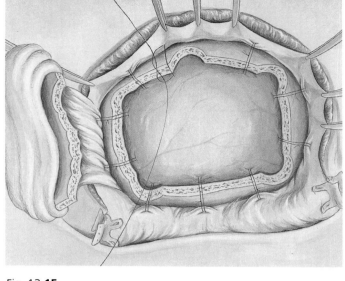

Fig. 13.**15**

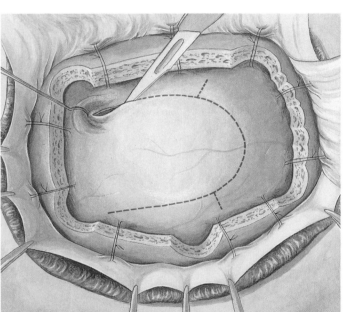

Fig. 13.**16**

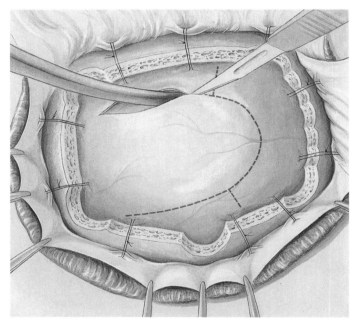

Fig. 13.**17**

(Fig. 13.**14** and 13.**15**). These tack–up sutures serve to control dural bleeding and keep postoperative epidural bleeding from transcending the boundaries of the craniotomy. The cutaneous and bony margins are covered with moist gauze. Then the dura is picked up with a sharp hook and incised with a scalpel (Fig. 13.**16**). The dural opening is extended with a scalpel or scissors while the underlying brain is protected with a grooved probe or spatula (Fig. 13.**17**). The dural flap is always based toward the sinus. Small bleeding points on the cut edge of the dura, which can be identified more clearly

by gently irrigating the dural edge with clear fluid, are cauterized with bipolar forceps. Veins bridging from the brain to the dural sinuses should be preserved if possible. Bleeding from pacchionian granulations or the dural sinuses can generally be controlled by applying strips of gelatin sponge or by temporary compression. The sponge may have to be tacked to the bleeding sinus with sutures. Figures 13.**18** and 13.**19** illustrate how a tear in the wall of the sagittal sinus can be patched with a stamp of muscle tissue or gelatin sponge. Rarely, sinus bleeding is so heavy that it may be neces-

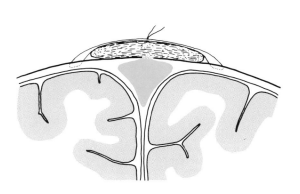

Fig. 13.**18**

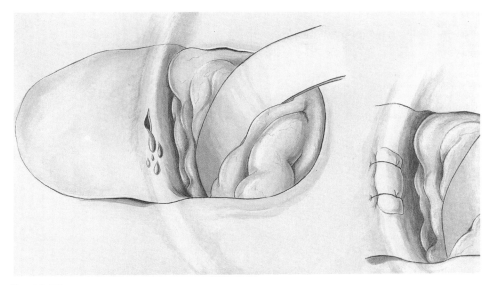

Fig. 13.**19**

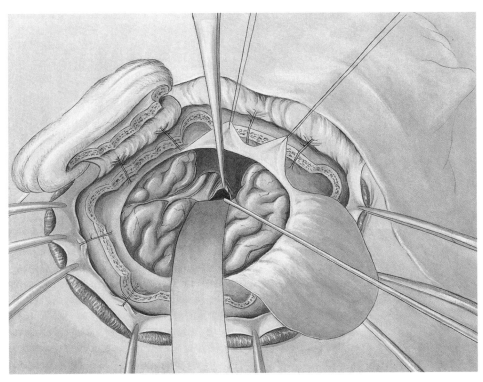

Fig. 13.**20**

sary to underrun and ligate the sinus. The superior sagittal sinus can be ligated in its anterior third without deleterious effects, but ligation at more posterior sites generally leads to severe neurologic deficits due to the obstruction of venous outflow. Extracerebral lesions are exposed by retracting the brain with self–retaining retractors. Cotton patties or gelatin sponges are placed between the retractor and brain to protect the brain from injury. Figure 13.20 illustrates a left–sided frontal craniotomy. Following elevation of the dural flap, the dissection proceeds toward the subfrontal area, and cere-

brospinal fluid (CSF) is aspirated from the opened basal cisterns. The left optic nerve and, lateral to it, the left internal carotid artery are visible within the opened cistern. Removing CSF by aspirating it from the basal cisterns or by lumbar drainage can gain valuable space for exposure of the lesion. The intravenous administration of hypertonic solutions can also facilitate the exposure of intracranial, extracranial lesions. Large lesions deep within the brain are manifested by widening of the overlying gyri, and many can be located by palpating the cerebral cortex with the moistened gloved finger.

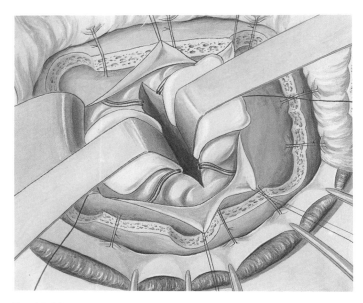

Fig. 13.**21**

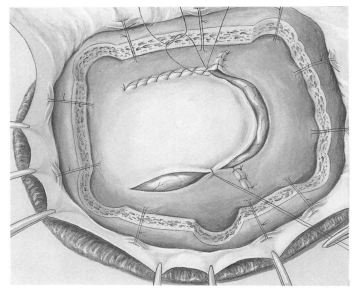

Fig. 13.**22**

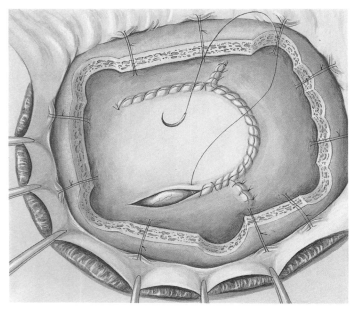

Fig. 13.**23**

Small, nonpalpable lesions can be located intraoperatively with ultrasound probes or preoperatively by the stereotactic insertion of a guide cannula.

The tumor is generally approached by the most direct route, using bipolar coagulation to expose the lesion while preserving larger blood vessels and surrounding tissues. To preserve cortical tissue, the arachnoid is first incised along a gyrus, then very fine self–retaining retractors are inserted into the subarachnoid space down to the mass, which is approached practically on an extracerebral plane. The adjacent cortex is protected with cotton strips. If cortical vessels must be divided, they are first cauterized with the bipolar forceps. Further dissection within the white matter is performed bluntly, using brain retractors to develop an adequate plane (Fig. 13.**21**). Bleeding sites in the white matter are cauterized. Moist cotton strips beneath the retractors compress bleeding capillaries and facilitate demarcation of the tissue during retraction. Patties placed in deeper areas are tagged with sutures that are brought out through the incision. Gentle irrigation of the surgical cavity with fluid warmed to 37 °C is helpful for detecting residual bleeding sites. If the ventricle is breached during the operation, the perforation site must be covered with cotton for the rest of the procedure; this will keep blood from entering the ventricular system and perhaps causing obstructive hydrocephalus. When the intracerebral surgery has been completed and all residual bleeding meticulously controlled, watertight closure of the dura is carried out (Figs. 13.**22** and 13.**23**).

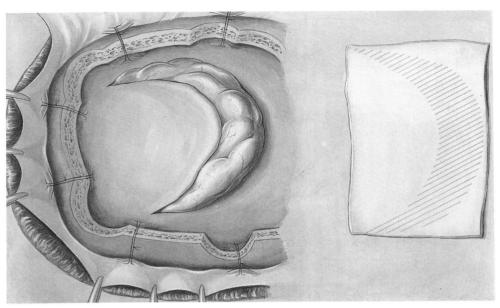

Fig. 13.**24**

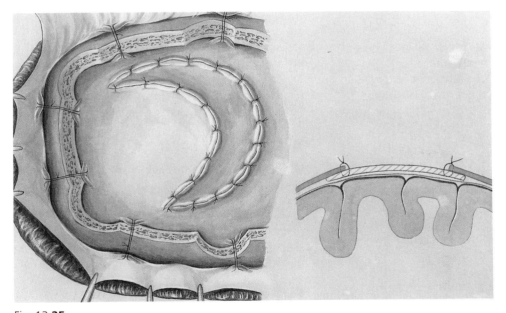

Fig. 13.**25**

If a dural defect has been created by the excision of involved dura or the laceration of very thin dura, or if dural decompression is required, the dural defect can be repaired using periosteum, fascia lata, lyophilized dura, or lyophilized equine pericardium. The principle of the duraplasty is illustrated in Figures 13.**24** and 13.**25**. A watertight dural closure is important for preventing leakage of CSF.

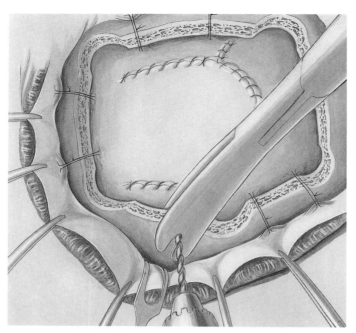

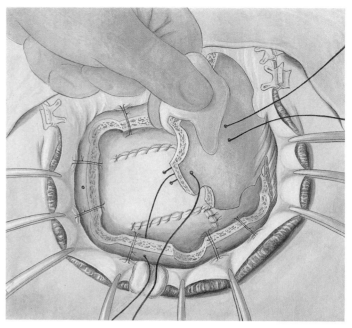

Fig. 13.**26**

Fig. 13.**27**

Drill holes are made at 3 to 5 sites in the craniotomy rim and in the bone flap for subsequent reattachment of the flap with Dexon or silk threads. The Okonek protector, shown in Figure 13.**26**, is placed beneath the bone margin to shield the dura from the drill bit. Following the placement of an epidural suction drain (not pictured), the bone flap is replaced and secured. In Figure 13.**27** the fixation sutures have been passed through the drill holes in the bone flap. Two additional holes have been drilled through the center of the bone flap for tacking the dura to the flap. This "tending suture" is tied after the bone flap has been secured in place (Fig. 13.**28**). If there is marked cerebral swelling, replacement of the bone flap may be deferred in order to relieve pressure. The bone flap is placed in sterile wrapping, deep frozen, and may be replaced later when swelling has subsided or can serve as a model for a methylmethacrylate cranioplasty. Cranial defects can also be reconstructed with stainless wire mesh. The soft–tissue wound is closed in layers (Fig. 13.**29**), using absorbable suture material for the muscle and subcutaneous tissue, and an adhesive dressing is applied.

Subtentorial Craniotomy

Before performing surgery in the posterior fossa, we generally place a burr hole in the right frontal area, open the dura, and coagulate the cerebral surface at one point. This prepares the way for a ventricular puncture to relieve obstructive hydrocephalus that may result from postoperative swelling or hemorrhage. Timely decompression can prevent the development of a potentially life–threatening midbrain herniation. The

posterior fossa is approached through a linear incision placed either on the midline (for centrally located lesions, Fig. 13.**30**) or adjacent to the midline (for more lateral lesions). A third possibility is the lateral retromastoid exposure for surgery in the area of the cerebellopontine angle (Fig. 13.**31**). This approach is described elsewhere in the book (see pages 313 ff).

The muscles are stripped aside from the occipital squama, and the bone over the cerebellar hemispheres is removed with ronguers after the placement of multiple burr holes. The foramen magnum and the posterior arch of the atlas are routinely removed as well (Fig. 13.**32**) to prevent postoperative impaction of the cerebellar tonsils in the foramen magnum.

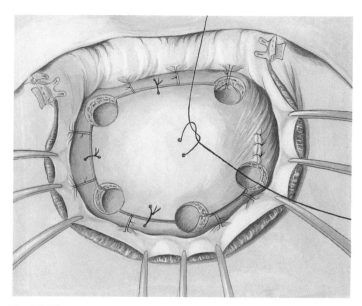

Fig. 13.**28**

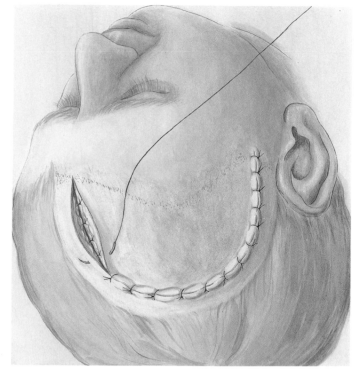

Fig. 13.**29**

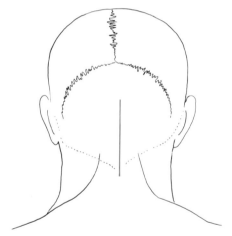

Fig. 13.**30**

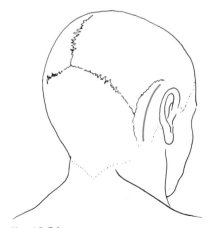

Fig. 13.**31**

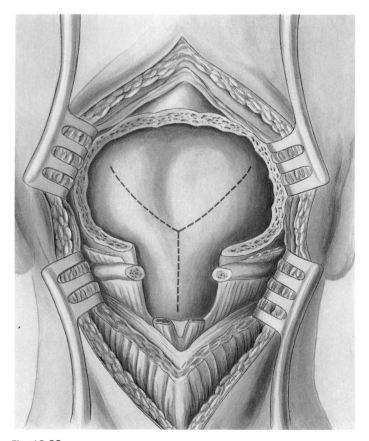

Fig. 13.**32**

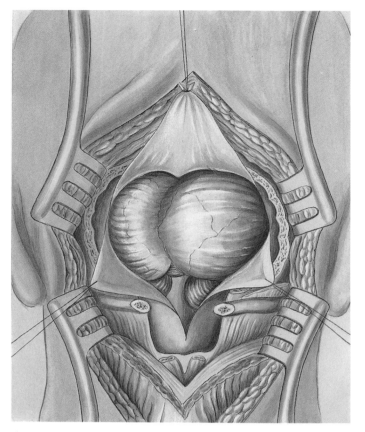

Fig. 13.**33**

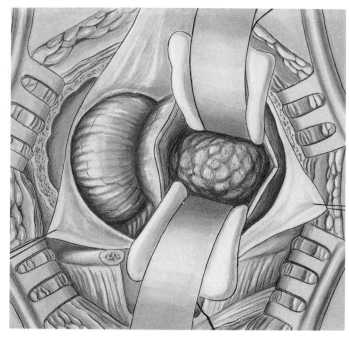

Fig. 13.**34**

The dura is opened with a Y–shaped incision (Fig. 13.**32**), and the dural leaves are retracted with stay sutures (Fig. 13.**33**) to expose the cerebellar hemispheres. The intracerebellar lesion in Figure 13.**33** is manifested by prominence of the right cerebellar hemisphere, a shift of the midline to the opposite side, and a low position of the right cerebellar tonsil. After incision of the cortex, the dissection proceeds deeply to expose and isolate the mass (Fig. 13.**34**). After the tumor has been removed, the dura is closed in a watertight fashion.

Notable risks associated with exposure of the posterior fossa are injury to the vertebral artery during removal of the arch of the atlas and tearing of the transverse and sigmoid sinuses or other major veins, which can lead to life–threatening air embolism. The prevention or early detection of these complications is aided by increasing the expiratory pressure, by repeated compression of the jugular veins, and by attaching an ultrasound probe at the level of the heart. Opening the mastoid air cells can provide a route for leakage of CSF through the middle ear via the eustachian tube, so any mastoid cells exposed during the operation should be occluded with wax or fascia and fibrin glue.

Burr Hole Trephination

Frontal burr holes (Fig. 13.**35**) provide access for the placement of an external ventricular drain, for relieving an acute obstruction to CSF circulation following surgery in the posterior fossa, for decompression, and for the implantation of valves. If possible, burr holes are placed on the side of the nondominant hemisphere, which is generally the right side. Enlarged burr holes can additionally be placed at any desired site (parietal, temporal, occipital, etc.) for the treatment of chronic subdural hematomas and intracranial abscesses (Fig. 13.**36**). In exceptional cases, an enlarged burr hole may be considered for the removal of circumscribed contusional hemorrhages. Frontal burr holes are positioned on or anterior to the coronal suture, 3–4 cm from the midline. Occipital burr holes are placed on the lambdoid suture 3–4 cm from the midline (Fig. 13.**37**). Parietal burr holes are placed at the level of the inion, and temporal burr holes may be placed above the ear or in the temporopolar area as required.

The incision is carried all the way to the bone, and the burr hole is cut (Fig. 13.**38**). The exposed dura is

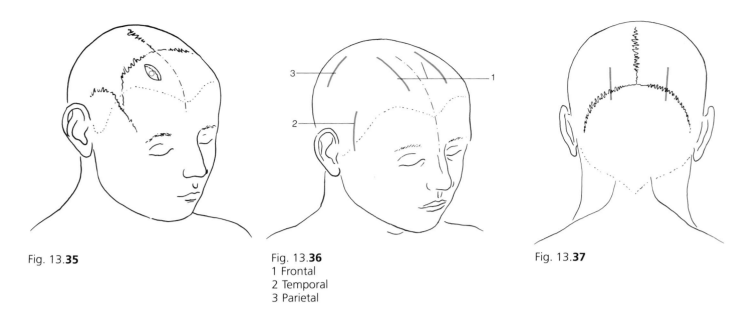

Fig. 13.**35**

Fig. 13.**36**
1 Frontal
2 Temporal
3 Parietal

Fig. 13.**37**

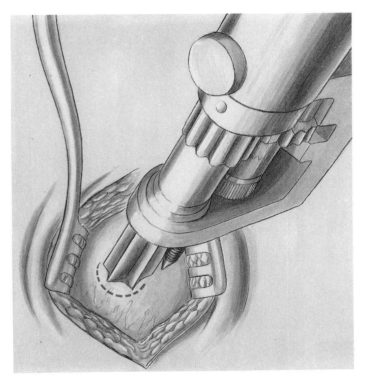

Fig. 13.**38**

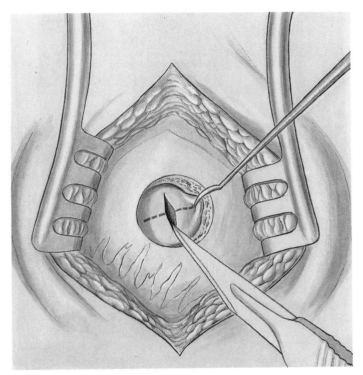

Fig. 13.**39**

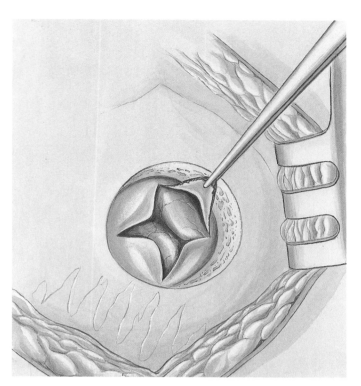

Fig. 13.**40**

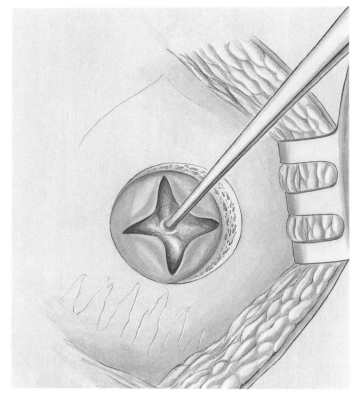

Fig. 13.**41**

opened with a cruciate incision (Fig. 13.**39**). After coagulation of the dural edges (Fig. 13.**40**), the cortex is superficially coagulated at one point (Fig. 13.**41**), simultaneously opening the arachnoid so that subsequent brain trauma will be minimal if ventricular puncture becomes necessary (Fig. 13.**42**). For drainage of the anterior horn, the ventricular catheter is inserted perpendicularly into the brain; for drainage of the posterior horn, the catheter is advanced along an imaginary line between the burr hole and the ipsilateral eye. The ventricular system is shown schematically in Figure 13.**43**. Figure 13.**44** illustrates closure of the soft tissues in layers.

A chronic subdural hematoma is generally evacuated through a parietal burr hole (Fig. 13.**45**) that is ronguered to approximately the size of a 50-cent piece (Fig. 13.**46**). The dura is opened in cruciate fashion and the leaves retracted with stay sutures (Fig. 13.**47**). Figure 13.**48** shows the dural retraction sutures and the incision of the hematoma capsule. The hematoma is then aspirated. Residual hematoma is washed out with Ringer's solution delivered into the subdural space through soft catheters.

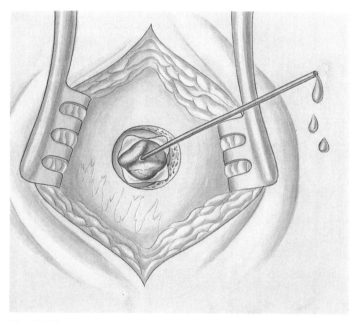

Fig. 13.**42**

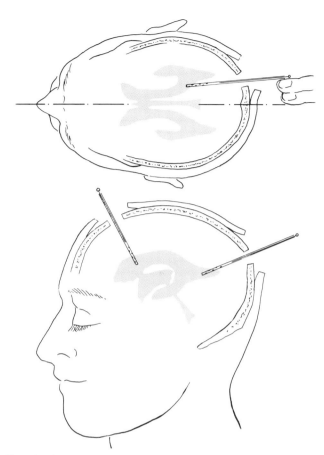

Fig. 13.**43**

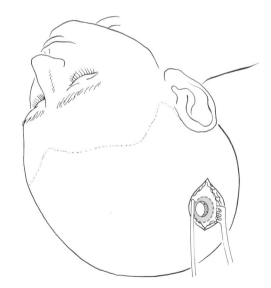

Fig. 13.**45**

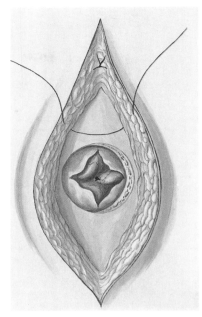

Fig. 13.**44**

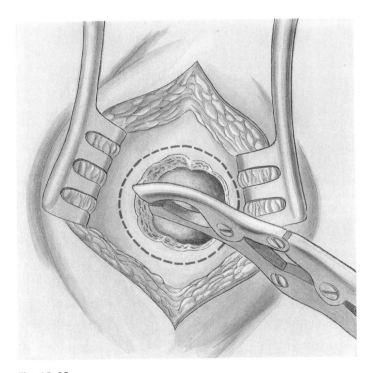

Fig. 13.**46**

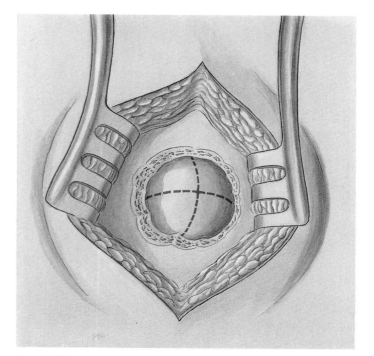

Fig. 13.**47**

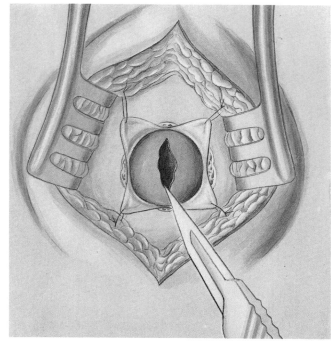

Fig. 13.**48**

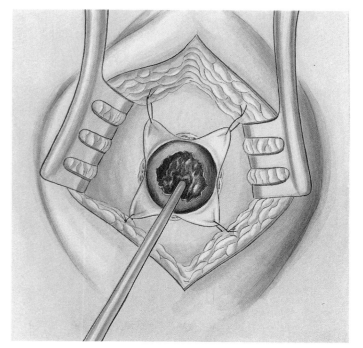

Fig. 13.**49**

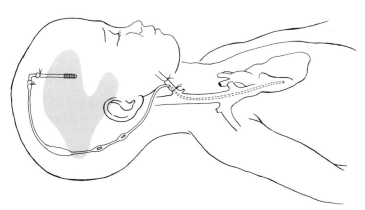

Fig. 13.**50**

Postoperative Care and Complications

Every patient who has undergone brain surgery requires observation in an intensive care unit with monitoring of blood pressure, heart rate, respiration, and temperature. There should be continual monitoring of consciousness level, pupil size, and focal neurologic signs. Unconscious patients should be watched for changes in responsiveness. Reoperation may become necessary in the immediate postoperative period due to a rise in intracranial pressure caused by postoperative hemorrhage or progressive brain edema. These complications are signaled by the appearance or aggravation of focal neurologic deficits, impairment of consciousness, and frequently by a broadening of the blood–pressure amplitude. They may culminate in an impending tentorial or bulbar herniation with pupillary dilation and extensor spasms and possible impairment of respiratory drive and circulatory failure. Measurement of the intracranial pressure has proven especially helpful in these cases. The objective pressure data provide a rational basis for the initiation of diagnostic and perhaps therapeutic measures, including the regulation of antiedematous therapy and decompression by CSF drainage. Besides intraventricular pressure measurements, other epidural and interstitial monitoring systems are currently available. Strict selection criteria are applied to the use of sensor probes due to the risk of infection, and the probes should be left indwelling for no more than 3–5 days. The leakage of CSF in the wound area indicates an inadequate dural closure. Given the associated risk of infection, secondary sutures should be placed to bolster the closure, and the CSF pressure should be reduced by periodic lumbar punctures or the placement of lumbar CSF drains. Persistent leaks should be definitively repaired by reexposing the dura and securing a watertight closure.

Current valve systems function by permitting CSF drainage to the heart only when the CSF pressure reaches a designated value that exceeds the opening pressure of the valve unit. Access to the anterior horn of the right lateral ventricle is gained through a frontal burr hole. A probe is inserted into the lateral ventricle, the intraventricular pressure is measured, and a valve unit for high, moderate, or low pressures is selected according to the measured pressure level. The ventricular catheter is then inserted into the lateral ventricle and connected to the valve unit, which is passed subcutaneously to the right side of the neck and connected to the cardiac catheter, which has been advanced into the right atrium via the facial and internal jugular veins (Fig. 13.**50**). Alternatively, the CSF may be drained into the peritoneum. The principal indication for valve implantation is hydrocephalus in children.

Specific Operations

Head Injuries

The primary damage inflicted by head injuries occurs immediately after the trauma as a result of direct or inertial deformation and shearing of the brain. The main primary effects are cerebral contusion, diffuse axonal damage, cranial fractures, and soft–tissue injuries. The secondary effects of head injuries include hematomas, reactive swelling, and infections, which may be associated with a rise of intracranial pressure and mass effect. Following the primary care of open injuries, the prompt recognition of secondary complications is important for avoiding further irreversible damage.

Once the circulation has been stabilized and a patent airway established, the clinical examination is carried out. Radiographs of the skull and cervical spine are obtained routinely. In patients with impaired consciousness and focal neurologic deficits, a cranial CT or MRI examination is performed (a noncontrast study should suffice). Unconscious patients are intubated prior to CT to avert hypoxic brain damage. Comatose patients with signs of midbrain herniation should additionally be hyperventilated and given dexamethasone (24 mg Decadron) and mannitol (1–2 g/kg) intravenously.

Some authors recommend prophylactic anticonvulsant medication (e.g., diphenylhydantoin, 18 mg/kg). Even with multiple injuries, cranial CT should be a priority study if the patient is hemodynamically stable.

To prevent infection, all open craniocerebral injuries are managed by primary operative treatment, taking care to secure a watertight dural closure. Isolated scalp wounds are also closed primarily. Prophylactic antibiotics are not recommended. Imprimated skull fractures are elevated only if the depression exceeds the width of the calvarium. The value of this measure in preventing posttraumatic seizures is controversial. Larger bone defects can be reconstructed at a later time to improve the cosmetic result.

Epidural Hematoma

The immediate removal of epidural hematomas is generally indicated. Surgery may be deferred only for very thin hematomas that appear "filmlike" on CT or MRI scans. Any secondary increase in the volume of the collection can be detected by frequent follow–up scans. Most epidural hematomas are temporal or frontotemporal, i.e., in close proximity to the damaged middle meningeal artery. The standard approach is through a frontotemporal craniotomy, which affords generous exposure of the sylvian fissure and its surroundings. The patient is positioned supine with the shoulder slightly elevated. The skin incision starts anterior to the tragus, curves frontally 2–3 cm behind the hairline, and terminates about 2 cm short of the midline. Following elevation and reflection of the bone flap hinged on the temporalis muscle, the clotted blood is removed, and the torn middle meningeal artery is identified and occluded. If the vascular injury has occurred at the foramen spinosum and the bleeding vascular stump cannot be coagulated, the foramen is occluded with bone wax. If this does not produce adequate hemostasis, the vascular stump must be exposed at a more proximal site by removing portions of the sphenoid wing. In critical cases involving a large space–occupying hematoma, it is wise first to debulk the hematoma through an enlarged burr hole. When cerebral pulsations have resumed, signifying a reduction of intracranial pressure, the craniotomy may be completed. If cerebral pulsations are not detected after hematoma removal and the dura remains tense, a limited dural opening is carried out to exclude subdural hemorrhage.

The postoperative course following removal of the epidural hematoma is generally marked by a rapid improvement of consciousness level. If progress is unsatisfactory, CT or MRI scans should be taken to exclude postoperative hemorrhage or incomplete evacuation of the hematoma.

Subdural Hematoma

Subdural hematomas are extracerebral collections of blood and serum, clotted or liquid, that usually do not involve the subarachnoid spaces.

Acute Subdural Hematoma

Acute subdural hematomas become evident shortly after the head injury and consist mainly of clotted blood. If the hematoma is very fresh, areas of liquid blood may be noted within the clot at operation. Accordingly, acute subdural hematomas can have varying presentations on CT scans. While the clotted portion appears hyperdense, liquid portions appear hypodense or isodense. The hematoma has a convex–concave configuration and generally extends over the entire hemisphere. Operative treatment is indicated if the hematoma has caused more than a 5–mm shift of the midline. The operative goals are to decompress the brain and secure hemostasis.

Typical sources of subdural hemorrhage are frontobasal and temporobasal contusions and injuries of the vein of Labbé and the cerebral veins passing to the superior sagittal sinus. A broad operative exposure is required. As in the treatment of epidural hematomas, immediate decompression can be effected through an initial burr hole if clinical signs are ominous. After completion of the craniotomy, the dura is opened, and the hematoma is progressively irrigated and lifted away from the underlying brain. Venous and arterial hemorrhages are controlled with bipolar coagulation. Hemostasis of diffuse cortical bleeding is obtained by the application of gelatin sponges, Tabotamp, or collagen powder. If severe brain swelling occurs during the operation, the patient's head and neck position should be checked for obstruction of jugular venous outflow. If an obstruction is not found, implying the presence of a swelling–related volume increase, mannitol is administered intraoperatively, and hyperventilation is initiated.

Chronic Subdural Hematoma

Chronic subdural hematomas generally have a liquid consistency and are weeks to months old. They are most common in elderly patients, and may result from a "trivial" injury in patients who may have an underlying coagulation disorder. Chronic subdural hematomas are frequently missed because of their isodense appearance on CT scans. Absence of an appreciable midline shift on CT suggests that a bilateral hematoma is present. Contrast–enhanced CT or MRI scans can help to confirm this suspicion.

Operative treatment is carried out under general anesthesia in patients who can tolerate it. Local anesthesia is used in high–risk patients. The hematoma is completely evacuated by irrigation through one or more burr holes. For a typical hematoma covering all of the affected hemisphere, the patient is placed in a lateral position. With bilateral hematomas, the larger collection should be evacuated first, but both should be removed in one sitting. Usually the burr hole is placed at a high parietal site, i.e., level with the greatest extent of the hematoma. If the hematoma is not completely liquid, or if it is loculated, a large craniotomy may be needed for sufficient access. An effort is made to avoid venous injury during incision of the dura, since bleeding from these vessels can be difficult to control. After the dura is opened, a greenish–brown capsule may be encountered if the hematoma is old, and this capsule must be opened before the liquid hematoma can be aspirated or washed out with soft silicone catheters. Great care is taken not to damage bridging veins or injure the brain surface. Following evacuation of the hematoma, the subdural space is filled with saline solution to expel significant subdural air accumulations. We insert a soft catheter into the subdural space to drain it externally, without suction, for 48–72 hours. Some authors dispense with postoperative drainage if the brain is sufficiently close to the dural surface following hematoma removal.

Postoperative follow–up CT scans demonstrate a gradual reapproximation of the brain surface to the inner table of the skull. Postoperative complications are rare. Postoperative subdural hemorrhage is a serious complication that necessitates immediate re–exploration through a large craniotomy. Also, extreme care should be taken to avoid injuring the arachnoid during the primary operation, as this can lead to CSF accumulations with a mass effect.

Cerebrospinal Rhinorrhea

The leakage of CSF through the nose is based on a fistulous communication from the subdural space through the dura and skull to the paranasal sinuses. Most cases have a traumatic etiology. Spontaneous, non-traumatic CSF rhinorrhea can result from congenital defects (encephalocele, persistent craniopharyngeal duct), tumors of the skull base, or pressure atrophy due to a prolonged, general rise in intracranial pressure. Traumatic CSF fistulae most commonly involve the cribriform plate or the posterior wall of the frontal sinus.

Traumatic CSF rhinorrhea may occur immediately after the injury or may be delayed. Occasionally the condition remains undiagnosed for years until a purulent pneumococcal meningitis supervenes. Discharge of CSF can be provoked by positioning the patient head–down and by compression of the jugular vein. CT or MRI can demonstrate intracranial air collections (pneumocephalus) as well as fractures and defects involving the skull base. Bone–window CT scans can generally demonstrate the site of the leak.

Given the risk of ascending infection, operative repair should be considered in all cases of persistent CSF rhinorrhea. While the neurosurgeon provides for broad intradural coverage of the fistula and manages the brain wound, the rhinosurgeon explores the paranasal sinuses and adjacent skull base (see Volume 1, Chapters 9 and 10). In patients with severe frontobasal injuries, the procedure is carried out no earlier than 2 weeks postinjury to allow time for regression of reactive changes. Experience has shown that there is virtually no risk of infection during this period, so prophylactic antibiotics are not administered. If olfactory function is intact, exploration of the skull base should be performed by the rhinosurgical route.

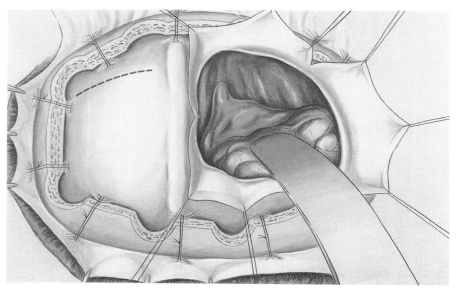

Fig. 13.**51**

Transcranial Intradural Approach

The operation is performed under general endotracheal anesthesia. A unilateral or occasionally bilateral frontal exposure provides the best access for exploring the anterior skull base. The putative site of the CSF leak is approached on the intradural plane, opening the basal cisterns (if posttraumatic adhesions permit) so that fluid can be drained and space gained for the frontobasal exposure. After adhesions have been cleared between contused brain and the basal dura, generally a nub of brain tissue will appear marking the perforation site (Fig. 13.**51**). In Figure 13.**52** the frontal brain has been retracted to expose a fistulous opening in the cribriform plate. The fistula can be repaired with a fascia lata autograft or a turnover flap. Figure 13.**53** shows closure of the fistula with a free graft (fascia) sutured to the basal dura. Figures 13.**54** and 13.**55** illustrate the principle of the turnover flap. A trapdoor incision is made in the falx cerebri, and the resulting flap is swung down over the fistulous opening and attached to the dura with simple interrupted sutures. Tissue adhesive also may be used.

Cranial Infections

Cranial Osteomyelitis

This may result from wound healing problems after brain surgery, hematogenous spread, or contiguous spread of infection from the paranasal sinuses or middle ear. The clinical manifestations include fever, severe headache, and local cutaneous swelling and red-

ness. Radiographs demonstrate typical bone destruction no earlier than 2–3 weeks after the onset of infection. Rhinosurgical aspects are discussed in Chapter 9, Volume 1.

All involved portions of the calvarium are broadly exposed through a craniotomy and resected into healthy tissue. A drain is left indwelling for several days. Concomitant infections (e.g., of the paranasal sinuses or middle ear) must be eradicated. Operative treatment is followed by a course of antibiotics that is continued for at least 3–4 weeks after florid infection has subsided. Larger bone defects can be reconstructed 6 months later by cranioplasty for cosmetic reasons or to protect the brain. See also Volume 1, Chapter 10.

Epidural Abscess

Epidural abscesses most commonly result from suppurative infections of neighboring structures such as the paranasal sinuses, middle ear, and calvarium (see Volume 1, Chapter 9). The predominant symptoms are fever, headache, a subgaleal pus collection, and possibly obtundation if there is a progressive mass effect. CT and MRI are helpful for establishing the diagnosis. Treatment begins with eradication of the focus in the paranasal sinuses or middle ear. The extradural space is then broadly exposed through the same approach and treated by external drainage. Further details are given in Chapter 9 and in Volume 1, Chapter 10.

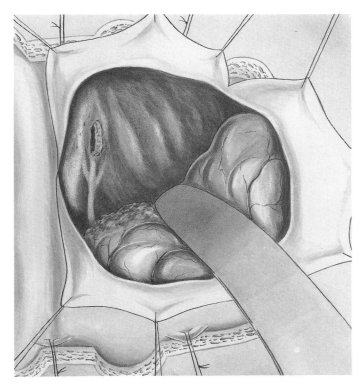

Fig. 13.**52**

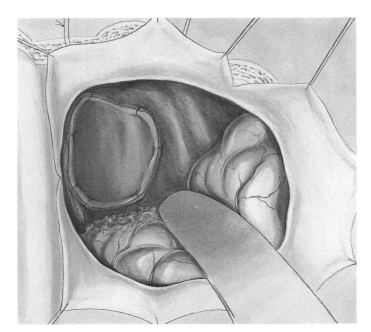

Fig. 13.**53**

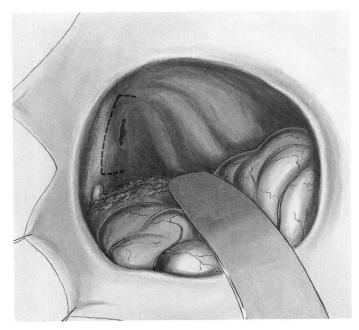

Fig. 13.**54**

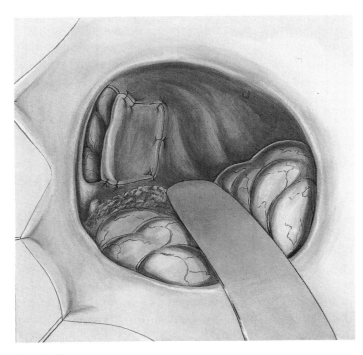

Fig. 13.**55**

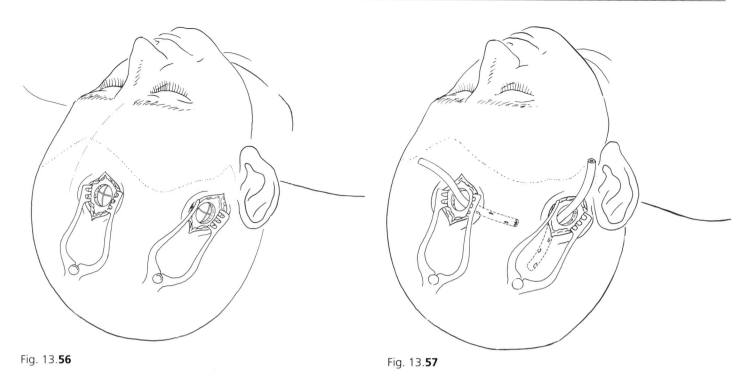

Fig. 13.**56**   Fig. 13.**57**

Subdural Abscess

Subdural abscesses can develop by the extension of infection from the frontal sinus, middle ear, or mastoid.
They occasionally arise as a complication following the
aspiration of subdural effusions in children. The symptoms of subdural abscess include nuchal stiffness and
focal seizures, which are rapidly followed by focal neurologic deficits and deterioration of consciousness. The
diagnosis is usually established by CT or magnetic resonance imaging (MRI).

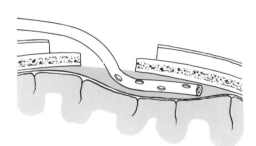

Fig. 13.**58**

The main goal of surgery is to drain the entire pus collection, leaving no residual pus behind. This can prove
difficult with a loculated abscess chamber. The result is
assessed by serial CT or MRI scans taken at frequent intervals after the operation. Surgical evacuation is
supplemented by drainage of the subdural space and
the administration of antibiotics.

The treatment of a subdural empyema covering the
entire hemisphere is illustrated in Figure 13.**56** to 13.**58**.
The placement of the two burr holes (frontal and temporal) is shown in Figure 13.**56**. In Figure 13.**57** the subdural empyema has been evacuated, and two tubes (rubber, silicone) are providing external drainage of the abscess cavity. The placement of the drainage tube is
shown schematically in Figure 13.**58**.

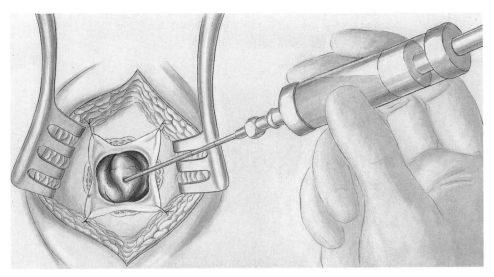

Fig. 13.**59**

Brain Abscess

Brain abscesses may develop by the direct extension of infection from the paranasal sinuses, middle ear, or mastoid (see Chapter 9 and Volume 1, Chapter 10), or they may be caused by metastatic or hematogenous dissemination, often originating from a pulmonary focus. A similar pathogenesis can occur in children with congenital heart defects, where a right–to–left shunt channels venous blood to the brain without prior filtration by the lung. Abscesses may also develop within the cerebral wound produced by intracranial surgery or an open head injury. Abscesses can form in the temporal lobe or cerebellum by the direct extension of otologic disease, or in the basal portion of the frontal lobe by the extension of paranasal sinus disease (see Chapter 9 and Volume 1, Chapter 10 for further details). Hematogenous seeding can produce multiple abscesses whose distribution generally follows that of the middle cerebral artery and its branches. Bacteriologic examination most commonly identifies streptococci as the causative organism, although *Staphylococcus aureus* and *E. coli* can also be demonstrated.

Brain abscess is manifested by the symptoms of an intracranial mass lesion and may initially produce focal neurologic signs. But this is very quickly followed by a general rise of intracranial pressure with headache, vomiting, and papilledema. Meningism is generally absent. CSF examination usually reveals a moderate pleocytosis of up to several 100/3 cells.

The principal diagnostic modalities are CT and MRI. The appearance of the abscess depends on its stage of development. Scans initially show an enhancing area consistent with a phlegmonous lesion, followed in the liquefaction stage by a zone of decreased density that fi-nally is bordered by an abscess capsule. Since the advent of the newer modalities, isotope brain scans and cerebral angiography have lost much of their diagnostic value.

The following treatment of brain abscess is described from the perspective of the neurosurgeon, whose central concern is the increasing, life–threatening rise of intracranial pressure. This means precise localization of the intracerebral lesion and selective operative decompression aimed at lowering the intracranial pressure as rapidly as possible. Eradication of the extracranial focus is a secondary priority once the life–treatening situation has been brought under control. The alternative to this approach, favored by head and neck surgeons, is to eliminate the nasal or otologic focus and then follow the pathway of infection to attack the brain abscess (see Chapter 9 and Volume 1, Chapter 10 for further details).

The basic goal is total removal of the abscess. A lesser goal should be considered only in patients who are poor candidates for major surgery or already exhibit symptoms of midbrain or cerebellar tonsillar impaction in the foramen magnum. In these cases a burr hole should be cut for immediate aspiration of the abscess. In all other cases we prefer primary extirpation.

The burr hole is placed directly over the abscess and enlarged with ronguers to about the size of a 50–cent piece. After the dura has been opened with a cruciate incision and the edges tacked up, the abscess is punctured with a blunt Cushing needle (Fig. 13.**59**). Resistance will be felt as the needle pierces the abscess capsule. Following aspiration of the pus, the cavity is flushed with Ringer's solution, and a broad–spectrum antibiotic is instilled. Once the contents of the abscess are sterile, extirpation of the capsule can be performed via a craniotomy.

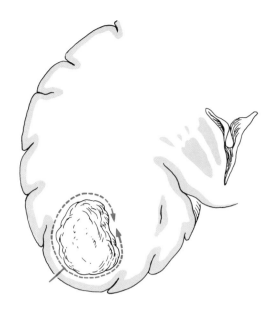

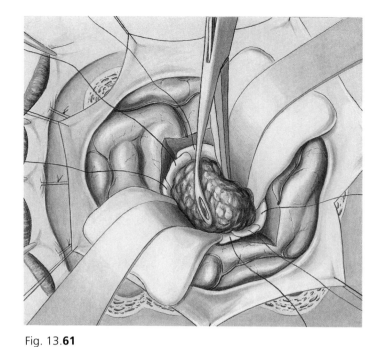

Fig. 13.**60**

Fig. 13.**61**

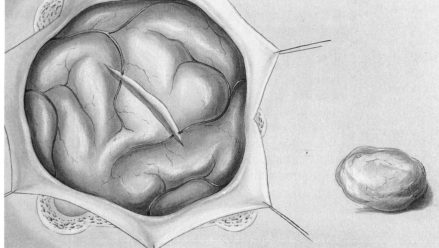

Fig. 13.**62**

Extirpation of a Brain Abscess

After the bone flap has been elevated and the dura incised, the cortex is incised over the abscess or abscess capsule. The capsule is isolated within the edematous zone using brain retractors and patty dissection, and all of the capsule is removed. The principle of total brain abscess removal is shown schematically in Figure 13.**60**.

In Figure 13.**61** the cerebral cortex has been opened, and the abscess capsule has been identified in the edematous zone and partially isolated. Figure 13.**62** shows the brain following abscess removal along with the enucleated abscess with its capsule intact.

This method allows for primary closure of the wound. Antibiotic therapy (confirmed by sensitivity testing) is instituted or continued, and a search is made for the primary infectious focus.

Nerve Repair

Technique of Nerve Repair

A good clinical result following the repair of divided nerves relies critically on undisturbed regeneration and growth of the axons at the level of the repair. Axonal growth is negatively affected by neuromas and scarring in the juncture area, which can result from imprecise approximation of the nerve ends, excessive tension at the repair site, or inadequate resection of the traumatic neuroma and fast–growing epineurium.

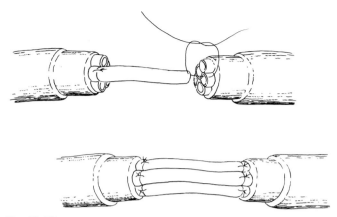

Fig. 13.**63**

A nerve repair may be classified as direct, involving epineural closure, or interfascicular, involving perineural closure. Microsurgical technique is routinely employed. See also Chapters 5 and 7 and Volume 1, Chapter 16.

Interfascicular (Perineural) Repair

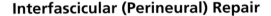

In most nerve repairs the stumps are separated by a defect that must be bridged by interposing a nerve graft. Various cutaneous nerves can be used as autogenous graft material, including the sural nerve, lateral femoral cutaneous nerve, and the intercostal nerves.

The interface is prepared by trimming back the epineurium about 0.5 cm from the nerve end. Then the individual fascicular bundles are dissected free (Fig. 13.**63**), and the scarred ends of the fasciculi are resected with a razor blade until the individual fascicular bundles can be identified. The defect between the cut ends is now measured, and one (e.g., facial nerve) or more grafts are interposed depending on the caliber of the nerve requiring repair. The grafts should have ample length to avoid tension at the repair site. A total of 2 or 3 fine interfascicular sutures (10-0 monofilament) are used. After the sutures have been placed and tied, the repair is reinforced with fibrin glue. The approximation of corresponding motor and sensory fascicles in both nerve ends is essential for a good postoperative result.

The sural nerve is harvested through a skin incision approximately 6–7 cm long made between the achilles tendon and lateral malleolus. The nerve courses below or alongside the saphenous vein. After the nerve is divided, a nerve stripper can be used to harvest a segment over 20 cm in length. If a stripper is not used, it will generally be necessary to make 2 additional skin incisions over the course of the nerve.

Perineural sutures and interposition grafting are used to repair facial nerve lesions in the area of the cerebellopontine angle.

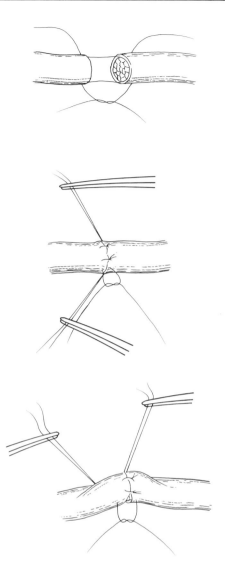

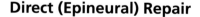

Fig. 13.**64**

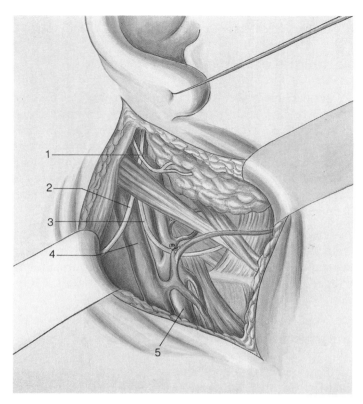

Fig. 13.**65**
1 Facial nerve
2 Accessory nerve
3 Hypoglossal nerve
4 Internal jugular vein
5 Common carotid artery

Direct (Epineural) Repair

A direct repair (Fig. 13.**64**) is feasible only if the nerve has been cleanly severed by a sharp object, so that the ends can be reapproximated without a defect and without significant tension. The strongest repair is obtained by passing the sutures through the epineurium. The anastomosis is performed with monofilament sutures of size 6-0 to 10-0, depending on the caliber of the damaged nerve. When the sutures are placed, care is taken to achieve a perfect coaptation of the nerve ends all about their circumference to prevent subsequent neuroma formation.

Epineural closure is also used for substitution anastomoses (e.g., hypoglossal–facial anastomosis) and for repairing the facial portion of the facial nerve by direct suture or by free grafting, since the very small caliber of the nerve may preclude resection of the epineurium at the nerve ends.

Autogenous Nerve Bypass (Dott's Technique)

Following surgery in the cerebellopontine angle, the free graft from the sural nerve or lateral femoral cutaneous nerve is sutured to the central stump of the facial nerve. It is brought out through the craniotomy opening and tunneled through the muscle to the retromandibular fossa. In a second operation, which Dott (1936) delayed for 90 days but other authors perform successfully just a few days after the cerebellopontine angle surgery, the facial nerve is identified at the stylomastoid foramen, and the divided distal limb of the nerve is anastomosed to the graft. See also Chapters 7 and 11.

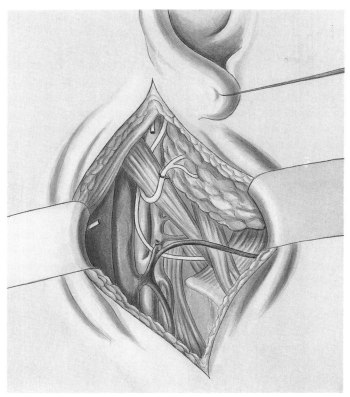

Fig. 13.**66**

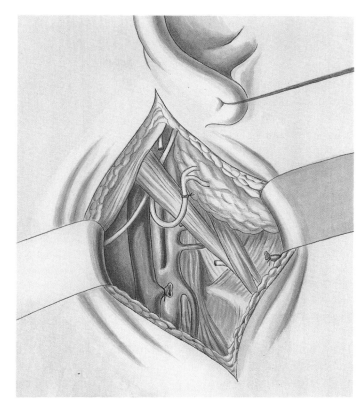

Fig. 13.**67**

Cranial Nerve Anastomoses

The hypoglossal (and occassionally the accessory) nerve are used for anastomosis to the facial nerve. Figure 13.**65** shows a schematic representation of these nerves in the sternocleidomastoid region. Through an incision from the tip of the mastoid process to the anterior border of the sternocleidomastoid muscle, the facial nerve is identified and snared at the stylomastoid foramen. The accessory nerve is identified in the retromandibular fossa, where it passes between the posterior belly of the digastric muscle and the sternocleidomastoid muscle. It is divided proximal to its entry into the sternocleidomastoid and anastomosed to the distal end of the divided facial nerve using epineural sutures (Fig. 13.**66**).

The hypoglossal nerve is exposed in the carotid triangle below the posterior belly of the digastric muscle, divided distal to the origin of the ascending branch of the hypoglossal nerve, and anastomosed to the peripheral facial nerve. The principle of this anastomosis is shown in Fig. 13.**67**.

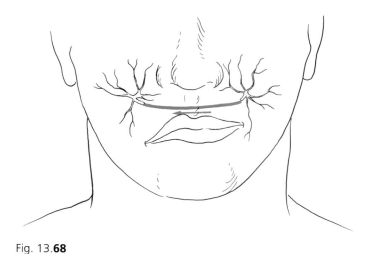

Fig. 13.**68**

Cross–Facial Nerve Grafting

The facial nerve branches supplying paretic facial muscles can be anastomosed to their contralateral, normally functioning counterparts using fascicular nerve autografts from the thigh or lower leg. Buccal–zygomatic reinnervation is especially useful for restoring function to the area of the upper lip and eye.

A skin incision approximately 5 cm long is made on both sides of the face parallel to the nasolabial folds. Identification of the nerve plexus in that area can be aided by electrical stimulation. One or two branches are divided on each side and anastomosed by fascicular suture to an autogenous sural or lateral femoral cutaneous nerve graft that is tunneled subcutaneously through the upper lip. The principle is shown in Fig. 13.**68**.

Tumors of the Skull Base

These tumors are of particular interdisciplinary interest because they may necessitate a team approach. Most common are nasopharyngeal fibromas, chordomas, chondromas, basal cell carcinomas, and meningiomas.

CT and MRI have assumed major importance in the evaluation of these tumors. Coronal projections are particularly useful for demonstrating intra– and extracranial extent.

With heavily vascularized lesions, noninvasive studies are supplemented by selective angiography of both carotid arteries, including the external carotid system. These studies are also useful if subsequent tumor devascularization by embolization is proposed. Treatment planning additionally requires biopsy to establish a tissue diagnosis.

For radical extirpation of the tumor, the subfrontal transcranial–transbasal approach has proven an effective adjunct to the anterior ENT approach (see also Volume 1, Chapter 9). It provides access to the entire anterior cranial fossa and large portions of the middle fossa. The excellent exposure of the optic foramen, superior orbital fissure, and the foramina rotundum and ovale allows for preservation of the corresponding cranial nerves except for the olfactory nerve.

The transcranial approach is made through a frontal or bifrontal craniotomy. To minimize the need for frontal lobe retraction to expose the skull base, the operation is preceded by lumbar drainage of CSF. Because surgical procedures in the anterior fossa always entail a risk of postoperative CSF leak, a periosteal flap is prepared and elevated during the exposure for subsequent lining of the skull base. The craniotomy is placed as far basally as possible, close to the orbital margin. The breached frontal sinus is appropriately managed. Whether the rest of the approach is extradural or transdural depends on the extent of the tumor. The crista galli is resected, and the olfactory nerves traversing the cribriform plate are coagulated and divided. Infiltrated portions of the dura are progressively resected at the tumor margin. If the tumor has a soft consistency, it can first be debulked with the ultrasonic aspirator. The procedure at the skull base requires often the use of the microdrill.

The main complication of this surgery is basal CSF leakage to the paranasal sinuses with risk of meningitis. For this reason antibiotics are administered preoperatively, and lumbar drainage of CSF is continued for 1–2 days after the operation. The decision whether to remove the tumor in 1or 2 sittings depends on the size of the dural defect created during the frontal approach. The extracranial part of the procedure is done in the same sitting only if complete closure of the dural defect has been achieved. Otherwise the second stage of the tumor resection is performed several weeks later. Larger defects can be repaired with the periosteal flap prepared during the craniotomy or with fascia lata. Less common alternatives are lyophilized dura and equine pericardium.

Endovascular Procedures

Devascularization of Highly Vascular Tumors

The devascularization of highly vascular neoplasms by embolization of the feeding arterial vessels is usually done as a prelude to surgical removal or to control intractable tumor hemorrhage in the upper respiratory tract. Another application is tumor devascularization, possibly combined with radiotherapy, for palliative arrest of tumor growth in inoperable cases. These tumors consist chiefly of nasopharyngeal fibromas, glomus tumors, and carcinomas of the skull base and paranasal sinuses.

The blood supply to the tumor is mapped by selective, bilateral angiography of the internal and external carotid circulations. Vertebral angiography is additionally performed for the evaluation of glomus jugulare tumors.

The embolization technique essentially follows the original technique described by Djindjian (1973). The goal of the procedure is the superselective catheterization and occlusion of the tumor supply vessels. The devascularization should be accomplished as close to the tumor as possible to eliminate supply from peripheral collaterals.

Superselective catheterization of the target vessels is generally done by the percutaneous transfemoral route. The transcarotid route can also be used. The very fine catheters currently available can negotiate vessels as small as 1 mm in diameter.

The embolic material may consist of fine particles that can be accurately calibrated (polyvinyl alcohol-Ivalon) or a polymerizing liquid (such as 2-methyl-2-cyanoacrylate Bucrylate). A very small quantity of the material, along with liquid contrast medium, is delivered into the catheterized vessel.

The progress of the embolization is closely followed using monitor and serial digital–subtraction angiograms. Bilateral embolization is indicated for tumors located in the midline (e.g., nasopharyngeal fibroma).

Embolization is followed immediately by pain and cutaneous swelling in the corresponding vascular territories. Postembolization symptoms rarely last more than 2–3 days and are well controlled with analgesics and dexamethasone. Potential complications of embolization in the external carotid system include ischemic facial nerve paralysis and even cerebral infarction if the embolic material enters the internal carotid or vertebral artery. This would contraindicate the embolization of an occipital artery, for example, that has substantial collateral connections with the vertebral artery via its muscular branches.

Traumatic Carotid Cavernous Fistula

Traumatic carotid cavernous fistulas result from injury to the carotid artery within the cavernous sinus. One effect of the consequent pressure rise in the venous circulation is a pulsatile exophthalmos, which dominates the clinical presentation.

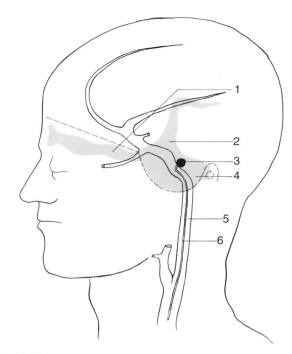

Fig. 13.**69**
1 Ophthalmic vein
2 Fistula
3 Balloon
4 Cavernous sinus
5 Internal carotid artery
6 Balloon catheter

Traumatic carotid cavernous fistula can also result from iatrogenic manipulations in the area of the cavernous sinus such as an internal carotid endarterectomy near the siphon, a retroganglionic rhizotomy for relief of trigeminal neuralgia, or the biopsy of tumors involving the skull base and sphenoid sinus.

The hemodynamics of the fistula are investigated by selective, bilateral angiographic examination of the internal and external carotid arteries and of the vertebrobasilar system. These studies can determine, for example, whether the shunt involves the internal carotid artery alone or there is concomitant involvement of the external carotid artery.

Combined intra– and extracranial occlusion of the internal carotid artery — first intracranial below the posterior communicating artery and then extracranial at the cervical level ("trapping operation") — was the preferred treatment method for decades. By the mid-1970s, success was achieved in directly occluding the fistula and preserving the internal carotid artery by operative exposure of the fistula and by electrothrombosis.

Today, endovascular occlusion of the fistula with a detachable balloon has become the procedure of choice (Fig. 13.**69**). Selective occlusion of the fistula with preservation of the internal carotid artery is achieved in 80–90% of cases. If the transarterial approach is unsuccessful, a transvenous route can be taken via the jugular vein and petrous sinus. If selective occlusion fails, both the shunt and the internal carotid artery can be occluded by positioning the balloon at the level of the fistula. This is acceptable, however, only if the patient has previously tolerated a trial carotid occlusion of approximately 40 minutes duration. Also, measurements of regional cerebral blood flow and of arterial pressure distal to the occlusion site provide valuable information on the quality of the natural collateral circulation. If the collateral supply is deficient, an extracranial–intracranial bypass is performed before the definitive operation, and occlusion testing is repeated. With few exceptions, the endovascular procedure is performed under local anesthesia. The balloon is maneuvered through the fistula into the cavernous sinus, inflated with a polymerizing liquid, and detached from the catheter tip (Fig. 13.**69**). (See also Chapter 15.)

Serious ischemic complications can arise if the balloon is dislodged and swept into the cerebral vessels. However, the balloon can be successfully retrieved by immediate surgical exposure of the affected vessels.

Bibliography

Baethmann A, Lanksch W, Schmiedek P. Formation and treatment of cerebral edema. Neurochirurgia 1974; 17:37.
Ballantine H T, Shealy C N. The role of radical surgery in the treatment of abscess of the brain. Surg Gynec Obstet 1959; 109:370.
Becker D P, Miller J D, Young H F, et al. Diagnosis and treatment of head injury in adults. In: Youmans JR (ed). Neurological Surgery. Philadelphia: W B Saunders, 1982.
Bettag W. Der derzeitige Stand von Klinik und Behandlung der otogenen und rhinogenen Hirnkomplikationen. Neurochirurgische Betrachtungen. HNO-Wegw 1972; 20:47.
Bucy P C. Exposure of the posterior or cerebellar fossa. J Neurosurg 1966; 14:820.
Dandy W E. Treatment of rhinorrhea and otorrhea. Arch Surg 1944; 49:75.
Debrun G, Lacour P, Vinuela F, et al. Treatment of 54 traumatic carotid cavernous fistulas. J Neurosurg 1981; 55:678.
Derome P Y. The transbasal approach to tumors invading the base of the skull. In. Operative neurosurgical techniques. Orlando: Grune & Stratton, 1988.
Dietz H. Die frontobasale Schädelhirnverletzung. Berlin: Springer, 1970.
Dott N M. Facial paralysis-restitution by extrapetrous nerve graft. Proc Roy Soc Med 1958; 51:900.
Drake C G. Acoustic neurinoma. Repair of facial nerve with autogenous graft. J Neurosurg 1960; 17:836.
Drake C G. Surgical treatment of acoustic neuroma with preservation or reconstruction of the facial nerve. J Neurosurg 1967; 26:459.
Epstein M H. Surgical management of hydrocephalus. In: Operative neurosurgical techniques. Orlando: Grune & Stratton, 1988.

Gerlach J. Grundriß der Neurochirurgie. Darmstadt: Steinkopf, 1967.
Gianotta S L, Weiss M H, Apuzzo M I J, et al. High dose glucocorticoids in the management of head injury. Neurosurgery 1984; 15:497.
Gratzl O, Marguth F. Dringliche Neurochirurgie. Monatskurse ärztl Fortbild 1969; 19:301.
Gurdjian E S, Thomas L M. Operative Neurosurgery, 3rd edn, Baltimore: Williams & Wilkins, 1970.
Hakim S, Burton J D. Flow through CSF shunts. J Neurosurg 1973; 39:127.
Horwitz N H, Rizzolli H V. Postoperative complications in neurosurgical practice. Recognition, prevention and management. Baltimore: Williams & Wilkins, 1967.
Horwitz N H, Rizzoli H V. Postoperative complications of intracranial surgery. Baltimore: Williams & Wilkins, 1982.
Kempe L G. Operative Neurosurgery. Berlin: Springer, 1968/1970.
Kessel F K, Guttmann L, Maurer G. Neuro-Traumatologie mit Einschluß der Grenzgebiete. München: Urban & Schwarzenberg, 1969.
Kurze T. Microtechniques in neurological surgery. Clin Neurosurg 1964; 11:128.
Light R U. Hemostasis in neurosurgery. J Neurosurg 1945; 2:414.
Loew F, Kivelitz R. Surgical reconstruction of intracranial lesions of cranial nerves. In: Advances of Neurosurgery, Vol. I. Berlin: Springer, 1973.
Matson D D, Salam M. Brain abscess in congenital heart disease. Pediatrics 1961; 27:772.
Merrem G, Goldhahn W E. Neurochirurgische Operationen. München: Barth, 1966.
Miehlke A. Surgery of the facial nerve. Philadelphia: Saunders, 1973.
Miller, J D, Becker D P. General principles and pathophysiology of head injury. In: Youmans J R (ed). Neurological surgery. Philadelphia: WB Saunders, 1982.
Mullan, S. Treatment of carotid cavernous fistula by cavernous sinus occlusion. J Neurosurg 1981; 55:678.
Nulsen F E, Spitz E B. Treatment of hydrocephalus by direct shunt from ventricle to jugular vein. Surg Forum 2 1951; 2:399.
Parkinson D, Downs A R, Whitehead L L, et al. Carotid cavernous fistula: Direct repair with preservation of carotid. Surgery 1974; 76:882.
Poppen J L. An atlas of neurosurgical technic. Philadelphia: Saunders, 1960.
Pudenz R H. The ventriculo-atrial shunt. J Neurosurg 1966; 25:602.
Ray B S, Bergland R M. Cerebrospinal fluid fistula: Clinical aspects, techniques of localization and methods of closure. J Neurosurg 1969; 30:399.
Seddon H J. Three types of nerve injury. Brain 1943; 66:238.
Smith J W. Advances in facial nerve repair. Surg Clin N Amer 1972; 52:1287.
Sundaresan N, Sachdev V, Krol G J. Craniofacial resection for anterior skull base tumors. In: Operative neurosurgical techniques. Orlando: Grune & Stratton, 1988.
Tönnis W K, Frowein A, Loew F, Grote W, Hemmer R, Klug W, Finkemeyer H. Organisation der Behandlung schwerer Schädel-Hirn-Verletzungen. Stuttgart: Thieme, 1968.
Yasargil M G. Mircosurgery Applied to Neurosurgery. Stuttgart: Thieme, 1969.

14 Cochlear Implant

Bruce J. Gantz

The development of reliable and effective cochlear implant systems (Fig. 14.1) has restored the sensation of sound and in many instances speech perception to profoundly deaf individuals. To date the devices have been most effective in persons who have lost their hearing after learning language (postlingual deafness). However, some congenitally deafened children (prelingual deafness) implanted with multichannel cochlear implant systems have been able to improve their speech perception and production skills. It must be kept in mind that the present generation of devices do not restore normal hearing. Ongoing research continues to search for the keys to improving speech perception. Implants are continuing to evolve as are the indications for their use. This chapter will review the work–up and indications for using a cochlear implant and describe in detail the operative techniques that have been most useful. Reviews detailing differences in cochlear implant designs and speech coding can be found elsewhere (Gantz, 1987; Pfingst, 1986).

Diagnosis and Preoperative Evaluation

A team of specialists is essential for the appropriate preoperative evaluation of candidates as well as for providing the necessary postoperative rehabilitation. The team should consist of audiologists, aural rehabilitation specialists, psychologists and otolaryngologists. If a child is being evaluated for an implant, deaf educators and speech therapists must be included in the selection process. It is helpful to involve the child's teacher in the initial visits. Continued teamwork is essential for effective rehabilitation on all levels.

The preoperative work–up should be prefaced by sending the candidate or family general information about cochlear implants. A recent audiogram should also be requested in order to establish that the candidate is bilaterally profoundly deaf. The work–up at the

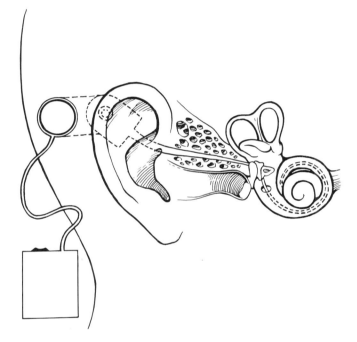

Fig. 14.**1** Basics of a cochlear implant system. Microphone in speech processor picks up acoustic signal. The acoustic signal is changed into electronic signal by speech processor. External coil transmits information to internal receiver coil. Electronic signal delivered to specific electrodes in the cochlea which activates cochlear nerve.

implant center should include an extensive audiologic evaluation, a medical evaluation, imaging studies, and in certain instances, electrophysiologic testing. Audiologic testing should be the first evaluation obtained to establish if the subject's hearing level is appropriate for an implant prior to proceeding with costly imaging studies.

Indications

Audiologic

In general, most cochlear implant systems specify similar guidelines for candidate selection. Cochlear implantation is limited to bilaterally profoundly deaf individuals. The average hearing thresholds for pure tone stimuli at 500 Hz, 1 kHz, and 2 kHz should be 90 dB hearing level (HL) or poorer. There should be no word understanding with an appropriate hearing aid or aids. A comprehensive hearing aid evaluation is mandatory. If the subject can detect speech at 65 dB sound pressure level (SPL), a series of tests are performed aided in a sound field at 65 dB SPL. The tests depend on the mother language of the patient and include a sound field audiogram, recorded W–22 monosyllabic word test, recorded NU-6 (Northwestern University) word list, and a recorded sentence test. Our center uses the Iowa Sentence Test without context laser video disc in a sound only condition (Tyler et al., 1986). Presently, we exclude candidates if they score better than 4% on the monosyllabic word tests or greater than 10% on the sentence test, both presented sound only in a sound field with appropriate hearing aids. These criteria have been established based on our experience with over 200 cochlear implant subjects. Eighty-seven percent of our multichannel cochlear implant subjects score better than 10% on the Iowa Sentence Test with their implant (average 31%, plus/minus 5.7%, range 0–92%, N = 39). All of the above subjects had no word understanding preoperatively with hearing aids. It can be argued that if candidates understand less than 10% on the Iowa Sentence Test without context in a sound field with a hearing aid, they have almost a 90% chance of improving their performance with a multichannel cochlear implant. Further changes in audiologic criteria are now under investigation. Similar tests are employed in other countries depending on the mother language.

The audiologic criteria for implantation of young children are also continuing to evolve. At this time, a child has to be at least two years of age to be considered for a cochlear implant. However, most audiologists agree that assessment of the benefit of conventional amplification is difficult at this young age. By 2½ years of age most children can be conditioned and tested using the House Ear Institute DAT test (discrimination after training test) (Thielemeir, 1982). At our center, appropriately fitted conventional or tactile aids are monitored for at least six months before final determination regarding implantation is made. If a candidate is unable to detect speech in a sound field at 60 dB HL or greater, he or she is considered for an implant.

Children capable of detecting a speech signal at 60 dB HL or better are administered speech recogni-

tion tests to assess the benefits of conventional amplification. These tests include the Monosyllable Trochee Spondee test (MTS), Word Intelligibility Picture Inventory (WIPI) (Ross et al., 1971), CID 12 choice Spondee and Monosyllables, and Matrix Test. Children with less sophisticated language and cognitive abilities are assessed using the DAT without training, the CID Low Verbal Test Battery, and the Body Parts test. Subjects failing to score above chance on two tests appropriate to the child's language and cognitive abilities would be considered as meeting the audiologic criteria for implantation. The tests used in other countries of necessity vary.

Medical

The medical history should address the general health of the candidates and assess their ability to undergo general anesthesia. In addition, certain biographic details such as onset of profound deafness, educational environment, previous chronic ear disease and surgery are helpful. The etiology of deafness is important in those individuals with a history of meningitis, as will be discussed.

The onset of profound deafness has an impact on performance in both adults and children. Postlingually deafened adults and children have received the greatest benefit from the present generation of cochlear implants. Open–set word understanding (speech perception without the aid of lipreading) has been generally limited to this group. Prelingual adults (profoundly deaf before development of language), however, have obtained only modest improvement in their communication skills with either single channel (Eisenberg, 1982) or multichannel (Brimacombe, 1988) implants. Subjects educated in a manual, or mostly manual, communication setting have the greatest difficulty using the auditory information delivered by cochlear implants. In some instances, prelingually deafened adults have not been able to identify the signal as auditory information. Careful counseling is especially important with this group, since some prelingual adults discontinue using their devices. The preliminary results in prelingual children using multichannel implants have been more encouraging. Some young prelingual children (4–6 years of age) have demonstrated limited open–set word understanding after 2 years of experience with their device. There appears to be a critical learning period when the central auditory system is most receptive to new auditory information. The age boundaries of this critical period, however, are not known, but it is suspected that implantation of prelingual children should be performed prior to puberty for best results.

The performance with a cochlear implant has been thought to be related to the etiology of the acquired deafness. Attempts to correlate performance with both single channel and multichannel cochlear implants and etiology of hearing loss have failed to demonstrate a relationship. Profound deafness following meningitis or labyrinthitis, however, should be considered as exceptions if labyrinthine imaging reveals ossification in the cochlea. In addition, meningitis is one of the only conditions that can result in near total loss of auditory nerve ganglion cells, and cases with labyrinthitis ossificans are at a higher risk for ganglion cell depletion. Candidates displaying cochlear ossification should undergo preoperative electrical stimulation to determine the integrity of the auditory nerve. The history of temporal bone trauma resulting in profound deafness also requires electrical stimulation to determine if the auditory nerve is intact. A diagnosis of otosclerosis should alert the surgeon to the possibility of distortion of the cochlear anatomy and loss of landmarks during implantation. A previous stapedectomy or iatrogenic labyrinthine injury resulting in deafness is also important information. There have been several anecdotal cases in which this type of injury has resulted in the inability to place an intracochlear electrode due to fibrous tissue obstruction. Imaging studies in these cases may be normal.

In children, recurrent acute or chronic otitis media must be controlled prior to proceeding with implantation. There have been implants placed with ventilation tubes in place. However, one should proceed with caution in this situation. Over 15 cases of acute otitis media in implanted ears have been reported, one occurred 3 weeks following implantation (House et al., 1985). To date, there have been no reports of labyrinthitis or intracranial infection in subjects with cochlear implants.

The duration of profound deafness has been found to have some effect on performance with an implant. The House Ear Institute and Cochlear Corporation data have identified age and duration of deafness as accounting for 9 to 20% of the variance in their subjects. In our series of 39 multichannel implants duration of profound deafness was strongly correlated with open-set word understanding ($r = -0.45$, $p = 0.002$) (Gantz et al., 1988). This information must be interpreted with care since some patients who have been profoundly deaf for over 20 years still achieved limited open-set word understanding. In contrast, some recently deafened individuals performed poorly.

Another important historic feature to note in postlingual subjects is whether one ear was deaf from birth. In this situation, the congenitally deafened ear may perform similarly to the prelingual adult subjects. The medical history can identify potential problems that can result in less than effective use of the cochlear implant. This information should be considered when counseling the candidate and planning rehabilitation.

Rarely is a subject eliminated as a candidate for an implant based on historic information.

The physical examination should assess the ability to undergo general anesthesia and determine if the ear to be implanted is free of disease. The ear should be dry and without evidence of infection. Large perforations should be repaired prior to proceeding with implantation. Small perforations can be repaired during implantation. If chronic eustachian tube dysfunction is encountered, the middle ear and eustachian tube can be obliterated prior to placing an implant. Previous open cavity mastoidectomies can be obliterated with temporalis muscle flaps at the time of implantation.

able to hear sound using the round window technique. The cause of deafness in both subjects was meningitis and they exhibited extensive ossification on their CT scans. One individual was implanted, but had a severely restricted dynamic range which limited the usefulness of the device. Even though preoperative electrical stimulation is not predictive of performance level with an implant, it does appear that if a perception of sound is obtained with round window stimulation that sufficient auditory nerve is present to proceed with implantation. It is suggested that all candidates with extensive labyrinthine ossification, temporal bone trauma, and previous acoustic tumor excision undergo preoperative electrical stimulation prior to implantation.

The selection of the ear to implant differs from center to center. Some physicians select the poorer hearing ear. Our philosophy has always been to implant the better hearing, most recently deafened side. We select the ear that responds to the greatest number of frequencies, subjectively sounds better with a hearing aid, and has the widest dynamic range on electrical testing. Other criteria include the side with least ossification, noncongenital hearing loss, and the ear that has not been iatrogenically deafened.

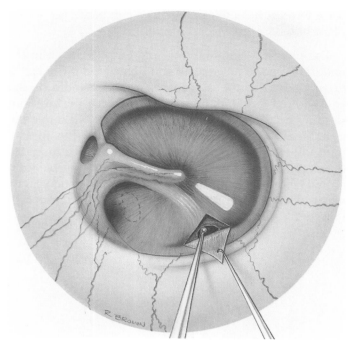

Fig. 14.**2**

Imaging

High resolution computed axial tomography is the most effective imaging procedure for evaluating cochlear patency. Ossification within the cochlea is usually apparent, but we have encountered bony changes when the CT scan appears normal. Ossification is not necessarily a contraindication to implantation. Cochleas with basilar turn obstructions have been successfully implanted with long intracochlear electrodes (Balkany et al., 1988), and techniques, to be described, for implanting multichannel electrode arrays in near totally obliterated ears have been developed (Gantz et al., 1988). Drilling away bone within the scala tympani does not appear to induce a progressive deterioration of performance. Subjects who have required extensive bone removal for placement of an electrode have maintained stable current and performance levels for over 3 years.

Electrophysiology

An accurate preoperative assessment of the functional integrity of the residual auditory nerve is difficult to obtain. Several promontory and round window electrical tests have been devised. However, responses have been inconsistent and have not correlated with outcome measures. Stimulation at the round window (Fig. 14.**2**) has successfully resulted in the perception of sound in over 80 candidates in our series. Two subjects were not

Goal of the Operation

The objectives of the operation are to 1) place the stimulating electrode in close proximity to the cochlear nerve and 2) implant the components in such a way that minimizes chances of future extrusion and/or infection. The scala tympani is the most effective site for placement of the present generation of stimulating electrodes. The facial recess or posterior tympanotomy has provided safe access to the inner ear. Endaural access and placement of electrodes along the external auditory canal has resulted in eventual exposure of electrodes and led to explantation.

A postauricular skin flap is designed to accommodate the electronics package. The facial recess is reached through a partial mastoidectomy. The round window is exposed, a cochleostomy created, and the electrode array is advanced into the scala tympani. The electronic package is then secured and the wound is closed.

Anesthesia

General anesthesia through an endotracheal tube is the preferred anesthesia technique. As in any tympanomastoid operation muscle paralytic agents should be avoided in order to monitor facial nerve function if desired by the surgeon. The Xomed nerve integrity monitor-2 is used (Fig. 14.**3a**).

Preoperative Preparation

The patient is positioned supine on the operating table. Hair is shaved 8–10 cm above the ear and 8–10 cm post-auricularly. The entire hemiface and side of the head is prepped with a povidine–iodine solution. A ground electrode is inserted in the procerus muscle (Fig. 14.**3b**). Facial nerve monitoring electrodes, if desired, are placed in the orbicularis oculi and orbicularis oris muscles (Fig. 14.**3c**). It is recommended that the entire hemiface be draped to allow visual observation during the procedure. A large transparent plastic drape is used for this purpose. Standard sterile draping techniques similar to a tympanomastoidectomy procedure complete the preoperative preparation.

Instruments

Instrumentation is similar to a routine tympanomastoid procedure. Several additional instruments should be available including small angled picks, 0.2 mm Fisch footplate hook, Farrior rasp, angled and straight "claw" electrode inserters (Cochlear Corporation), 0.6 mm, 0.8 mm, and 1.0 mm diamond burrs with long tapered shafts. The long tapered shafts on the micro burrs are necessary to visualize structures while working through the facial recess. A suction–irrigation system should be used during bone removal.

Operative Technique

Skin Incision

The outline and position of the skin incision is dependent on the type of implant system to be used. In general, the incision should be drawn at least one centimeter peripheral to the implanted electronics package or percutaneous pedestal. The incision should not be in contact with any of the implanted components, i.e. antenna or electrode wires. The importance of skin flap design cannot be over emphasized because the most common complication reported with cochlear implants is skin flap breakdown (Cohen et al., 1988). The skin flap must be designed to incorporate the superficial temporal and/or occipital arterial blood supplies and adhere to appropriate width–length ratios (Fig. 14.**4**).

We have used a large C–shaped flap design in over 200 subjects with five different cochlear implant electrode packages without skin flap complications.

A template of the specific implant is placed in the posterosuperior postauricular area. The antenna or external components must be placed in a position as to not interfere with the auricle. The incision is positioned to incorporate blood supply from the superficial tem-

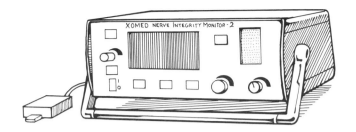

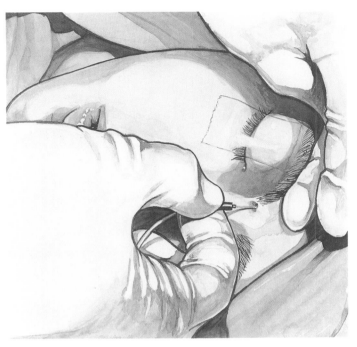

Fig. 14.**3b**

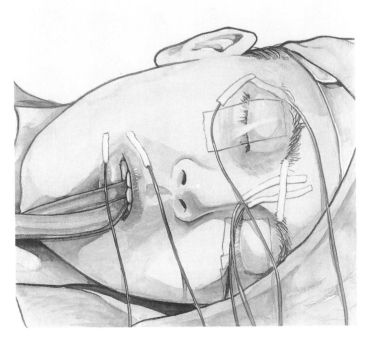

Fig. 14.**3c**

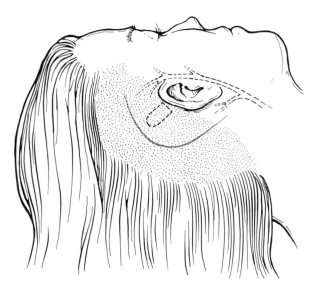

Fig. 14.**4**

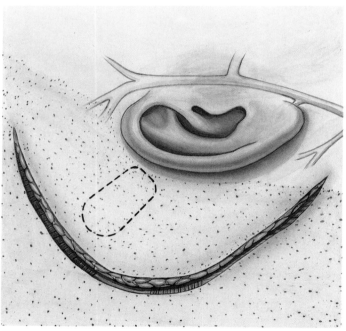

Fig. 14.**5**

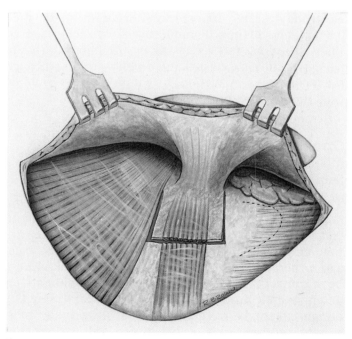

Fig. 14.**6**

poral artery as well as the suboccipital artery. Since a complete mastoidectomy is not necessary, the incision can be oriented more superiorly. The superior limb of the incision should be 4–5 cm above the superior attachment of the auricle, and extend posteriorly at least 1 cm behind the internal package and inferoposterior to the mastoid tip (Fig. 14.**5**). To induce vasoconstriction, 1:100,000 epinephrine is injected along the incision line. The skin incision is started superiorly and carried to the depth of the temporalis fascia.

Flaps

Inferior to the temporal line, the skin flap is elevated at the same depth leaving a layer of subcutaneous tissue and pericranium. The entire skin flap is elevated anteriorly to approximately the postauricular crease. A rectangular anteriorly based pericranial flap is fashioned to expose the mastoid cortex (Fig. 14.**6**). The upper incision is made at the temporal line. The flap is approximately 2½ cm wide and 3 cm long.

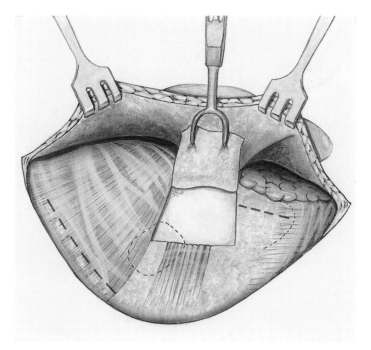

Fig. 14.**7**

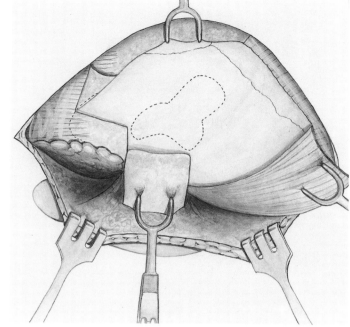

Fig. 14.**8**

A Lempert periosteal elevator is used to elevate the flap anteriorly to the spine of Henle (Fig. 14.**7**). The posterior external canal skin should not be elevated away from the canal wall. Finally, a broad posterior–based pericranial flap is elevated to expose the bone in the area of the implant electronic package or pedestal. The second pericranial flap is created by making a vertical superior incision through the temporalis muscle and an inferior incision posteroinferior from the previous mastoid cortex flap through the suboccipital muscles (Fig. 14.**8**). The pericranium is elevated to create a pocket to hold the implant. If an implant with a percutaneous pedestal is to be used, this flap is used to cover the pedestal base, as will be described. Self–retaining retractors are placed.

A limited mastoidectomy is carried out by exposing the mastoid antrum, lateral semicircular canal, and fossa incudis. An overhang of the superior mastoid cortex is left to anchor and protect the electrode bundle (Fig. 14.**9**). It is important to thin the posterior canal wall (anterior mastoid wall) to allow visualization of the round window through the facial recess. This is necessary because the direction of vision of the round window is parallel to the external canal wall. Two holes are drilled in the cortical overhang to anchor the electrode. Next, a seat or bed to hold the implant package is created. Each implant system has its own specifications. In general, the outer cortex and diploe bone are removed leaving the inner cortex of the skull. With some implants, part of the electronic package can be placed

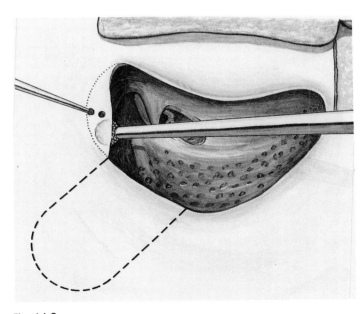

Fig. 14.**9**

in the mastoid. However, attention to the position of the connecting system (percutaneous or transcutaneous) should avoid contact with the auricle.

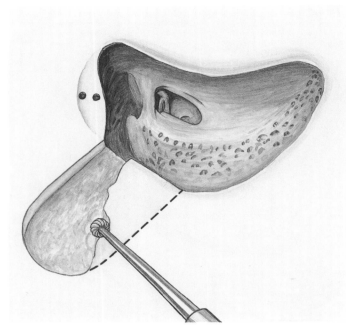

Fig. 14.**10**

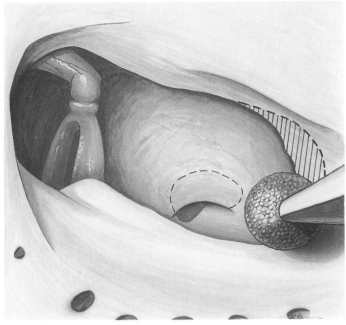

Fig. 14.**11**

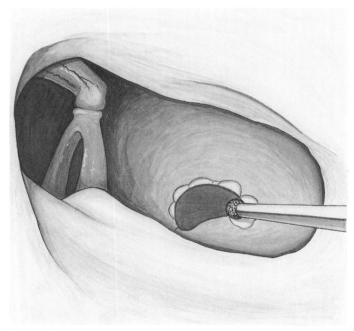

Fig. 14.**12**

The facial recess (posterior tympanotomy) is opened by first skeletonizing the superior descending mastoid segment of the facial nerve (Fig. 14.**10**). A layer of bone should be left over the nerve to prevent injury which can occur due to the rotating shaft of the burr as the more anterior cochleostomy is created. The chorda tympani nerve can usually be spared. However, in some cases, the position of the nerve and location of the

round window requires removal of the chorda tympani. Care is taken not to disrupt the anulus of the tympanic membrane and posterior external canal skin. Upon opening the facial recess, the stapes and stapedius tendon are seen (Fig. 14.**11**). Approximately 1 to 1.5 mm inferior to the stapedius muscle tendon the round window niche is identified.

Scala Tympani Cochleostomy

The round window is usually not directly visualized until the lip or superior overhang of the round window niche is removed with a 1 to 1.5 mm diamond burr (Fig. 14.**12**). The round window has a banana–like shape with a superior–anterior orientation. Several short electrodes have been placed through the round window. For longer intracochlear electrodes, creation of a separate cochleostomy anteroinferior to the anulus of the round window membrane provides the most direct access to the basilar turn of the scala tympani (Fig. 14.**13**). A cochleostomy eliminates maneuvering around the hook created by the crista fenestrae. The cochleastomy is created using a 0.8 mm to 1 mm diamond burr. The drilling proceeds until a blue area of the cochlea is visualized. The final thin layer of endosteum is removed with 0.2 mm footplate hooks or small Farrior rasp (Fig. 14.**14**). Prior to placing the electrode, the monopolar diathermy system is removed from the operative field (Fig. 14.**15**). Monopolar cautery can damage the implanted electronics or intracochlear structures when the electrode is in the scala tympani. A bipolar cautery system can be used after the implant is in place.

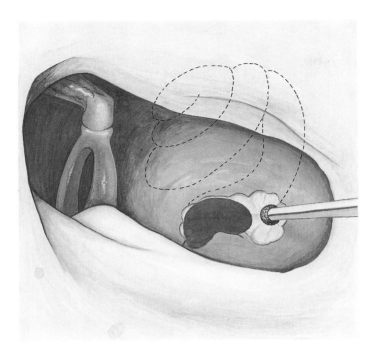

Fig. 14.**13**

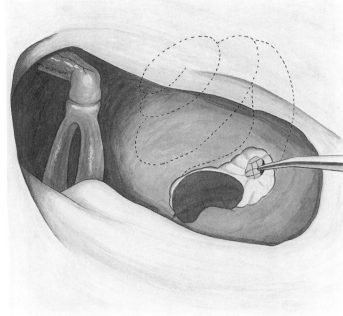

Fig. 14.**14**

Electrode Placement

The electrode wires are directed through the facial recess and into the scala tympani. Metal instruments should not directly contact the exposed active electrodes. An alligator forceps can be used to guide the electrode but should contact only the insulated portions. Some implant manufacturers have designed specific instruments for advancing electrodes (i.e. claws: Cochlear Corporation, inserter: Mini–Med). The electrode array usually can be easily passed through the first turn, a distance of approximately 8–10 mm (Fig. 14.**16 a**). Upon meeting resistance, the electrode is withdrawn 1 mm and slowly advanced and turned in the direction of the cochlear spiral (counter–clockwise AD, clockwise AS). Most electrodes can be slowly advanced 23–25 mm into the scala tympani. If continued resistance is encountered it is best to secure the electrode at that point to prevent kinking or bunching up the remaining portion within the basal cochlea.

The electrode is secured to the mastoid cortex overhang with a 4-0 nylon suture or dacron ties provided by some manufacturers (Fig. 14.**16 b**). A piece of temporalis fascia is placed around the electrode at the cochleostomy to seal the scala tympani. A second piece of fascia is placed in the facial recess between the electrode and the facial nerve. The implant package is placed in the previously created cortical seat and covered with the posterior based pericranial flap (Fig. 14.**16 c**). If a percutaneous pedestal is used, the pedestal is secured with screws as in Figure 14.**16 b**. If sutures are used to secure a magnet system, ensure that

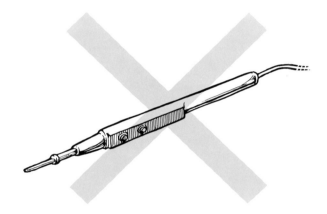

Fig. 14.**15**

the sutures to do not lie on the magnet. The Palva flap is placed along the posterior canal wall in the mastoid or used to cover the implanted electronics. The wound is drained by placing a ¹/₄ inch penrose in the mastoid defect. The skin flap is closed in layers and a mastoid pressure dressing is placed. The drain is removed on the first or second postoperative day and skin sutures removed on the seventh postoperative day.

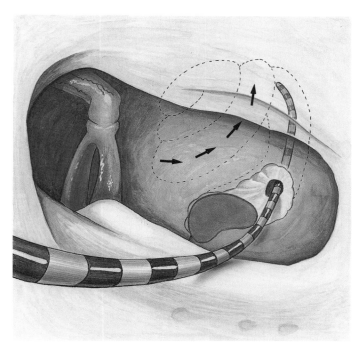

Fig. 14.**16 a**

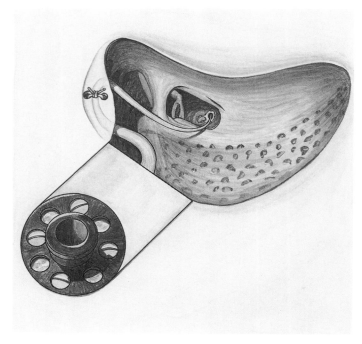

Fig. 14.**16 b**

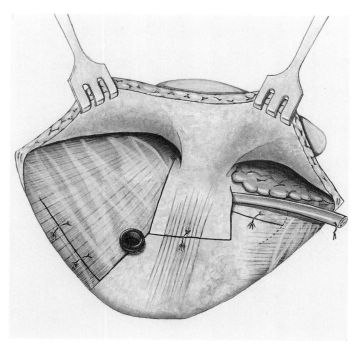

Fig. 14.**16 c**

Modifications

Diseases that cause deafness (i.e. meningitis, otosclerosis) can induce intracochlear changes ranging from fibrosis to total labyrinthitis ossificans. High resolution computed tomography can identify calcified irregularities in the cochlear lumen. However, fibrous alterations cannot be detected by imaging studies at this time.

In most instances, new bone formation is limited to the basilar turn and can be removed by extending the cochleostomy more anteriorly. The new bone formation has a whiter appearance than the yellowish otic capsule bone. Usually, the bone is soft and can be removed with small hooks. When perilymph is encountered the cochleostomy is enlarged and the electrode passed similar to an unobstructed cochlea. This technique has been used successfully in many cases (Balkany et al., 1988).

If the entire cochlea is involved in the obliterative process a trough can be drilled along the inferior basilar turn and up to 10 electrodes can be placed in the trough. We have developed an alternative procedure that has allowed placement of long intracochlear electrodes in severely obliterated cochleas (Gantz et al., 1988). It is remarkable that some subjects have been able to achieve open–set word understanding following an extensive cochlear drill–out procedure. This technique should only be performed if the subject is able to perceive auditory sensations on preoperative round window or promontory stimulation.

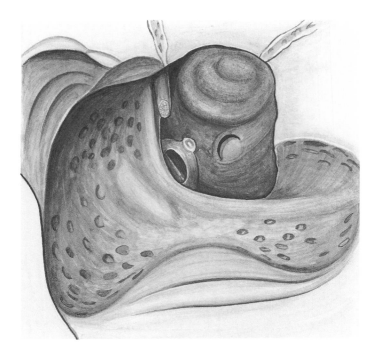

Fig. 14.**17**

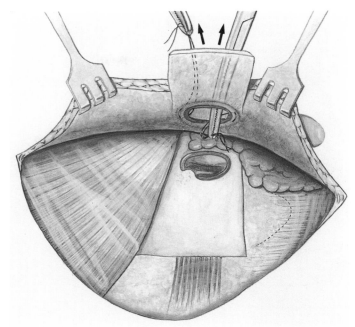

Fig. 14.**18 a**

The extended cochlear drill–out procedure requires a more radical surgical approach. The ascending basal turn cannot be reached through the facial recess and thus a more anterolateral exposure is created by performing a radical mastoidectomy (Fig. 14.**17**). The tympanic membrane, anulus, malleus, and incus are removed. The eustachian tube is obliterated, anterior canal prominence thinned, and the external auditory canal closed (Fig. 14.**18 a**, **b**). A diamond burr is used to remove all the mucosa within the mesotympanum and eustachian tube entrance and the eustachian tube is obliterated with muscle and fascia. The tensor tympani muscle is also removed as the helicotrema may lie medial to the muscle.

After the above is completed the exposure of the cochlea is begun by removing the round window niche to identify the round window membrane using a 1 mm diamond burr. The round window region may be distorted. If it is obliterated, the exposure is begun 1 mm inferior to the stapedius muscle tendon. The scala tympani can be identified as it usually contains bone that is whiter in color than the surrounding yellowish–white otic capsule bone (Fig. 14.**19**). This color differentiation is used as a "road–map" for locating the position of the previous scala tympani. A trough is created by removing the outermost perimeter of the otic capsule bone. Diamond burrs with irrigation are required to continue to differentiate the scala tympani bone from the otic capsule. Care is taken to remove only the outermost bone in an attempt to preserve the modiolus containing the cochlear nerve fibers. Drilling proceeds anterosupe-

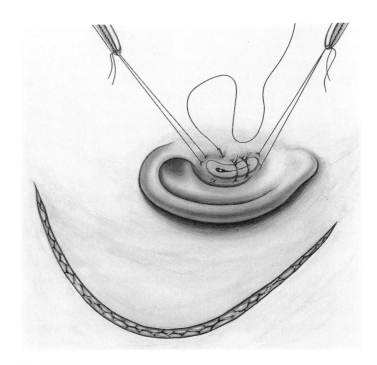

Fig. 14.**18 b**

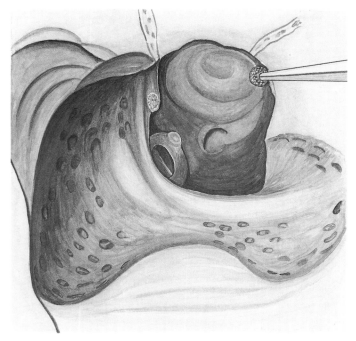

Fig. 14.**19**

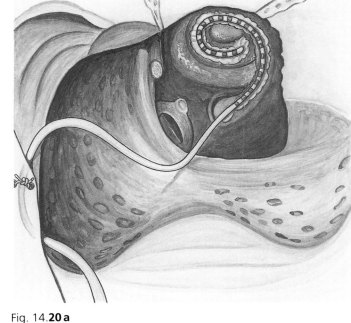

Fig. 14.**20 a**

riorly along the inferior basilar turn. As the basal turn curves upward the internal carotid artery is encountered. The distance between the cochlea and the artery can be variable. The ascending basal turn can be medial to the artery. Complete removal of the outer ascending basal turn wall can be difficult if the cochlea is tipped severely anterior. The superior segment of the basal turn is opened by first identifying the posterior descending portion and working anterosuperiorly.

Facial nerve monitoring is an absolute necessity since the labyrinthine segment of the facial nerve is immediately superior to this portion of the cochlea. Bone is then removed from the lateral arc of the second turn of the cochlea. Finally, bone around the modiolus is thinned leaving a faint blue layer of bone separating the auditory nerve and cerebrospinal fluid from the trough. The cochlear implant is coiled around the modiolus (Fig. 14.**20 a**). In certain instances, while drilling along the ascending basilar turn, one encounters perilymph and an open scala tympani and the full electrode can be freely passed (Fig. 14.**20 b**). A piece of temporalis fascia is positioned over the trough to hold the electrode in place (Fig. 14.**21**). The electrode is anchored to the mastoid cortex and the electrode package secured as previously described. A penrose drain is placed in the mastoid cavity. The wound is closed in layers and a mastoid pressure dressing placed. The penrose is left in place for 48 to 72 hours depending on drainage. The skin sutures are removed at seven days.

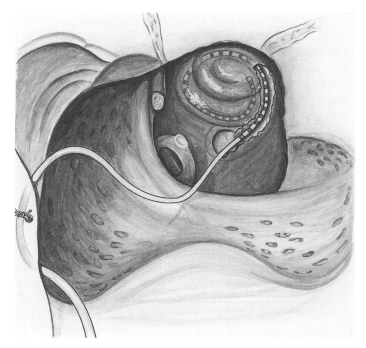

Fig. 14.**20 b**

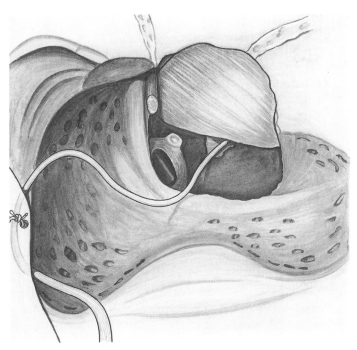

Fig. 14.**21**

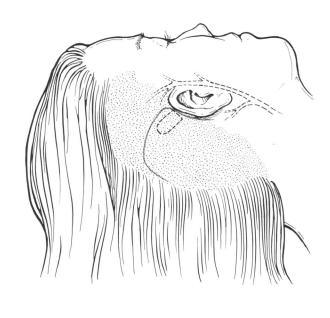

Fig. 14.**22**

The long–term results following the extensive bone removal have been encouraging. Subjects have maintained sound only open set word understanding without a change in stimulating current for over 6 years.

Incision Modifications

Previous postauricular skin incisions may compromise the use of large C–shaped skin flaps. An inverted "U" incision has been proposed in the Cochlear Corporation manual (Fig. 14.**22**). Another design that has been used successfully by us is shown in Figure 14.**23**. A posterior–based skin incision is elevated. The pericranial flap is anteriorly based and is used to cover the implanted components. It is important that the skin flap and pericranial flap incision are overlapping and thus prevent exposure of the device.

Reimplantation

Device failure and the ability to upgrade original cochlear implant electrode systems have been of concern. Unfortunately, all of the implant systems now in use have experienced some component failure requiring replacement. In most instances, removal of short single channel electrodes and long multichannel arrays and replacement with similar or different systems has not resulted in a deterioration in auditory performance. At the same time, upgrading from a single channel system to a multichannel device does not guarantee enhanced performance.

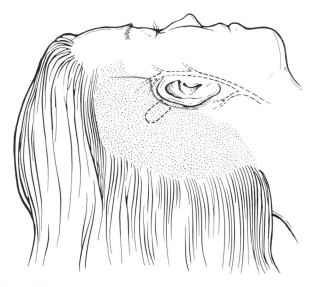

Fig. 14.**23**

The original skin incision should be used for exposure. The skin flap is elevated anteriorly to identify the implant package. The package will likely be encased in a thick fibrous capsule. The fibrous capsule also surrounds the electrode. Sharp dissection is required to free the electrode without dislodging it from the cochlea. New cortical bone may partially encase the lateral extent of the electrode. The medial mastoid and facial recess are usually open. Facial nerve monitoring should be used when freeing the electrode from the facial ridge as an exposed nerve may adhere to the electrode. On exposure of the round window and

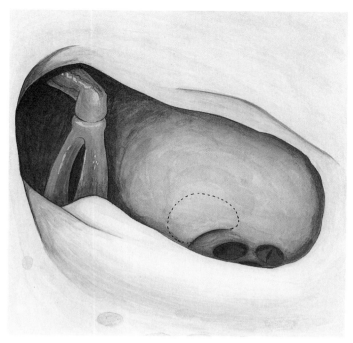

Fig. 14.**24**

cochleostomy, the electrode can be slowly removed from the cochlea. The cochleostomy may require enlargement with a small diamond drill to remove ball–type electrodes (House 3M, Ineraid). If a ball becomes dislodged, do not attempt to retrieve it as it has not affected reinsertion or the electrical field, in our experience.

After removal, the cochleostomy should be slightly enlarged to remove obstructing soft tissue and a replacement device inserted. Bone and/or soft tissue obstruction has not prevented replacement of the same size or longer implants in our series (Gantz et al., 1989).

Postoperative Care

The postoperative care following placement of a cochlear implant is similar to an intact canal wall mastoidectomy. The mastoid pressure dressing is changed during the first postoperative day. If there is a moderate drainage, the penrose drain is left in place and the pressure dressing replaced. The drain is removed by 48 hours (except in the canal wall down extended drillout procedure). A light dressing can be placed by 72 hours. The skin sutures are removed at one week. Stimulation and implant programming usually occur one month after placement of the electrode.

Complications

Placement of cochlear implants has resulted in few complications. The most common surgical complication has been associated with skin–flap breakdown and exposure of the implant (Cohen et al., 1988). Facial nerve injury, prolonged vestibular disturbance, and infections necessitating removal of implants are rare. There have been no reported cases of meningitis following otitis media in an implanted ear in either children or adults.

Skin–flap failure can be prevented by appropriate design. It is important to incorporate the superficial temporal artery and/or occipital artery distribution in the outline. Known width–length ratios for skin flaps must be taken into consideration. The flap should be handled minimally and kept moist with a gauze sponge during the procedure.

Facial nerve injury is best prevented by direct observation of the course of the nerve during surgical exposure and use of facial nerve monitoring equipment. Copious irrigation and diamond burrs are used to open the facial recess. A thin layer of bone should be left over the nerve. During creation of the cochleostomy anterior to the nerve, the shaft of the burr should not come in contact with the facial ridge. Heat from friction can induce severe injury to the nerve.

Misplacement of the electrodes has also occurred. Occasionally, a large retrocochlear air cell is present inferior to the round window. High resolution CT imaging studies will demonstrate the position of such a feature. The round window is 1 to 1.5 mm inferior to the pyramidal eminence. If an opening is inferior to this distance, a retrocochlear air cell may have been exposed (Fig. 14.**24**). There is almost always excessive fluid drainage from the scala tympani when the endosteal layer is penetrated. A dry scala should alert the surgeon that an air cell has been exposed.

Kinking of the electrode array during insertion can be averted by slow introduction into the scala tympani. If resistance is encountered, the array is withdrawn 1 or 2 mm, turned in the direction of the cochlear spiral, and advanced. If continued resistance prevents insertion, repeat one or two times, then leave the electrode in its most forward position. Do not continue to advance the system, as bunching of the electrodes may short out the entire system.

If a transcutaneous system or percutaneous transmission system becomes exposed, a procedure is performed to close the defect. Closure should incorporate both a scalp rotation advancement design, and a separate pericranial rotation advancement flap (Fig. 14.**25 a, b**). Rarely is explantation of a system required.

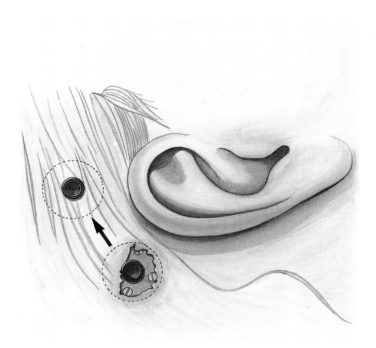

Fig. 14.**25 a**

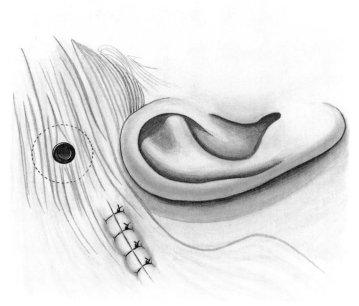

Fig. 14.**25 b**

Conclusions

The clinical results have been reported elsewhere (Gantz et al., 1988; Tye-Murray et al., 1992). In summary, multichannel implant systems provide more useful information and have provided word recognition without the aid of speach reading in most postlingual adults. There are subjects who only achieve enhanced speech reading and sound awareness with all systems. Evaluation of different multichannel designs has shown little overall difference using different numbers of electrodes and speech coding strategies. There are, however, great individual differences in performance within groups of subjects using similar implant design. A newer, faster alternating pulsatile speech coding algorithm has been shown to greatly enhance speech understanding in some postlingual adults (Wilson et al., 1989). Newly designed implant systems are incorporating this coding strategy.

Bibliography

Balkany T, Gantz B, Nadol J. Multichannel Cochlear Implants in Partially Ossified Cochleas. Ann Otol Rhinol Laryngol (Suppl) 1988; 135:3.

Brimacombe J A. Cochlear Implant Results in Pre/Perilinguistically Deafened Adults. Presented at 92nd Annual Meeting of American Academy Otolaryngology-Head and Neck Surgery, Washington, DC, September 28, 1988.

Cohen N L, Hoffman R A, Strochein M. Medical or Surgical Complications Related to the Nucleus Multichannel Cochlear Implant. Ann Otol Rhinol Laryngol (Suppl) 1988; 135.

Eisenberg L S. Use of the Cochlear Implant by the Prelingually Deaf. In House WF, Berliner KT (Eds): Cochlear Implants: Progress and Perspectives. Ann Otol Rhinol Laryngol (Suppl) 1982; 91:62.

Gantz B J: Cochlear Implants: An Overview. In: Adv Otolaryngol Head Neck Surg 1987; 1:171.

Gantz B J, Lowder M W, McCabe B F. Audiologic Results Following Reimplantation of Cochlear Implants. Ann Otol Rhinol Laryngol (Suppl) 1989; 142:12.

Gantz B J, McCabe B F, Tyler R S. Use of Multichannel Cochlear Implants in Obstructed and Obliterated Cochleas. Otolaryngol Head Neck Surg 1988; 98:72.

Gantz B J, Tyler R S, Knutson J F, Woodworth G, et al. Evaluation of 5 Different Cochlear Implant Designs. Laryngoscope 1988; 98:1100.

House W F, Luxford W M, Courtney B. Otitis Media in Children Following Cochlear Implant. Ear & Hear (Suppl) 1986; 3:245.

Pfingst B. Stimulation and Encoding Strategies for Cochlear Prostheses. Otolaryngologic Clinics North America 1986; 19:219.

Ross M, Lerman J. Word Intelligibility By Picture Identification. Pittsburgh: Stansix House, Inc., 1971.

Thielemeir M A. Discrimination After Training Test. House Ear Institute, 1982.

Tye-Murray N, Tyler R, Woodworth G, Gantz B. Performance Over Time With a Nucleus or Ineraid Cochlear Implant. Speech Hearing, 1992; 13:200.

Tyler R S, Preece J, Tye-Murray N. The Laser Video-disc Sentence Test, Laser Videodisc. The University of Iowa, Department of Otolaryngology-Head and Neck Surgery, Iowa City, IA, 1986.

Wilson B S, Finley C C, Lawson D T. Speech Processors for auditory prosthesis. First Quarter Report, May 1-July 31, 1989. NIH Prosthesis Program, Grant NO1-DC-9-2401.

15 Interventional Neuroradiology for Tumors of the Temporal Bone

Anton Valavanis

Introduction to Embolization Techniques

Interventional neuroradiology uses the technique of embolization to achieve preoperative devascularization of hypervascular tumors of the temporal bone and adjacent areas of the skull base. Recent advances in interventional technology such as the introduction of steerable, highly flexible microcatheters and appropriate embolic materials along with an improved understanding of the functional vascular anatomy of the head and neck allow today a sophisticated endovascular exploration and efficient devascularization of complex, hypervascular tumors of the temporal bone and skull base, with a morbidity near zero (Valavanis, 1990).

This chapter describes the indications, principles, techniques as well as dangers and potential complications of preoperative embolization of tumors involving the temporal bone and its adjacent skull base area.

Indications

The main indications for embolization of tumors of the temporal bone and the surrounding skull base include neoplasms which are known to be hypervascular and others which are shown by CT and MRI to possess significant hypervascularity. The following list includes tumors which represent an indication for embolization:

- Glomus tumors of the temporal bone;
- Meningiomas:
  - posterior surface of temporal bone,
  - cerebellopontine angle,
  - petroclival area,
  - jugular foramen,
  - within the temporal bone (very rare);
- Neurinomas:
  - cerebellopontine angle,
  - jugular foramen,
  - hypoglossal canal,
  - trigeminal root;
- Hemangiomas of the temporal bone;
- Neurofibromas in conjunction with neurofibromatosis;
- Hemangiopericytoma;

Since glomus tumors of the temporal bone represent by far the most common and most important indication for preoperative embolization, this chapter will deal specifically with the principles, techniques as well as dangers and potential complications of embolization of glomus tumors of the temporal bone. These techniques apply also to the other, more rare, tumor types of the temporal bone.

Pretherapeutic Neuroradiologic Evaluation

A thorough neuroradiologic evaluation of the tumor prior to embolization and surgery is essential for planning the embolization technique and the surgical approach. Computed tomography (CT) and magnetic resonance imaging (MRI) represent complementary imaging techniques for the evaluation of glomus tumors as well as of other hypervascular lesions of the temporal bone. High resolution CT provides essential information concerning the relationship of the tumor to the surrounding bony structures, specifically the jugular foramen, the carotid canal, the facial nerve canal, the hypoglossal canal and the infralabyrinthine and labyrinthine compartments of the temporal bone.

Gadolinium-enhanced, multiplanar, thin section, T1-weighted MRI is used to assess the intrinsic soft tissue morphology of the tumor, the degree of its vascularity, any intracranial extradural or intradural tumor extension as well as invasion of the adventitia of the petrous portion of the internal carotid artery (Valavanis, 1990).

Goal and Principles of Embolization

The goal of embolization of glomus tumors of the temporal bone as well as of any other tumor of the head and neck is selective obliteration of the pathologic intratumoral vasculature while preserving the normal supply to surrounding tissues. This devascularization of the tumor facilitates subsequent operative removal by improving the intraoperative conditions in terms of blood loss, almost bloodless tumor exposure and therefore easy identification of surgically important or critical structures such as cranial nerves and the wall of the internal carotid artery (Lasjaunias and Berenstein, 1987 b; Valavanis, 1988). If tumor devascularization is properly performed, then it contributes significantly to shortening of the overall operation time, increasing the rate of radicality and reducing the surgical complication rate (Valavanis, 1990).

The basic principles of embolization of tumors in the head and neck is based on superselective angiographic exploration of the tumor, identification of the supplying arteries to the tumor, arteries supplying normal tissue around the tumor, and the selection of the appropriate embolic material.

It must be stressed, however, that embolization of tumors represents a purely preoperative measure and not an alternative to surgery. Its role is not to cure neoplasms, but to assist the surgeon in treating his patients harboring hypervascular and challenging tumors. However, in exceptional situations, where general anaesthesia or operation cannot be performed due to severe medical conditions, embolization can be performed as a palliative measure in order to reduce temporarily the size and thus the mass effect of the tumor as well as related symptoms.

General Techniques of Embolization

Angiographic investigation of the tumor and its subsequent embolization should preferably by performed under general anaesthesia. This provides optimal working conditions for the interventional neuroradiologist and in addition it minimizes the risk of arterial spasm in the sensitive external carotid artery. The patient should be prepared and premedicated for general anaesthesia the night before the procedure.

All procedures should be performed through the femoral artery because this approach allows catheterization of both internal carotid arteries, both external carotid arteries, and both vertebral arteries from a single puncture site and provides in addition optimal irradiation protection for the interventional neuroradiologist. Angiography should be performed with the digital subtraction technique which provides instantaneously subtracted images, has an inherent higher contrast resolution than conventional film angiography, and permits the use of reduced amounts of diluted iodinated contrast material.

Selective angiographic exploration of the tumor should be performed with polyethylene, medium–sized catheters of a diameter of 5.5 French. Such catheters are flexible enough and have a sufficient torque control to permit catheterization of individual feeding arteries in the head and neck area. Furthermore, their relatively thin wall permits the coaxial insertion of microcatheters for subsequent superselective angiography and embolization. Variable stiffness microcatheters (Tracker Microcatheter, Target Therapeutics, Los Angeles) are usually used for that purpose. These microcatheters can be advanced over tortuous or angulated arterial segments and allow catheterization of the distal portion of feeding arteries, very close to the tumoral vascular bed.

Among the available embolic materials including various types of microparticles, polymerizing and not-polymerizing fluid materials, detachable balloons, and various types of microcoils, microparticles of polyvinyl alcohol foam (Ivalon, Contour) are usually preferred in preoperative tumor embolization (Lasjaunias and Berenstein, 1987 b). Microparticles of polyvinyl alcohol foam are available in different sizes ranging from 45–500 mu. As a general rule, the smallest available size in the range of 45–150 mu should be used in tumor embolization (Valavanis, 1990).

Microparticles of this size easily reach the intratumoral vascular bed and are ideal for preoperative tumor devascularization. Since there is no diastolic flow in the territory of the external carotid artery, injection of the microparticles diluted in contrast material should be performed during systole. This is performed with intermittent injections of small amounts of embolic material under fluoroscopic control during the systolic peak, as seen on the electrocardiogram.

In exceptional cases, fluid materials, specifically N-butyl–2–cyanoacrylate (NBCA) can be used. This material should only be used in tumors characterized by high arterial flow and intratumoral av-shunts. The polymerization time can be delayed if one adds oily iodinated contrast material (Pantopaque). NBCA is made radiopaque and visible fluoroscopically by the addition of a small amount of tantalum powder. For tumor embolization, the mixture of NBCA and Pantopaque should be such that the polymerization is significantly delayed in order for the NBCA to penetrate into the distal intratumoral vascular bed. NBCA is a dangerous embolic material because it can penetrate distally into vascular territories and cause ischemia of vital tissues and it may polymerize rapidly, thus gluing the catheter tip within the arterial lumen. Therefore, its use requires considerable expertise in interventional neuroradiology (Lasjaunias and Berenstein, 1987 b).

Balloon Occlusion of the Internal Carotid Artery

Tumors of the temporal bone, specifically glomus tumors, may exhibit an intimate relationship to the adventitia of the internal carotid artery. Invasion of the adventitia of the internal carotid artery or significant arterial supply from branches of the internal carotid artery arising from its cavernous or petrous segments represent major limiting factors for safe and radical removal of such tumors (Lasjaunias et al., 1987).

Attempts at removal of pericarotid tumor portions attached to the adventitia may lead to laceration of the wall of the internal carotid artery with uncontrollable hemorrhage and thus to significant morbidity and mortality. The introduction of the technique of preoperative permanent balloon occlusion of the internal carotid artery contributed to safe and complete removal of extensive skull base tumors and especially extensive glomus tumors of the temporal bone involving the adventitia of the internal carotid artery. This technique contributed to increasing the rate of radical tumor removal and decreasing both the recurrence rate and the intraoperative complication rate (Valavanis, 1988).

In contrast to the transarterial embolization procedure, the procedure of permanent balloon occlusion of the internal carotid artery should be performed with the patient awake, so that the neurologic condition can be continuously controlled. Prior to permanent balloon occlusion, an angiographic tolerance test has to demonstrate an adequate collateral supply to the cerebral hemisphere ipsilateral to the internal carotid artery to be sacrificed and the absence of any neurologic deficit occurring during the test period. This test is performed by temporary endoluminal inflation of a non–detachable balloon at the level of the cavernous segment of the internal carotid artery and injection of contrast material into the contralateral internal carotid artery as well as into the dominant vertebral artery. Sufficient collaterals at the level of the circle of Willis are present when there is rapid and complete filling of the middle and anterior cerebral arteries on the side of the temporarily

occluded internal carotid artery as well as when there is simultaneous appearance of the venous phase, on both sides.

For permanent balloon occlusion of the internal carotid artery, a non–tapered 7 French catheter is placed transfemorally into the proximal segment of the internal carotid artery. A latex microballoon attached to a microcatheter system is inserted coaxially through the guiding catheter into the internal carotid artery and advanced towards the cavernous segment of the internal carotid artery. The balloon should be inflated with isotonic iodinated contrast material until the lumen of the internal carotid artery is occluded. The inflated balloon should be positioned distal to the origin of the inferolateral trunk of the cavernous segment of the internal carotid artery but proximal to the origin of the ophthalmic artery. This will prevent anterograde thromboembolism from thrombus formed distal to the balloon and dislodged by inflow through the inferolateral trunk. The balloon is detached by gently pulling on the microcatheter to which it is attached. In cases with extensive supply of the tumor from the internal carotid artery branches, the pericarotid portions of the tumor can be embolized with microparticles injected through the guiding catheter into the internal carotid artery and flow carried into the supplying branches, after balloon detachment. In order to prevent distal migration of the first balloon in case it should deflate prematurely, and in order to prevent extensive thrombus formation within the proximal internal carotid artery carrying the risk of ophthalmic artery embolism through the external carotid artery system, the procedure should be terminated by detaching a second balloon within the proximal segment of the internal carotid artery (Lasjaunias and Berenstein, 1987 b; Valavanis, 1990).

Following this procedure the patient should be monitored closely for at least 12 hours in an intensive care unit with special attention to the clinical neurologic condition of the patient and continuous monitoring of the blood pressure. Blood pressure below the systolic level of 100 mm Hg may cause ischemia in the cerebral hemisphere ipsilateral to the occluded internal carotid artery. In these cases volume expanders (Dextran) should be infused.

Embolization Technique for Glomus Tumors of the Temporal Bone

Glomus tumors of the temporal bone comprise approximately 48% of all glomus tumors in the head and neck area. In approximately 10% of cases multifocal glomus tumors are encountered. Familial cases do occur and have a high incidence of approximately 30% for multifocal tumors. Five percent of glomus tumors exhibit secretory activity causing hypertensive crises, palpitations, and headaches (Zak and Lawson, 1982).

Glomus tumors of the temporal bone are usually benign but are characterized by local invasiveness, and a high degree of vascularity. They may arise from glomus bodies distributed in the middle ear cavity (i.e. glomus tympanicum tumors) or in the jugular fossa (i.e. glomus jugulare tumors).

In 1982 Fisch introduced a detailed classification of glomus tumors of the temporal bone which was later further refined in order to incorporate the experience of neuroradiologic imaging techniques, interventional neuroradiology, and otoneuromicrosurgical techniques. This classification proved useful both for planning the embolization and for selecting the appropriate surgical approach. According to this classification glomus tumors of the temporal bone are categorized as follows (Fisch and Mattox, 1988):

Class A:
Glomus tympanicum tumors confined to the tympanic cavity;

Class B:
Glomus tympanicum tumors extending into the mastoid bone but leaving the cortical outline of the jugular bulb intact;

Class C:
Glomus jugulare tumors with variable degrees of extension into the infralabyrinthine portion of the temporal bone and along the petrous carotid canal. Class C tumors are further categorized according to the degree of involvement of the carotid canal, i.e.:

Class C1:
Glomus tumors with minimal erosion of the vertical segment of the carotid canal;

Class C2:
Glomus tumors with extensive erosion of the vertical segment of the carotid canal;

Class C3:
Glomus tumors with additional erosion of the horizontal segment of the carotid canal;

Class C4:
Glomus tumors with extension into the foramen lacerum and into the cavernous sinus;

Class D:
Glomus jugulare tumors with intracranial extension. Depending on the intra- or extradural location of the intracranial extension these tumors are further subdivided into:

Del-De3
extradural extension of the tumor with variable sizes;

Dil-Di3
tumors with intradural extension and variable sizes.

The complementary use of high–resolution CT and gadolinium–enhanced MRI provides the correct tumor classification. This is followed by the angiographic work–up of the tumor. This is performed according to a specific protocol elaborated for each individual tumor according to the class of tumor present.

Angiographically, glomus tumors of the temporal bone have a pathognomonic appearance consisting of enlarged feeding arteries (ascending pharyngeal artery as well as other branches of the external carotid artery, petrous and cavernous branches of the internal carotid artery, dural and pial branches of the vertebro–basilar system), an early, intense, slightly inhomogeneous tumor blush, and early appearing draining veins (Fig. 15.1). The angiographic exploration of glomus tumors of the temporal bone should identify all supplying arteries (Figs. 15.1 to 15.7) (arising from the external carotid artery, internal carotid artery, and/or vertebral artery), the presence of any dangerous anastomoses between feeding arteries and the internal carotid artery or vertebral artery, cranial nerve supply provided by the feeding arteries (the lower cranial nerves are supplied by the neuromeningeal branch of the ascending pharyngeal artery), and finally the vascular composition of the tumor. It is also very important that

Fig. 15.**1** Common carotid angiography demonstrating medium–sized glomus jugulare tumor with intense tumor blush. Several dilated branches of the external carotid artery supply the tumor. The tumor drains retrograde into the sigmoid sinus.

Fig. 15.**2** Selective catheterization of the inferior tympanic branch of the ascending pharyngeal artery showing the tympanic portion of the tumor.

Fig. 15.**3** Selective catheterization of the neuromeningeal trunk of the ascending pharyngeal artery showing the jugular portion of the tumor.

Fig. 15.**4** Occipital artery angiography showing supply of the tumor from the stylomastoid branch.

Fig. 15.**5** Superselective injection of the stylomastoid branch showing the posterior tympanic and mastoid extension of the tumor, draining into suboccipital veins.

Fig. 15.**6** Selective injection of the posterior auricular artery.

Fig. 15.**7** Selective injection of the middle meningeal artery showing supply of the superior compartment of the tumor from the petrosal branch.

Fig. 15.**8** Common carotid angiography after embolization of all identified feeding arteries with macroparticles of Ivalon of the size of 45–100 mu. This control angiogram shows complete devascularization of the tumor.

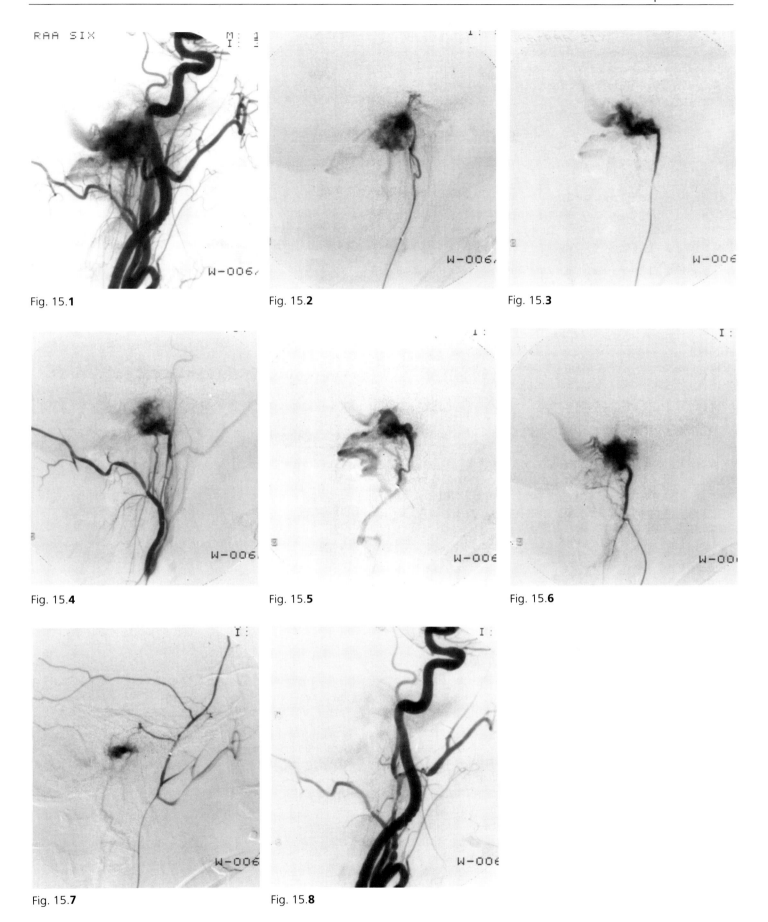

Fig. 15.**1**

Fig. 15.**2**

Fig. 15.**3**

Fig. 15.**4**

Fig. 15.**5**

Fig. 15.**6**

Fig. 15.**7**

Fig. 15.**8**

the relationship of the tumor mass to the internal jugular vein and the adjacent dural sinuses is identified. This is best done by analysis of the venous phase of the ipsilateral vertebral artery angiography performed in frontal projection, in conjunction with the information obtained previously by CT and MRI. With this technique, identification of obstruction of the internal jugular vein and extraluminal compression or intraluminal tumor extension can be reliably identified. Angiographically, 2/3 of glomus temporale tumors exhibit a multicompartmental composition and 1/3 are composed of a single compartment. In monocompartmental tumors embolization of the entire tumor can be performed through one main feeding artery (Valavanis, 1986).

Initially, all glomus temporale tumors receive their supply from branches of the ascending pharyngeal artery. Glomus tympanicum tumors are supplied by the inferior tympanic branch of the ascending pharyngeal artery. Glomus jugulare tumors are supplied by the neuromeningeal branch of the ascending pharyngeal artery. Since glomus jugulare tumors frequently extend into the tympanic cavity, they receive also supply from the inferior tympanic branch of the ascending pharyngeal artery. Larger tumors extending posterolaterally into the tympano–mastoid area receive additional supply from the stylomastoid branch of the occipital artery. If these tumors reach the intracranial extradural space, they receive additional supply from the mastoid branch of the occipital artery which supplies the dura on the posterior part of the posterior surface of the petrous bone and mastoid area.

Anterior intratemporal extensions of the tumor along the carotid canal receive supply from the carotico–tympanic branch of the internal carotid artery which classically arises from the bend of the vertical to the horizontal segment of the internal carotid artery. Further supply of the anterior tumor portion is provided by the anterior tympanic artery arising from the proximal superficial temporal artery or from the distal external carotid artery trunk. Superior tumor extensions into the superior tympanic area and the supralabyrinthine compartment of the temporal bone are supplied by the petrosal branch of the middle meningeal artery. Intracranial extradural tumor extensions receive supply from the lateral clival branch of the internal carotid artery, arising from the proximal cavernous segment of this vessel. More posteriorly located extradural extensions receive supply from dural branches of the vertebral artery. Intracranial intradural tumor extensions are in close contact to the pia mater of the cerebellar and pontine surface and are by definition supplied from the distal pial branches of the anterior and posterior inferior cerebellar arteries (AICA, PICA) (Valavanis, 1986).

Embolization of the tumor is carried out step by step following catheterization of each individual feeding artery of the external carotid artery (Figs. 15.**1** to 15.**8**). If the tumor receives additional supply from the internal carotid artery, the microcatheters available today allow in a high percentage of cases superselective catheterization and embolization of these branches. If, however, this is not possible because of the small size of these internal carotid artery feeding branches, temporary balloon occlusion of the internal carotid artery distal to the origin of these branches and free flow embolization through the microcatheter placed in a more proximal position within the internal carotid artery represents an equally efficient alternative technique (Valavanis, 1990). Before balloon deflation, repeated aspiration of blood through the microcatheter should be performed in order to retrieve any microparticles remaining in the lumen of the internal carotid artery (Theron et al., 1986). The newer types of microcatheters allow also distal catheterization of the branches of AICA and PICA and embolization of the intradural extension of the tumor in selected cases. This, however, requires significant experience with interventional neuroradiologic techniques. As mentioned earlier, embolization of the tumor should be carried out with the smallest available microparticles of polyvinyl–alcohol foam which are usually of a size of 45–100 mu.

Large glomus tumors of the temporal bone exhibiting intracranial extension may require preoperative permanent balloon occlusion of the internal carotid artery, as mentioned earlier in this chapter. This technique should be considered in the following situations (Valavanis 1990):

• tumors with extensive destruction of the horizontal segment of the carotid canal as seen on high–resolution CT;
• all class C4 tumors with extension into the cavernous sinus, as seen on gadolinium–enhanced MRI;
• tumors with erosion of the carotid canal as seen on high–resolution CT and extensive supply from the carotico–tympanic and cavernous branches of the internal carotid artery as seen on selective angiography.

Dangers and Complications

The main dangers of embolization of glomus tumors of the temporal bone include reflux of embolic material from the external carotid into the internal carotid artery, passage of embolic material through arterio–arterial anastomoses from the external carotid artery into the internal carotid artery or vertebral artery, occlusion of external carotid artery branches supplying cranial nerves, and finally occlusion of cutaneous branches of the external carotid artery.

If embolization is being properly performed, reflux of embolic material from the external carotid artery into the internal carotid artery is a very rare event. Distal catheterization of the supplying branches and injection of the embolic material synchronously with the heart beat and thereby during the systolic pulswave of the arterial blood stream avoids reflux (Lasjaunias and Berenstein, 1987b).

It is of utmost importance that the interventional neuroradiologist performing embolization in the external carotid artery territory identifies any arterio–arterial anastomoses. When dealing with glomus tumors of the temporal bone, the most frequently encountered arterio–arterial anastomoses are the following (Lasjaunias and Berenstein, 1987a):

- anastomoses between the ascending pharyngeal artery and the cavernous segment of the internal carotid artery;
- anastomoses between the ascending pharyngeal artery and the petrous segment of the internal carotid artery;
- anastomoses between the ascending pharyngeal artery and the vertebral artery;
- anastomoses between the occipital artery and the vertebral artery;
- anastomoses between the proximal or distal internal maxillary artery and the internal carotid artery.

The presence of an anastomosis does not represent an absolute contraindication to embolization. The following techniques can be used to protect the internal carotid artery or vertebral artery territory in the presence of an anastomosis (Valavanis, 1990):

- the use of particles which are larger in size than the diameter of the anastomotic artery,
- positioning of the catheter tip distal to the origin of the anastomotic artery,
- protection of the internal carotid artery or vertebral artery with a temporarily inflated balloon at the level of entry of the anastomotic artery,
- temporary occlusion of the anastomosing artery by a large reabsorbable piece of embolic material such as gelfoam.

Cranial nerve palsies may occur after embolization of glomus tumors of the temporal bone if the branches of the external carotid artery supplying the cranial nerves are embolized with permanently occluding embolic materials. Knowledge of the normal supply to the transcranial segments of the cranial nerves by branches of the external carotid artery and the use of microparticulate materials instead of polymerizing fluids help to avoid lower cranial nerve palsies during embolization of glomus tumors of the temporal bone.

Since embolization of glomus tumors of the temporal bone is followed by the operative removal of the tumor, occlusion of cutaneous branches of the external carotid artery may cause postoperative wound healing retardation and infection. For this reason occlusion of cutaneous branches of the external carotid artery should be avoided. Cutaneous branches of the external carotid artery that supply the skin in the area of craniotomy in cases of glomus tumors of the temporal bone include the superficial temporal artery and its branches, the posterior auricular artery, and the cutaneous branches of the occipital artery (Lasjaunias and Berenstein, 1987a).

Postembolization Follow-Up

Embolization of glomus tumors of the temporal bone proved to be highly efficient in devascularizing most of these challenging neoplasms. In experienced hands preoperative embolization of glomus tumors is associated with a very low complication rate and without mortality. The effectiveness of embolization is best appreciated on postembolization MRI which shows extensive intratumoral necroses and size reduction of the tumor. Since the great majority of embolizations of glomus tumors of the temporal bone are performed with microparticulate materials, the operation should be performed within 1 to 2 weeks after embolization in order to avoid revascularization of the tumor.

Bibliography

Fisch U, Mattox D. Microsurgery of the skull base. New York: Thieme Medical, 1988.

Lasjaunias P, Berenstein A. Surgical neuroangiography, Volume I: Functional anatomy of craniofacial arteries. Berlin, Heidelberg, New York: Springer, 1987a.

Lasjaunias P. Berenstein A. Surgical neuroangiography, Volume II: Endovaseular treatment of craniofacial lesions. Berlin, Heidelberg, New York: Springer, 1987b.

Lasjaunias P, TerBrugge K, Chin M, Lopez Ibor L. Embolization and balloon–occlusion techniques in the management of cranial base tumors. In: Sekhar L, Schramm Jr, V L (eds). Tumors of the cranial base: diagnosis and treatment. New York: Futura Mount Kisco, 1987.

Théron J, Cosgrove R, Melanson D, Ethier R. Embolization with temporary balloon occlusion of the internal carotid or vertebral arteries. Neuroradiology 1986; 28:246.

Valavanis A. Preoperative embolization of the head and neck: indications, patient selection, goals and precautions. AJNR 1986; 7:943.

Valavanis A. Interventional neuroradiology of skull base tumors. In: Fisch U, Mattox D (eds). Microsurgery of the skull base. New York: Thieme Medical, 1988.

Valavanis A. Interventional neuroradiology for head and neck surgery. In: Cummings C W, Fredrickson J M, Harker L A, Krause C J, Schuller D E (eds). Otolaryngology — head and neck surgery. Update II. St. Louis: Mosby Year Book, 1990.

Zak, F G, Lawson W. The paraganglionic chemoreceptor system: Physiology, pathology and clinical medicine. Berlin, Heidelberg, New York: Springer, 1982.

Index

A

Abscess(es)
  brain 363
  cerebellar 268
  epidural 360
  episinus 263
  extradural 263, 266
    diagnosis 264
  otogenic brain 267
  otogenic cerebellar 268
  otogenic extradural 263
  subdural 362
  temporal lobe 268
Accessory nerve 367
Acoustic neuroma/tumor 171, 301
  diagnosis 301, 313
  indications for surgery 301, 313
  MRI 313
    gadolinium enhanced 313
  preoperative evaluation 301, 313
  radiotherapy 311
    gamma knife 311
    linear accelerator 311
  removal 301, 313
    anesthesia 302
    incision of dura 304
    middle fossa approach 311, 313
      anesthesia 318
      exposure of internal auditory canal
        322
      incision 318
      indications for surgery 313
      instruments 315
      operative technique 318
      postoperative complications 327
    opening of internal auditory canal 304
    patient position 302
    postoperative complications 310
    retrosigmoid (lateral suboccipital) ap-
      proach 301
      operative technique 303
    translabyrinthine approach 311, 313, 328
      anesthesia 328
      indications 328
      operative technique 328
      patient selection 328
      postoperative complications 339
Acromegaly 230
Adipose tissue
  middle ear 44

AIDS 126
Allergic reactions
  local anesthesia of ear 3
Anastomosis(es)
  hypoglossofacial nerve 153
  spinal accessory to facial nerve 153
Anatomy
  temporal bone 67
Anesthesia
  acoustic neuroma removal 302
    middle fossa approach 318
    translabyrinthine approach 328
  antral drainage 80
  antrotomy 80
  cochlear implants 374
  congenital aural atresia 54
  congenital ear malformations 40
  congenital microtia 22
    auricular reconstruction 22
  congenital stenosis 54
  ear
    allergic reactions 3
    infiltration technique 2
    local 1
    premedication 2
  earlobe reconstruction 31
  endolymphatic sac surgery 277
  external ear canal surgery 132
  external meatus surgery 69
  facial nerve reconstruction 216
  fenestration 254
  helix reconstruction 18
  labyrinthectomy 283
  local 1
    of ear 1
  lop ear correction 14
  mastoid 1
    injuries 155
  mastoidectomy 80
  middle ear 1
  otogenic intracranial complications 265
  otogenic sinus thrombosis 271
  otoplasty 6
  radical mastoid cavity 87
  stapedectomy 232
  subtotal petrosectomy 180
  total petrosectomy 180
  translabyrinthine neurectomy 293
  transtemporal neurectomy 286
  tympanic cholesteatoma 107
  tympanic sclerosis 105

  tympanosclerosis 102
Angiography
  digital subtraction 388
Anotia 14
Antral drainage 80
  anesthesia 80
  operative technique 82
Antritis 80
Antrotomy 77, 80
  anesthesia 80
  indications 80
  operative technique 82
Antrum 80
Arachnoid cyst 101, 166
  external meatus 68
    removal 73
Aseptic bone necrosis 73
  external meatus 73
Ataxia
  cerebellar 268
Atelectasis
  tympanic 108
Atresia
  aural 38
    bilateral 22
Atropine 2
Atticoantrotomy 84
Atticotomy 46
Audiologic evaluation/testing
  congenital ear malformations 38
  congenital microtia 22
  facial nerve injuries 147
  stapedectomy 230
Audiometric evaluation
  congenital aural atresia 51
  congenital stenosis 51
  ossicular chain injuries 139
  temporal bone trauma 132
  tympanic membrane injuries 136
Auditory brain stem response 309
  audiometry 313
  test 50, 51
Auditory canal
  benign tumors 159
  external 159
    tumors 159
      CT 159
      diagnosis 162
      operative technique 160
      tympanic membrane involvement 162
  malignant tumors 159

Aural atresia 38, 50, 54
  congenital 50
    anesthesia 54
    audiometric evaluation 51
    auditory brainstem response test 51
    CT of temporal bone 51
    diagnosis 50
    indications for surgery 52
    operative technique 54
Auricle
  angle to head 6
  hypoplasia 14
  plastic surgery 5
  reconstruction 5, 22
    congenital microtia 22
  sensory nerves 2
Auricular defects 14
  Tanzer's classification 14
Autogenous nerve bypass (Dott's technique) 366
Axonotmesis 210, 218

B

Balloon occlusion
  internal carotid artery 389
Barotrauma 136
Basal cell carcinoma 368
Battle's sign 154
  mastoid injuries 154
Bell's palsy 207, 216, 220
Bell's phenomenon 145
Bellucci classification 110
Bezold's mastoiditis 85
Bill's bar 323,324, 333
Bill's island 331, 332
Body parts test 372
Brain abscess 100, 363
  diagnosis 363
  extirpation 364
  otogenic 267
  rhinogenic 267
  surgical treatment 363
  symptoms 363
Brain herniation 154
Brainstem audiometry 208, 277, 309
Brainstem auditory evoked potentials 309
Brent's technique 23, 31
  auricular reconstruction for congenital
    microtia 23
  earlobe reconstruction 31
Burr hole trephination 352
Buttock sign 56

C

Carhart's notch 230, 261
Carotid artery 38
  anomalous internal 38
Carotid cavernous fistula 369
  traumatic 369
    endovascular occlusion 369
    hemodynamics 369
    trapping operation 369
Carticaine 1
Cartilage
  tympanic membrane reconstruction 114
Catheter
  urethral 40
Celestamine 79
Cerebellar abscess 268

Cerebellopontine angle 220, 221, 339, 387
  hematoma 339
  meningioma 387
  neurinoma 387
Cerebral prolapse 101, 270
Cerebrospinal fluid (CSF) 136
  examination 264
  fistula 281
    traumatic 359
  otorrhea 138, 154
  rhinorrhea 359
    paradoxical 310
    persistent 359
    spontaneous nontraumatic 359
    transcranial intradural approach 360
    traumatic 359
Ceruminoma 166
Cervical plexus 212
  nerve grafts 212
Chemosis 145
  periorbital 145
Chest wall 30
  deformities 30
Children
  tests for cochlear implant 372
Cholesteatoma 52, 88, 110, 134, 135, 154,
  161, 216
  bacterially infected 263
  closed technique 85
  congenital 38
  invasion of labyrinth 98
  invasion of petrous apex 98, 171
  open technique 85
  petrous apex 98,171
  primary 124
  recurrence 101
  treatment options 85
  true (epidermoid) 171
Cholesterol granuloma 80, 88, 101, 105
Chondritis 13, 30
Chondroma 368
Chorda tympani 114
  nerve, abnormal 47
Chordoma 368
Choristoma 44
CID low verbal test battery 372
Ciprofloxicin 49
Cleft deformities 77
  ventilation tube 77
Cochlea 374
  patency 374
Cochlear function 39
Cochlear implant(s) 371
  anesthesia 374
  audiologic prerequisites 372
  complications 384
    electrode misplacement 384
    facial nerve injury 384
  electrophysiology 374
  imaging 374
  indications 372
  medical prerequisites 372
  operative technique 375
    electrode replacement 379
    limited mastoidectomy 377
    posterior tympanotomy 378
    radical mastoidectomy 381
    reimplantation 383
    scala tympani cochleostomy 378
    skin flaps 376
    skin incision 375
  postoperative care 384
  preoperative evaluation 371

selection of ear 374
Cochlear nerve 301, 374
  preservation 301
Cochleostomy 378
  scala tympani 378
Cochleovestibular neurectomy 299
Computed tomography (CT)
  external auditory canal tumors 162
  facial nerve paralysis 208
  glomus tumor of temporal bone 387
  high resolution
    cochlear patency 374
    mastoid injuries 154
    temporal bone fractures 147
  temporal bone 38, 51, 132, 387
    congenital aural atresia 51
    congenital stenosis 51
    glomus tumors 387
    trauma 132
Conchal cartilage 9
  excision 9
Conductive hearing loss 65, 171
  progressive 65
Congenital ear malformations 35
  anesthesia 40
  audiologic evaluation 38
  classification 35
  CT of temporal bones 38
  indications for surgery 39
  minor 35
  operative technique 42
    endaural approach 47
    postauricular approach 42
  surgical management 35
Congenital microtia 22
  audiologic evaluation 22
  auricular reconstruction 22
    anesthesia 22
    Brent's technique 23
    indications 22
    operative technique 23
    postoperative complications 30
    rib graft 24
  classification 22
Congenital stapes ankylosis 40
Converse technique 12
Cosman technique 15
  lop ear correction 15
Cranial infections 360
Cranial nerve(s) 194, 367, 393
  anastomosis 367
  palsy 393
Cranial osteomyelitis 360
  operative treatment 360
Craniectomy 342
Craniopharyngeal duct 359
  persistent 359
Craniotomy 303, 342, 350
  subtentorial 350
  supratentorial 342
Cross-facial grafting 368
  nerve repair 368
Cryptotia 14
CSF, see cerebrospinal fluid
CT, see computed tomography
Cup ear 14

D

Deafness
  postlingual 371
  prelingual 371

Dermatitis 161
Devascularization 368, 387
   highly vascularized skull base tumors 368
   hypervascular temporal bone tumors 387
Diabetes mellitus 310
Diazepam 2
Digital subtraction angiography 388
Disequilibrium 277
   surgery of internal auditory canal 277
   surgery of the labyrinth 277
Diversification concept of Stennert 211
Dizziness 313
Dott's technique 366
   autogenous nerve bypass 366
Down syndrome 40
Dura
   incision 304
Dysdiadochokinesia 268

E

Ear(s)
   anesthesia 1
   lop, see lop ears
   pinching 13
   protruding 5
      correction 5
Ear canal
   removal of exostoses 70
Earlobe
   reconstruction 30
      anesthesia 31
      Brent's technique 31
      diagnosis 30
      Gavellos technique 32
      operative technique 31
      reduction 30, 32
Ectactic jugular bulb 168
Electrical testing 208
   facial nerve paralysis 208
Electrocochleography 277
Electrodiagnostic tests 147
   facial nerve injuries 147
Electromyography 148, 208
   evoked 208
   facial nerve injuries 148
   facial nerve paralysis 208
Electroneuro(no)graphy 148, 208
   facial nerve injuries 148
   facial nerve paralysis 208
Electrophysiology
   cochlear implants 374
Embolic materials 388
   N-butyl-2-cyanoacrylate (NBCA) 388
   detachable balloons 388
   microcoils 388
   microparticles 388
   non-polymerizing fluids 388
   polymerizing fluids 388
   polyvinyl alcohol foam microparticles 388
Embolization 388
   general technique 388
   glomus tumors of temporal bone 388
   highly vascular skull base tumors 368
Empyema
   subdural 267, 362
Encephalocele 359
Endarterectomy 369
   internal carotid 369
Endolymphatic hydrops 277
Endolymphatic sac surgery 277
   anesthesia 277

indications 277
   operative technique 278
Epidural abscess 360
Epidural hematoma 358
   surgical management 358
Epinephrine 1
Epineural nerve repair 366
Episinus abscess 263
ESR, increased 80
Eustachian tube 76, 105, 108, 230
   bony stenosis 106
   mucous plug removal 76
   occlusion 105, 108
   patency 230
   stenosis 108
Evoked electromyography 208
   facial nerve paralysis 208
Exophthalmos 369
   pulsatile 369
Exostoses 69, 70
   ear canal 70
      removal 70
   obliterative 69
   pedunculated 70
External auditory canal 131
   indications for surgery 132
   injuries 131
   stenosis 132
External carotid artery 388
External ear canal 132
   bony stenosis 132
   removal of bone fragments 132
   soft tissue stenosis 132
      recurrence 135
   surgery 132
      anesthesia 132
      operative technique 132
External meatus 67, 68, 69, 70, 73
   arachnoid cysts 68, 73
      removal 73
   aseptic bone necrosis 73
   foreign bodies 68
      removal 68
         operative technique 70
   infection 72
   inflammatory lesions 69
   partial resection 73
   polyps 68
      removal 68
         operative technique 70
   reactive lesions 69
   surgery 67
      anesthesia 69
      indications 68
      operative technique 70
Extradural abscess 263, 266
   diagnosis 264

F

Facial nerve 115, 144
   aberrant 124
   decompression 216
      transmastoid 214
         operative technique 216
   displaced 44, 56
   dissection 336
   electromyography test 301
   end-to-end anastomosis in cerebellopon-
      tine angle 221
   function, grafting 146
   identification 336

immediate reconstruction 307
infranuclear (peripheral) lesions 207
injuries
   anastomosis 151
   audiologic testing 147
   cochlear implants 384
   diagnosis 145
      physical examination 145
   electrodiagnostic tests 147
   electromyography 148
   electroneuronography 148
   etiology 144
   imaging 147
   incidence 144
   indications for surgery 148
   intraoperative 209
   maximal stimulation test 147
   nerve excitability test 147
   neurological status 149
   operative technique 149
      transmastoid-extralabyrinthine 149
   pathology 144
   Schirmer's test 147
   stapedius reflex 147
   surgical treatment 144
intracranial-intratemporal anastomosis 221
intracranial portion 211
   lesions 211
      surgical options 211
   proximal to stylomastoid foramen 207
intratemporal-extratemporal reconstruction 226
   operative technique 226
intratemporal portion 221
   lesions 211
      surgical options 211
meatolabyrinthine-tympanomastoid exposure 220
   indications 220
   operative technique 220
monitoring 48
motor evoked potentials test
neuroma 166, 168, 171
palsy 118, 284
paralysis 48, 64, 138, 144, 146, 209
   classification 146
   CT 208
   electrical testing 208
   electromyography 208
   electroneuronography 208
   indications for surgery 209
   MRI 208
   otitis media 210
   postoperative 209
   posttraumatic 209
   site-of-lesion determination 208
   traumatic 144
   radiology 208
preservation 301
reconstruction 212, 214, 215, 216, 222
   anesthesia 216
   grafts 212
   indications for surgery 215
   in internal auditory canal 222
   operative technique 214
supranuclear (central) lesions 207
surgery 144, 222, 224
   from cerebellopontine angle to sty-
      lomastoid foramen 220
      operative technique 220
   for injuries 144
      translabyrinthine approach 224
         operative technique 224

Facial surgery
    transtemporal extradural approach 222
      operative technique 222
    surgical segmental anatomy 212
    transposition 180
    tympanomastoid reconstruction 225
    vascular decompression 220
      in cerebellopontine angle 220
    weakness 48
Facial paralysis 37, 143, 207
    see also facial nerve paralysis
    House-Brackmann grading system 207
    idiopathic 207
    Stennert's paresis score 207
    Stennert's residual defect score 207
Femoral artery 388
Fenestration 48, 229, 254
    anesthesia 254
    indications 254
    operative technique 254
      one-stage endaural procedure 254
    postoperative complications 261
    promontory 126
    standard 259
Fibroma 368
    nasopharyngeal 368
Fisch classification 178, 390
    glomus tumors of temporal bone 390
    middle ear tumors 178
Fisch type C infratemporal fossa approach
    197
Floating footplate 248
Fluctuating hearing 49
Footplate 127, 143, 245, 248
    floating 248
    fractures 143
    thick 245
Foreign bodies 68, 70
    external meatus 68
      removal 70
        operative technique 70
Fossa triangularis 12
Frankfurt horizontal 303

G

Gavello's technique 32
    earlobe reconstruction 32
Geniculate ganglion
    decompression through auditory canal
    218
      anesthesia 218
      operative technique 219
Gentamycin 282
    partial destruction of vestibular labyrinth
    282
Glomus tumor(s)
    jugulare 38
    middle ear 171
    radiation therapy 180
    temporal bone 387
      balloon occlusion of internal carotid
        artery 389
      dangers of embolization 392
      embolization principles 388
      embolization technique 388, 389
      Fisch classification 390
      postembolization follow-up 393
      pretherapeutic neuroradiologic evalua-
        tion 387
    tympanicum 38, 166
Glomus tympanicum tumor 38, 166

Greater auricular nerve 152
    grafts 152
Greater petrosal nerve 191
Griesinger's sign 154
    mastoid injuries 154
Grunert's operation 275
Gunshot wounds 154, 155
    mastoid injuries 154
Gushers 248

H

Head injuries 358
    surgical management 358
Hearing device 49
Hearing loss 49, 105, 277
    bilateral conductive 105
    fluctuating 277
    sensorineural 49
Heermann's cartilage reconstruction tech-
    nique 108
Heermann dilatation technique 105
Heermann's palisade technique 114, 116
Helix 14, 18
    constricted 14
    reconstruction 18
      anesthesia 18
      indications 18
      operative technique 18
Hemangioma 387
    temporal bone 387
Hemangiopericytoma 387
Hematoma 339, 358, 359
    acute subdural 358
    cerebellopontine angle 339
    chronic subdural 359
    epidural 358
Herpes zoster 264
High jugular bulb 166
House-Brackmann grading system, facial
    paralysis 207
House Ear Institute DAT (discrimination
    after training) test 372
House/Urban dissector 335
House/Urban middle fossa retractor 317
Hydrocephalus 268, 271
    otitic 268
Hypertension 268
    otogenic intracranial 268
Hypertrophic scarring 30
Hyperventilation 155
Hypoglossal canal 387
    neurinoma 387
Hypoglossal nerve 367
Hypoplasia 14
    of auricle 14

I

Ice-cream cone appearance 139
    incudomallear joint 139
Incudomallear joint 139
    ice-cream cone appearance 139
Incudostapedial joint 88, 139
    disruption 139
    Y sign 139
Incus 44, 120, 127
    abnormality 38
    absent 121
      malleus absent 122
    autograft 123

    displaced 138, 141
      removal 141
    fixation 46
    fractured/dislocated 142
      and stapes fractured/dislocated 142
    homograft 123, 142
    intact 142
      and stapes fractured 142
    interposition 142
    long arm 58
      piggyback appearance 58
    remnant 124
    superstructure 124
Incus/malleus 56
    fused 56
Index for defective hearing 146
    Stennert's 146
Index for paresis 146
    Stennert's 146
Infection
    external meatus 72
    middle ear 76
Infiltration technique
    local anesthesia of ear 2
Inner ear
    abnormalities 39
Instruments
    acoustic tumor removal 314
      middle fossa approach 314
    House/Urban dissector 335
    House/Urban middle fossa retractor 317
    myringotomy tubes 77
    otogenic sinus thrombosis 271
    otoplasty 7
    stapedectomy 231
    Zimmer dermatome 53
Interfascicular nerve repair 365
Internal auditory canal
    dissection 332
    exposure 322
    facial nerve reconstruction 222
    surgery for disequilibrium 277
Internal carotid artery 180, 388, 389
    balloon occlusion 389
    transposition 180
Interventional neuroradiology 387
    temporal bone tumors 387
      indications 387
Iowa sentence test 372

J

Jakob-Creuzfeldt disease 126
Jansen's intact canal wall technique 96
Jansen-type posterior tympanotomy 106
Jugular bulb 38, 180, 27, 2741
    high 38, 307
      uncovered 38
    irrigation 274
    resection 180
    surgery 274
Jugular foramen 387
    meningioma 387
    neurinoma 387
Jugular vein 274
    ligation 274

K

Keratitis 145
Klippel-Feil syndrome 40

L

Labyrinth 98, 277
  cholesteatoma invasion 98
  surgery for disequilibrium 277
Labyrinthectomy 171, 283, 330
  anesthesia 283
  indications 283
  operative technique 283
Labyrinthine fistula 98
  closure 98
Labyrinthine function 117
  assessment 117
Labyrinthine windows 44, 59
Labyrinthitis 85, 263, 267, 373, 380
  cochlear implants 373
  ossificans 380
  purulent 263, 267
Lacrimation 147
  reduced 147
lateral skull base 159
  tumors 159
    surgical treatment 159
Leptomeningitis 263
Lop ear(s) 14, 15, 16
  correction 14,15,16
    anesthesia 14
    Cosman technique 15
    indications 14
    Weerda technique 16

M

Magnetic resonance imaging
  facial nerve paralysis 208
  gadolinium-enhanced 313
    acoustic tumor 313
  glomus tumor of temporal bone 387
Malleostapedopexy 120
  with wire 120
Malleus 44
  absent 122
    and incus absent 122
Malleus bar 36, 46
Malleus handle 36, 120, 127
  absent 120
  curved 36
    imprint on ear drum 36
  encased by cholesteatoma 120
  encroaching on anterior ear canal wall 36
  fractured 120
  shortened 120
  tip 36
    tenting tympanic membrane 36
Malleus head 46
  fixation 46
Mandible 40
  hypoplastic 40
Mannitol 155
Mastoid 80, 154
  anesthesia 1, 155
  bony defect of roof 100
    closure 100
  cavity 260
  injuries 154
    anesthesia 155
    Battle's sign 154
    blunt trauma 154
    causes 154
    diagnosis 154
    Griesinger's sign 154
    imaging 154

  incidence 154
  indications for surgery 154
  surgical treatment 80, 154
Mastoidectomy 80, 81, 155, 162, 330, 337, 381
  anesthesia 80
  complete simple 330
  cortical 330
  indications 80
  limited 377
  operative technique 81
    postauricular approach 81
  radical 381
  simple 155
Mastoiditis 80, 83, 85, 210, 263
  Bezold's 85
  suppurative 85
  purulent 83
Maximal stimulation test 147, 208
  facial nerve injuries 147
  facial nerve paralysis 208
Meatal stenosis 65, 73
Meatoplasty 62
Ménière's disease 77, 231, 277, 282, 285, 299
Ménière-like vestibulocochlear dysfunction 220
Meningioma 368, 387
  cerebellopontine angle 387
  jugular foramen 387
  petroclival area 387
  posterior surface of temporal bone 387
Meningitis 79, 138, 143, 153, 154, 156, 266, 327, 339, 368, 372, 380, 384
  diagnosis 264
  early 263
  labyrinthogenic 265
  otogenic 263
  pneumococcal 264
  potential development routes 263
  purulent 310
  purulent pneumococcal 359
  viral 264
Meperidine 2
Microsomia 40
  hemifacial 40
Microtia 14
  congenital 22, 50
Middle ear
  anesthesia 1
  congenital anomalies 254
  curative surgery 67
  deficient function 126
  effusion 75
    seromucous 75
  glomus tumors 171
  infection 76
  malformations 35
  malignant tumors 196
    indications for surgery 196
    operative technique 197
  opening 112
  reconstructive surgery 67, 110
  sensory nerves 2
  tumors 159, 166
    diagnosis 166
    Fisch classification 178
    indications for surgery 166
    operative technique 166
    surgical treatment 159, 166
  vascular malformations 38
  ventilation tube 75, 77
    operative technique 78

Middle fossa
  dura 84
  exploration 151
    permission 149
Monosyllable Trochee Spondess test (MTS) 372
MRI, see magnetic resonance imaging
Myringoplasty 110, 127
  indications 110
  operative technique 110
Myringosclerosis 102, 116
Myringotomy 75
  ventilation tubes 77

N

Nasopharynx
  inspection 77
Neck
  short and thick 40
Nerve(s)
  anastomosis technique 214
  excitability test 147
    facial nerve injuries 147
  repair techniques 365
    autogenous nerve bypass (Dott's technique) 366
    cranial nerve anastomosis 367
    cross-facial grafting 368
    direct (epineural) 366
    interfascicular (perineural) 365
Neurectomy 283, 285
  cochleovestibular 299
  translabyrinthine 293
  transtemporal 285
Neurinoma
  cerebellopontine angle 387
  hypoglossal canal 387
  jugular foramen 387
  trigeminal root 387
Neurofibroma
  and neurofibromatosis 387
Neurofibromatosis
  and neurofibroma 387
Neuroma
  acoustic, see acoustic neuroma
Neurosurgery
  instruments 341
  operative techniques 342
  preoperative preparation 341
  principles 341
  procedures in head region 341
Neurotmesis 210
Neutapraxia 218
Newborn
  congenital microtia 50
Nitrous oxide 40
NU-6 (Northwestern University) word list 372
Nystagmus 49, 145, 268

O

Onlay technique
  tympanic membrane reconstruction 118
Oozers 248
Oral cavity
  small 40
Ossicular chain 44, 114, 119, 139, 247, 248
  congenital anomalies 248
  fixation at several points 247

Ossicular chain
  injuries 139
    audiometry 139
    causes 139
    diagnosis 139
    imaging 139
    incidence 139
    indications for surgery 140
    operative technique 140
    otoscopy 139
    surgical repair 139
    inspection 141, 236
  lesions 138
  reconstruction 119
    grafts 128
    implants 128
    indications
    operative technique 119
Ossicular landmarks
  abnormal 38
Ossicular prosthesis 119
  PORP 119, 142
  TORP 119
Ossiculoplasty 44, 119
Osteogenesis imperfecta 230
Osteomyelitis
  cranial 360
Otitic hydrocephalus 271
Otitis
  bacterial 264
  externa 68
    malignant 67, 73
    necrotizing 216
  media 115
    acute 79, 210, 216
      cochlear implants 373
    bacterial 263
    chronic 210, 216, 373
      suppurative 80, 103
    facial nerve paralysis 210
    recurrent acute 373
  pneumococcal 264
Otobar 76
Otogenic brain abscess 267
  causes 267
  indications for surgery 268
  location 267
  operative technique 269
    closed treatment 269
    open drainage 269
  pathogenesis 267
  preoperative evaluation 267
Otogenic cerebellar abscess 267
Otogenic extradural abscess 263
Otogenic intracranial complications 263
  anesthesia 265
  indications for surgery 264
  operative technique 265
  surgical management 263
Otogenic sinus thrombosis 271
  anesthesia 272
  indications for surgery 271
  operative technique 271
    aspiration from sinus lumen 273
    evacuation of sinus 273
    jugular bulb irrigation 271
    jugular bulb surgery 274
    jugular vein ligation 274
  preoperative evaluation 271
  signs of sepsis 271
  special instruments 272
Otoplasty
  anesthesia 6

indications 5
  operative technique 8
  postoperative complications 12
Otorrhea
  cerebrospinal fluid 138
  fetid 110
Otosclerosis 45, 86, 229, 380
  around round window 246
  bilateral 230
  malignant juvenile obliterating 254
  unilateral 230
Otoscopy
  ossicular chain injuries 139
Otovent 76
Outer ear
  curative surgery 67
  reconstructive surgery 67, 110
Oval window 44, 48
  complete obstruction 254
  congenital absence 35
  niche
    inaccessible 126
    narrow 246
    obliterated 245
  recurrent closure 250

P

Pachymenigitis
  external 263
Paget's disease 230
Palisade technique of Heermann 114,
  116
Pantopaque 388
Paracentesis 75, 106
Paralysis, facial, 37
  see also facial paralysis
Partial ossicular replacement prosthesis
  (PORP) 119, 142
Pentazocine 2
Perichondritis 101, 161
Perichondrium
  tympanic membrane reconstruction
    114
Perilymph(atic) fistula 49, 140, 248, 250
  closure 140, 142
Perilymphatic gusher 38, 39, 48
Perineural nerve repair 365
Persistent craniopharyngeal duct 359
Persistent stapedial artery 254
Petroclival area
  meningioma 387
Petrosectomy
  subtotal 166, 178
    anesthesia 180
    indications for surgery 178
    operative techniques 180
    with facial nerve resection 178
    with facial nerve transposition 178
    with internal carotid artery transposi-
      tion 178
    with labyrinth preservation 166
  supralabyrinthine subtotal 171
    indications 171
    operative technique 172
    with labyrinth preservation 171
    with labyrinthectomy 171
  total 178
    anesthesia 180
    indications for surgery 178
    operative techniques 180
    with facial nerve resection 178

with facial nerve transposition 178
    with internal carotid artery transposi-
      tion 178
Petrositis 263
Petrous apex
  cholesteatoma invasion 98
Petrous bone
  see temporal bone
Petrous pyramid
  tumor invasion 159
Pierre Robin syndrome 40
Piggyback appearance
  incus long arm 58
Pitanguy technique 10
Plester's promontorial window 47
Pneumocephalus 359
Pneumomediastinum 30
Pneumothorax 30
Pogany cell 217
Polyposis 101
Polyps
  external meatus 68
    removal 70
      operative technique 70
PORP (partial ossicular replacement pros-
  thesis) 119, 142
Positive end expiratory pressure (PEEP)
  ventilation 302
Postlingual deafness 371
Prelingual deafness 371
Prolapse
  cerebral 270
Promethazine 2
Prominent ear 14
Promontorial window 47
Promontory
  fenestration 126
  overhanging wall 246
Prosthesis
  alloplastic 123
  ossicular 119, 142
Protruding ears
  correction 5
Pseudomonas aeruginosa 49, 73
Pure tone audiometry 301, 313
Pyramidal petrous sinus 271

R

Raccoon sign 145
Radiation therapy
  glomus tumors 180
Radical mastoid cavity 85
  anesthesia 87
  indications 86
  operative technique 87
  reduction 91
Radiology
  facial nerve paralysis 208
Retrocochlear air cell 384
Retrosigmoid (lateral suboccipital) approach 301
  acoustic neuroma removal 301
Rhizotomy
  retroganglionic 369
Ribs
  anatomy 23
  dissection 24
  graft for auricular reconstruction 24
Round window
  otosclerosis 246
  reflex 115

S

Salivary glands
  ectopic tissue 44
Scala tympani cochleosotomy 378
Schirmer's test 147, 208
  facial nerve injuries 147
Schüller X-ray projections
  temporal bone 68
Schwann cells 301
Schwannoma
  vestibular 301
Semicircular canal
  dissection 260
Semisitting position
  venous air embolism 302
Sensorineural hearing loss 65, 143, 171
  unilateral 313
Sigmoid sinus 84, 271, 338
  thrombosis 154
Sinus thrombosis 85
Skull base
  fracture 145
  tumors 368
    diagnosis 368
    endovascular procedures 368
    highly vascularized 368
      devascularization 368
    surgical management 368
      subfrontal transcranial-transbasal approach 368
Snuffle ear 102
Sound pressure level 372
Speech audiometry 313
Spinal fluid gusher 38
Stapedectomy 46, 142
  anesthesia 232
  audiological criteria 230
  complete 229, 231, 240
    operative technique 240
  contraindications 231
  indications 230
  instruments 231
  operative technique 233
  partial 229, 231, 238
    removal of posterior third of footplate
      238
  postoperative complications 261
  preoperative evaluation 230
Stapedial ankylosis 229
  surgery 229
Stapedial artery
  persistent 38
Stapedial operations
  complications 248
  early granuloma 249
  facial paralysis 249
  incorrect prosthesis position 250
  long prosthesis 250
  loose prosthesis 249
  revision surgery 248
    indications 248
  subluxation of ossicular chain 249
Stapediovestibular joint
  subluxation 143
Stapedius muscle
  ossified tendon 248
Stapedius reflex test 147, 208
  facial nerve injuries 147
Stapedotomy 46, 240
  operative technique 240
Stapes 44
  capitulum 124

congenital absence 35
  fixation 45
  footplate
    fixation 35
  intact
    and incus dislocated 142
  isolated arch defect 124
  operation 229
  superstructure 124
Stapes/facial nerve axis 35
Stapes-to-malleus reconstruction 120
Staphylococcus aureus 48
Stennert's diversification concept 211
Stennert's index for defective hearing 146
Stennert's index for paresis 146, 207
  facial paralysis 207
Stennert's residual defect score 207
  facial paralysis 207
Stenosis
  congenital 50
    anesthesia 54
    audiometric evaluation 51
    auditory brainstem response test 51
    CT of temporal bone 51
    diagnosis 50
    indications for surgery 52
    operative technique 54
  eustachian tube 108
Stenvers X-ray projections
  temporal bone 68
Stitch abscess 13
Stylomastoid foramen 221
Subdural abscess 362
  surgical management 362
Subdural empyema 267, 362
Subdural hematoma
  acute 358
    surgical management 358
  chronic 359
    surgical management 359
Sulfur hexafluoride 77
Suprameatal spine 84
Suprarenin 1
Sural nerve graft 212, 365
Synkinesis 153

T

Tanzer's classification
  auricular defects 14
Tegmen
  exposure 155
Telephone deformity 12, 13
Temporal bone
  CT 38, 51, 132, 147
    congenital aural atresia 51
    congenital stenosis 51
  curative surgery 67
  fractures 144
    longitudinal 144
    neurological status 149
    oblique 145
    transverse 144
  glomus tumor 387
    balloon occlusion of internal carotid
      artery 389
    dangers of embolization 392
    embolization principles 388
    embolization technique 388, 389
    Fisch classification 390
    postembolization follow-up 393

pretherapeutic neuroradiologic evaluation 387
    hemangioma 387
    imaging 147
    meningioma on posterior surface 387
    reconstructive surgery 67, 110
    Schüller X-ray projections 68
    Stenvers X-ray projections 68
    surgical anatomy 67
    trauma 131
      audiometric evaluation 132
      diagnosis 131
    tumors 387
      interventional neuroradiology 387
      indications 387
Temporal lobe abscess 268
Temporalis fascia
  removal 110
Temporomandibular joint 65, 134
  dysfunction 135
  swelling 65
Thrombosis
  sigmoid sinus 154
Tinnitus 153, 171, 230, 253, 277
  unilateral 313
TORP (total ossicular replacement prosthesis) 119, 142
Translabyrinthine neurectomy 293
  anesthesia 293
  indications 293
  operative technique 293
  postoperative complications 299
Transmastoid facial nerve decompression
  operative technique 216
Transtemporal neurectomy 285
  anesthesia 286
  indications 285
  operative technique 286
  postoperative complications 292
Transtympanic air insufflation 77
Trapping operation
  traumatic carotid cavernous fistula 369
Trauma
  blunt
    mastoid injuries 154
    temporal bone 131
      audiometric evaluation 132
      diagnosis 131
Treacher Collins syndrome 40
Trigeminal nerve 192
Trigeminal root neurinoma 387
Tullio phenomenon 261
Tympanic atelectasis 108
  operative technique 108
  surgical treatment 108
    indications 108
Tympanic bone
  remnant 55
Tympanic cavity 80
  epidermal overgrowth 108
  surgical procedures 80
Tympanic cholesteatoma 106
  anesthesia 107
  indications 107
  operative technique 107
Tympanic fibrosis 105
  anesthesia 105
  surgical treatment 105
    indications 105
Tympanic membrane 75, 116, 127
  atrophy 77, 108, 116
  defects 116
  exposure of region 111

Tympanic membrane
  homograft 118
  injuries 136
    audiometric evaluation 136
    causes 136
    incidence 136
  inspection 36
  perforated 121, 136
  physical examination 136
  reconstruction 112
    graft material 114
    onlay technique 118
  small 38
  surgical procedures 75
    indications 75
    operative technique 76
  surgical repair 136
    indications 136
    operative technique 137
  thermal burns 136
Tympanic membrane-ossicular chain homograft 126
Tympanic sclerosis
  operative technique 105
Tympanoplasty 110
  type II 120
  type III 115, 120
  type IV 126
  Wullstein type I 110
Tympanosclerosis 102, 124, 230, 254
  anesthesia 102
  operative technique 103
  special forms 125
  surgical treatment 102
    indications 102

Tympanotomy
  Jansen-type posterior 106
  posterior 83, 378
Tympanum
  empty 126

U

Ultracain 1
Urethral catheter 40

V

van der Hoeve-de Kleyn syndrome 230
van der Hoeves syndrome 124
Venous air embolism
  semisitting position 302
Ventilation tube 106, 108
  cleft deformities 77
  middle ear 75, 77
    operative technique 78
Vertebral artery 388
Vertigo 48, 277, 281, 283, 285
  persistent 49
Vestibular labyrinth
  partial destruction 282
    gentamycin 282
Vestibular nerve 301
Vestibular schwannoma 301
Vestibular testing 301
Vestibule 127
Vestibulocochlear dysfunction 301
  Ménière-like 220

Vestibulotomy 47
Vestibulotoxic drugs
  gentamycin 282

W

W-22 monosyllabic word test 372
Weerda technique
  lop ear correction 16
White blood count
  elevated 80
Wire prosthesis 48
Word intelligibility picture test (WIPI) 372
Wound healing problems 118
Wullstein type I tympanoplasty 110
Wullstein Type III tympanoplasty 120

X

Xylocaine 18

Y
Y sign
  incudostapedial joint 139

Z

Zimmer dermatome 53
Zygomaticitis 85